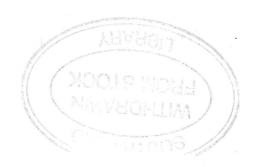

Plastic Surgery

THIRD EDITION

Volume Five

Breast

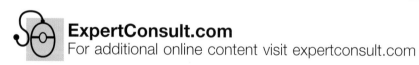

ExpertConsult.com
For additional online content visit expertconsult.com

Content Strategists: Sue Hodgson, Belinda Kuhn
Content Development Specialists: Louise Cook, Poppy Garraway, Alexandra Mortimer
Content Coordinators: Emma Cole, Trinity Hutton, Sam Crowe
Project Managers: Caroline Jones, Cheryl Brant
Design: Stewart Larking, Miles Hitchen
Illustration Manager: Jennifer Rose
Illustrator: Antbits
Marketing Manager: Helena Mutak
Technical Copyeditors: Darren Smith, Colin Woon
Video Reviewers: Leigh Jansen, James Saunders
Artwork Reviewer: Priya Chadha

Plastic Surgery

THIRD EDITION

Volume Five

Breast

Editor in Chief

Peter C. Neligan
MB, FRCS(I), FRCSC, FACS
Professor of Surgery
Department of Surgery, Division of Plastic Surgery
University of Washington
Seattle, WA, USA

Volume Editor

James C. Grotting
MD, FACS
Clinical Professor of Plastic Surgery
University of Alabama at Birmingham;
The University of Wisconsin, Madison, WI;
Grotting and Cohn Plastic Surgery
Birmingham, AL, USA

Video editor:

Allen L. Van Beek
MD, FACS
Adjunct Professor
University Minnesota School of Medicine
Division Plastic Surgery
Minneapolis, MN, USA

ELSEVIER
SAUNDERS London, New York, Oxford, St Louis, Sydney, Toronto

ELSEVIER
SAUNDERS

SAUNDERS an imprint of Elsevier Inc

First edition 1990
Second edition 2006
Third edition 2013

Notices

Knowledge and best practice in this field are constantly changing. As new research and experience broaden our understanding, changes in research methods, professional practices, or medical treatment may become necessary.

Practitioners and researchers must always rely on their own experience and knowledge in evaluating and using any information, methods, compounds, or experiments described herein. In using such information or methods they should be mindful of their own safety and the safety of others, including parties for whom they have a professional responsibility.

With respect to any drug or pharmaceutical products identified, readers are advised to check the most current information provided (i) on procedures featured or (ii) by the manufacturer of each product to be administered, to verify the recommended dose or formula, the method and duration of administration, and contraindications. It is the responsibility of practitioners, relying on their own experience and knowledge of their patients, to make diagnoses, to determine dosages and the best treatment for each individual patient, and to take all appropriate safety precautions.

To the fullest extent of the law, neither the Publisher nor the authors, contributors, or editors, assume any liability for any injury and/or damage to persons or property as a matter of products liability, negligence or otherwise, or from any use or operation of any methods, products, instructions, or ideas contained in the material herein.

Volume 5 ISBN: 978-1-4557-1056-0
Volume 5 Ebook ISBN: 978-1-4557-4039-0
6 volume set ISBN: 978-1-4377-1733-4

ELSEVIER your source for books, journals and multimedia in the health sciences
www.elsevierhealth.com

Working together to grow
libraries in developing countries
www.elsevier.com | www.bookaid.org | www.sabre.org
ELSEVIER   **BOOK AID International**   Sabre Foundation

Printed in China
Last digit is the print number: 9 8 7 6 5 4 3 2 1

The publisher's policy is to use **paper manufactured from sustainable forests**

Contents

Volume Six: Hand and Upper Extremity

James Chang

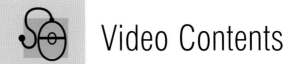

Video Contents

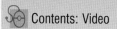

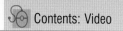

Foreword

In many ways, a textbook defines a particular discipline, and this is especially true in the evolution of modern plastic surgery. The publication of Zeis's *Handbuch der Plastischen Chirurgie* in 1838 popularized the name of the specialty but von Graefe in his monograph *Rhinoplastik*, published in 1818, had first used the title "plastic". At the turn of the last century, Nélaton and Ombredanne compiled what was available in the nineteenth century literature and published in Paris a two volume text in 1904 and 1907. A pivotal book, published across the Atlantic, was that of Vilray Blair, entitled *Surgery and Diseases of the Jaws* (1912). It was, however, limited to a specific anatomic region of the human body, but it became an important handbook for the military surgeons of World War I. Gillies' classic *Plastic Surgery of the Face* (1920) was also limited to a single anatomic region and recapitulated his remarkable and pioneering World War I experience with reconstructive plastic surgery of the face. Davis' textbook, *Plastic Surgery: Its Principles and Practice* (1919), was probably the first comprehensive definition of this young specialty with its emphasis on plastic surgery as ranging from the "top of the head to the soles of the feet." Fomon's *The Surgery of Injury and Plastic Repair* (1939) reviewed all of the plastic surgery techniques available at that time, and it also served as a handbook for the military surgeons of World War II. Kazanjian and Converse's *The Surgical Treatment of Facial Injuries* (1949) was a review of the former's lifetime experience as a plastic surgeon, and the junior author's World War II experience. The comprehensive plastic surgery text entitled *Plastic and Reconstructive Surgery*, published in 1948 by Padgett and Stephenson, was modeled more on the 1919 Davis text.

The lineage of the Neligan text began with the publication of Converse's five volume *Reconstructive Plastic Surgery* in 1964. Unlike his co-authored book with Kazanjian 15 years earlier, Converse undertook a comprehensive view of plastic surgery as the specialty existed in mid-20th century. Chapters were also devoted to pertinent anatomy, research and the role of relevant specialties like anesthesiology and radiology. It immediately became the bible of the specialty. He followed up with a second edition published in 1977, and I was the Assistant Editor. The second edition had grown from five to seven volumes (3970 pages) because the specialty had also grown. I edited the 1990 edition which had grown to eight volumes and 5556 pages; the hand section was edited by J. William Littler and James W. May. I changed the name of the text from *Reconstructive Plastic Surgery* to *Plastic Surgery* because in my mind I could not fathom the distinction between both titles. To the mother of a child with cleft lip, the surgery is "cosmetic," and many of the facelift procedures at that time were truly reconstructive because of the multiple layers at which the facial soft tissues were being readjusted. The late Steve Mathes edited the 2006 edition in eight volumes. He changed the format somewhat and V.R. Hentz was the hand editor. At that time, the text had grown to more than 7000 pages.

The education of the plastic surgeon and the reference material that is critically needed are no longer limited to the printed page or what is described in modern parlance as "hard copy". Certainly, Gutenberg's invention of movable type printing around 1439 allowed publication and distribution of the classic texts of Vesalius (*Fabrica*, 1543) and Tagliacozzi (*De Curtorum Chirurgia Per Insitionem* (1597) and for many years, this was the only medium in which surgeons could be educated. However, by the nineteenth century, travel had become easier with the development of reliable railroads and oceangoing ships, and surgeons conscientiously visited different surgical centers and attended organized meetings. The American College of Surgeons after World War II pioneered the use of operating room movies, and this was followed by videos. The development of the internet has, however, placed almost all information at the fingertips of surgeons around the world with computer access. In turn, we now have virtual surgery education in which the student or surgeon sitting at a computer is interactive with a software program containing animations, intraoperative videos with sound overlay, and access to the world literature on a particular subject. We are rapidly progressing from the bound book of the Gutenberg era to the currently ubiquitous hand held device or tablet for the mastery of surgical/knowledge.

The Neligan text continues this grand tradition of surgical education by bringing the reader into the modern communications world. In line with advances of the electronic era, there is extra online content such as relevant history, complete reference lists and videos. The book is also available as an e-book. It has been a monumental task, consuming hours of work by the editor and all of its participants. The "text" still defines the specialty of plastic surgery. Moreover, it ensures that a new generation of plastic surgeons will have access to all that is known. They, in turn, will not only carry this information into the future but will also build on it. Kudos to Peter Neligan and his colleagues for continuing the chronicle of the plastic surgery saga that has been evolving over two millennia.

Joseph G. McCarthy, MD
2012

Preface

I have always loved textbooks. When I first started my training I was introduced to Converse's *Reconstructive Plastic Surgery*, then in its second edition. I was over-awed by the breadth of the specialty and the expertise contained within its pages. As a young plastic surgeon in practice I bought the first edition of this book, *Plastic Surgery*, edited by Dr. Joseph McCarthy and found it an invaluable resource to which I constantly referred. I was proud to be asked to contribute a chapter to the second edition, edited by Dr. Stephen Mathes and never thought that I would one day be given the responsibility for editing the next edition of the book. I consider this to be the definitive text on our specialty so I took that responsibility very seriously. The result is a very changed book from the previous edition, reflecting changes in the specialty, changes in presentation styles and changes in how textbooks are used.

In preparation for the task, I read the previous edition from cover to cover and tried to identify where major changes could occur. Inevitably in a text this size, there is some repetition and overlap. So the first job was to identify where the repetition and overlap occurred and try to eliminate it. This allowed me to condense some of the material and, along with some other changes, enabled me to reduce the number of volumes from 8 to 6. Reading the text led me to another realization. That is that the breadth of the specialty, impressive when I was first introduced to it, is even more impressive now, 30 years later and it continues to evolve. For this reason I quickly realized that in order to do this project justice, I could not do it on my own. My solution was to recruit volume editors for each of the major areas of practice as well as a video editor for the procedural videos. Drs. Gurtner, Warren, Rodriguez, Losee, Song, Grotting, Chang and Van Beek have done an outstanding job and this book truly represents a team effort.

Publishing is at a crossroads. The digital age has made information much more immediate, much more easy to access and much more flexible in how it is presented. We have tried to reflect that in this edition. The first big change is that everything is in color. All the illustrations have been re-drawn and the vast majority of patient photographs are in color. Chapters on anatomy have been highlighted with a red tone to make them easier to find as have pediatric chapters which have been highlighted in green. Reflecting on the way I personally use textbooks, I realized that while I like access to references, I rarely read the list of references at the end of a chapter. When I do though, I frequently pull some papers to read. So you will notice that we have kept the most important references in the printed text but we have moved the rest to the web. However, this has allowed us to greatly enhance the usefulness of the references. All the references are hyperlinked to PubMed and expertconsult facilitates a search across all volumes. Furthermore, while every chapter has a section devoted to the history of the topic, this is again something I like to be able to access but rarely have the leisure to read. That section in each of the chapters has also been moved to the web. This not only relieved the pressure on space in the printed text but also allowed us to give the authors more freedom in presenting the history of the topic. As well, there are extra illustrations in the web version that we simply could not accommodate in the printed version. The web edition of the book is therefore more complete than the printed version and owning the book, automatically gets one access to the web. A mouse icon has been added to the text to mark where further content is available online. In this digital age, video has become a very important way to impart knowledge. More than 160 procedural videos contributed by leading experts around the world accompany these volumes. These videos cover the full scope of our specialty. This text is also available as an e-Book.

This book then is very different from its predecessors. It is a reflection of a changing age in communication. However I will be extremely pleased if it fulfils its task of defining the current state of knowledge of the specialty as its predecessors did.

Peter C. Neligan, MB, FRCS(I), FRCSC, FACS
2012

List of Contributors

Neta Adler, MD
Senior Surgeon
Department of Plastic and Reconstructive
Surgery
Hadassah University Hospital
Jerusalem, Israel
*Volume 3, Chapter 40 Congenital melanocytic
nevi*

Ahmed M. Afifi, MD
Assistant Professor of Plastic Surgery
University of Winsconsin
Madison, WI, USA
Associate Professor of Plastic Surgery
Cairo University
Cairo, Egypt
*Volume 3, Chapter 1 Anatomy of the head and
neck*

Maryam Afshar, MD
Post Doctoral Fellow
Department of Surgery (Plastic and
Reconstructive Surgery)
Stanford University School of Medicine
Stanford, CA, USA
*Volume 3, Chapter 22 Embryology of the
craniofacial complex*

Jamil Ahmad, MD, FRCSC
Staff Plastic Surgeon
The Plastic Surgery Clinic
Mississauga, ON, Canada
*Volume 2, Chapter 18 Open technique
rhinoplasty*
*Volume 5, Chapter 8.3 Superior or medial
pedicle*

Hee Chang Ahn, MD, PhD
Professor
Department of Plastic and Reconstructive
Surgery
Hanyang University Hospital, School of
Medicine
Seoul, South Korea
Volume 6, Chapter 22 Ischemia of the hand
*Volume 6, Video 22.01 Radial artery periarterial
sympathectomy*
*Volume 6, Video 22.02 Ulnar artery periarterial
sympathectomy*
*Volume 6, Video 22.03 Digital artery periarterial
sympathectomy*

Tae-Joo Ahn, MD
Jeong-Won Aesthetic Plastic Surgical Clinic
Seoul, South Korea
*Volume 2, Video 10.01 Eyelidplasty non-
incisional method*
Volume 2, Video 10.02 Incisional method

Lisa E. Airan, MD
Assistant Clinical Professor
Department of Dermatology
Mount Sinai Hospital
Aesthetic Dermatologist
Private Practice
New York, NY, USA
Volume 2, Chapter 4 Soft-tissue fillers

Sammy Al-Benna, MD, PhD
Specialist in Plastic and Aesthetic Surgery
Department of Plastic Surgery
Burn Centre, Hand Centre, Operative
Reference Centre for Soft Tissue Sarcoma
BG University Hospital Bergmannsheil, Ruhr
University Bochum
Bochum, North Rhine-Westphalia, Germany
*Volume 4, Chapter 18 Acute management of
burn/electrical injuries*

Amy K. Alderman, MD, MPH
Private Practice
Atlanta, GA, USA
*Volume 1, Chapter 10 Evidence-based medicine
and health services research in plastic surgery*

Robert J. Allen, MD
Clinical Professor of Plastic Surgery
Department of Plastic Surgery
New York University Medical Centre
Charleston, SC, USA
*Volume 5, Chapter 18 The deep inferior
epigastric artery perforator (DIEAP) flap*
*Volume 5, Chapter 19 Alternative flaps for breast
reconstruction*
*Volume 5, Video 18.02 DIEP flap breast
reconstruction*

Mohammed M. Al Kahtani, MD, FRCSC
Clinical Fellow
Division of Plastic Surgery
Department of Surgery
University of Alberta
Edmonton, AB, Canada
*Volume 1, Chapter 33 Facial prosthetics in
plastic surgery*

Faisal Al-Mufarrej, MB, BCh
Chief Resident in Plastic Surgery
Division of Plastic Surgery
Department of Surgery
Mayo Clinic
Rochester, MN, USA
*Volume 6, Chapter 20 Osteoarthritis in the hand
and wrist*

Gary J. Alter, MD
Assistant Clinical Professor
Division of Plastic Surgery
University of Califronia at Los Angeles School
of Medicine
Los Angeles, CA, USA
Volume 2, Chapter 31 Aesthetic genital surgery

Al Aly, MD, FACS
Director of Aesthetic Surgery
Professor of Plastic Surgery
Aesthetic and Plastic Surgery Institute
University of California
Irvine, CA, USA
Volume 2, Chapter 27 Lower bodylifts

Khalid Al-Zahrani, MD, SSC-PLAST
Assistant Professor
Consultant Plastic Surgeon
King Khalid University Hospital
King Saud University
Riyadh, Saudi Arabia
Volume 2, Chapter 27 Lower bodylifts

Kenneth W. Anderson, MD
Marietta Facial Plastic Surgery & Aesthetics
Center
Mareitta, GA, USA
Volume 2, Video 23.04 FUE FOX procedure

Alice Andrews, PhD
Instructor
The Dartmouth Institute for Health Policy and
Clinical Practice
Lebanon, NH, USA
*Volume 5, Chapter 12 Patient-centered health
communication*

Louis C. Argenta, MD
Professor of Plastic and Reconstructive Surgery
Department of Plastic Surgery
Wake Forest Medical Center
Winston Salem, NC, USA
*Volume 1, Chapter 27 Principles and applications
of tissue expansion*

Charlotte E. Ariyan, MD, PhD
Surgical Oncologist
Gastric and Mixed Tumor Service
Memorial Sloan-Kettering Cancer Center
New York, NY, USA
Volume 3, Chapter 14 Salivary gland tumors

Stephan Ariyan, MD, MBA
Clinical Professor of Surgery
Plastic Surgery
Otolaryngology Yale University School of
Medicine Associate Chief
Department of Surgery
Yale New Haven Hospital Director
Yale Cancer Center Melanoma Program
New Haven, CT, USA
Volume 1, Chapter 31 Melanoma
Volume 3, Chapter 14 Salivary gland tumors

Bryan S. Armijo, MD
Plastic Surgery Chief Resident
Department of Plastic and Reconstructive
Surgery
Case Western Reserve/University Hospitals
Cleveland, OH, USA
*Volume 2, Chapter 20 Airway issues and the
deviated nose*

Eric Arnaud, MD
Chirurgie Plastique et Esthétique
Chirurgie Plastique Crânio-faciale
Unité de chirurgie crânio-faciale du
departement de neurochirurgie
Hôpital Necker Enfants Malades
Paris, France
Volume 3, Chapter 32 Orbital hypertelorism

Christopher E. Attinger, MD
Chief, Division of Wound Healing
Department of Plastic Surgery
Georgetown University Hospital
Georgetown, WA, USA
Volume 4, Chapter 8 Foot reconstruction

Tomer Avraham, MD
Resident, Plastic Surgery
Institute of Reconstructive Plastic Surgery
NYU Medical Center
New York, NY, USA
*Volume 1, Chapter 12 Principles of cancer
management*

Kodi K. Azari, MD, FACS
Associate Professor of Orthopaedic Surgery
Plastic Surgery Chief
Section of Reconstructive Transplantation
Department of Orthopaedic Surgery and
Surgery
David Geffen School of Medicine at UCLA
Los Angeles, CA, USA
*Volume 6, Chapter 15 Benign and malignant
tumors of the hand*

Sérgio Fernando Dantas de Azevedo, MD
Member
Brazilian Society of Plastic Surgery
Volunteer Professor of Plastic Surgery
Department of Plastic Surgery
Federal University of Pernambuco
Permambuco, Brazil
Volume 2, Chapter 26 Lipoabdominoplasty
*Volume 2, Video 26.01 Lipobdominoplasty
(including secondary lipo)*

Daniel C. Baker, MD
Professor of Surgery
Insitiue of Reconstructive Plastic Surgery
New York University Medical Center
Department of Plastic Surgery
New York, NY, USA
*Volume 2, Chapter 11.5 Facelift: Lateral
SMASectomy*

Steven B. Baker, MD, DDS, FACS
Associate Professor and Program Director
Co-director Inova Hospital for Children
Craniofacial Clinic
Department of Plastic Surgery
Georgetown University Hospital
Georgetown, WA, USA
*Volume 3, Chapter 30 Cleft and craniofacial
orthognathic surgery*

Karim Bakri, MD, MRCS
Chief Resident
Division of Plastic Surgery
Mayo Clinic
Rochester, MN, USA
*Volume 6, Chapter 20 Osteoarthritis in the hand
and wrist*

Carla Baldrighi, MD
Staff Surgeon
Reconstructive Microsurgery Unit
Azienda Ospedaliera Universitaria Careggi
Florence, Italy
*Volume 6, Chapter 30 Growth considerations in
pediatric upper extremity trauma and
reconstruction*
*Volume 6, Video 30.01 Epiphyseal transplant
harvesting technique*

Jonathan Bank, MD
Resident, Section of Plastic and Reconstructive
Surgery
Department of Surgery
Pritzker School of Medicine
University of Chicago Medical Center
Chicago, IL, USA
*Volume 4, Chapter 12 Abdominal wall
reconstruction*

A. Sina Bari, MD
Chief Resident
Division of Plastic and Reconstructive Surgery
Stanford University Hospital and Clinics
Stanford, CA, USA
*Volume 1, Chapter 16 Scar prevention,
treatment, and revision*

Scott P. Bartlett, MD
Professor of Surgery
Peter Randall Endowed Chair in Pediatric
Plastic Surgery
Childrens Hospital of Philadelphia, University of
Philadelphia
Philadelphia, PA, USA
*Volume 3, Chapter 34 Nonsyndromic
craniosynostosis*

Fritz E. Barton, Jr., MD
Clinical Professor
Department of Plastic Surgery
University of Texas Southwestern Medical
Center
Dallas, TX, USA
*Volume 2, Chapter 11.7 Facelift: SMAS with skin
attached – the "high SMAS" technique*
*Volume 2, Video 11.07.01 The High SMAS
technique with septal reset*

Bruce S. Bauer, MD, FACS, FAAP
Director of Pediatric Plastic Surgery, Clinical
Professor of Surgery
Northshore University Healthsystem
University of Chicago, Pritzker School of
Medicine, Highland Park Hospital
Chicago, IL, USA
*Volume 3, Chapter 40 Congenital melanocytic
nevi*

Ruediger G.H. Baumeister, MD, PhD
Professor of Surgery Emeritus
Consultant in Lymphology
Ludwig Maximilians University
Munich, Germany
*Volume 4, Chapter 3 Lymphatic reconstruction of
the extremities*

Leslie Baumann, MD
CEO
Baumann Cosmetic and Research Institute
Miami, FL, USA
*Volume 2, Chapter 2 Non surgical skin care and
rejuvenation*

Adriane L. Baylis, PhD
Speech Scientist
Section of Plastic and Reconstructive Surgery
Nationwide Children's Hospital
Columbus, OH, USA
*Volume 3, Chapter 28 Velopharyngeal
dysfunction*
*Volume 3, Video 28 Velopharyngeal
incompetence (1-3)*

Elisabeth Beahm, MD, FACS
Professor
Department of Plastic Surgery
University of Texas MD Anderson Cancer
Center
Houston, TX, USA
*Volume 5, Chapter 10 Breast cancer: Diagnosis
therapy and oncoplastic techniques*
*Volume 5, Video 10.01 Breast cancer: diagnosis
and therapy*

Michael L. Bentz, MD, FAAP, FACS
Professor of Surgery Pediatrics and
Neurosurgery Chairman
Chairman of Clinical Affairs
Department of Surgery
Division of Plastic Surgery Vice
University of Winconsin School of Medicine and
Public Health
Madison, WI, USA
Volume 3, Chapter 42 Pediatric tumors

Aaron Berger, MD, PhD
Resident
Division of Plastic Surgery, Department of Surgery
Stanford University Medical Center
Palo Alto, CA, USA
Volume 1, Chapter 31 Melanoma

Pietro Berrino, MD
Teaching Professor
University of Milan
Director
Chirurgia Plastica Genova SRL
Genoa, Italy
Volume 5, Chapter 23 Poland's syndrome

Valeria Berrino, MS
In Training
Chirurgia Plastica Genova SRL
Genoa, Italy
Volume 5, Chapter 23 Poland's syndrome

Miles G. Berry, MS, FRCS(Plast)
Consultant Plastic and Aesthetic Surgeon
Institute of Cosmetic and Reconstructive Surgery
London, UK
Volume 2, Chapter 11.3 Facelift: Platysma-SMAS plication
Volume 2, Video 11.03.01 Facelift – Platysma SMAS plication

Robert M. Bernstein, MD, FAAD
Associate Clinical Professor
Department of Dermatology
College of Physicians and Surgeons
Columbia University
Director
Private Practice
Bernstein Medical Center for Hair Restoration
New York, NY, USA
Volume 2, Video 23.04 FUE FOX procedure
Volume 2, Video 23.02 Follicular unit hair transplantation

Michael Bezuhly, MD, MSc, SM, FRCSC
Assistant Professor
Department of Surgery, Division of Plastic and Reconstructive Surgery
IWK Health Centre, Dalhousie University
Halifax, NS, Canada
Volume 6, Chapter 23 Nerve entrapment syndromes
Volume 6, Video 23.01-04 Carpal tunnel and cubital tunnel releases in the same patient in one procedure with field sterility – local anaesthetic and surgery

Sean M. Bidic, MD, MFA, FAAP, FACS
Private Practice
American Surgical Arts
Vineland, NJ, USA
Volume 6, Chapter 16 Infections of the hand

Phillip N. Blondeel, MD, PhD, FCCP
Professor of Plastic Surgery
Department of Plastic and Reconstructive Surgery
University Hospital Gent
Gent, Belgium
Volume 5, Chapter 18 The deep inferior epigastric artery perforator (DIEAP) Flap
Volume 5, Chapter 19 Alternative flaps for breast reconstruction
Volume 5, Video 18.02 DIEP flap breast reconstruction

Sean G. Boutros, MD
Assistant Professor of Surgery
Weill Cornell Medical College (Houston)
Clinical Instructor
University of Texas School of Medicine (Houston)
Houston Plastic and Craniofacial Surgery
Houston, TX, USA
Volume 3, Video 7.02 Reconstruction of acquired ear deformities

Lorenzo Borghese, MD
Plastic Surgeon
General Surgeon
Department of Plastic and Maxillo Facial Surgery
Director of International Cooperation South East Asia
Pediatric Hospital "Bambino Gesu'"
Rome, Italy
Volume 4, Chapter 19 Extremity burn reconstruction
Volume 4, Video 19.01 Extremity burn reconstruction

Trevor M. Born, MD, FRCSC
Lecturer
Division of Plastic and Reconstructive Surgery
The University of Toronto
Toronto, Ontario, Canada
Attending Physician
Lenox Hill Hospital
New York, NY, USA
Volume 2, Chapter 4 Soft-tissue fillers

Gregory H. Borschel, MD, FAAP, FACS
Assistant Professor
University of Toronto Division of Plastic and Reconstructive Surgery
Assistant Professor
Institute of Biomaterials and Biomedical Engineering
Associate Scientist
The SickKids Research Institute
The Hospital for Sick Children
Toronto, ON, Canada
Volume 6, Chapter 35 Free functioning muscle transfer in the upper extremity

Kirsty U. Boyd, MD, FRCSC
Clinical Fellow – Hand Surgery
Department of Surgery – Division of Plastic Surgery
Washington University School of Medicine
St. Louis, MO, USA
Volume 1, Chapter 22 Repair and grafting of peripheral nerve
Volume 6, Chapter 33 Nerve transfers

James P. Bradley, MD
Professor of Plastic and Reconstructive Surgery
Department of Surgery
University of California, Los Angeles David Geffen School of Medicine
Los Angeles, CA, USA
Volume 3, Chapter 33 Craniofacial clefts

Burton D. Brent, MD
Private Practice
Woodside, CA, USA
Volume 3, Chapter 7 Reconstruction of the ear

Mitchell H. Brown, MD, Med, FRCSC
Associate Professor of Plastic Surgery
Department of Surgery
University of Toronto
Toronto, ON, Canada
Volume 5, Chapter 3 Secondary breast augmentation

Samantha A. Brugmann, PHD
Postdoctoral Fellow
Department of Surgery
Stanford University
Stanford, CA, USA
Volume 3, Chapter 22 Embryology of the craniofacial complex

Terrence W. Bruner, MD, MBA
Private Practice
Greenville, SC, USA
Volume 2, Chapter 28 Buttock augmentation
Volume 2, Video 28.01 Buttock augmentation

Todd E. Burdette, MD
Staff Plastic Surgeon
Concord Plastic Surgery
Concord Hospital Medical Group
Concord, NH, USA
Volume 1, Chapter 36 Robotics, simulation, and telemedicine in plastic surgery

Renee M. Burke, MD
Attending Plastic Surgeon
Department of Plastic Surgery
St. Alexius Medical Center
Hoffman Estates, IL, USA
Volume 3, Chapter 8 Acquired cranial and facial bone deformities
Volume 3, Video 8.01 Removal of venous malformation enveloping intraconal optic nerve

Charles E. Butler, MD, FACS
Professor, Department of Plastic Surgery
The University of Texas MD Anderson Cancer
Center
Houston, TX, USA
Volume 1, Chapter 32 Implants and biomaterials

Peter E. M. Butler, MD, FRCSI, FRCS,
FRCS(Plast)
Consultant Plastic Surgeon
Honorary Senior Lecturer
Royal Free Hospital
London, UK
Volume 1, Chapter 34 Transplantation in plastic
surgery

Yilin Cao, MD
Director, Department of Plastic and
Reconstructive Surgery
Shanghai 9th People's Hospital
Vice-Dean
Shanghai Jiao Tong University Medical School
Shanghai, The People's Republic of China
Volume 1, Chapter 18 Tissue graft, tissue repair,
and regeneration
Volume 1, Chapter 20 Repair, grafting, and
engineering of cartilage

Joseph F. Capella, MD, FACS
Chief, Post-Bariatric Body Contouring
Division of Plastic Surgery
Hackensack University Medical Center
Hackensack, NJ, USA
Volume 2, Chapter 29 Upper limb contouring
Volume 2, Video 29.01 Upper limb contouring

Brian T. Carlsen, MD
Assistant Professor of Plastic Surgery
Department of Surgery
Mayo Clinic
Rochester, MN, USA
Volume 6, Chapter 20 Osteoarthritis in the hand
and wrist

Robert C. Cartotto, MD, FRCS(C)
Attending Surgeon
Ross Tilley Burn Centre
Health Sciences Centre
Toronto, ON, Canada
Volume 4, Chapter 23 Management of patients
with exfoliative disorders, epidermolysis bullosa,
and TEN

Giuseppe Catanuto, MD, PhD
Research Fellow
The School of Oncological Reconstructive
Surgery
Milan, Italy
Volume 5, Chapter 14 Expander/implant breast
reconstructions
Volume 5, Video 14.01 Mastectomy and
expander insertion: first stage
Volume 5, Video 14.02 Mastectomy and
expander insertion: second stage

Peter Ceulemans, MD
Assistant Professor
Department of Plastic Surgery
Ghent University Hospital
Ghent, Belgium
Volume 4, Chapter 13 Reconstruction of male
genital defects

Rodney K. Chan, MD
Staff Plastic and Reconstructive Surgeon
Burn Center
United States Army Institute of Surgical
Research
Fort Sam
Houston, TX, USA
Volume 3, Chapter 19 Secondary facial
reconstruction

David W. Chang, MD, FACS
Professor
Department of Plastic Surgery
MD. Anderson Centre
Houston, TX, USA
Volume 4, Chapter 3 Lymphatic reconstruction of
the extremities
Volume 4, Video 3.01 Lymphatico-venous
anastomosis
Volume 6, Chapter 15 Benign and malignant
tumors of the hand

Edward I. Chang, MD
Assistant Professor
Department of Plastic Surgery
The University of Texas M.D. Anderson Cancer
Center
Houston, TX, USA
Volume 3, Chapter 17 Carcinoma of the upper
aerodigestive tract

James Chang, MD
Professor and Chief
Division of Plastic and Reconstructive Surgery
Stanford University Medical Center
Stanford, CA, USA
Volume 6, Introduction: Plastic surgery
contributions to hand surgery
Volume 6, Chapter 1 Anatomy and biomechanics
of the hand
Volume 6, Video 11.01 Hand replantation
Volume 6, Video 12.01 Debridement technique
Volume 6, Video 19.01 Extensor tendon rupture
and end-side tendon transfer
Volume 6, Video 29.01 Addendum pediatric
trigger thumb release

Robert A. Chase, MD
Holman Professor of Surgery – Emeritus
Stanford University Medical Center
Stanford, CA, USA
Volume 6, Chapter 1 Anatomy and biomechanics
of the hand

Constance M. Chen, MD, MPH
Plastic and Reconstructive Surgeon
Division of Plastic and Reconstructive Surgery
Lenox Hill Hospital
New York, NY, USA
Volume 3, Chapter 9 Midface reconstruction

Philip Kuo-Ting Chen, MD
Director
Department of Plastic and Reconstructive
Surgery
Chang Gung Memorial Hospital and Chang
Gung University
Taipei, Taiwan, The People's Republic of China
Volume 3, Chapter 23 Repair of unilateral cleft lip

Yu-Ray Chen, MD
Professor of Surgery
Department of Plastic and Reconstructive
Surgery
Chang Gung Memorial Hospital
Chang Gung University
Tao-Yuan, Taiwan, The People's Republic of
China
Volume 3, Chapter 15 Tumors of the facial
skeleton: Fibrous dysplasia

Ming-Huei Cheng, MD, MBA, FACS
Professor and Chief, Division of Reconstructive
Microsurgery
Department of Plastic and Reconstructive
Surgery
Chang Gung Memorial Hospital
Chang Gung Medical College
Chang Gung University
Taoyuan, Taiwan, The People's Republic of
China
Volume 3, Chapter 12 Oral cavity, tongue, and
mandibular reconstructions
Volume 3, Video 12.02 Ulnar forearm flap for
buccal reconstruction

You-Wei Cheong, MBBS, MS
Consultant Plastic Surgeon
Department of Surgery
Faculty of Medicine and Health Sciences,
University of Putra Malaysia
Selangor, Malaysia
Volume 3, Chapter 15 Tumors of the facial
skeleton: Fibrous dysplasia

Armando Chiari Jr., MD, PhD
Adjunct Professor
Department of Surgery
School of Medicine of the Federal University of
Minas Gerais
Belo Horzonti, Minas Gerais, Brazil
Volume 5, Chapter 8.5 The L short scar
mammaplasty

Ernest S. Chiu, MD, FACS
Associate Professor of Plastic Surgery
Department of Plastic Surgery
New York University
New York
USA
Volume 2, Chapter 9 Secondary blepharoplasty:
Techniques

Hong-Lim Choi, MD, PhD
Jeong-Won Aesthetic Plastic Surgical Clinic
Seoul, South Korea
Volume 2, Video 10.01 Eyelidplasty non-incisional method
Volume 2, Video 10.02 Incisional method

Jong Woo Choi, MD, PhD
Associate Professor
Department of Plastic and Reconstructive
Surgery
Asan Medical Center
Ulsan University
College of Medicine
Seoul, South Korea
Volume 2, Chapter 10 Asian facial cosmetic surgery

**Alphonsus K. Chong, MBBS, MRCS,
MMed(Orth), FAMS(Hand Surgery)**
Consultant Hand Surgeon
Department of Hand and Reconstructive
Microsurgery
National University Hospital
Assistant Professor
Department of Orthopaedic Surgery
Yong Loo Lin School of Medicine
National University of Singapore
Singapore
Volume 6, Chapter 3 Diagnostic imaging of the hand and wrist
Volume 6, Video 3.01 Diagnostic imaging of the hand and wrist – Scaphoid lunate dislocation

David Chwei-Chin Chuang, MD
Senior Consultant, Ex-President, Professor
Department of Plastic Surgery
Chang Gung University Hospital
Tao-Yuan, Taiwan, The People's Republic of
China
Volume 6, Chapter 36 Brachial plexus injuries-adult and pediatric
Volume 6, Video 36.01-02 Brachial plexus injuries

Kevin C. Chung, MD, MS
Charles B. G. de Nancrede, MD Professor
Section of Plastic Surgery, Department of
Surgery
Assistant Dean for Faculty Affairs
University of Michigan Medical School
Ann Arbor, MI, USA
Volume 6, Chapter 8 Fractures and dislocations of the carpus and distal radius
Volume 6, Chapter 19 Rheumatologic conditions of the hand and wrist
Volume 6, Video 8.01 Scaphoid fixation
Volume 6, Video 19.01 Silicone MCP arthroplasty

Juan A. Clavero, MD, PhD
Radiologist Consultant
Radiology Department
Clínica Creu Blanca
Barcelona, Spain
Volume 5, Chapter 13 Imaging in reconstructive breast surgery

Mark W. Clemens, MD
Assistant Professor
Department of Plastic Surgery
Anderson Cancer Center University of Texas
Houston, TX, USA
Volume 4, Chapter 8 Foot reconstruction
Volume 5, Chapter 15 Latissimus dorsi flap breast reconstruction
Volume 5, Video 15.01 Latissimus dorsi flap technique

Steven R. Cohen, MD
Senior Clinical Research Fellow, Clinical
Professor
Plastic Surgery
University of California
San Diego, CA
Director
Craniofacial Surgery
Rady Children's Hospital, Private Practice,
FACES+ Plastic Surgery, Skin and Laser Center
La Jolla, CA, USA
Volume 2, Chapter 5 Facial skin resurfacing

Sydney R. Coleman, MD
Clinical Assistant Professor
Department of Plastic Surgery
New York University Medical Center
New York, NY, USA
Volume 2, Chapter 14 Structural fat grafting
Volume 2, Video 14.01 Structural fat grafting of the face

John Joseph Coleman III, MD
James E. Bennett Professor of Surgery,
Department of Dermatology and Cutaneuous
Surgery
University of Miami Miller School of Medicine
Miami, FA
Chief of Plastic Surgery
Department of Surgery
Indiana University School of Medicine
Indianapolis, IN, USA
Volume 3, Chapter 16 Tumors of the lips, oral cavity, oropharynx, and mandible

Lawrence B. Colen, MD
Associate Professor of Surgery
Eastern Virginia Medical School
Norfolk, VA, USA
Volume 4, Chapter 8 Foot reconstruction

E. Dale Collins Vidal, MD, MS
Chief
Section of Plastic Surgery
Dartmouth-Hitchcock Medical Center
Professor of Surgery
Dartmouth Medical School
Director of the Center for Informed Choice
The Dartmouth Institute (TDI) for Health Policy
and Clinical Practice
Hanover, NH, USA
Volume 1, Chapter 10 Evidence-based medicine and health services research in plastic surgery
Volume 5, Chapter 12 Patient-centered health communication

Shannon Colohan, MD, FRCSC
Clinical Instructor, Plastic Surgery
Department of Plastic Surgery
University of Texas Southwestern Medical
Center
Dallas, TX, USA
Volume 4, Chapter 2 Management of lower extremity trauma

Mark B. Constantian, MD, FACS
Active Staff
Saint Joseph Hospital
Nashua, NH (private practice)
Assistant Clinical Professor of Plastic Surgery
Division of Plastic Surgery
Department of Surgery
University of Wisconsin
Madison, WI, USA
Volume 2, Chapter 19 Closed technique rhinoplasty

Peter G. Cordeiro, MD, FACS
Chief
Plastic and Reconstructive Surgery
Memorial Sloan-Kettering Cancer Center
Professor of Surgery
Weill Cornell Medical College
New York, NY, USA
Volume 3, Chapter 9 Midface reconstruction
Volume 4, Chapter 14 Reconstruction of acquired vaginal defects

Christopher Cox, MD
Chief Resident
Department of Orthopaedic Surgery
Stanford University Medical School
Stanford, CA, USA
Volume 6, Chapter 5 Principles of internal fixation as applied to the hand and wrist
Volume 6, Video 5.01 Dynamic compression plating and lag screw technique

Albert Cram, MD
Professor Emeritus
University of Iowa
Iowa City Plastic Surgery
Coralville, IO, USA
Volume 2, Chapter 27 Lower bodylifts

Catherine Curtin, MD
Assistant Professor
Department of Surgery Division of Plastic
Stanford University
Stanford, CA, USA
*Volume 6, Chapter 37 Restoration of upper
extremity function*
*Volume 6, Video 37.01 1 Stage grasp IC 6 short
term*
*Volume 6, Video 37.02 2 Stage grasp release
outcome*

Lars B. Dahlin, MD, PhD
Professor and Consultant
Department of Clinical Sciences, Malmö-Hand
Surgery
University of Lund
Malmö, Sweden
*Volume 6, Chapter 32 Peripheral nerve injuries of
the upper extremity*
Volume 6, Video 32.01 Digital Nerve Suture
Volume 6, Video 32.02 Median Nerve Suture

Dai M. Davies, FRCS
Consultant and Institute Director
Institute of Cosmetic and Reconstructive
Surgery
London, UK
*Volume 2, Chapter 11.3 Facelift: Platysma-SMAS
plication*
*Volume 2, Video 11.03.01 Platysma SMAS
plication*

**Michael R. Davis, MD, FACS, LtCol,
USAF, MC**
Chief
Reconstructive Surgery and Regenerative
Medicine
Plastic and Reconstructive Surgeon
San Antonio Military Medical Center
Houston, TX, USA
*Volume 5, Chapter 1 Anatomy for plastic surgery
of the breast*

Jorge I. De La Torre, MD
Professor and Chief
Division of Plastic Surgery
University of Alabama at Birmingham
Birmingham, AL, USA
*Volume 5, Chapter 1 Anatomy for plastic surgery
of the breast*

A. Lee Dellon, MD, PhD
Professor of Plastic Surgery
Professor of Neurosurgery
Johns Hopkins University
Baltimore, MD, USA
*Volume 4, Chapter 6 Diagnosis and treatment of
painful neuroma and of nerve compression in the
lower extremity*
*Volume 4, Video 6.01 Diagnosis and treatment
of painful neuroma and of nerve compression in
the lower extremity*

Sara R. Dickie, MD
Resident, Section of Plastic and Reconstructive
Surgery
Department of Surgery
University of Chicago Medical Center
Chicago, IL, USA
*Volume 4, Chapter 9 Comprehensive trunk
anatomy*

Joseph J. Disa, MD, FACS
Attending Surgeon
Plastic and Reconstructive Surgery in the
Department of Surgery
Memorial Sloan Kettering Cancer Center
New York, NY, USA
Volume 3, Chapter 9 Midface reconstruction
*Volume 4, Chapter 14 Reconstruction of
acquired vaginal defects*

Risal Djohan, MD
Head of Regional Medical Practice
Department of Plastic Surgery
Cleveland Clinic
Cleveland, OH, USA
*Volume 3, Chapter 1 Anatomy of the head and
neck*

Erin Donaldson, MS
Instructor
Department of Otolaryngology
New York Medical College
Valhalla, NY, USA
*Volume 1, Chapter 36 Robotics, simulation, and
telemedicine in plastic surgery*

Amir H. Dorafshar, MBChB
Assistant Professor
Department of Plastic and Reconstructive
surgery
John Hopkins Medical Institute
John Hopkins Outpatient Center
Baltimore, MD, USA
Volume 3, Chapter 3 Facial fractures

Ivica Ducic, MD, PhD
Professor – Plastic Surgery
Director – Peripheral Nerve Surgery Institute
Department of Plastic Surgery
Georgetown University Hospital
Washington, DC, USA
*Volume 6, Chapter 23 Complex regional pain
syndrome in the upper extremity*

Gregory A. Dumanian, MD, FACS
Chief of Plastic Surgery
Division of Plastic Surgery, Department of
Surgery
Northwestern Feinberg School of Medicine
Chicago, IL, USA
*Volume 4, Chapter 11 Reconstruction of the soft
tissues of the back*
*Volume 6, Chapter 40 Treatment of the upper
extremity amputee*
*Volume 6, Video 40.01 Targeted muscle
reinnervation in the transhumeral amputee –
Surgical technique and guidelines for restoring
intuitive neural control*

William W. Dzwierzynski, MD
Professor and Program Director
Department of Plastic Surgery
Medical College of Wisconsin
Milwaukee, WI, USA
*Volume 6, Chapter 11 Replantation and
revascularization*

L. Franklyn Elliott, MD
Assistant Clinical Professor
Emory Section of Plastic Surgery
Emory University
Atlanta, GA, USA
*Volume 5, Chapter 16 The bilateral pedicled
TRAM flap*
*Volume 5, Video 16.01 Pedicle TRAM breast
reconstruction*

Marco Ellis, MD
Chief Resident
Division of Plastic Surgery
Northwestern Memorial Hospital
Northwestern University, Feinberg School of
Medicine
Chicago, IL, USA
Volume 2, Chapter 8 Blepharoplasty
Volume 2, Video 8.01 Periorbital rejuvenation

Dino Elyassnia, MD
Associate Plastic Surgeon
Marten Clinic of Plastic Surgery
San Francisco, CA, USA
*Volume 2, Chapter 12 Secondary deformities
and the secondary facelift*

Surak Eo, MD, PhD
Chief, Associate Professor
Plastic and Reconstructive Surgery
DongGuk University Medical Center
DongGuk University Graduate School of
Medicine
Gyeonggi-do, South Korea
*Volume 6, Video 34.01 EIP to EPL tendon
transfer*

Elof Eriksson, MD, PhD
Chief
Department of Plastic Surgery
Joseph E. Murray Professor of Plastic and
Reconstructive Surgery
Brigham and Women's Hospital
Boston, MA, USA
*Volume 1, Chapter 11 Genetics and prenatal
diagnosis*

Simon Farnebo, MD, PhD
Consultant Hand Surgeon
Department of Plastic Surgery, Hand Surgery
and Burns
Institution of Clinical and Experimental
Medicine, University of Linköping
Linköping, Sweden
*Volume 6, Chapter 32 Peripheral nerve injuries of
the upper extremity*
Volume 6, Video 32.01 Digital Nerve Suture
Volume 6, Video 32.02 Median Nerve Suture

Jeffrey A. Fearon, MD
Director
The Craniofacial Center
Medical City Children's Hospital
Dallas, TX, USA
Volume 3, Chapter 35 Syndromic craniosynostosis

John M. Felder III, MD
Resident Physician
Department of Plastic Surgery
Georgetown University Hospital
Washington, DC, USA
Volume 6, Chapter 23 Complex regional pain syndrome in the upper extremity

Evan M. Feldman, MD
Chief Resident
Division of Plastic Surgery
Baylor College of Medicine
Houston, TX, USA
Volume 3, Chapter 29 Secondary deformities of the cleft lip, nose, and palate
Volume 3, Video 29.01 Complete takedown
Volume 3, Video 29.02 Abbé flap
Volume 3, Video 29.03 Thick lip and buccal sulcus deformities
Volume 3, Video 29.04 Alveolar bone grafting
Volume 3, Video 29.05 Definitive rhinoplasty

Julius Few Jr., MD
Director
The Few Institute for Aesthetic Plastic Surgery
Clinical Associate
Division of Plastic Surgery
University of Chicago
Chicago, IL, USA
Volume 2, Chapter 8 Blepharoplasty
Volume 2, Video 8.01 Periorbital rejuvenation

Alvaro A. Figueroa, DDS, MS
Director
Rush Craniofacial Center
Rush University Medical Center
Chicago, IL, USA
Volume 3, Chapter 27 Orthodontics in cleft lip and palate management

Neil A. Fine, MD
Associate Professor of Clinical Surgery
Department of Surgery
Northwestern University
Chicago, IL, USA
Volume 5, Chapter 5 Endoscopic approaches to the breast
Volume 5, Video 5.01 Endoscopic transaxillary breast augmentation
Volume 5, Video 5.02 Endoscopic approaches to the breast
Volume 5, Video 11.02 Partial breast reconstruction with a latissimus D

Joel S. Fish, MD, MSc, FRCSC
Medical Director Burn Program
Department of Surgery, University of Toronto,
Division of Plastic and Reconstructive Surgery
Hospital for Sick Children
Toronto, ON, Canada
Volume 4, Chapter 23 Management of patients with exfoliative disorders, epidermolysis bullosa, and TEN

David M. Fisher, MB, BCh, FRCSC, FACS
Medical Director, Cleft Lip and Palate Program
Division of Plastic and Reconstructive Surgery
The Hospital for Sick Children
Toronto, ON, Canada
Volume 3, Video 23.02 Unilateral cleft lip repair – anatomic subunit approximation technique

Jack Fisher, MD
Department of Plastic Surgery
Vanderbilt University
Nashville, TN, USA
Volume 2, Chapter 23 Hair restoration
Volume 5, Chapter 8.1 Reduction mammaplasty
Volume 5, Chapter 8.2 Inferior pedicle breast reduction

James W. Fletcher, MD, FACS
Chief Hand Surgery
Department Plastic and Hand Surgery
Regions Hospital
Assistant Prof. U MN Dept of Surgery and Dept Orthopedics
St. Paul, MN, USA
Volume 6, Video 20.01 Ligament reconstruction tendon interposition arthroplasty of the thumb CMC joint

Joshua Fosnot, MD
Resident
Division of Plastic Surgery
The University of Pennsylvania Health System
Philadelphia, PA, USA
Volume 5, Chapter 17 Free TRAM breast reconstruction
Volume 5, Video 17.01 The muscle sparing free TRAM flap

Ida K. Fox, MD
Assistant Professor of Plastic Surgery
Department of Surgery
Washington University School of Medicine
Saint Louis, MO, USA
Volume 6, Chapter 33 Nerve transfers
Volume 6, Video 33.01 Nerve transfers

Ryan C. Frank, MD, FRCSC
Attending Surgeon
Plastic and Craniofacial Surgery
Alberta Children's Hospital
University of Calgary
Calgary, AB, Canada
Volume 2, Chapter 5 Facial skin resurfacing

Gary L. Freed, MD
Assistant Professor Plastic Surgery
Dartmouth-Hitchcock Medical Center
Lebanon, NH, USA
Volume 5, Chapter 12 Patient-centered health communication

Jeffrey B. Friedrich, MD
Assistant Professor of Surgery, Orthopedics and Urology (Adjunct)
Department of Surgery, Division of Plastic Surgery
University of Washington
Seattle, WA, USA
Volume 6, Chapter 13 Thumb reconstruction (non microsurgical)

Allen Gabriel, MD
Assitant Professor
Department of Plastic Surgery
Loma Linda University Medical Center
Chief of Plastic Surgery
Southwest Washington Medical Center
Vancouver, WA, USA
Volume 5, Chapter 2 Breast augmentation
Volume 5, Chapter 4 Current concepts in revisionary breast surgery
Volume 5, Video 4.01 Current concepts in revisionary breast surgery

Günter Germann, MD, PhD
Professor of Plastic Surgery
Clinic for Plastic and Reconstructive Surgery
Heidelberg University Hospital
Heidelberg, Germany
Volume 6, Chapter 10 Extensor tendon injuries and reconstruction

Goetz A. Giessler, MD, PhD
Plastic Surgeon, Hand Surgeon, Associate Professor of Plastic Surgery, Fellow of the European Board of Plastic Reconstructive and Aesthetic Surgery
BG Trauma Center Murnau
Murnau am Staffelsee, Germany
Volume 4, Chapter 4 Lower extremity sarcoma reconstruction
Volume 4, Video 4.01 Management of lower extremity sarcoma reconstruction

Jesse A. Goldstein, MD
Chief Resident
Department of Plastic Surgery
Georgetown University Hospital
Washington, DC, USA
Volume 3, Chapter 30 Cleft and craniofacial orthognathic surgery

Vijay S. Gorantla, MD, PhD
Associate Professor of Surgery
Department of Surgery, Division of Plastic and
Reconstructive Surgery
University of Pittsburgh Medical Center
Administrative Medical Director
Pittsburgh Reconstructive Transplantation
Program
Pittsburgh, PA, USA
*Volume 6, Chapter 38 Upper extremity
composite allotransplantation*
*Volume 6, Video 38.01 Upper extremity
composite allotransplantation*

Arun K. Gosain, MD
DeWayne Richey Professor and Vice Chair
Department of Plastic Surgery
University Hospitals Case Medical Center
Chief, Pediatric Plastic Surgery
Rainbow Babies and Children's Hospital
Cleveland, OH, USA
Volume 3, Chapter 38 Pierre Robin sequence

Lawrence J. Gottlieb, MD, FACS
Professor of Surgery
Director of Burn and Complex Wound Center
Director of Reconstructive Microsurgery
Fellowship
Section of Plastic and Reconstructive Surgery
Department of Surgery
University of Chicago
Chicago, IL, USA
*Volume 3, Chapter 41 Pediatric chest and trunk
defects*

Barry H. Grayson, DDS
Associate Professor of Surgery (Craniofacial
Orthodontics)
New York University Langone Medical Centre
Institute of Reconstructive Plastic Surgery
New York, NY, USA
Volume 3, Chapter 36 Craniofacial microsomia
Volume 3, Video 24.01 Repair of bilateral cleft lip

Arin K. Greene, MD, MMSc
Associate Professor of Surgery
Department of Plastic and Oral Surgery
Children's Hospital Boston
Harvard Medical School
Boston, MA, USA
Volume 1, Chapter 29 Vascular anomalies

James C. Grotting, MD, FACS
Clinical Professor of Plastic Surgery
University of Alabama at Birmingham;
The University of Wisconsin, Madison, WI;
Grotting and Cohn Plastic Surgery
Birmingham, AL, USA
Volume 5, Chapter 7 Mastopexy
Volume 5, Chapter 8.7 Sculpted pillar vertical
*Volume 5, Video 8.7.01 Marking the sculpted
pillar breast reduction*
Volume 5, Video 8.7.02 Breast reduction surgery

Ronald P. Gruber, MD
Associate Adjunct Clinical Professor
Division of Plastic and Reconstructive Surgery
Stanford University
Associate Clinical Professor
Division of Plastic and Reconstructive Surgery
University of California, San Francisco
San Francisco, CA, USA
Volume 2, Chapter 21 Secondary rhinoplasty

**Mohan S. Gundeti, MB, MCh, FEBU,
FRCS, FEAPU**
Associate Professor of Urology in Surgery and
Pediatrics, Director Pediatric Urology, Director
Centre for Pediatric Robotics and Minimal
Invasive Surgery
University of Chicago and Pritzker Medical
School Comer Children's Hospital
Chicago, IL, USA
*Volume 3, Chapter 44 Reconstruction of
urogenital defects: Congenital*
*Volume 3, Video 44.01 First stage hypospadias
repair with free inner preputial graft*
*Volume 3, Video 44.02 Second stage
hypospadias repair with tunica vaginalis flap*

Eyal Gur, MD
Head
Department of Plastic and Reconstructive
Surgery
The Tel Aviv Sourasky Medical Center
The Tel Aviv University School of Medicine
Tel Aviv, Israel
Volume 3, Chapter 11 Facial paralysis
Volume 3, Video 11.01 Facial paralysis

Geoffrey C. Gurtner, MD, FACS
Professor and Associate Chairman
Stanford University Department of Surgery
Stanford, CA, USA
*Volume 1, Chapter 13 Stem cells and
regenerative medecine*
*Volume 1, Chapter 35 Technology innovation in
plastic surgery*

Bahman Guyuron, MD
Kiehn-DesPrez Professor and Chairman
Department of Plastic Surgery
Case Western Reserve University School of
Medicine
Cleveland, OH, USA
*Volume 2, Chapter 20 Airway issues and the
deviated nose*
*Volume 3, Chapter 21 Surgical management of
migraine headaches*
Volume 2, Video 3.02 Botulinum toxin

Steven C. Haase, MD
Clinical Associate Professor
Department of Surgery, Section of Plastic
Surgery
University of Michigan Health
Ann Arbor, MI, USA
*Volume 6, Chapter 8 Fractures and dislocations
of the carpus and distal radius*

Robert S. Haber, MD, FAAD, FAAP
Assistant Professor, Dermatology and
Pediatrics
Case Western Reserve University School of
Medicine
Director
University Hair Transplant Center
Cleveland, OH, USA
*Volume 2, Video 23.08 Strip harvesting the
haber spreader*

Florian Hackl, MD
Research Fellow
Division of Plastic Surgery
Brigham and Women's Hospital
Harvard Medical School
Boston, MA, USA
*Volume 1, Chapter 11 Genetics and prenatal
diagnosis*

Phillip C. Haeck, MD
Private Practice
Seattle, WA, USA
*Volume 1, Chapter 4 The role of ethics in plastic
surgery*

Bruce Halperin, MD
Adjunct Associate Clinical Professor of
Anesthesia
Department of Anesthesia
Stanford University School of Medicine
Palo Alto, CA, USA
*Volume 1, Chapter 8 Patient safety in plastic
surgery*

Moustapha Hamdi, MD, PhD
Professor and Chairman of Plastic and
Reconstructive Surgery
Department of Plastic Surgery
Brussels University Hospital
Brussels, Belgium
*Volume 5, Chapter 21 Local flaps in partial
breast reconstruction*

Warren C. Hammert, MD
Associate Professor of Orthopaedic and
Plastic Surgery
Department of Orthopaedic Surgery
University of Rochester Medical Center
Rochester, NY, USA
*Volume 6, Chapter 7 Hand fractures and joint
injuries*

Dennis C. Hammond, MD
Clinical Assistant Professor
Department of Surgery
Michigan State University College of Human
Medicine
East Lansing
Associate Program Director
Plastic and Reconstructive Surgery
Grand Rapids Medical Education and Research
Center for Health Professions
Grand Rapids, MI, USA
*Volume 5, Chapter 8.4 Short scar periareolar
inferior pedicle reduction (SPAIR) mammaplasty*
Volume 5, Video 8.4.01 Spair technique

Scott L. Hansen, MD, FACS
Assistant Professor of Plastic and
Reconstructive Surgery
Chief, Hand and Microvascular Surgery
University of California, San Francisco
Chief, Plastic and Reconstructive Surgery
San Francisco General Hospital
San Francisco, CA, USA
*Volume 1, Chapter 24 Flap classification and
applications*

James A. Harris, MD
Cosmetic Surgeon
Private Practice
Hasson & Wong Aesthetic Surgery
Vancouver, BC, Canada
Volume 2, Video 23.05 FUE Harris safe system

Isaac Harvey, MD
Clinical Fellow
Department of Paediatric Plastic and
Reconstructive Surgery
Hospital for Sick Kids
Toronto, ON, Canada
*Volume 6, Chapter 35 Free functional muscle
transfers in the upper extremity*

Victor Hasson, MD
Cosmetic Surgeon
Private Practice
Hasson & Wong Aesthetic Surgery
Vancouver, BC, Canada
*Volume 2, Video 23.07 Perpendicular angle
grafting technique*

Theresa A Hegge, MD, MPH
Resident of Plastic Surgery
Division of Plastic Surgery
Southern Illinois University
Springfield, IL, USA
*Volume 6, Chapter 6 Nail and fingertip
reconstruction*

Jill A. Helms, DDS, PhD
Division of Plastic and Reconstructive Surgery
Department of Surgery
School of Medicine
Stanford University
Stanford, CA, USA
*Volume 3, Chapter 22 Embryology of the
craniofacial complex*

Ginard I. Henry, MD
Assistant Professor of Surgery
Section of Plastic Surgery
University of Chicago Medical Center
Chicago, IL, USA
*Volume 4, Chapter 1 Comprehensive lower
extremity anatomy, embryology, surgical exposure*

Vincent R. Hentz, MD
Emeritus Professor of Surgery and Orthopedic
Surgery (by courtesy)
Stanford University
Stanford, CA, USA
*Volume 6, Chapter 1 Anatomy and biomechanics
of the hand*
*Volume 6, Chapter 37 Restoration of upper
extremity function in tetraplegia*
*Volume 6, Video 37.01 1 Stage grasp IC 6 short
term*
*Volume 6, Video 37.02 2 Stage grasp release
outcome*

**Rebecca L. von der Heyde, PhD,
OTR/L, CHT**
Associate Professor
Program in Occupational Therapy
Maryville University
St. Louis, MO, USA
Volume 6, Chapter 39 Hand therapy
*Volume 6, Video 39.01 Hand therapy
Goniometric measurement*
Volume 6, Video 39.02 Threshold testing
*Volume 6, Video 39.03 Fabrication of a
synergistic splint*

Kent K. Higdon, MD
Former Aesthetic Fellow
Grotting and Cohn Plastic Surgery;
Current Assistant Professor
Vanderbilt University
Nashville, TN, USA
Volume 5, Chapter 7 Mastopexy
Volume 5, Chapter 8.1 Reduction mammaplasty
*Volume 5, Chapter 8.7 Sculpted pillar vertical
mammaplasty*

John Hijjawi, MD, FACS
Assistant Professor
Department of Plastic Surgery, Department of
General Surgery
Medical College of Wisconsin
Milwaukee, WI, USA
*Volume 4, Chapter 20 Cold and chemical injury
to the upper extremity*

Jonay Hill, MD
Clinical Assistant Professor
Anesthesiology Department
Anesthesia and Critical Care
Stanford University School of Medicine
Stanford, CA, USA
*Volume 6, Chapter 4 Anesthesia for upper
extremity surgery*

Piet Hoebeke, MD, PhD
Full Senior Professor of Paediatric Urology
Department of Urology
Ghent University Hospital
Ghent, Belgium
*Volume 4, Chapter 13 Reconstruction of male
genital defects*
*Volume 4, Video 13.01 Complete and partial
penile reconstruction*

William Y. Hoffman, MD
Professor and Chief
Division of Plastic and Reconstructive Surgery
University of California, San Francisco
San Francisco, CA, USA
Volume 3, Chapter 25 Cleft palate

Larry H. Hollier Jr., MD, FACS
Professor and Program Director
Division of Plastic Surgery
Baylor College of Medicine and Texas
Children's Hospital
Houston, TX, USA
*Volume 3, Chapter 29 Secondary deformities of
the cleft lip, nose, and palate*
Volume 3, Video 29.01 Complete takedown
Volume 3, Video 29.02 Abbé flap
*Volume 3, Video 29.03 Thick lip and buccal
sulcus deformities*
Volume 3, Video 29.04 Alveolar bone grafting
Volume 3, Video 29.05 Definitive rhinoplasty

Joon Pio Hong, MD, PhD, MMM
Chief and Associate Professor
Department of Plastic Surgery
Asian Medical Center University of Ulsan
School of Medicine
Seoul, Korea
*Volume 4, Chapter 5 Reconstructive surgery:
Lower extremity coverage*

Richard A. Hopper, MD, MS
Chief
Division of Pediatric Plastic Surgery
University of Washingtion
Surgical Director
Craniofacial Center
Seattle Childrens Hospital
Associate Professor
Division of Plastic Surgery
Seattle, WA, USA
Volume 3, Chapter 26 Alveolar clefts
Volume 3, Chapter 36 Craniofacial microsomia

Philippe Houtmeyers, MD
Resident
Plastic Surgery
Ghent University Hospital
Ghent, Belgium
*Volume 4, Chapter 13 Reconstruction of male
genital defects*
*Volume 4, Video 13.01 Complete and partial
penile reconstruction*

Steven E.R. Hovius, MD, PhD
Head
Department of Plastic, Reconstructive and
Hand Surgery
ErasmusmMC
University Medical Center
Rotterdam, The Netherlands
*Volume 6, Chapter 28 Congenital hand IV
disorders of differentiation and duplication*

Michael A. Howard, MD
Clinical Assistant Professor of Surgery
Division of Plastic Surgery
University of Chicago, Pritzker School of
Medicine
Northbrook, IL, USA
*Volume 4, Chapter 9 Comprehensive trunk
anatomy*

Jung-Ju Huang, MD
Assistant Professor
Division of Microsurgery
Plastic and Reconstructive Surgery
Chang Gung Memorial Hospital
Taoyuan, Taiwan, The People's Republic of
China
*Volume 3, Chapter 12 Oral cavity, tongue, and
mandibular reconstructions*
*Volume 3, Video 12.01 Fibula
osteoseptocutaneous flap for composite
mandibular reconstruction*
*Volume 3, Video 12.02 Ulnar forearm flap for
buccal reconstruction*

C. Scott Hultman, MD, MBA, FACS
Ethel and James Valone Distinguished
Professor of Surgery
Division of Plastic Surgery
University of North Carolina
Chapel Hill, NC, USA
*Volume 1, Chapter 5 Business principles for
plastic surgeons*

Leung-Kim Hung, MChOrtho (Liv)
Professor
Department of Orthopaedics and Traumatology
Faculty of Medicine
The Chinese University of Hong Kong
Hong Kong, The People's Republic of China
*Volume 6, Chapter 29 Congenital hand V
disorders of overgrowth, undergrowth, and
generalized skeletal deformities*

Gazi Hussain, MBBS, FRACS
Clinical Senior Lecturer
Macquarie Cosmetic and Plastic Surgery
Macquarie University
Sydney, Australia
Volume 3, Chapter 11 Facial paralysis

Marco Innocenti, MD
Director Reconstructive Microsurgery
Department of Oncology
Careggi University Hospital
Florence, Italy
*Volume 6, Chapter 30 Growth considerations in
pediatric upper extremity trauma and
reconstruction*
*Volume 6, Video 30.01 Epiphyseal transplant
harvesting technique*

Clyde H. Ishii, MD, FACS
Assistant Clinical Professor of Surgery
John A. Burns School of Medicine
Chief, Department of Plastic Surgery
Shriners Hospital
Honolulu Unit
Honolulu, HI, USA
*Volume 2, Chapter 10 Asian facial cosmetic
surgery*

Jonathan S. Jacobs, DMD, MD
Associate Professor of Clinical Plastic Surgery
Eastern Virginia Medical School
Norfolk, VA, USA
*Volume 2, Chapter 16 Anthropometry,
cephalometry, and orthognathic surgery*
*Volume 2, Video 16.01 Anthropometry,
cephalometry, and orthognathic surgery*

Jordan M.S. Jacobs, MD
Craniofacial Fellow
Department of Plastic Surgery
New York University Langone Medical Center
New York, NY, USA
*Volume 2, Chapter 16 Anthropometry,
cephalometry, and orthognathic surgery*
*Volume 2, Video 16.01 Anthropometry,
cephalometry, and orthognathic surgery*

**Ian T. Jackson, MD, DSc(Hon), FRCS,
FACS, FRACS (Hon)**
Emeritus Surgeon
Surgical Services Administration
William Beaumont Hospitals
Royal Oak, MI, USA
*Volume 3, Chapter 18 Local flaps for facial
coverage*

Oksana Jackson, MD
Assistant Professor of Surgery
Division of Plastic Surgery
University of Pennsylvania School of Medicine
Clinical Associate
The Children's Hospital of Philadelphia
Philadelphia, PA, USA
Volume 3, Chapter 43 Conjoined twins

Jeffrey E. Janis, MD, FACS
Associate Professor
Program Director
Department of Plastic Surgery
University of Texas Southwestern Medical
Center
Chief of Plastic Surgery
Chief of Wound Care
President-Elect
Medical Staff
Parkland Health and Hospital System
Dallas, TX, USA
Volume 4, Chapter 16 Pressure sores

Leila Jazayeri, MD
Resident
Stanford University Plastic and Reconstructive
Surgery
Stanford, CA, USA
*Volume 1, Chapter 35 Technology innovation in
plastic surgery*

Elizabeth B. Jelks, MD
Private Practice
Jelks Medical
New York, NY, USA
*Volume 2, Chapter 9 Secondary blepharoplasty:
Techniques*

Glenn W. Jelks, MD
Associate Professor
Department of Ophthalmology
Department of Plastic Surgery
New York University School of Medicine
New York, NY, USA
*Volume 2, Chapter 9 Secondary blepharoplasty:
Techniques*

Mark Laurence Jewell, MD
Assistant Clinical Professor of Plastic Surgery
Oregon Health Science University
Jewell Plastic Surgery Center
Eugene, OR, USA
*Volume 2, Chapter 11.4 Facelift: Facial
rejuvenation with loop sutures, the MACS lift and
its derivatives*

Andreas Jokuszies, MD
Consultant Plastic, Aesthetic and Hand
Surgeon
Department of Plastic, Hand and
Reconstructive Surgery
Hanover Medical School
Hanover, Germany
*Volume 1, Chapter 15 Skin wound healing:
Repair biology, wound, and scar treatment*

Neil F. Jones, MD, FRCS
Chief of Hand Surgery
University of California Medical Center
Professor of Orthopedic Surgery
Professor of Plastic and Reconstructive Surgery
University of California Irvine
Irvine, CA, USA
Volume 6, Chapter 22 Ischemia of the hand
*Volume 6, Chapter 34 Tendon transfers in the
upper extremity*
*Volume 6, Video 34.01 EIP to EPL tendon
transfer*

David M. Kahn, MD
Clinical Associate Professor of Plastic Surgery
Department of Surgery
Stanford University School of Medicine
Stanford, CA, USA
Volume 2, Chapter 21 Secondary rhinoplasty

Ryosuke Kakinoki, MD, PhD
Associate Professor
Chief of the Hand Surgery and Microsurgery
Unit
Department of Orthopedic Surgery and
Rehabilitation Medicine
Graduate School of Medicine
Kyoto University
Kyoto, Japan
*Volume 6, Chapter 2 Examination of the upper
extremity*
*Volume 2, Video 2.01-2.17 Examination of the
upper extremity*

Alex Kane, MD
Associate Professor of Surgery
Washington University School of Medicine
St. Louis, WO, USA
Volume 3, Chapter 23 Repair of unilateral cleft lip

Gabrielle M. Kane, MBBCh, EdD, FRCPC
Medical Director, Associate Professor
Department of Radiation Oncology
Associate Professor
Department of Medical Education and
Biomedical Informatics
University of Washington School of Medicine
Seattle, WA, USA
*Volume 1, Chapter 28 Therapeutic radiation:
Principles, effects, and complications*

Michael A. C. Kane, MD
Attending Surgeon Manhattan Eye, Ear and
Throat Institute
Department of Plastic Surgery
New York, NY, USA
Volume 2, Chapter 3 Botulinum toxin (BoNT-A)

Dennis S. Kao, MD
Hand Fellow
Department of Plastic Surgery
Medical College of Wisconsin
Milwaukee, WI, USA
*Volume 4, Chapter 20 Cold and chemical injury
to the upper extremity*

Sahil Kapur, MD
Resident, Plastic and Reconstructive Surgery
Department of Surgery, Division of Plastic and
Reconstructive Surgery
University of Wisconsin
Madison, WI, USA
Volume 3, Chapter 42 Pediatric tumors

Leila Kasrai, MD, MPH, FRCSC
Head, Division of Plastic Surgery
St Joseph's Hospital
Toronto, ON, Canada
Volume 2, Video 22.01 Setback otoplasty

Abdullah E. Kattan, MBBS, FRCS(C)
Clinical Fellow
Division of Plastic Surgery
Department of Surgery
University of Toronto
Toronto, ON, Canada
*Volume 4, Chapter 23 Management of patients
with exfoliative disorders, epidermolysis bullosa,
and TEN*

David L. Kaufman, MD, FACS
Private Practice Plastic Surgery
Aesthetic Artistry Surgical and Medical Center
Folsom, CA, USA
Volume 2, Chapter 21 Secondary rhinoplasty

Lindsay B. Katona, BA
Research Associate
Thayer School of Engineering
Dartmouth College
Hanover, NH, USA
*Volume 1, Chapter 36 Robotics, simulation, and
telemedicine in plastic surgery*

Henry K. Kawamoto, Jr., MD, DDS
Clinical Professor
Division of Plastic Surgery
University of California at Los Angeles
Los Angeles, CA, USA
Volume 3, Chapter 33 Craniofacial clefts

Jeffrey M. Kenkel, MD, FACS
Professor and Vice-Chairman
Rod J Rohrich MD Distinguished Professorship
in Wound Healing and Plastic Surgery
Department of Plastic Surgery
Southwestern Medical School
Director
Clinical Center for Cosmetic Laser Treatment
Dallas, TX, USA
*Volume 2, Chapter 24 Liposuction: A
comprehensive review of techniques and safety*

Carolyn L. Kerrigan, MD, MSc
Professor of Surgery
Section of Plastic Surgery
Dartmouth Hitchcock Medical Center
Lebanon, NH, USA
*Volume 1, Chapter 10 Evidence-based medicine
and health services research in plastic surgery*

Marwan R. Khalifeh, MD
Instructor of Plastic Surgery
Department of Plastic Surgery
Johns Hopkins University School of Medicine
Washington, DC, USA
*Volume 4, Chapter 12 Abdominal wall
reconstruction*

Jae-Hoon Kim, MD
April 31 Aesthetic Plastic Surgical Clinic
Seoul, South Korea
*Volume 2, Video 10.03 Secondary rhinoplasty:
septal extension graft and costal cartilage strut
fixed with K-wire*

**Timothy W. King, MD, PhD, MSBE,
FACS, FAAP**
Assistant Professor of Surgery and Pediatrics
Director of Research
Division of Plastic Surgery, Department of
Surgery
University of Wisconsin School of Medicine and
Public Health
Madison, WI, USA
Volume 1, Chapter 32 Implants and biomaterials

Brian M. Kinney, MD, FACS, MSME
Clinical Assistant Professor of Plastic Surgery
University of Southern California School of
Medicine
Los Angeles, CA, USA
*Volume 1, Chapter 7 Photography in plastic
surgery*

Richard E. Kirschner, MD
Chief, Section of Plastic and Reconstructive
Surgery
Director, Ambulatory Surgical Services
Director, Cleft Lip and Palate Center
Co-Director Nationwide Children's Hospital
Professor of Surgery and Pediatrics
Senior Vice Chair, Department of Plastic Surgery
The Ohio State University College of Medicine
Columbus, OH, USA
Volume 3, Chapter 28 Velopharyngeal dysfunction
*Volume 3, Video 28.01-28.03 Velopharyngeal
incompetence*

Elizabeth Kiwanuka, MD
Division of Plastic Surgery
Brigham and Women's Hospital
Harvard Medical School
Boston, MA, USA
*Volume 1, Chapter 11 Genetics and prenatal
diagnosis*

Grant M. Kleiber, MD
Plastic Surgery Resident
Section of Plastic and Reconstructive Surgery
University of Chicago Medical Center
Chicago, IL, USA
*Volume 4, Chapter 1 Comprehensive lower
extremity anatomy, embryology, surgical exposure*

Mathew B. Klein, MD, MS
David and Nancy Auth-Washington Research
Foundation Endowed Chair for Restorative
Burn Surgery
Division of Plastic Surgery
University of Washington
Program Director and Associate Professor
Division of Plastic Surgery
Harborview Medical Center
Seattle, WA, USA
Volume 4, Chapter 22 Reconstructive burn surgery

Kyung S Koh, MD, PhD
Professor of Plastic Surgery
Asan Medical Center, University of Ulsan
School of Medicine
Seoul, Korea
*Volume 2, Chapter 10 Asian facial cosmetic
surgery*

John C. Koshy, MD
Postdoctoral Research Fellow
Division of Plastic Surgery
Baylor College of Medicine
Houston, TX, USA
*Volume 3, Chapter 29 Secondary deformities of
the cleft lip, nose, and palate*
Volume 3, Video 29.01 Complete takedown
Volume 3, Video 29.02 Abbé flap
*Volume 3, Video 29.03 Thick lip and buccal
sulcus deformities*
Volume 3, Video 29.04 Alveolar bone grafting
Volume 3, Video 29.05 Definitive rhinoplasty

Evan Kowalski, BS
Section of Plastic Surgery
University of Michigan Health System
Ann Arbor, MI, USA
Volume 6, Video 19.02 Silicone MCP arthroplasty

Stephen J. Kovach, MD
Assistant Professor of Surgery
Division of Plastic and Reconstructive Surgery
University of Pennsylvannia Health System
Assistant Professor of Surgery
Department of Orthopaedic Surgery
University of Pennsylvannia Health System
Philadelphia, PA, USA
Volume 4, Chapter 7 Skeletal reconstruction

Steven J. Kronowitz, MD, FACS
Professor, Department of Plastic Surgery
MD Anderson Cancer Center
The University of Texas
Houston, TX, USA
*Volume 1, Chapter 28 Therapeutic radiation
principles, effects, and complications*

Todd A. Kuiken, MD, PhD
Director
Center for Bionic Medicine
Rehabilitation Institute of Chicago
Professor
Department of PMandR
Fienberg School of Medicine
Northwestern University
Chicago, IL, USA
*Volume 6, Chapter 40 Treatment of the upper
extremity amputee*
*Volume 6, Video 40.01 Targeted muscle
reinnervation in the transhumeral amputee*

Michael E. Kupferman, MD
Assistant Professor
Department of Head and Neck Surgery
Division of Surgery
The University of Texas MD Anderson Cancer
Center
Houston, TX, USA
*Volume 3, Chapter 17 Carcinoma of the upper
aerodigestive tract*

Robert Kwon, MD
Plastic Surgeon
Regional Plastic Surgery Center
Richardson, TX, USA
Volume 4, Chapter 16 Pressure sores

**Eugenia J. Kyriopoulos, MD, MSc, PhD,
FEBOPRAS**
Attending Plastic Surgeon
Department of Plastic Surgery and Burn Center
Athens General Hospital "G. Gennimatas"
Athens, Greece
*Volume 5, Chapter 21 Local flaps in partial
breast reconstruction*

Donald Lalonde, BSC, MD, MSc, FRCSC
Professor Surgery
Division of Plastic Surgery
Saint John Campus of Dalhousie University
Saint John, NB, Canada
*Volume 6, Chapter 24 Nerve entrapment
syndromes*
*Volume 6, Video 24.01 Carpal tunnel and cubital
tunnel releases*

Wee Leon Lam, MB, ChB, M Phil, FRCS
Microsurgery Fellow
Department of Plastic and Reconstructive
Surgery
Chang Gung Memorial Hospital
Taipei, Taiwan, The People's Republic of China
*Volume 6, Chapter 14 Thumb and finger
reconstruction – microsurgical techniques*
Volume 6, Video 14.01 Trimmed great toe
Volume 6, Video 14.02 Second toe for index
*Volume 6, Video 14.03 Combined second and
third toe for metacarpal hand*

Julie E. Lang, MD, FACS
Assistant Professor of Surgery
Department of surgery
Director of Breast Surgical Oncology
University of Arizona
Tucson, AZ, USA
*Volume 5, Chapter 10 Breast cancer: Diagnosis
therapy and oncoplastic techniques*
*Volume 5, Video 10.01 Breast cancer: diagnosis
and therapy*

Patrick Lang, MD
Plastic Surgery Resident
University of California
San Francisco, CA, USA
*Volume 1, Chapter 24 Flap classification and
applications*

Claude-Jean Langevin, MD, DMD
Assistant Professor University of Central Florida
Department of Surgery MD Anderson Cancer
Center
Plastic and Reconstructive Surgeon
University of Central Florida
Orlando, FL, USA
Volume 2, Chapter 13 Neck rejuvenation

Laurent Lantieri, MD
Department of Plastic Surgery
Hôpital Européen Georges Pompidou
Assistance Publique Hôpitaux de Paris
Paris Descartes University
Paris, France
Volume 3, Chapter 20 Facial transplant
Volume 3, Video 20.1 and 20.2 Facial transplant

Michael C. Large, MD
Urology Resident
Department of Surgery, Division of Urology
University of Chicago Hospitals
Chicago, IL, USA
*Volume 3, Chapter 44 Reconstruction of
urogenital defects: Congenital*
*Volume 3, Video 44.01 First stage hypospadias
repair with free inner preputial graft*
*Volume 3, Video 44.02 Second stage
hypospadias repair with tunica vaginalis flap*

Don LaRossa, MD
Emeritus Professor of Surgery
Division of Plastic and Reconstructive Surgery
Perelman School of Medicine
University of Pennsylvania
Philadelphia, PA, USA
Volume 3, Chapter 43 Conjoined twins

Caroline Leclercq, MD
Consultant Hand Surgeon
Institut de la Main
Paris, France
*Volume 6, Chapter 17 Management of
Dupuytren's disease*

Justine C. Lee, MD, PhD
Chief Resident
Section of Plastic and Reconstructive Surgery
Department
University of Chicago Medical Center
Chicago, IL, USA
*Volume 3, Chapter 41 Pediatric chest and trunk
defects*

W. P. Andrew Lee, MD
The Milton T. Edgerton, MD, Professor and
Chairman
Department of Plastic and Reconstructive
Surgery
Johns Hopkins University School of Medicine
Baltimore, MD, USA
*Volume 1, Chapter 34 Transplantation in plastic
surgery*
*Volume 6, Chapter 38 Upper extremity
composite allotransplantation*
*Volume 6, Video 38.01 Upper extremity
composite tissue allotransplantation*

Valerie Lemaine, MD, MPH, FRCSC
Assistant Professor of Plastic Surgery
Department of Surgery
Division of Plastic Surgery
Mayo Clinic
Rochester, MN, USA
*Volume 1, Chapter 10 Evidence-based medicine
and health services research in plastic surgery*

**Ping-Chung Leung, SBS, OBE, JP, MBBS,
MS, DSc, Hon DSocSc, FRACS, FRCS,
FHKCOS, FHKAM (ORTH)**
Professor Emeritus
Orthopaedics and Traumatology
The Chinese University of Hong Kong
Hong Kong, The People's Republic of China
*Volume 6, Chapter 29 Congenital hand V
disorders of overgrowth, undergrowth, and
generalized skeletal deformities*

Benjamin Levi, MD
Post Doctoral Research Fellow
Division of Plastic and Reconstructive Surgery
Stanford University
Stanford, CA
House Officer
Division of Plastic and Reconstructive Surgery
University of Michigan
Ann Arbor, MI, USA
*Volume 1, Chapter 13 Stem cells and
regenerative medicine*

L. Scott Levin, MD, FACS
Chairman of Orthopedic Surgery
Department of Orthopaedic Surgery
University of Pennsylvania School of Medicine
Philadelphia, PA, USA
Volume 4, Chapter 7 Skeletal reconstruction

Bradley Limmer, MD
Assistant Clinical Professor
Department of Internal Medicine
Division of Dermatology
Associate Clinical Professor
Department of Plastic and Reconstructive
Surgery
Surgeon, Private Practice
Limmer Clinic
San Antonio, TX, USA
*Volume 2, Video 23.02 Follicular unit hair
transplantation*

Bobby L. Limmer, MD
Professor of Dermatology
University of Texas
Surgeon, Private Practice
Limmer Clinic
San Antonio, TX, USA
*Volume 2, Video 23.02 Follicular unit hair
transplantation*

Frank Lista, MD, FRCSC
Medical Director
Burn Program
The Plastic Surgery Clinic
Mississauga, ON, Canada
*Volume 5, Chapter 8.3 Superior or medial
pedicle*

Wei Liu, MD, PhD
Professor of Plastic Surgery
Associate Director of National Tissue
Engineering Research Center
Department of Plastic and Reconstructive
Surgery
Shanghai 9th People's Hospital
Shanghai Jiao Tong University School of
Medcine
Shanghai, The People's Republic of China
*Volume 1, Chapter 18 Tissue graft, tissue repair,
and regeneration*
*Volume 1, Chapter 20 Repair, grafting, and
engineering of cartilage*

Michelle B. Locke, MBChB, MD
Honourary Lecturer
University of Auckland Department of Surgery
Auckland City Hospital Support Building
Grafton, Auckland, New Zealand
*Volume 2, Chapter 1 Managing the cosmetic
patient*

Sarah A. Long, BA
Research Associate
Thayer School of Engineering
Dartmouth College
San Mateo, CA, USA
*Volume 1, Chapter 36 Robotics, simulation, and
telemedicine in plastic surgery*

Michael T. Longaker, MD, MBA, FACS
Deane P. and Louise Mitchell Professor and
Vice Chair
Department of Surgery
Stanford University
Stanford, CA, USA
*Volume 1, Chapter 13 Stem cells and
regenerative medicine*

Peter Lorenz, MD
Chief of Pediatric Plastic Surgery, Director
Craniofacial Surgery Fellowship
Department of Surgery, Division of Plastic
Surgery
Stanford University School of Medicine
Stanford, CA, USA
*Volume 1, Chapter 16 Scar prevention,
treatment, and revision*

Joseph E. Losee, MD, FACS, FAAP
Professor of Surgery and Pediatrics
Chief, Division Pediatric Plastic Surgery
Children's Hospital of Pittsburgh
University of Pittsburgh Medical Center
Pittsburgh, PA, USA
Volume 3, Chapter 31 Pediatric facial fractures

Albert Losken, MD, FACS
Associate Professor Program Director
Emory Division of Plastic and Reconstructive
Surgery
Emory University School of Medicine
Atlanta, GA, USA
*Volume 5, Chapter 11 The oncoplastic approach
to partial breast reconstruction*

Maria M. LoTempio, MD
Assistant Professor in Plastic Surgery
Medical University of South Carolina
Charleston, SC
Adjunct Assistant Professor in Plastic Surgery
New York Eye and Ear Infirmary
New York, NY, USA
*Volume 5, Chapter 19 Alternative flaps for breast
reconstruction*

Otway Louie, MD
Assistant Professor
Division of Plastic and Reconstructive Surgery
Department of Surgery
University of Washington Medical Center
Seattle, WA, USA
Volume 4, Chapter 17 Perineal reconstruction

David W. Low, MD
Professor of Surgery
Division of Plastic Surgery
University of Pennsylvania School of Medicine
Clinical Associate
The Children's Hospital of Philadelphia
Philadelphia, PA, USA
Volume 3, Chapter 43 Conjoined twins

Nicholas Lumen, MD, PhD
Assistant Professor of Urology
Urology
Ghent University Hospital
Ghent, Belgium
*Volume 4, Chapter 13 Reconstruction of male
genital defects*
*Volume 4, Video 13.01 Complete and partial
penile reconstruction*

Antonio Luiz de Vasconcellos Macedo, MD
General Surgery
Director of Robotic Surgery
President of Oncology
Board of Albert Einstein Hospital
Sao Paulo, Brazil
*Volume 5, Chapter 20 Omentum reconstruction
of the breast*

Gustavo R. Machado, MD
University of California Irvine Medical Center
Department of Orthopaedic Surgery, Orange,
CA, USA
*Volume 6, Video 34.01 EIP to EPL tendon
transfer*

Susan E. Mackinnon, MD
Sydney M. Shoenberg, Jr. and Robert H.
Shoenberg Professor
Department of Surgery, Division of Plastic and
Reconstructive Surgery
Washington University School of Medicine
St. Louis, MO, USA
*Volume 1, Chapter 22 Repair and grafting of
peripheral nerve*
Volume 6, Chapter 33 Nerve transfers
Volume 6, Video 33.01 Nerve transfers

Ralph T. Manktelow, BA, MD, FRCS(C)
Professor
Department of Surgery
University of Toronto
Toronto, ON, Canada
Volume 3, Chapter 11 Facial paralysis

Paul N. Manson, MD
Professor of Plastic Surgery
University of Maryland Shock Trauma Unit
University of Maryland and Johns Hopkins
Schools of Medicine
Baltimore, MD, USA
Volume 3, Chapter 3 Facial fractures

Daniel Marchac, MD
Professor
Plastic, Reconstructive and Aesthetic
College of Medicine of Paris Hospitals
Paris, France
Volume 3, Chapter 32 Orbital hypertelorism

Malcom W. Marks, MD
Professor and Chairman
Department of Plastic Surgery
Wake Forest University School of Medicine
Winston-Salem, NC, USA
*Volume 1, Chapter 27 Principles and applications
of tissue expansion*

Timothy J. Marten, MD, FACS
Founder and Director
Marten Clinic of Plastic Surgery
Medical Director
San Francisco Center for the Surgical Arts
San Francisco, CA, USA
*Volume 2, Chapter 12 Secondary deformities
and the secondary facelift*

Mario Marzola, MBBS
Private Practice
Norwood, SA, Australia
Volume 2, Video 23.01 Donor closure tricophytic technique

Alessandro Masellis, MD
Plastic Surgeon
Department of Plastic Surgery and Burn Therapy
Ospedale Civico ARNAS Palermo
Palermo, Italy
Volume 4, Chapter 19 Extremity burn reconstruction

Mioholo Macollic, MD, PhD
Plastic Surgeon
Former Chief
Professor Emeritus
Department of Plastic Surgery and Burn Unit
ARNAS Civico Hospital
Palermo, Italy
Volume 4, Chapter 19 Extremity burn reconstruction

Jaume Masia, MD, PhD
Professor and Chief
Plastic Surgery Department
Hospital de la Santa Creu i Sant Pau
Universidad Autónoma de Barcelona
Barcelona, Spain
Volume 5, Chapter 13 Imaging in reconstructive breast surgery

David W. Mathes, MD
Associate Professor of Surgery
Department of Surgery, Division of Plastic and Reconstructive Surgery
University of Washington School of Medicine
Chief of Plastic Surgery
Puget Sound Veterans Affairs Hospital
Seattle, WA, USA
Volume 1, Chapter 34 Transplantation in plastic surgery

Evan Matros, MD
Assistant Attending Surgeon
Department of Surgery
Memorial Sloan-Kettering Cancer Center
Assistant Professor of Surgery (Plastic)
Weill Cornell University Medical Center
New York, NY, USA
Volume 1, Chapter 12 Principles of cancer management

G. Patrick Maxwell, MD, FACS
Clinical Professor of Surgery
Department of Plastic Surgery
Loma Linda University Medical Center
Loma Linda, CA, USA
Volume 5, Chapter 2 Breast augmentation
Volume 5, Chapter 4 Current concepts in revisionary breast surgery

Isabella C. Mazzola
Milan, Italy
Volume 1, Chapter 2 History of reconstructive and aesthetic surgery

Riccardo F. Mazzola, MD
Professor of Plastic Surgery
Postgraduate School Plastic Surgery
Maxillo-Facial and Otolaryngolog
Department of Specialistic Surgical Science
School of Medicine
University of Milan
Milan, Italy
Volume 1, Chapter 2 History of reconstructive and aesthetic surgery

Steven J. McCabe, MD, MSc
Assistant Professor
Department of Bioinformatics and Biostatistics
University of Louisville School of Public Health and Information Sciences
Louisville, KY, USA
Volume 6, Chapter 18 Occupational hand disorders

Joseph G. McCarthy, MD
Lawrence D. Bell Professor of Plastic Surgery,
Director Institute of Reconstructive Plastic Surgery and Chair
Department of Plastic Surgery
New York University Langone Medical Center
New York, NY, USA
Volume 3, Chapter 36 Craniofacial microsomia

Mary H. McGrath, MD, MPH
Plastic Surgeon
Division of Plastic Surgery
University of California San Francisco
San Francisco, CA, USA
Volume 1, Chapter 3 Psychological aspects of plastic surgery

Kai Megerle, MD
Research Fellow
Division of Plastic and Reconstructive Surgery
Stanford Medical Center
Stanford, CA, USA
Volume 6, Chapter 10 Extensor tendon injuries

Babak J. Mehrara, MD, FACS
Associate Member, Associate Professor of Surgery (Plastic)
Memorial Sloan-Kettering Cancer Center
Weil Cornell University Medical Center
New York, NY, USA
Volume 1, Chapter 12 Principles of cancer management

Bryan Mendelson, FRCSE, FRACS, FACS
Private Plastic Surgeon
The Centre for Facial Plastic Surgery
Melbourne, Australia
Volume 2, Chapter 6 Anatomy of the aging face

Constantino G. Mendieta, MD, FACS
Private Practice
Miami, FL, USA
Volume 2, Chapter 28 Buttock augmentation
Volume 2, Video 28.01 Buttock augmentation

Frederick J. Menick, MD
Private Practitioner
Tucson, AZ, USA
Volume 3, Chapter 6 Aesthetic nasal reconstruction
Volume 3, Video 6.01 Aesthetic reconstruction of the nose – The 3-stage folded forehead flap for cover and lining,
Volume 3, Video 6.02 Aesthetic reconstruction of the nose-First stage transfer and intermediate operation

Ursula Mirastschijski, MD, PhD
Assistant Professor
Department of Plastic, Hand and Reconstructive Surgery, Burn Center Lower Saxony, Replantation Center
Hannover Medical School
Hannover, Germany
Volume 1, Chapter 15 Skin wound healing: Repair biology, wound, and scar treatment

Takayuki Miura, MD
Emeritus Professor of Orthopedic Surgery
Department of Orthopedic Surgery
Nagoya University School of Medicine
Nagoya, Japan
Volume 6, Chapter 29 Congenital hand V: Disorders of overgrowth, undergrowth, and generalized skeletal deformities

Fernando Molina, MD
Professor of Plastic, Aesthetic and Reconstructive Surgery
Reconstructive and Plastic Surgery
Hospital General "Dr. Manuel Gea Gonzalez"
Universidad Nacional Autonoma de Mexico
Mexico City, Mexico
Volume 3, Chapter 39 Treacher-Collins syndrome

Stan Monstrey, MD, PhD
Professor in Plastic Surgery
Department of Plastic Surgery
Ghent University Hospital
Ghent, Belgium
Volume 4, Chapter 13 Reconstruction of male genital defects
Volume 4, Video 13.01 Complete and partial penile reconstruction

Steven L. Moran, MD
Professor and Chair of Plastic Surgery
Division of Plastic Surgery, Division of Hand and Microsurgery
Professor of Orthopedics
Rochester, MN, USA
Volume 6, Chapter 20 Management of osteoarthritis of the hand and wrist

Luis Humberto Uribe Morelli, MD
Resident of Plastic Surgery
Unisanta Plastic Surgery Department
Sao Paulo, Brazil
Volume 2, Chapter 26 Lipoabdominoplasty
Volume 2, Video 26.01 Lipobdominoplasty
(including secondary lipo)

Robert J. Morin, MD
Plastic Surgeon and Craniofacial Surgeon
Department of Plastic Surgery
Hackensack University Medical Center
Hackensack, NJ
New York Eye and Ear Infirmary
New York, NY, USA
Volume 3, Chapter 8 Acquired cranial and facial bone deformities

Steven F. Morris, MD, MSc, FRCS(C)
Professor of Surgery
Professor of Anatomy and Neurobiology
Dalhousie University
Halifax, NS, Canada
Volume 1, Chapter 23 Vascular territories

Colin Myles Morrison, MSc (Hons), FRCSI (Plast)
Consultant Plastic Surgeon
Department of Plastic and Reconstructive Surgery
St. Vincent's University Hospital
Dublin, Ireland
Volume 2, Chapter 13 Neck rejuvenation
Volume 5, Chapter 18 The deep inferior epigastric artery perforator (DIEAP) flap

Wayne A. Morrison, MBBS, MD, FRACS
Director
O'Brien Institute
Professorial Fellow
Department of Surgery
St Vincent's Hospital
University of Melbourne
Plastic Surgeon
St Vincent's Hospital
Melbourne, Australia
Volume 1, Chapter 19 Tissue engineering

Robyn Mosher, MS
Medical Editor/Project Manager
Thayer School of Engineering (contract)
Dartmouth College
Norwich, VT, USA
Volume 1, Chapter 36 Robotics, simulation, and telemedicine in plastic surgery

Dimitrios Motakis, MD, PhD, FRCSC
Plastic and Reconstructive Surgeon
Private Practice
University Lecturer
Department of Surgery
University of Toronto
Toronto, ON, Canada
Volume 2, Chapter 4 Soft-tissue fillers

A. Aldo Mottura, MD, PhD
Associate Professor of Surgery
School of Medicine
National University of Córdoba
Cordoba, Argentina
Volume 1, Chapter 9 Local anesthetics in plastic surgery

Hunter R. Moyer, MD
Fellow
Department of Plastic and Reconstructive Surgery
Emory University, Atlanta, GA, USA
Volume 5, Chapter 16 The bilateral Pedicled TRAM flap

Gustavo Muchado, MD
Plastic surgeon
Division of Plastic and Reconstructive Surgery and Department of Orthopaedic Surgery
University of California Irvine Medical Center
Orange, CA, USA
Volume 6, Video 34.01 EIP to EPL tendon transfer

Reid V. Mueller, MD
Associate Professor
Division of Plastic and Reconstructive Surgery
Oregon Health and Science University
Portland, OR, USA
Volume 3, Chapter 2 Facial trauma: soft tissue injuries

John B. Mulliken, MD
Director, Craniofacial Centre
Department of Plastic and Oral Surgery
Children's Hospital
Boston, MA, USA
Volume 1, Chapter 29 Vascular anomalies
Volume 3, Chapter 24 Repair of bilateral cleft lip

Egle Muti, MD
Associate Professor of Plastic Reconstructive and Aesthetic Surgery
Department of Plastic Surgery
University of Turin School of Medicine
Turin, Italy
Volume 5, Chapter 23.1 Congenital anomalies of the breast
Volume 5, Video 23.01.01 Congenital anomalies of the breast: An example of tuberous breast type 1 corrected with glandular flap type 1

Maurice Y. Nahabedian, MD
Associate Professor Plastic Surgery
Department of Plastic Surgery
Georgetown University and Johns Hopkins University
Northwest, WA, USA
Volume 5, Chapter 22 Reconstruction of the nipple-areola complex
Volume 5, Video 11.01 Partial breast reconstruction using reduction mammaplasty
Volume 5, Video 11.03 Partial breast reconstruction with a pedicle TRAM

Foad Nahai, MD, FACS
Clinical Professor of Plastic Surgery
Department of Surgery
Emory University School of Medicine
Atlanta, GA, USA
Volume 2, Chapter 1 Managing the cosmetic patient

Fabio X. Nahas, MD, PhD
Associate Professor
Division of Plastic Surgery
Federal University of São Paulo
São Paulo, Brazil
Volume 2, Video 24.01 Liposculpture

Deepak Narayan, MS, FRCS (Eng), FRCS (Edin)
Associate Professor of Surgery
Yale University School of Medicine
Chief
Plastic Surgery
VA Medical Center
West Haven, CT, USA
Volume 3, Chapter 14 Salivary gland tumors

Maurizio B. Nava, MD
Chief of Plastic Surgery Unit
Istituto Nazionale dei Tumori
Milano, Italy
Volume 5, Chapter 14 Expander/implant reconstruction of the breast
Volume 5, Video 14.01 Mastectomy and expander insertion: first stage
Volume 5, Video 14.02 Mastectomy and expander insertion: second stage

Carmen Navarro, MD
Plastic Surgery Consultant
Plastic Surgery Department
Hospital de la Santa Creu i Sant Pau
Universidad Autónoma de Barcelona
Barcelona, Spain
Volume 5, Chapter 13 Imaging in reconstructive breast surgery

Peter C. Neligan, MB, FRCS(I), FRCSC, FACS
Professor of Surgery
Department of Surgery, Division of Plastic Surgery
University of Washington
Seattle, WA, USA
Volume 1, Chapter 1 Plastic surgery and innovation in medicine
Volume 1, Chapter 25 Flap pathophysiology and pharmacology
Volume 3, Chapter 10 Cheek and lip reconstruction
Volume 4, Chapter 3 Lymphatic reconstruction of the extremities
Volume 3, Video 11.01-03 (1) Facial paralysis (2) cross fact graft, (3) gracilis harvest
Volume 3, Video 18.01 Facial artery perforator flap
Volume 4, Video 3.02 Charles Procedure
Volume 5, Video 18.01 SIEA
Volume 5, Video 19.01-19.03 Alternative free flaps

Jonas A Nelson, MD
Integrated General/Plastic Surgery Resident
Department of Surgery
Division of Plastic Surgery
Perelman School of Medicine
University of Pennsylvania
Philadelphia, PA, USA
Volume 5, Video 17.01 The muscle sparing free TRAM flap

David T. Netscher, MD
Clinical Professor
Division of Plastic Surgery
Baylor College of Medicine
Houston, TX, USA
Volume 6, Chapter 21 The stiff hand and the spastic hand

Michael W. Neumeister, MD
Professor and Chairman
Division of Plastic Surgery
SIU School of Medicine
Springfield, IL, USA
Volume 6, Chapter 6 Nail and fingertip reconstruction

M. Samuel Noordhoff, MD, FACS
Emeritus Superintendent
Chang Gung Memorial Hospitals
Taipei, Taiwan, The People's Republic of China
Volume 3, Chapter 23 Repair of unilateral cleft lip

Christine B. Novak, PT, PhD
Research Associate
Hand Program, Division of Plastic and Reconstructive Surgery
University Health Network, University of Toronto
Toronto, ON, Canada
Volume 6, Chapter 39 Hand therapy

Daniel Nowinski, MD, PhD
Director
Department of Plastic and Maxillofacial Surgery
Uppsala Craniofacial Center
Uppsala University Hospital
Uppsala, Sweden
Volume 1, Chapter 11 Genetics and prenatal diagnosis

Scott Oates, MD
Professor
Department of Plastic Surgery
The University of Texas MD Anderson Cancer Center
Houston, TX, USA
Volume 6, Chapter 15 Benign and malignant tumors of the hand

Kerby Oberg, MD, PhD
Associate Professor
Department of Pathology and Human Anatomy
Loma Linda University School of Medicine
Loma Linda, CA, USA
Volume 6, Chapter 25 Congenital hand 1: embryology, classification, and principles

James P. O'Brien, MD, FRCSC
Associate Professor of Surgery
Dalhousie University
Halifax Nova Scotia
Clinical Associate Professor of Surgery
Memorial University
St. John's Newfoundland
Vice President Research
Innovation and Development
Horizon Health Network
New Brunswick, NB, Canada
Volume 6, Chapter 24 Nerve entrapment syndromes

Andrea J. O'Connor, BE(Hons), PhD
Associate Professor of Chemical and Biomolecular Engineering
Department of Chemical and Biomolecular Engineering
University of Melbourne
Melbourne, VIC, Australia
Volume 1, Chapter 19 Tissue engineering

Rei Ogawa, MD, PhD
Associate Professor
Department of Plastic
Reconstructive and Aesthetic Surgery Nippon Medical School
Tokyo, Japan
Volume 1, Chapter 30 Benign and malignant nonmelanocytic tumors of the skin and soft tissue

Dennis P. Orgill, MD, PhD
Professor of Surgery
Division of Plastic Surgery, Brigham and Women's Hospital
Harvard Medical School
Boston, MA, USA
Volume 1, Chapter 17 Skin graft

Cho Y. Pang, PhD
Senior Scientist
Research Institute
The Hospital for Sick Children
Professor
Departments of Surgery/Physiology
University of Toronto
Toronto, ON, Canada
Volume 1, Chapter 25 Flap pathophysiology and pharmacology

Ketan M. Patel, MD
Resident Physician
Department of Plastic Surgery
Georgetown University Hospital
Washington DC, USA
Volume 5, Chapter 22 Reconstruction of the nipple-areola complex

William C. Pederson, MD, FACS
President and Fellowship Director
The Hand Center of San Antonio
Adjunct Professor of Surgery
The University of Texas Health Science Center at San Antonio
San Antonio, TX, USA
Volume 6, Chapter 12 Reconstructive surgery of the mutilated hand

José Abel de la Peña Salcedo, MD
Secretario Nacional
Federación Iberolatinoamericana de Cirugía Plástica, Estética y Reconstructiva
Director del Instituto de Cirugia Plastica, S.C.
Hospital Angeles de las Lomas
Col.Valle de las Palmas
Huixquilucan, Edo de Mexico, Mexico
Volume 2, Chapter 28 Buttock augmentation
Volume 2, Video 28.01 Buttock augmentation

Angela Pennati, MD
Assistant Plastic Surgeon
Unit of Plastic Surgery
Istituto Nazionale dei Tumori
Milano, Italy
Volume 5, Chapter 14 Expander/implant breast reconstructions
Volume 5, Video 14.01 Mastectomy and expander insertion: first stage
Volume 5, Video 14.02 Mastectomy and expander insertion: second stage

Joel E. Pessa, MD
Clinical Associate Professor of Plastic Surgery
UTSW Medical School
Dallas, TX
Hand and Microsurgery Fellow
Christine M. Kleinert Hand and Microsurgery
Louisville, KY, USA
Volume 2, Chapter 17 Nasal analysis and anatomy

Walter Peters, MD, PhD, FRCSC
Professor of Surgery
Department of Plastic Surgery
University of Toronto
Toronto, ON, Canada
Volume 5, Chapter 6 Iatrogenic disorders following breast surgery

Giorgio Pietramaggiori, MD, PhD
Plastic Surgery Resident
Department of Plastic and Reconstructive Surgery
University Hospital of Lausanne
Lausanne, Switzerland
Volume 1, Chapter 17 Skin graft

John W. Polley, MD
Professor and Chairman
Rush University Medical Center
Department of Plastic and Reconstructive Surgery
John W. Curtin – Chair
Co-Director, Rush Craniofacial Center
Chicago, IL, USA
Volume 3, Chapter 27 Orthodontics in cleft lip and palate management

Bohdan Pomahac, MD
Assistant Professor
Harvard Medical School
Director
Plastic Surgery Transplantation
Medical Director
Burn Center
Division of Plastic Surgery
Brigham and Women's Hospital
Boston, MA, USA
Volume 1, Chapter 11 Genetics and prenatal diagnosis

Julian J. Pribaz, MD
Professor of Surgery Harvard Medical School
Division of Plastic Surgery
Brigham and Women's Hospital
Boston, MA, USA
Volume 3, Chapter 19 Secondary facial reconstruction

Andrea L. Pusic, MD, MHS, FRCSC
Associate Attending Surgeon
Department of Plastic and Reconstructive
Memorial Sloan-Kettering Cancer Center
New York, NY, USA
Volume 1, Chapter 10 Evidence-based medicine and health services research in plastic surgery
Volume 4, Chapter 14 Reconstruction of acquired vaginal defects

Oscar M. Ramirez, MD, FACS
Adjunct Clinical Faculty
Plastic Surgery Division
Cleveland Clinic Florida
Boca Raton, FL, USA
Volume 2, Chapter 11.8 Facelift: Subperiosteal facelift
Volume 2, Video 11.08.01 Facelift: Subperiosteal mid facelift endoscopic temporo-midface

William R. Rassman, MD
Director
Private Practice
New Hair Institution
Los Angeles, CA, USA
Volume 2, Video 23.04 FUE FOX procedure

Russell R. Reid, MD, PhD
Assistant Professor of Surgery, Bernard Sarnat Scholar
Section of Plastic and Reconstructive Surgery
University of Chicago
Chicago, IL, USA
Volume 1, Chapter 21 Repair and grafting of bone
Volume 3, Chapter 41 Pediatric chest and trunk defects

Neal R. Reisman, MD, JD
Chief of Plastic Surgery, Clinical Professor
Plastic Surgery
St. Luke's Episcopal Hospital
Baylor College of Medicine
Houston, TX, USA
Volume 1, Chapter 6 Medico-legal issues in plastic surgery

Dominique Renier, MD, PhD
Pediatric Neurosurgeon
Service de Neurochirurgie Pédiatrique
Hôpital Necker-Enfants Malades
Paris, France
Volume 3, Chapter 32 Orbital hypertelorism

Dirk F. Richter, MD, PhD
Clinical Director
Department of Plastic Surgery
Dreifaltigkeits-Hospital Wesseling
Wesseling, Germany
Volume 2, Chapter 25 Abdominoplasty procedures
Volume 2, Video 25.01 Abdominoplasty

Thomas L. Roberts III, FACS
Plastic Surgery Center of the Carolinas
Spartanburg, SC, USA
Volume 2, Chapter 28 Buttock augmentation
Volume 2, Video 28.01 Buttock augmentation

Federico Di Rocco, MD, PhD
Pediatric Neurosurgery
Hôpital Necker Enfants Malades
Paris, France
Volume 3, Chapter 32 Orbital hypertelorism

Natalie Roche, MD
Associate Professor
Department of Plastic Surgery
Ghent University Hospital
Ghent, Belgium
Volume 4, Chapter 13 Reconstruction of male genital defects
Volume 4, Video 13.01 Complete and partial penile reconstruction

Eduardo D. Rodriguez, MD, DDS
Chief, Plastic Reconstructive and Maxillofacial Surgery, R Adams Cowley Shock Trauma Center
Professor of Surgery
University of Maryland School of Medicine
Baltimore, MD, USA
Volume 3, Chapter 3 Facial fractures

Thomas E. Rohrer, MD
Director, Mohs Surgery
SkinCare Physicians of Chestnut Hill
Clinical Associate Professor
Department of Dermatology
Boston University
Boston, MA, USA
Volume 2, Video 5.02 Facial resurfacing

Rod J. Rohrich, MD, FACS
Professor and Chairman Crystal Charity Ball
Distinguished Chair in Plastic Surgery
Department of Plastic Surgery
Professor and Chairman Betty and Warren
Woodward Chair in Plastic and Reconstructive Surgery
University of Texas Southwestern Medical Center at Dallas
Dallas, TX, USA
Volume 2, Chapter 17 Nasal analysis and anatomy
Volume 2, Chapter 18 Open technique rhinoplasty

Joseph M. Rosen, MD
Professor of Surgery
Division of Plastic Surgery, Department of Surgery
Dartmouth-Hitchcock Medical Center
Lyme, NH, USA
Volume 1, Chapter 36 Robotics, simulation, and telemedicine in plastic surgery

E. Victor Ross, MD
Director of Laser and Cosmetic Dermatology
Scripps Clinic
San Diego, CA, USA
Volume 2, Chapter 5 Facial skin resurfacing

Michelle C. Roughton, MD
Chief Resident
Section of Plastic and Reconstructive Surgery
University of Chicago Medical Center
Chicago, IL, USA
Volume 4, Chapter 10 Reconstruction of the chest

Sashwati Roy, PhD
Associate Professor of Surgery
Department of Surgery
The Ohio State University Medical Center
Columbus, OH, USA
Volume 1, Chapter 14 Wound healing

J. Peter Rubin, MD, FACS
Chief of Plastic Surgery
Director, Life After Weight Loss Body Contouring Program
University of Pittsburgh
Pittsburgh, PA, USA
Volume 2, Chapter 30 Post-bariatric reconstruction
Volume 2, Video 30.01 Post bariatric reconstruction – bodylift procedure
Volume 5, Chapter 25 Contouring of the arms, breast, upper trunk, and male chest in the massive weight loss patient
Volume 5, Video 25.01 Brachioplasty part 1: contouring of the arms
Volume 5, Video 25.02 Bracioplasty part 2: contouring of the arms

Alesia P. Saboeiro, MD
Attending Physician
Private Practice
New York, NY, USA
Volume 2, Chapter 14 Structural fat grafting
Volume 2, Video 14.01 Structural fat grafting of
the face

Justin M. Sacks, MD
Assistant Professor
Department of Plastic and Reconstructive
Surgery
The Johns Hopkins University School of
Medicine
Baltimore, MD, USA
Volume 3, Chapter 17 Carcinoma of the upper
aerodigestive tract
Volume 6, Chapter 15 Benign and malignant
tumors of the hand

Hakim K. Said, MD
Assistant Professor of Surgery
Division of Plastic Surgery
University of Washington
Seattle, WA, USA
Volume 4, Chapter 17 Perineal reconstruction

Michel Saint-Cyr, MD, FRCSC
Associate Professor Plastic Surgery
Department of Plastic Surgery
University of Texas Southwestern Medical
Center
Dallas, TX, USA
Volume 4, Chapter 2 Management of lower
extremity trauma
Volume 4, Video 2.01 Alternative flap harvest

Cristianna Bonneto Saldanha, MD
Resident
General Surgery Department
Santa Casa of Santos Hospital
São Paulo, Brazil
Volume 2, Chapter 26 Lipoabdominoplasty
Volume 2, Video 26.01 Lipobdominoplasty
(including secondary lipo)

Osvaldo Ribeiro Saldanha, MD
Chairman of Plastic Surgery
Unisanta
Santos
Past President of the Brazilian Society of
Plastic Surgery (SBCP)
International Associate Editor of Plastic and
Reconstructive Surgery
São Paulo, Brazil
Volume 2, Chapter 26 Lipoabdominoplasty
Volume 2, Video 26.01 Lipobdominoplasty
(including secondary lipo)

Osvaldo Ribeiro Saldanha Filho, MD
São Paulo, Brazil
Volume 2, Chapter 26 Lipoabdominoplasty
Volume 2, Video 26.01 Lipobdominoplasty
(including secondary lipo)

Douglas M. Sammer, MD
Assistant Professor of Plastic Surgery
Department of Plastic Surgery
University of Texas Southwestern Medical
Center
Dallas, TX, USA
Volume 6, Chapter 19 Rheumatologic conditions
of the hand and wrist

Joao Carlos Sampaio Goes, MD, PhD
Director Instituto Brasileiro Controle Cancer
Chairman
Department Plastic Surgery and Mastology of
IBCC
Sao Paulo, Brazil
Volume 5, Chapter 8.6 Periareolar technique with
mesh support
Volume 5, Chapter 20 Omentum reconstruction
of the breast

Michael Sauerbier, MD, PhD
Chairman and Professor
Department for Plastic, Hand and
Reconstructive Surgery
Cooperation Hospital for Plastic Surgery of the
University Hospital Frankfurt
Academic Hospital University of Frankfurt a.
Main
Frankfurt, Germany
Volume 4, Chapter 4 Lower extremity sarcoma
reconstruction
Volume 4, Video 4.01 Management of lower
extremity sarcoma reconstruction

Hani Sbitany, MD
Plastic and Reconstructive Surgery
Assistant Professor of Surgery
University of California
San Francisco, CA, USA
Volume 1, Chapter 24 Flap classification and
applications

Tim Schaub, MD
Private Practice
Arizona Center for Hand Surgery, PC
Phoenix, AZ, USA
Volume 6, Chapter 16 Infections of the hand

Loren S. Schechter, MD, FACS
Assistant Professor of Surgery
Chief, Division of Plastic Surgery
Chicago Medical School
Chicago, IL, USA
Volume 4, Chapter 15 Surgery for gender identity
disorder

Stephen A. Schendel, MD
Professor Emeritus of Surgery and Clinical
Adjunct Professor of Neurosurgery
Department of Surgery and Neurosurgery
Stanford University Medical Center
Stanford, CA, USA
Volume 3, Chapter 4 TMJ dysfunction and
obstructive sleep apnea

Saja S. Scherer-Pietramaggiori, MD
Plastic Surgery Resident
Department of Plastic and Reconstructive
Surgery
University Hospital of Lausanne
Lausanne, Switzerland
Volume 1, Chapter 17 Skin graft

Clark F. Schierle, MD, PhD
Vice President
Aesthetic and Reconstructive Plastic Surgery
Northwestern Plastic Surgery Associates
Chicaho, IL, USA
Volume 5, Chapter 5 Endoscopic approaches to
the breast

Stefan S. Schneeberger, MD
Visiting Associate Professor of Surgery
Department of Plastic Surgery
Johns Hopkins Medical University
Baltimore, MD, USA
Associate Professor of Surgery
Center for Operative Medicine
Department for Viszeral
Transplant and Thoracic Surgery
Innsbruck Medical University
Innsbruck, Austria
Volume 6, Chapter 38 Upper extremity
composite allotransplantation

Iris A. Seitz, MD, PhD
Director of Research and International
Collaboration
University Plastic Surgery
Rosalind Franklin University
Clinical Instructor of Surgery
Chicago Medical School
University Plastic Surgery, affiliated with
Chicago Medical School, Rosalind Franklin
University
Morton Grove, IL, USA
Volume 1, Chapter 21 Repair and grafting of
bone

Chandan K. Sen, PhD, FACSM, FACN
Professor and Vice Chairman (Research) of
Surgery
Department of Surgery
The Ohio State University Medical Center
Associate Dean
Translational and Applied Research
College of Medicine
Executive Director
OSU Comprehensive Wound Center
Columbus, OH, USA
Volume 1, Chapter 14 Wound healing

Subhro K. Sen, MD
Clinical Assistant Professor
Division of Plastic and Reconstructive Surgery
Robert A. Chase Hand and Upper Limb
Center, Stanford University Medical Center
Palo Alto, CA, USA
Volume 1, Chapter 14 Wound healing
Volume 6, Chapter 4 Anesthesia for upper
extremity surgery
Volume 6, Video 4.01 Anesthesia for upper
extremity surgery

Joseph M. Serletti, MD, FACS
Henry Royster – William Maul Measey
Professor of Surgery and Chief
Division of Plastic Surgery
Vice Chair (Finance)
Department of Surgery
University of Pennsylvania
Philadelphia, PA, USA
Volume 5, Chapter 17 Free TRAM breast
reconstruction
Volume 5, Video 17.01 The muscle sparing free
TRAM flap

Randolph Sherman, MD
Vice Chair
Department of Surgery
Cedars-Sinai Medical Center
Los Angeles, CA, USA
Volume 6, Chapter 12 Reconstructive surgery of
the mutilated hand

Kenneth C. Shestak, MD
Professor of Plastic Surgery
Division of Plastic Surgery
University of Pittsburgh
Pittsburgh, PA, USA
Volume 5, Chapter 9 Revision surgery following
breast reduction and mastopexy
Volume 5, Video 7.01 Circum areola mastopexy

Lester Silver, MD, MS
Professor of Surgery
Department of Surgery/Division of Plastic
Surgery
Mount Sinai School of Medicine
New York, NY, USA
Volume 3, Chapter 37 Hemifacial atrophy

Navin K. Singh, MD, MSc
Assistant Professor of Plastic Surgery
Department of Plastic Surgery
Johns Hopkins University School of Medicine
Washington, DC, USA
Volume 4, Chapter 12 Abdominal wall
reconstruction

Vanila M. Singh, MD
Clinical Associate Professor
Stanford University Medical Center
Department of Anesthesiology and Pain
Management
Stanford, CA, USA
Volume 6, Chapter 4 Anesthesia for upper
extremity surgery

Carla Skytta, DO
Resident
Department of Surgery
Doctors Hospital
Columbus, OH, USA
Volume 3, Chapter 5 Scalp and forehead
reconstruction

Darren M. Smith, MD
Resident
Division of Plastic Surgery
University of Pittsburgh Medical Center
Pittsburgh, PA, USA
Volume 3, Chapter 31 Pediatric facial fractures

Gill Smith, MB, BCh, FRCS(Ed),
FRCS(Plast)
Consultant Hand, Plastic and Reconstructive
Surgeon
Great Ormond Street Hospital
London, UK
Volume 6, Chapter 26 Congenital hand II Failure
of formation (transverse and longitudinal arrest)

Paul Smith, MBBS, FRCS
Honorary Consultant Plastic Surgeon
Great Ormond Street Hospital London, UK
Volume 6, Chapter 26 Congenital hand II Failure
of formation (transverse and longitudinal arrest)

Laura Snell, MSc, MD, FRCSC
Assistant Professor
Division of Plastic Surgery
University of Toronto
Toronto, ON, Canada
Volume 4, Chapter 14 Reconstruction of
acquired vaginal defects

Nicole Z. Sommer, MD
Assistant Professor of Plastic Surgery
Southern Illinois University School of Medicine
Springfield, IL, USA
Volume 6, Chapter 6 Nail and fingertip
reconstruction

David H. Song, MD, MBA, FACS
Cynthia Chow Professor of Surgery
Chief, Section of Plastic and Reconstructive
Surgery
Vice-Chairman, Department of Surgery
The University of Chicago Medicine & Biological
Sciences
Chicago, IL, USA
Volume 4, Chapter 10 Reconstruction of the
chest

Andrea Spano, MD
Senior Assistant Plastic Surgeon
Unit of Plastic Surgery
Istituto Nazionale dei Tumori
Milano, Italy
Volume 5, Chapter 14 Expander/implant breast
reconstructions
Volume 5, Video 14.01 Mastectomy and
expander insertion: first stage
Volume 5, Video 14.02 Mastectomy and
expander insertion: second stage

Scott L. Spear, MD, FACS
Professor and Chairman
Department of Plastic Surgery
Georgetown University Hospital
Georgetown, WA, USA
Volume 5, Chapter 15 Latissimus dorsi flap
breast reconstruction
Volume 5, Chapter 26 Fat grafting to the breast
Volume 5, Video 15.01 Latissimus dorsi flap
technique

Robert J. Spence, MD
Director
National Burn Reconstruction Center
Good Samaritan Hospital
Baltimore, MD, USA
Volume 4, Chapter 21 Management of facial
burns
Volume 4, Video 21.01 Management of the
burned face intra-dermal skin closure
Volume 4, Video 21.02 Management of the
burned face full-thickness skin graft defatting
technique

Samuel Stal, MD, FACS
Professor and Chief
Division of Plastic Surgery, Baylor College of
Medicine and Texas Children's Hospital
Houston, TX, USA
Volume 3, Chapter 29 Secondary deformities of
the cleft lip, nose, and palate
Volume 3, Video 29.01 Complete takedown
Volume 3, Video 29.02 Abbé flap
Volume 3, Video 29.03 Thick lip and buccal
sulcus deformities
Volume 3, Video 29.04 Alveolar bone grafting
Volume 3, Video 29.05 Definitive rhinoplasty

Derek M. Steinbacher, MD, DMD
Assistant Professor
Plastic and Carniomaxillofacial Surgery
Yale University, School of Medicine
New Haven, CT, USA
Volume 3, Chapter 34 Nonsyndromic
craniosynostosis

Douglas S. Steinbrech, MD, FACS
Gotham Plastic Surgery
New York, NY, USA
Volume 2, Chapter 9 Secondary blepharoplasty:
Techniques

Lars Steinstraesser, MD
Heisenberg-Professor for Molecular Oncology
and Wound Healing
Department of Plastic and Reconstructive
Surgery, Burn Center
BG University Hospital Bergmannsheil, Ruhr
University
Bochum, North Rhine-Westphalia, Germany
Volume 4, Chapter 18 Acute management of
burn/electrical injuries

Phillip J. Stephan, MD
Clinical Instructor
Department of Plastic Surgery
University of Texas Southwestern
Wichita Falls, TX, USA
Volume 2, Chapter 24 Liposuction: A comprehensive review of techniques and safety

Laurie A. Stevens, MD
Associate Clinical Professor of Psychiatry
Columbia University College of Physicians and Surgeons
New York, NY, USA
Volume 1, Chapter 3 Psychological aspects of plastic surgery

Alexander Stoff, MD, PhD
Senior Fellow
Department of Plastic Surgery
Dreifaltigkeits-Hospital Wesseling
Wesseling, Germany
Volume 2, Chapter 25 Abdominoplasty procedures
Volume 2, Video 25.01 Abdominoplasty

Dowling B. Stough, MD
Medical Director
The Dermatology Clinic
Clinical Assistant Professor
Department of Dermatology
University of Arkansas for Medical Sciences
Little Rock, AR, USA
Volume 2, Video 23.09 Tension donor dissection

James M. Stuzin, MD
Associate Professor of Surgery (Plastic)
Voluntary
University of Miami Leonard M. Miller School of Medicine
Miami, FL, USA
Volume 2, Chapter 11.6 Facelift: The extended SMAS technique in facial rejuvenation
Volume 2, Video 11.06.01 Facelift – Extended SMAS technique in facial shaping

John D. Symbas, MD
Plastic and Reconstructive Surgeon
Private Practice
Marietta Plastic Surgery
Marietta, GA, USA
Volume 5, Chapter 16 The bilateral pedicled TRAM flap
Volume 5, Video 16.01 Pedicle TRAM breast reconstruction

Amir Taghinia, MD
Instructor in Surgery
Harvard Medical School
Staff Surgeon
Department of Plastic and Oral Surgery
Children's Hospital
Boston, MA, USA
Volume 6, Chapter 27 Congenital hand III disorders of formation – thumb hypoplasia
Volume 6, Video 27.01 Congenital hand III disorders of formation – thumb hypoplasia
Volume 6, Video 31.01 Vascular anomalies of the upper extremity

David M.K. Tan, MBBS
Consultant
Department of Hand and Reconstructive Microsurgery
National University Hospital
Yong Loo Lin School of Medicine
National University Singapore
Kent Ridge, Singapore
Volume 6, Chapter 3 Diagnostic imaging of the hand and wrist
Volume 6, Video 3.01 Diagnostic imaging of the hand and wrist – Scaphoid lunate dislocation

Jin Bo Tang, MD
Professor and Chair
Department of Hand Surgery
Chair
The Hand Surgery Research Center
Affiliated Hospital of Nantong University
Nantong, The People's Republic of China
Volume 6, Chapter 9 Flexor tendon injuries and reconstruction
Volume 6, Video 9.01 Flexor tendon injuries and reconstruction – Partial venting of the A2 pulley
Volume 6, Video 9.02 Flexor tendon injuries and reconstruction – Making a 6-strand repair
Volume 6, Video 9.03 Complete flexor-extension without bowstringing

Daniel I. Taub, DDS, MD
Assistant Professor
Oral and Maxillofacial Surgery
Thomas Jefferson University Hospital
Philadelphia, PA, USA
Volume 2, Chapter 16 Anthropometry, cephalometry, and orthognathic surgery
Volume 2, Video 16.01 Anthropometry, cephalometry, and orthognathic surgery

Peter J. Taub, MD, FACS, FAAP
Associate Professor, Surgery and Pediatrics
Division of Plastic and Reconstructive Surgery
Mount Sinai School of Medicine
New York, NY, USA
Volume 3, Chapter 37 Hemifacial atrophy

Sherilyn Keng Lin Tay, MBChB, MRCS, MSc
Microsurgical Fellow
Department of Plastic Surgery
Chang Gung Memorial Hospital
Taoyuan, Taiwan, The People's Republic of China
Specialist Registrar
Department of Reconstructive and Plastic Surgery
St George's Hospital
London, UK
Volume 1, Chapter 26 Principles and techniques of microvascular surgery

G. Ian Taylor, AO, MBBS, MD, MD (HonBrodeaux), FRACS, FRCS (Eng), FRCS (Hon Edinburgh), FRCSI (Hon), FRSC (Hon Canada), FACS (Hon)
Professor
Deparment of Plastic Surgery
Royal Melbourne Hospital
Professor
Department of Anatomy
University of Melbourne
Melbourne, Australia
Volume 1, Chapter 23 Vascular territories

Oren M. Tepper, MD
Assistant Professor
Plastic and Reconstructive Surgery
Montefiore Medical Center
Albert Einstein College of Medicine
New York, NY, USA
Volume 3, Chapter 36 Craniofacial microsomia

Chad M. Teven, BS
Research Associate
Section of Plastic and Reconstructive Surgery
University of Chicago
Chicago, IL, USA
Volume 1, Chapter 21 Repair and grafting of bone

Brinda Thimmappa, MD
Adjunct Assistant Professor
Department of Plastic and Reconstructive Surgery
Loma Linda Medical Center
Loma Linda, CA
Plastic Surgeon
Division of Plastic and Maxillofacial Surgery
Southwest Washington Medical Center
Vancouver, WA, USA
Volume 3, Chapter 4 TMJ dysfunction and obstructive sleep apnea

Johan Thorfinn, MD, PhD
Senior Consultant of Plastic Surgery, Burn Unit
Co-Director
Department of Plastic Surgery, Hand Surgery, and Burns
Linköping University Hospital
Linköping, Sweden
Volume 6, Chapter 32 Peripheral nerve injuries of the upper extremity
Volume 6, Video 32.01-02 Peripheral nerve injuries (1) Digital Nerve Suture (2) Median Nerve Suture

Charles H. Thorne, MD
Associate Professor of Plastic Surgery
Department of Plastic Surgery
NYU School of Medicine
New York, NY, USA
Volume 2, Chapter 22 Otoplasty

Michael Tonkin, MBBS, MD, FRACS (Orth), FRCS Ed Orth
Professor of Hand Surgery
Department of Hand Surgery and Peripheral
Nerve Surgery
Royal North Shore Hospital
The Childrens Hospital at Westmead
University of Sydney Medical School
Sydney, Australia
*Volume 6, Chapter 25 Congenital hand 1
Principles, embryology, and classification*
*Volume 6, Chapter 29 Congenital hand V
Disorders of Overgrowth, Undergrowth, and
Generalized Skeletal Deformities (addendum)*

Patrick L Tonnard, MD
Coupure Centrum Voor Plastische Chirurgie
Ghent, Belgium
*Volume 2, Video 11.04.01 Loop sutures MACS
facelift*

Kathryn S. Torok, MD
Assistant Professor
Division of Pediatric Rheumatology
Department of Pediatrics
Univeristy of Pittsburgh School of Medicine
Childrens Hospital of Pittsburgh
Pittsburgh, PA, USA
Volume 3, Chapter 37 Hemifacial atrophy

Ali Totonchi, MD
Assistant Professor of Surgery
Division of Plastic Surgery
MetroHealth Medical Center
Case Western Reserve University
Cleveland, OH, USA
*Volume 3, Chapter 21 Surgical management of
migraine headaches*

Jonathan W. Toy, MD
Body Contouring Fellow
Division of Plastic and Reconstructive Surgery
University of Pittsburgh
University of Pittsburgh Medical Center Suite
Pittsburg, PA, USA
*Volume 2, Chapter 30 Post-bariatric
reconstruction*
*Volume 5, Chapter 25 Contouring of the arms,
breast, upper trunk, and male chest in the
massive weight loss patient*

Matthew J. Trovato, MD
Dallas Plastic Surgery Institute
Dallas, TX, USA
Volume 2, Chapter 29 Upper limb contouring
Volume 2, Video 29.01 Upper limb contouring

Anthony P. Tufaro, DDS, MD, FACS
Associate Professor of Surgery and Oncology
Departments of Plastic Surgery and Oncology
Johns Hopkins University
Baltimore, MD, USA
*Volume 3, Chapter 16 Tumors of the lips, oral
cavity, oropharynx, and mandible*

Joseph Upton III, MD
Clinical Professor of Surgery
Department of Plastic Surgery
Children's Hospital Boston
Shriner's Burn Hospital Boston
Beth Israel Deaconess Hospital
Harvard Medical School
Boston, MA, USA
*Volume 6, Chapter 27 Congenital hand III
disorders of formation – thumb hypoplasia*
*Volume 6, Chapter 31 Vascular anomalies of the
upper extremity*
*Volume 6, Video 27.01 Congenital hand III
disorders of formation – thumb hypoplasia*
*Volume 6, Video 31.01 Vascular anomalies of
the upper extremity*

Walter Unger, MD
Clinical Professor
Department of Dermatology
Mount Sinai School of Medicine
New York, NY
Associate Professor (Dermatology)
University of Toronto
Private Practice
New York, NY, USA
Toronto, ON, Canada
Volume 2, Video 23.06 Hair transplantation

Francisco Valero-Cuevas, PhD
Director
Brain-Body Dynamics Laboratory
Professor of Biomedical Engineering
Professor of Biokinesiology and Physical
Therapy
By courtesy Professor of Computer Science
and Aerospace and Mechanical Engineering
The University of Southern California
Los Angeles, CA, USA
*Volume 6, Chapter 1 Anatomy and biomechanics
of the hand*

Allen L. Van Beek, MD, FACS
Adjunct Professor
University Minnesota School of Medicine
Division Plastic Surgery
Minneapolis, MN, USA
Volume 2, Video 3.01 Botulinum toxin
Volume 2, Video 4.01 Soft tissue fillers
Volume 2, Video 5.01 Chemical peel
*Volume 2, Video 18.01 Open technique
rhinoplasty*

Nicholas B. Vedder
Professor of Surgery and Orthopaedics
Chief of Plastic Surgery Vice Chair, Department
of Surgery
University of Washington
Seattle, WA, USA
*Volume 6, Chapter 13 Thumb reconstruction:
non microsurgical techniques*

Valentina Visintini Cividin, MD
Assistant Plastic Surgeon
Unit of Plastic Surgery
Istituto Nazionale dei Tumori
Milano, Italy
*Volume 5, Chapter 14 Expander/implant
reconstruction of the breast*
*Volume 5, Video 14.01 Mastectomy and
expander insertion: first stage*
*Volume 5, Video 14.02 Mastectomy and
expander insertion: second stage*

Peter M. Vogt, MD, PhD
Professor and Chairman
Department of Plastic Hand and Reconstructive
Surgery
Hannover Medical School
Hannover, Germany
*Volume 1, Chapter 15 Skin wound healing:
Repair biology, wound, and scar treatment*

Richard J. Warren, MD, FRCSC
Clinical Professor
Division of Plastic Surgery
University of British Columbia
Vancouver, BC, Canada
Volume 2, Chapter 7 Forehead rejuvenation
Volume 2, Chapter 11.1 Facelift: Principles
*Volume 2, Chapter 11.2 Facelift: Introduction to
deep tissue techniques*
Volume 2, Video 7.01 Modified Lateral Brow Lift
*Volume 2, Video 11.1.01 Parotid masseteric
fascia*
Volume 2, Video 11.1.02 Anterior incision
Volume 2, Video 11.1.03 Posterior Incision
Volume 2, Video 11.1.04 Facelift skin flap
Volume 2, Video 11.1.05 Facial fat injection

Andrew J. Watt, MD
Plastic Surgeon
Department of Surgery
Division of Plastic and Reconstructive Surgery
Stanford University Medical Center
Stanford University Hospital and Clinics
Palo Alto, CA, USA
*Volume 6, Chapter 17 Management of
Dupuytren's disease*
*Volume 6, Video 17.01 Management of
Dupuytren's disease*

Simeon H. Wall, Jr., MD, FACS
Private Practice
The Wall Center for Plastic Surgery
Gratis Faculty
Division of Plastic Surgery
Department of Surgery
LSU Health Sciences Center at Shreveport
Shreveport, LA, USA
Volume 2, Chapter 21 Secondary rhinoplasty

Derrick C. Wan, MD
Assistant Professor
Department of Surgery
Stanford University School of Medicine
Stanford, CA, USA
*Volume 1, Chapter 13 Stem cells and
regenerative medicine*

Renata V. Weber, MD
Assistant Professor Surgery (Plastics)
Division of Plastic and Reconstructive Surgery
Albert Einstein College of Medicine
Bronx, NY, USA
Volume 1, Chapter 22 Repair and grafting of peripheral nerve

Fu Chan Wei, MD
Professor
Department of Plastic Surgery
Chang Gung Memorial Hospital
Taoyuan, Taiwan, The People's Republic of China
Volume 1, Chapter 26 Principles and techniques of microvascular surgery
Volume 6, Chapter 14 Thumb and finger reconstruction – microsurgical techniques
Volume 6, Video 14.01 Trimmed great toe
Volume 6, Video 14.02 Second toe for index
Volume 6, Video 14.03 Combined second and third toe for metacarpal hand

Mark D. Wells, MD, FRCS, FACS
Clinical Assistant Professor of Surgery
The Ohio State University
Columbus, OH, USA
Volume 3, Chapter 5 Scalp and forehead reconstruction

Gordon H. Wilkes, MD
Clinical Professor and Divisional Director
Division of Plastic Surgery
University of Alberta Faculty of Medicine
Alberta, AB, Canada
Volume 1, Chapter 33 Facial prosthetics in plastic surgery

Henry Wilson, MD, FACS
Attending Plastic Surgeon
Private Practice
Plastic Surgery Associates
Lynchburg, VA, USA
Volume 5, Chapter 26 Fat grafting to the breast

Scott Woehrle, MS, BS
Physician Assistant
Department of Plastic Surgery
Jospeh Capella Plastic Surgery
Ramsey, NJ, USA
Volume 2, Chapter 29 Upper limb contouring
Volume 2, Video 29.01 Upper limb contouring

Johan F. Wolfaardt, BDS, MDent (Prosthodontics), PhD
Professor
Division of Otolaryngology-Head and Neck Surgery
Department of Surgery
Faculty of Medicine and Dentistry
Director of Clinics and International Relations
Institute for Reconstructive Sciences in Medicine
University of Alberta
Covenant Health Group
Alberta Health Services
Alberta, AB, Canada
Volume 1, Chapter 33 Facial prosthetics in plastic surgery

S. Anthony Wolfe, MD
Chief
Division of Plastic Surgery
Miami Children's Hospital
Miami, FL, USA
Volume 3, Chapter 8 Acquired cranial and facial bone deformities
Volume 3, Video 8.01 Removal of venous malformation enveloping intraconal optic nerve

Chin-Ho Wong, MBBS, MRCS, MMed (Surg), FAMS (Plast. Surg)
Consultant
Department of Plastic Reconstructive and Aesthetic Surgery
Singapore General Hospital
Singapore
Volume 2, Chapter 6 Anatomy of the aging face

Victor W. Wong, MD
Postdoctoral Research Fellow
Department of Surgery
Stanford University
Stanford, CA, USA
Volume 1, Chapter 13 Stem cells and regenerative medecine

Jeffrey Yao, MD
Assistant Professor
Department of Orthopaedic Surgery
Stanford University Medical Center
Palo Alto, CA, USA
Volume 6, Chapter 5 Principles of internal fixation as applied to the hand and wrist

Akira Yamada, MD
Assistant Professor
Department of Plastic and Reconstructive Surgery
Osaka Medical College
Osaka, Japan
Volume 3, Video 7.01 Microtia: auricular reconstruction

Michael J. Yaremchuk, MD, FACS
Chief of Craniofacial Surgery-Massachusetts General Hospital
Program Director-Plastic Surgery Training Program
Massachusetts General Hospital
Professor of Surgery
Harvard Medical School
Boston, MA, USA
Volume 2, Chapter 15 Skeletal augmentation
Volume 2, Video 15.01 Midface skeletal augmentation and rejuvenation

David M. Young, MD
Professor of Plastic Surgery
Department of Surgery
University of California
San Francisco, CA, USA
Volume 1, Chapter 24 Flap classification and applications

Peirong Yu, MD
Professor
Department of Plastic Surgery
The University of Texas M.D. Anderson Cancer Center
Houston, TX, USA
Volume 3, Chapter 13 Hypopharyngeal, esophageal, and neck reconstruction
Volume 3, Video 13.01 Reconstruction of pharyngoesophageal defects with the anterolateral thigh flap

James E. Zins, MD
Chairman
Department of Plastic Surgery
Dermatology and Plastic Surgery Institute
Cleveland Clinic
Cleveland, OH, USA
Volume 2, Chapter 13 Neck rejuvenation

Christopher G. Zochowski, MD
Chief Resident
Department of Plastic and Reconstructive Surgery
Case Western Reserve University
Cleveland, OH, USA
Volume 3, Chapter 38 Pierre Robin sequence

Elvin G. Zook, MD
Professor Emeritus
Division of Plastic Surgery
Southern Illinois University School of Medicine
Springfield, IL, USA
Volume 6, Chapter 6 Nail and fingertip reconstruction

Ronald M. Zuker, MD, FRCSC, FACS, FRCSEd(Hon)
Staff Plastic Surgeon
The Hospital for Sick Children
Professor of Surgery
Department of Surgery
The University of Toronto
Toronto, ON, Canada
Volume 3, Chapter 11 Facial paralysis

Acknowledgments

Editing a textbook such as this is an exciting, if daunting job. Only at the end of the project, over 4 years later, does one realize how much work it entailed and how many people helped make it happen. Sue Hodgson was the Commissioning Editor who trusted me to undertake this. Together, over several weekends in Seattle and countless e-mails and phone calls, we planned the format of this edition and laid the groundwork for a planning meeting in Chicago that included the volume editors and the Elsevier team with whom we have worked. I thank Drs. Gurtner, Warren, Rodriguez, Losee, Song, Grotting, Chang and Van Beek for tirelessly ensuring that each volume was as good as it could possibly be.

I had a weekly call with the Elsevier team as well as several visits to the offices in London. I will miss working with them. Louise Cook, Alexandra Mortimer and Poppy Garraway have been professional, thorough, and most of all, fun to work with. Emma Cole and Sam Crowe helped enormously with video content. Sadly, Sue Hodgson has left Elsevier, however Belinda Kuhn ably filled her shoes and ensured that we kept to our timeline, didn't lose momentum, and that the final product was something we would all be proud of.

Several residents helped, in focus groups to define format and style as well as specifically engaging in the editing process. I thank Darren Smith and Colin Woon for their help as technical copyeditors. Thanks to James Saunders and Leigh Jansen for reviewing video content and thanks also to Donnie Buck for all of his help with the electronic content. Of course we edited the book, we didn't write it. The writers were our contributing authors, all of whom engaged with enthusiasm. I thank them for defining Plastic Surgery, the book and the specialty.

Finally, I would like to thank my residents and fellows, who challenge me and make work fun. My partners in the Division of Plastic Surgery at the University of Washington, under the leadership of Nick Vedder, are a constant source of support and encouragement and I thank them. Finally, my family, Kate and David and most of all, my wife Gabrielle are unwavering in their love and support and I will never be able to thank them enough.

Peter C. Neligan, MB, FRCS(I), FRCSC, FACS
2012

I would like to express my appreciation to Dr. Peter Neligan for his confidence in selecting me to assemble this volume. I truly believe that consolidating all the information on breast surgery into one volume makes this project considerably more valuable to the reader. I would like to thank all my international expert contributors who have made sure the information in these pages is the most up-to-date available. I want to particularly thank Dr. Kent (Kye) Higdon, my trusted fellow from 2010-11, without whose careful combing of these chapters for content and organization, this volume would not have been nearly as good. Finally, I want to thank my office staff and the excellent leadership for the project at Elsevier for shepherding this volume to completion.

James C. Grotting, MD, FACS
2012

Dedicated to the memory of Stephen J. Mathes

Anatomy for plastic surgery of the breast

Jorge I. de la Torre and Michael R. Davis

SYNOPSIS

- Size, symmetry, proportionality and the location of the breast and its landmarks on the chest wall all play a role in the attractiveness of the breast.
- Knowledge of breast anatomy, in particular, the vascular pedicle and location of the nerves, facilitates safe and effective surgical management.
- Any pre-existing asymmetries, spinal curvature, or chest wall deformities must be recognized and demonstrated to the patient, as these may be difficult to correct and can become noticeable in the postoperative period.

Introduction

To successfully address the vast array of aesthetic and reconstructive procedures requires a thorough understanding of breast development and anatomy. Surgical techniques including breast augmentation, post-mastectomy reconstruction, mastopexy and reduction mammaplasty require comprehensive understanding of both the normal or ideal anatomy as well as pathologic or variant presentations. The normal appearance of the breast is a vital aspect of the female form. Knowledge of breast anatomy facilitates safe and effective surgical management.

Ideal breast architecture

The appearance of the ideal breast is somewhat subjective. Each patient has their own opinion as to the aesthetics of their breasts, which should be given consideration with any operative alteration of the breast. Reconstruction or cosmetic enhancement of the breast encompasses not only the way the breast looks, but also how it feels to the touch. Size, symmetry, proportionality and the location of the breast and its landmarks on the chest wall all play a role in the attractiveness of the breast. Statistical standards for the dimensions of the breast have been analyzed and reported by various authors *(Fig. 1.1)*.[1–7] The distance from the sternal notch to the nipple and the distance from the midclavicular line are each 19–21 cm. The distance from nipple to the inframammary fold is 5–7 cm *(Fig. 1.1)*. The distance from the nipple to the midline is 9–11 cm. These measurements offer guidelines for altering the breast, which must be individualized, based on proportionality, variances in chest wall anatomy, posture and patient preference *(Fig. 1.2)*.

The breast mound is situated over the pectoralis major muscle between the second and sixth ribs in the nonptotic state. Important landmarks include the upper pole, location of the nipple areolar complex, inframammary fold and lateral breast fold. The upper pole of the breast extends from just below the clavicle to the level

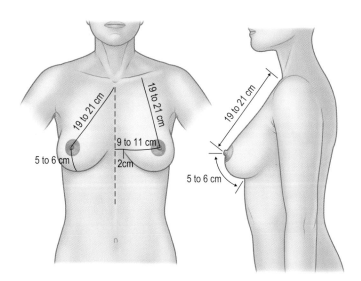

Fig. 1.1 Statistical standards for the dimensions of the breast.

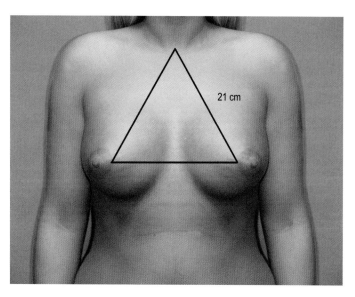

Fig. 1.2 AP image: ideal breast dimensions demonstrating symmetry and projection.

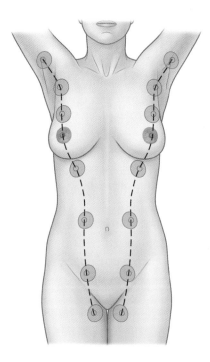

Fig. 1.3 The milk lines. (Reproduced with permission from Standring S, ed. Gray's anatomy, 40th edn. London: Churchill Livingstone; 2008.)

Development of the breast

The breast originates from the ectoderm, the germinal layer which forms the initial breast bud. The connective tissue is derived from the mesoderm. A group of glands, derived from the epidermis, develops within the dermis and underlying fascia. Breast development occurs along the milk line, which extends from the axilla to the groin. The normal breast develops at the level of the fourth intercostal space on the antero-lateral chest wall. Supernumerary breast formation can occur anywhere along the milk line *(Fig. 1.3)*. The most common location of supernumerary breast formation is at the inframammary crease on the left side, but additional breast formation can occur in the axilla as well.

Following a brief period of activity shortly after birth in response to maternal hormones, breast development is quiescent until puberty. Onset of puberty occurs at approximately 9 years of age *(Fig. 1.4)*. Typically, by age 14, parenchymal growth has extended to its mature borders. These include the clavicle at the superior border, the sternum at the medial border, the inframammary fold for the inferior border and the anterior border of the latissimus dorsi for the lateral border. Breast tissue can extend beyond the borders particularly medially and inferiorly. The breast tissue that extends laterally through the axillary fascia into the axillary fat pad

of the nipple. The contour should be neither concave nor convex, but a plane that extends out to the point of maximum projection of the breast at the level of the nipple. In the ideal breast form, the nipple areolar complex should be cephalad to the level of the inframammary fold.

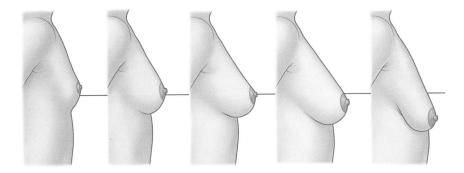

Fig. 1.4 Stages in breast development. Pre-and post-pubertal development and structure of the female breast, demonstrating changes in the contour of the breast. (Reproduced with permission from Standring S, ed. Gray's anatomy, 40th edn. London: Churchill Livingstone; 2008.)

is referred to as the "tail of Spence." Mature breast morphology projects from the chest wall in a conical fashion with its greatest point of projection at the nipple areolar complex *(Fig. 1.5)*.

Development of breast shape is dependent on many factors, including fat content, volume, muscular and skeletal contour and skin and connective tissue compliment. In particular, the Cooper's ligaments provide structural support for the breast parenchyma. These structures combine to provide the final breast shape; it is dependent in large part on heredity and will change with age as the suspensory structure become lax and the breast becomes more ptotic *(Fig. 1.6)*.

Parenchyma

The glandular tissue of the breast is dispersed through a significant amount of adipose tissue.[8] The glands themselves consist of millions of lobules clustered together into 20–25 lobes. Interlobular ducts join to form approximately 20 primary lactiferous ducts that open onto the nipple areolar complex. The lactiferous ducts converge into a specialized ductile network, which stores the milk prior to lactation. The glandular parenchymal ducts are lined with cuboidal cells which transition to stratified squamous epithelium in the ductile and sinus network *(Fig. 1.5)*.

The functioning parenchyma produces milk in the post-partum period. Adipose tissue comprises a significant amount of the breast volume, representing 50–70% of the breast volume. With age and the hormonal changes of menopause, the glandular tissue of the breast

involutes, increasing the adipose to parenchymal tissue ratio. The consistency of the breast softens with the increased fatty tissue accumulation.

An intricate fascial layer supports the breast tissue. The parenchyma is fixed in placed by the superficial fascial system, which extends cephalad from the abdomen, diverges into a superficial and deep component enveloping the breast tissue and maintaining its attachment to the breast wall *(Fig. 1.7)*. The superficial fascial layer is an extension of Scarpa's fascia, which envelopes the glandular tissue deep to the dermal layer. The superficial fascial layer and the dermis can be difficult to distinguish. Subcutaneous fatty tissue between the dermis and the superficial fascia distinguish the two layers. The deep layer diverges at the level of the sixth rib, where the inframammary fold is the inferior border of the parenchyma.

The Cooper's ligaments provide numerous interconnections between the deep and superficial fascial layers. These ligaments pass through ad invest in the breast parenchyma securing to the pectoralis fascia. With attenuation of these support structures, breast ptosis will develop (see *Fig. 1.14*). Regnault delineated a classification system for mammary ptosis describing the relative positions of the nipple and the inframammary fold.[9]

- Mild (*first-degree*) ptosis is described when the nipple lies at the level of the inframammary fold.
- Moderate (*second-degree*) ptosis is a descent of the nipple lies below the level of the inframammary fold but it remains above the most projected portion of the breast.

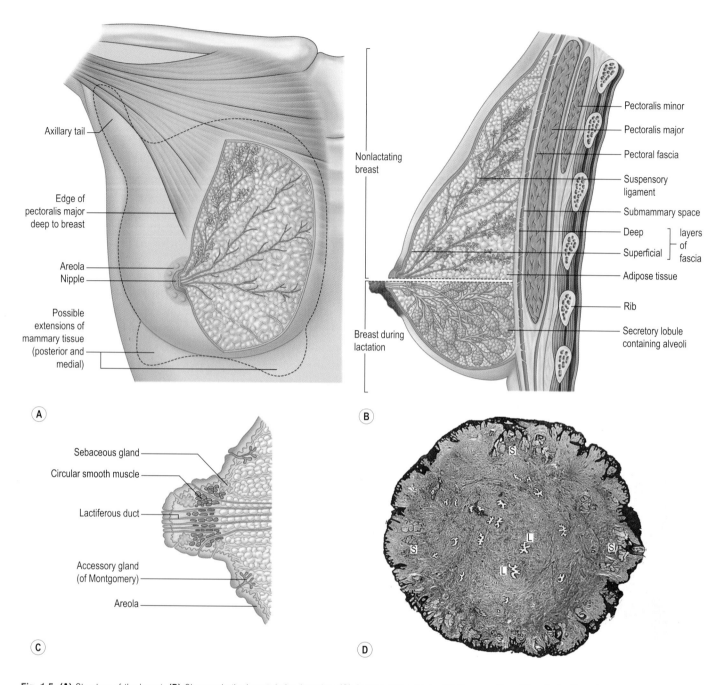

Fig. 1.5 (A) Structure of the breast. **(B)** Changes in the breast during lactation. **(C)** Section of the nipple. **(D)** Cross-section of the nipple. There is a corrugated layer of stratified squamous keratinized epithelium over the nipple surface; 20 or more lactiferous ducts **(L)** open onto the surface; sebaceous glands **(S)** are deep to the epidermis. (A–C, Reproduced with permission from Standring S, ed. Gray's anatomy, 40th edn. London: Churchill Livingstone; 2008; D, from Kerr JB. Atlas of functional histology. London: Mosby; 1999, with permission from Dr JB Kerr, Monash University.)

- Severe (*third-degree*) ptosis is present when the nipple lies below the inframammary fold at the lower contour of the breast and skin brassiere.
- A separate variant, *pseudoptosis* is present when the inferior pole of the breast descends, but the nipple lies above the level of the inframammary fold. The areola-to-inframammary fold distance is increased. Pseudoptosis can occur naturally as well as when bottoming out of a reduced breast occurs.

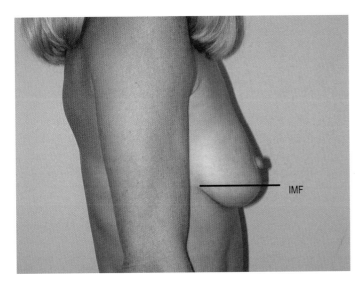

Fig. 1.6 Lateral pseudo ptosis. IMF, inframammary fold.

- Other descriptions of ptosis include the morphologic varieties and how they affect appropriate surgical management. These include the previously mentioned true ptosis, pseudoptosis as well as glandular ptosis.

Some authors have reported a distinct anatomic entity holding the inframammary fold in place, however surgically, this ligamentous structure is not readily apparent. The circumference of the dermis at this level does however, contribute to the effect of allowing the tissue of the breast to drop over at the level of the inframammary fold.

Nipple areola complex

The nipple areola complex is the primary landmark of the breast. As previously stated, it is located at the prominence of the breast mound. The nipple itself may project as much as ≥1 cm, with a diameter of approximately 4–7 mm. The areola consists of pigmented skin surrounding the nipple proper and is on average approximately 4.2–4.5 cm in diameter. The areola consists of keratinized, stratified epithelium and contains not only the lactiferous sinus openings, but also sebaceous glands and the Montgomery glands. The Montgomery glands are intermediate in their nature with characteristics of both the lactiferous gland and the sebaceous gland.

The lactiferous glands extend from their opening on the surface of the nipple down to the parenchyma. The lining of the ducts transition from stratified epithelium on the surface to cuboidal cells within the ducts, and ultimately to columnar cells of the lactiferous gland itself. The nipple and areolar have a network of connecting myoepithelial cells arranged surrounding the sinus opening. This myoepithelium lies between the surface epithelium and the basal lamina. In addition, deep to the nipple and areolar there are smooth muscle fibers which are arranged circumferentially and radially. These fibers are attached to the thick connective tissue of the areola and are responsible for nipple erection.

Because the nipple is the focus of the breast, maximizing its location and maintaining its function are of critical importance when performing breast surgery of any type. Fortunately, the blood supply to the nipple, as with the breast parenchyma, is redundant and rich. The internal mammary perforator, lateral thoracic perforators, and the intercostal perforators from both the anterolateral and anteromedial origins all provide arterial supply to the subdermal plexus of the nipple.[10] Surgical pedicles employed for reduction mammoplasty, mastopexy or oncoplastic procedures are based on preservation of the vasculature of the nipple. Preservation of the underlying parenchyma, with its robust arterial contributions, will maintain the viability of the nipple, as well as help to preserve lactation function.

The nipple and areola have a dense sensory distribution. Branches of the lateral division of the fourth intercostal nerve provide the primary innervation of the nipple.[11] Innervation of the nipple is from the lateral cutaneous branch of the fourth intercostal nerve via two branches, one which passes superficial to the gland, and the other which passes through the retromammary space. Contributions from the third and fifth anterior cutaneous intercostals, as well as the fifth lateral cutaneous intercostals, may also provide some sensation of the nipple.

Skeletal support

Breast asymmetry and form are dependent on normal skeletal support. The breast overlies the anterolateral thorax principally the second through sixth ribs. Deformities of the chest wall such as pectus excavatum,

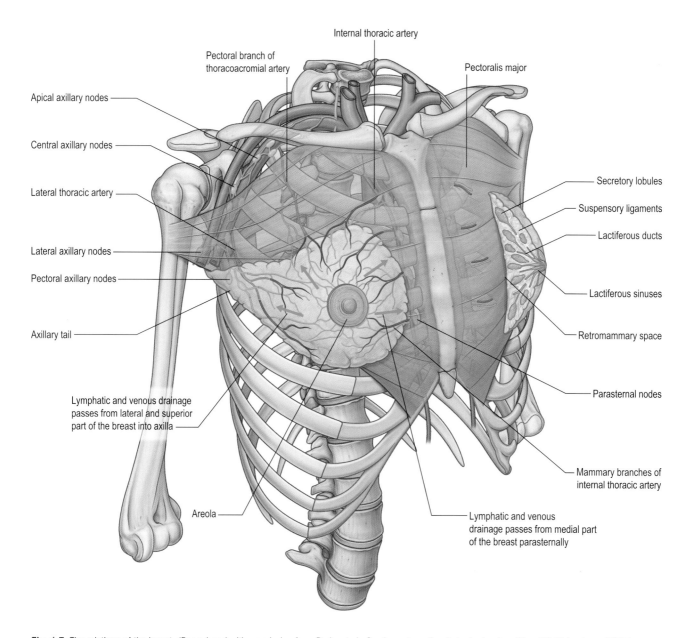

Internal thoracic artery

Pectoral branch of
thoracoacromial artery

Pectoralis major

Apical axillary nodes

Central axillary nodes

Lateral thoracic artery

Lateral axillary nodes

Pectoral axillary nodes

Axillary tail

Lymphatic and venous drainage
passes from lateral and superior
part of the breast into axilla

Areola

Secretory lobules

Suspensory ligaments

Lactiferous ducts

Lactiferous sinuses

Retromammary space

Parasternal nodes

Mammary branches of
internal thoracic artery

Lymphatic and venous
drainage passes from medial part
of the breast parasternally

Fig. 1.7 The relations of the breast. (Reproduced with permission from Drake *et al.*, Gray's anatomy for students. London: Churchill Livingstone; 2005.)

or pectus carinatum can lead to alterations in the projection of the breast. Even spinal abnormalities such as scoliosis can affect the appearance and symmetry of the breasts. Poland syndrome can lead to abnormalities of the structural foundation of the affected side, including the pectoralis muscle (see Ch. 23.2). Conditions which affect the normal alignment of the thoracic spine can also lead to alterations of the relative orientation of the two breast and cause perceived asymmetries of the inframammary fold and nipples.[12] While the breast itself is often fully analyzed, the abnormalities of the underlying chest wall may be more difficult to appreciate properly.

Vascularity

The breast has a rich vascular supply from multiple arterial sources *(Figs 1.8, 1.9)*. The primary arterial supply includes three main sources: the internal

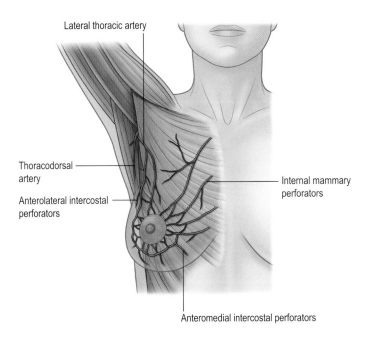

Fig. 1.8 Blood supply to the breast.

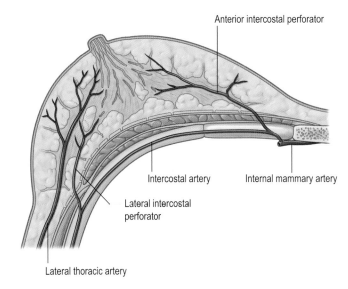

Fig. 1.9 Blood supply to the breast – cross-sectional view.

mammary perforators, lateral thoracic artery and the anterolateral intercostal perforators.[13,14] Additional arterial supply includes the thoracoacromial artery and its perforators and the vessels of the serratus anterior. The clinical implication of the redundancy in arterial supply is that division of the breast tissue is safe as long one or more of the vascular axes are preserved.

This collateralization provides redundant vascular supply to the breast parenchyma and ultimately the overlying skin. Because of the redundant vascularity the breast parenchymal flaps can be based on any of the various vascular pedicles. The skin also has a robust blood supply via the subdermal plexus which arises from the vessels within the breast parenchyma.

The internal mammary perforators enter the superior medial portion of the breast via the second through sixth intercostal spaces. The second and third perforators are the predominant of these perforating vessels. Because of their larger caliber the second or third perforators are the preferred recipient vessels for free tissue reconstruction using the internal mammary perforators. The internal mammary perforators provide approximately 60% of the vascular supply for the breast, although there is some variability in their configuration with relationship to the areola. The most common orientation involves the radial branches of the medial

perforators coalescing into a circumferential network of vessels around the areola that join with the intercostal perforators. This configuration is present approximately 75% of the time. Less commonly, occurring approximately 20% of the time, the radial branches of the medial perforators and the intercostal perforators will form a loop inferior to the areola with terminal branches investing in the nipple. In the less common orientation, the radial branches of the medial perforators can continue into the areola with separated radial branches emanating from the intercostal branches.

Supplying the superolateral aspect of the breast is the lateral thoracic or external mammary artery (*Figs 1.8, 1.9*). This vessel is a primary branch of the axillary artery and enters the breast after passing around the lateral border of the pectoralis major muscle at the inferior aspect of the axilla. It distributes its branches in the upper outer quadrant of the breast.

The lateral intercostal vessels represent an additional important blood supply of the breast. The lateral breast receives anterior intercostal arteries from the third through sixth interspaces. These vessels perforate the serratus anterior just lateral to the pectoral border. Lateral intercostal vessels enter the breast at the anterior margin of the latissimus dorsi to supply the lateral breast and overlying skin.

Medial intercostal perforators are responsible for direct supply of the inferior central portion of the breast inferior to the nipple areolar complex. These perforators

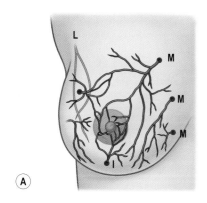
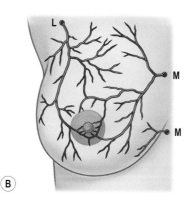
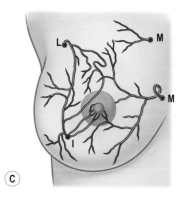

Fig. 1.10 (A–C) Variations in blood supply to the breast. M, internal mammary perforator; L, lateral thoracic artery; I, intercostal perforator.

pass from deep to superficial to supply the breast parenchyma as well as the nipple and nipple areolar complex.

Venous drainage of the breast is via two systems. The subdermal venous plexus above the superficial fascia is quite variable and represents the superficial system. The veins arise from the periareolar venous plexus within the parenchyma, the superficial systems anastomose with the deep system. The deep system parallels the arterial supply with the veins paired to their respective arteries. Venous perforators following the internal mammary perforators drain via the internal mammary vein to the innominate vein. The lateral thoracic veins drain via the azygos vein into the superior vena cava.

Vascular anatomy is also of importance with regard to the recipient site for microvascular anastomosis when free tissue transfer is used for breast reconstruction. Various clinical reports have described the use of the axillary and internal mammary vessels.[15,16] The thoracodorsal vessels have been used, particularly when the reconstruction is immediately postmastectomy. The thoracodorsal artery is often small (<2 mm) and may have insufficient flow. The more proximal circumflex scapular artery can provide a reliable anastomotic site, although a more demanding dissection. The axillary vessels can be technically difficult for the assistant, since they must operate across the chest. In addition, the axillary system may limit flap movement and shaping the breast.

The use of the internal mammary vessels as a recipient site facilitates shaping the medial portion of the breast.[17,18] However, the technique requires partial rib resection and eliminates the opportunity for a potential coronary artery bypass graft. Distal to the fourth rib, the internal mammary veins become smaller, <2 mm, and bifurcates, becoming unsuitable for anastomosis in microsurgical breast reconstruction. Therefore the third rib offers the appropriate level of access. The internal mammary vessel may be preferred in delayed cases, especially in patients who have had adjuvant radiation, as dissection of axillary vessels can be very difficult. Because the respiratory movement can present a challenge for microsurgical dissection, hand ventilation may be required.

The selection of suitable recipient vessels constitutes an important requirement for successful free tissue transfer *(Fig. 1.10)*.

Lymphatics

Lymphatic drainage of the breast has been studied extensively in particular for its role in the dissemination of breast cancer. The predominance of lymph drainage of the breast is via the interlobular lymphatic vessels to the subareolar plexus. Lymph is directed toward the axillary lymph nodes *(Fig. 1.11)*. This drainage is parallel to the venous drainage of the breast. Lateral lymphatics course around the edge of the pectoralis major toward the pectoral lymph nodes. Additional lymphatics course through the pectoral muscles to the apical lymph nodes. From the axillary lymph nodes, lymph drains into the subclavian and supraclavicular lymph nodes.

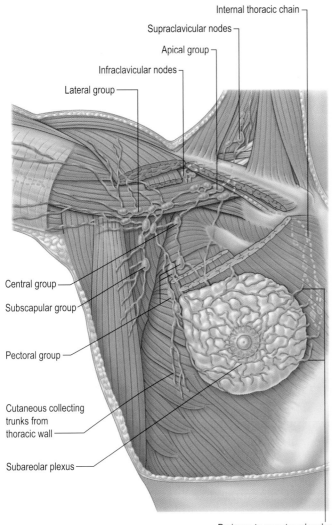

Internal thoracic chain

Supraclavicular nodes

Apical group

Infraclavicular nodes

Lateral group

Central group

Subscapular group

Pectoral group

Cutaneous collecting
trunks from
thoracic wall

Subareolar plexus

Drainage to parasternal nodes

Fig. 1.11 Lymph vessels of the breast and the axillary lymph nodes. (Reproduced with permission from Standring S, ed. Gray's anatomy, 40th edn. London: Churchill Livingstone; 2008.)

Innervation

Sensory innervation has three major nerve distributions which include the anterior lateral intercostals, the medial intercostals, and the cervical plexus. The anterior rami of the lateral cutaneous nerves of the intercostals provide sensation to the lateral portion of the breast extending to and including the nipple areolar complex. The breast demonstrates a dermatomal pattern derived from the anterolateral and anteromedial branches of the intercostal nerves (T3–T5).

Branches of the cervical plexus provide the superior medial sensory innervation. These fibers course superficially in the subcutaneous tissue and usually are undisturbed by the surgical elevation of the upper breast skin flap.

Intercostal segmental nerves contribute the remainder of the breast sensation and can be considered the primary sensory nerves. The third through sixth anterolateral intercostal nerves pass through the interdigitations of the serratus muscles to enter the lateral aspect of the breast.

Along the medial border of the breast, the second through sixth anteromedial intercostal nerves enter the breast parenchyma alongside the internal mammary perforating vessels. These sensory nerves provide innervation to the medial breast and nipple areolar complex.[19,20]

Musculature

When considering the musculature related to the breast, the anatomy of the muscles associated with breast reconstruction should be included. The muscles directly associated with the breast include the pectoralis major, serratus anterior, external oblique and the superior portion of the rectus abdominis *(Fig. 1.12)*.

The breast tissue is attached to the chest wall muscles, primarily the pectoralis major, but also the serratus anterior, external oblique, and the cephalad limit of the rectus abdominus.

Pectoralis major

The pectoralis minor lies between the pectoralis major and the chest wall. The pectoralis major muscle is a broad muscle that extends from its origin on the medial clavicle and lateral sternum to its insertion on the humerus. It has a primary blood supply based on the thoracoacromial artery and a secondary supply via the segmental intercostal perforators arising from the internal mammary artery *(Figs 1.13, 1.14)*.

The medial and lateral anterior thoracic nerves provide innervation for the muscle, entering posteriorly and laterally. The action of the pectoralis major is to flex, adduct, and rotate the arm medially.

The pectoralis major is extremely important in both aesthetic and reconstructive breast surgery, since it provides muscle coverage for the breast implant. In

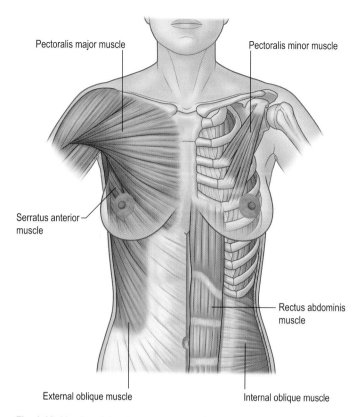

Fig. 1.12 Muscles of the chest wall.

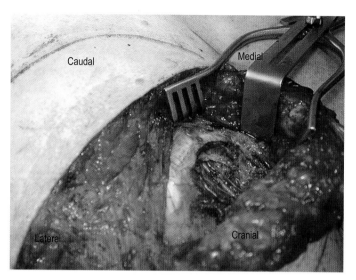

Fig. 1.13 Intraoperative photograph of the intercostal dissection for access to the internal mammary artery for microsurgical breast reconstruction. (From: Darcy *et al*. Surgical technique: The intercostal space approach to the internal mammary vessels in 463 microvascular breast reconstructions. J Plast Reconstr Aesthet Surg 2011; 64(1):58–62.)

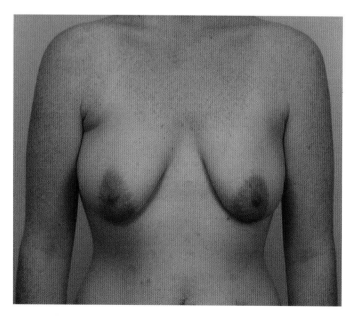

Fig. 1.14 Clinical example of a patient with moderate ptosis. The nipple areolar complex is below the level of the inframammary fold at the lower aspect of the breast.

reconstructive surgery, the pectoralis major muscle covers the implant, providing a decreased risk of exposure of the implant since the skin and underlying subcutaneous tissues are often thin following mastectomy. The muscle also provides additional tissue between the implant and skin, thus decreasing palpability of the implant. Placement of the implant beneath the muscle can cause the implant to be noticeable when the pectoralis is contracted. In these instances, it may be helpful to release the pectoralis muscle from its inferior and medial attachments to decrease the incidence of noticeable contractions. In addition, with inferior release of the pectoralis muscle, lower positioning of the implant can be achieved, resulting in a more aesthetically pleasing appearance.

Serratus anterior

The serratus anterior muscle is a broad muscle that runs along the anterolateral chest wall. Its origin is the outer surface of the upper borders of the first through eighth ribs, and its insertion is on the deep surface of the scapula. Its vascular supply is derived equally from the lateral thoracic artery and branches from the thoracodorsal artery. The long thoracic nerve serves to innervate the serratus anterior, which acts to rotate the scapula, raising the point of the shoulder and drawing the scapula forward toward the body. Transection of the long thoracic nerve is carefully avoided during an axillary lymph node dissection, since its loss results in "winging" as the scapula is released from the chest wall and moves upward and outward. Because the serratus anterior underlies the lateral aspect of the breast, in aesthetic surgery, blunt elevation of the pectoralis major laterally inadvertently elevates a small portion of the serratus muscle. To completely cover the implant with muscle in reconstructive surgery, often the serratus anterior must be elevated sharply to obtain a sufficient muscle layer to provide coverage.

Rectus abdominis

The rectus abdominis muscle demarcates the inferior border of the breast. It is an elongated muscle that runs from its origin at the crest of the pubis and interpubic ligament to its insertion at the xiphoid process and cartilages of the fifth through seventh ribs. It acts to compress the abdomen and flex the spine. The seventh through twelfth intercostal nerves provide sensation to overlying skin and innervate the muscle. Vascularity of the muscle is maintained through a network between the superior and inferior deep epigastric arteries.

When placing an implant for breast reconstruction, in attempting to achieve complete coverage with muscle, the rectus fascia must often be elevated to place the implant sufficiently caudal. This dense, thick fascia is often intimately adherent to the ribs below it. Once it is elevated and released, proper positioning and expansion of the implant can proceed.

External oblique

The external oblique muscle is a broad muscle that runs along the anterolateral abdomen and chest wall. Its origin is from the lower eight ribs, and its insertion is along the anterior half of the iliac crest and the aponeurosis of the linea alba from the xiphoid to the pubis. It acts to compress the abdomen, flex and laterally rotate the spine, and depress the ribs. The seventh through twelfth intercostal nerves serve to innervate the external oblique. A segmental blood supply is maintained through the inferior eight posterior intercostal arteries.

The external oblique muscle abuts the breast on the inferolateral aspect. Elevated along with the rectus

abdominis fascia to provide inferior coverage of the breast implant during reconstructive surgery, its fascia, like the fascia of the rectus abdominis muscle, must be released adequately to provide for proper placement and expansion of the implant. In aesthetic surgery, placement of the implant inferiorly is usually not below these fascial attachments. If the implant is placed behind the fascia, the implant often "rides too high" and may result in a "double bubble" effect, wherein the breast parenchyma slides over and off the implant.

Surgical indications

Indications for surgical alteration of the breast include breast size that is out of proportion to body and patient dissatisfaction with breast shape (see Chs 2, 7 and 8 for technical details specific to breast augmentation, breast reduction and mastopexy).[21] Inadequate size can be addressed by augmentation with prostheses or the use of autologous fat. Excess breast size requires resection of breast tissue or removal via suction lipectomy. Macromastia can result in disproportionate size and ill-fitting clothing as well as significant neck, shoulder and back pain secondary to the excess weight. Undesirable shape is most often related to ptosis as previously discussed. Correction includes addressing both the glandular changes as well as the excess skin in the lower pole. Repositioning of the parenchyma provides increased upper volume in an attempt to recreate an ideal shaped breast. Surgical approaches preserve the vascular supply to the nipple via vertical, horizontal, or medial pedicles.

Conclusion

Breast shape varies among patients, but knowing and understanding the anatomy of the breast ensures safe surgical planning. When the breasts are carefully examined, significant asymmetries are revealed in most patients. Any pre-existing asymmetries, spinal curvature, or chest wall deformities must be recognized and demonstrated to the patient, as these may be difficult to correct and can become noticeable in the postoperative period. Preoperative photographs with multiple views are obtained on all patients and maintained as part of the office record.

Access the complete references list online at **http://www.expertconsult.com**

1. Penn J. Breast reduction. *Br J Plast Surg.* 1955;7(4): 357–371.

   Penn defined the ideal measurements of the breasts with regard to the sternal notch, nipple and inframammary fold. He examined and recoded measurements in 150 female subjects, including 20 who he described as aesthetically perfect. He noted that the suprasternal notch and nipples form the corners of an equilateral triangle the limbs of which are approximately 21 cm in length. The average nipple-to-inframammary fold distance was 6.9 cm.

2. Liu YJ, Thomson JG. Ideal anthropomorphic values of the female breast: correlation of pluralistic aesthetic evaluations with objective measurements. *Ann Plast Surg.* 2011;67(1):7–11.

3. Tepper OM, Unger JG, Small KH, et al. Mammometrics: the standardization of aesthetic and reconstructive breast surgery. *Plast Reconstr Surg.* 2010;125(1):393–400.

4. Westreich M. Anthropomorphic breast measurement: protocol and results in 50 women with aesthetically perfect breasts and clinical application. *Plast Reconstr Surg.* 1997;100(2):468–479.

5. Vandeput JJ, Nelissen M. Considerations on anthropometric measurements of the female breast. *Aesthetic Plast Surg.* 2002;26(5):348–355.

6. Smith Jr DJ, Palin WE Jr, Katch VL, et al. Breast volume and anthropomorphic measurements: normal values. *Plast Reconstr Surg.* 1986;78(3):331–335.

8. Cruz-Korchin N, Korchin L, González-Keelan C, et al. Macromastia: how much of it is fat? *Plast Reconstr Surg.* 2002;109(1):64–68.

   The authors analyzed tissue samples taken from the central, lateral, and preaxillary areas of the breast taken from patients undergoing reduction mammoplasty. On average, the central breast area had only 7% gland and 29% connective tissue. The lateral and preaxillary areas of the breast had 1–3% gland and 5% connective tissue. Two separate methods of analysis were used and they concurred that the enlarged breasts consist primarily of fat with minimal glandular element.

10. Nakajima H, Imanishi N, Aiso S. Arterial anatomy of the nipple-areola complex. *Plast Reconstr Surg.* 1995;96(4):843–845.

    The blood supply to the nipple-areola complex was studied using radiographic analysis of cadaver dissections of five fresh cadavers that had been injected with lead oxide. The authors found that branches of the external and internal mammary arteries provide the dominant blood supply to the nipple-areola complex via small vessels that traverse the subcutaneous tissue.

11. Sarhadi NS, Shaw-Dunn J, Soutar DS. Nerve supply of the breast with special reference to the nipple and areola: Sir Astley Cooper revisited. *Clin Anat.* 1997;10(4):283–288.

    In 1840, Cooper provided the seminal description of innervation of the breast and nipple. Using advanced microsurgical dissecting techniques, the authors sought to confirm his work. They found that the innervation of the nipple was from the lateral cutaneous branch of the fourth intercostal nerve via two branches, one passing superficial to the gland, and the other through the retromammary space, as well as by variable lateral and medial additional branches from the second to fifth nerves. These branches are superficial and form a subdermal plexus under the areola.

12. Tsai FC, Hsieh MS, Liao CK, et al. Correlation between scoliosis and breast asymmetries in women undergoing augmentation mammaplasty. *Aesthetic Plast Surg.* 2010;34(3):374–380.

    The authors evaluated patients who were candidates for augmentation mammoplasty and looked at those with asymmetries as well as those with scoliosis of the back. The relationship between scoliosis and breast volume asymmetry was analyzed statistically. They found that the severity of scoliosis showed significant correlation with the breast volume asymmetry differences. Augmentation mammaplasty for breast asymmetries decreased not only the volume difference but also the difference in nipple levels.

2

Breast augmentation

G. Patrick Maxwell and Allen Gabriel

SYNOPSIS

- Breast augmentation is the most common aesthetic procedure performed in the United States, and perhaps in the world.
- In preparing for a breast augmentation, one must understand each patient's goals and expectations and see if they can be achieved.
- Three important variables have to be addressed prior to surgery: 1. *Incision length and placement* (inframammary, periareolar, transaxillary, transumbilical); 2. *Pocket plane* (subfascial, subglandular, submuscular, subpectoral with dual plane 1,2,3); 3. *Implant choice*: (saline vs silicone, round vs anatomic, smooth vs textured).
- Biodimensional planning may be utilized for optimal preoperative examination.

 Access the Historical Perspective section online at **http://www.expertconsult.com**

Introduction

Glandular hypomastia may occur as a developmental or involutional process and affects a significant number of women in the United States. Developmental hypomastia is often seen as primary mammary hypoplasia, or as a sequela of thoracic hypoplasia (Poland syndrome) or other chest wall deformity. Involutional hypomastia may develop in the postpartum setting and may be exacerbated by breast-feeding or significant weight loss. When compared to the norm, inadequate breast volume may lead to a negative body image, feelings of inadequacy and to low self-esteem.[1] These disturbances may adversely affect a patient's interpersonal relationships, sexual fulfillment, and quality of life.[2]

There has been a steady increase in breast augmentation surgery with the emerging importance of body image, changes in societal expectations, and the increasing acceptance of aesthetic surgery in the United States. Augmentation mammaplasty was performed 289 000 times in 2009, as the most frequently performed cosmetic surgical procedure in women in the United States.[3] In this chapter, we review the history of breast augmentation, operative planning and technique, and some perioperative and late complications of the procedure. The evolution of modern breast implants is described.

Basic science/disease process

Evolution of saline implants

The use of inflatable saline-filled breast implants was first reported in 1965 in France.[7] The saline-filled implant was developed in order to allow the non-inflated implant to be introduced through a relatively small incision, and then inflating the implant *in situ*.[8] Although the incidence of periprosthetic capsular contracture was lower with the saline-filled implants compared with the early silicone gel-filled implants, the deflation rate was initially quite high. The original saline-filled implants manufactured by Simiplast in France had a deflation rate of 75% at 3 years, and was subsequently withdrawn from the market. In 1968, the Heyer-Schulte Company introduced its version of the inflatable saline-filled breast implant (the Mentor 1-800) in the United States.

The thin, platinum-cured shell and the leaflet-style retention valve were two features of the early saline-filled implants that contributed to their high deflation rate.[11] The silicone elastomer shell of the saline-filled implant has been improved by making it thicker and by employing new room-temperature vulcanization (RTV) process. This process is used in the manufacture of all saline-filled implant shells currently available from Allergan (formerly INAMED and McGhan Medical) and from Ethicon/Mentor Corporation.

Saline-filled implants are manufactured with a range of recommended fill volumes. Mild breast asymmetry may be corrected by taking advantage of this range of recommended fill volumes during placement of the implants. Underfilling saline-filled implants may lead to increased deflation rates due to folding or friction subjected to the implant shell, and is not recommended. Underfilling saline-filled implants may also lead to a wrinkled appearance or *rippling* with the breast in certain positions. Saline-filled implants have historically performed better when slightly overfilled, and when placed under thicker soft tissue coverage. Although these implants may be slightly overfilled, aggressive overfilling may lead to a more spherical shape and *scalloping* along the implant edge with knuckle-like palpability and unnatural firmness. Another potential disadvantage of saline-filled implants, is that the consistency of these implants on palpation is similar to that of water instead of the more viscous feel of natural breast tissue. Several saline-filled breast prostheses are available from both manufacturers.

Silicone chemistry

Silicone is a mixture of semi-inorganic polymeric molecules composed of varying length chains of polydimethyl siloxane [$(CH_3)_2$-SiO] monomers. The physical properties of silicones are quite variable depending on the average polymer chain length and the degree of cross-linking between the polymer chains.[12] *Liquid* silicones are polymers with a relatively short average length and very little cross-linking. They have the consistency of an oily fluid and are frequently used as lubricants in pharmaceuticals and medical devices. Silicone *gels* can be produced of varying viscosity by progressively increasing the length of the polymer chains or the degree of cross-linking. The consistency of silicone gels may vary widely from a soft, sticky gel with fluid properties to a firm, cohesive gel exhibiting shape retention or *form-stability* depending upon the polymer chain length and the degree of cross-linking. Extensive chemical cross-linking of the silicone gel polymer will produce a solid form of silicone referred to as an *elastomer* with a flexible, rubber-like quality. Silicone elastomers are used for the manufacture of facial implants, tissue expanders, and the outer shell of all breast prostheses. The versatility of these compounds has made them indispensable in aerospace engineering, medical devices and the pharmaceutical industry.

Evolution of silicone implants

The first generation silicone gel-filled implant was the Cronin–Gerow implant, introduced in 1962 and manufactured by Dow Corning Corporation.[9] The shell of the first generation implant was constructed using a thick, smooth silicone elastomer as a two-piece envelope with a seam along the periphery. The shell was filled with a moderately viscous silicone gel. The implant was anatomically shaped (teardrop) and had several Dacron fixation patches on the posterior aspect to help maintain the proper position of the implant. Unfortunately, these early devices had a relatively high contracture rate that encouraged implant manufacturers to develop second-generation silicone gel-filled implants.

In the 1970s, the second-generation silicone implants were developed in an effort to reduce the incidence of capsular contracture with a thinner, seamless shell and without Dacron patches incorporated into the shell. These implants were round in shape and filled with a less viscous silicone gel to promote a *natural feel*. However, the second-generation breast implants were plagued by diffusion or *bleed* of small silicone molecules into the periprosthetic intra-capsular space due to their thin, permeable shell and low viscosity silicone gel filler. This diffused silicone may be encountered as an oily, sticky residue surrounding the implant within the periprosthetic capsule during explantation of older silicone-filled implants. The phenomenon of silicone bleed has *not* been shown to create significant local or systemic problems.[13]

The development of the third-generation silicone gel-filled implants in the 1980s focused on improving the strength and integrity of the shell in order to reduce silicone gel *bleed* from intact implants, and to reduce implant rupture and subsequent gel migration. Both manufactures (formerly INAMED and MENTOR) developed an implant shell, which consisted of multi layered silicone elastomer. These third-generation prostheses reduced gel bleed to an almost immeasurable level and significantly lowered device shell failure rate.

After the FDA required the temporary removal of third-generation silicone gel implants from the American market in 1992, the *fourth-generation* gel devices evolved for their market re-introduction. These silicone gel breast implants were designed under more stringent ASTM (American Society for Testing Methodology) and FDA-influenced criteria for shell thickness and gel cohesiveness. Furthermore, the fourth-generation devices were manufactured with improved quality control, and with a wider variety of surface textures and implant shapes. The fourth generation FDA approved gel devices are currently available from both breast implant manufactures in the united states.[14–18]

At the same time the concept of anatomically shaped implants with the evolution of the *fifth-generation* silicone gel implants, was introduced.[19] These anatomically-shaped (Style 410) implants are available with a range of volumes and any of the twelve combinations of low, moderate, and full *height* with low, moderate, full and extra *projection*. The Contour Profile® Gel (CPG) implant has been designed by the Mentor Corporation with a more rounded and projecting lower pole and a flatter, more sloping upper pole to yield a more natural breast shape in breast augmentation and reconstruction. These implants are currently under FDA review.

Interestingly, silicone-containing compounds are ubiquitous in everyday life. The general public has been exposed to them for over 50 years in consumer products such as hairsprays, suntan lotions, and moisturizing creams. Silicones are extremely resistant to the action of enzymes when implanted into living tissue largely due to their hydrophobic nature.[12] This makes silicone compounds extremely stable and inert. Silicones are often used in the consumer safety testing industry as the standard to which all other products are compared for biocompatibility.[12] While elemental silicon and silicone particles are detected in the periprosthetic tissues, the biological significance of this finding remains undetermined and uncharacterized.[20] In one study, no significant difference was found in levels of anti-silicone antibodies between patients who had silicone elastomer tissue expanders and control subjects.[21]

Several clinical studies have shown no difference in the incidence of autoimmune diseases in mastectomy patients receiving silicone gel implants compared to patients who had reconstruction with autogenous tissue.[22–28] Even meta-analysis research combining data from over 87 000 women has revealed no association between silicone breast implants and connective tissue diseases.[29,30] Notably, virtually all industrialized nations in the world except the United States use silicone gel implants almost exclusively for breast augmentation.

Diagnosis and patient presentation

The initial consultation for augmentation should begin with open-ended questions about the patient's goals and expectations for the procedure. Patients today have often spent some time researching the procedure either through friends or through the internet. The surgeon should be able to form an impression of the patient as a well-informed, psychiatrically stable person with appropriately realistic expectations for the procedure. Any concerns about the patient's level of understanding, unrealistic expectations, or self-esteem issues should be fully explored prior to proceeding with surgery. A careful medical history and physical examination is essential for the assessment of risk factors and candidacy for breast augmentation. Preoperative mammography is recommended for patients over 35 years of age or patients of any age with significant risk factors for breast cancer.

The *ideal* size and shape of the female breast is inherently subjective and relates to both personal preference and to cultural norms. However, most surgeons will agree that there are certain shared characteristics which represent the aesthetic ideal of the female breast form (*Fig. 2.1*). These characteristics include a profile with a sloping or full upper pole and a gently curved lower

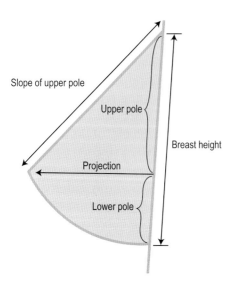

Fig. 2.1 The aesthetic breast form is composed of measurable parameters. The resultant breast form desired after surgical augmentation is determined by the dynamic interaction between the character and compliance of the soft tissue envelope; the quality, volume, and consistency of the breast parenchyma; and the dimensions, volume, and characteristics of the breast implant. This form can be attained by the careful planning and surgical performance of a breast augmentation.

pole with the nipple-areola complex at the point of maximal projection. The breast structure itself may be thought of as the breast parenchyma resting on the anterior chest wall surrounded by a soft tissue envelope made up of skin and subcutaneous adipose. Clearly, the resulting form of the breast after augmentation mammaplasty will be determined by the dynamic interaction of the breast implant, the parenchyma, and the soft tissue envelope.[31]

A thorough physical examination begins with observation and careful documentation of any signs of chest wall deformity or spinal curvature. It is imperative to document and draw attention to any asymmetry of breast size, nipple position, or inframammary fold (IMF) position. Careful palpation of all quadrants of the breast and axilla is required to rule out any dominant masses or suspicious lymph nodes. While palpating the breast, the surgeon should carefully assess the quantity and compliance of the parenchyma and soft tissue envelope. The soft tissue pinch test is useful method of assessment in which the superior pole of the breast is gathered between the examiner's thumb and index finger and measuring the thickness of the intervening tissue. In general, a pinch test result of <2 cm will often indicate a need for subpectoral placement of the implant. It is also important to characterize the amount, quality and

distribution of the breast parenchyma as it may be necessary to reshape or redistribute the parenchyma to achieve the desired shape of the breast mound. The elasticity of the skin should also be characterized by observing its resistance to deflection and noting any signs of skin redundancy or stretch marks. Both manufacturers have developed a preoperative planning system to facilitate patient assessment and implant selection. In addition, the authors utilize 4-D technology to asses both patient's chest wall and soft tissue abnormalities. Chest wall, soft tissue asymmetries, and combinations of both are important to identify preoperatively *(Figs 2.2–2.4)*. This tool is also utilized to understand patient's perception of the desired look by showing the outcomes of utilizing different size and style implants. This is also then projected in the operating room for surgical planning.[32]

Patient selection

Precise measurements must be taken using the IMF, the nipple-areola complex, and the suprasternal notch as key landmarks *(Fig. 2.5)*. The surgeon should measure the breast width (BW) at its widest point, the breast height (BH), and the distance from the nipple-areola complex to the inframammary fold (N:IMF). The distance from the suprasternal notch to the nipple areola complex (SSN:N) and the intermammary distance (IMD) should also be documented. It is often helpful to make markings on the patient in the seated position with a permanent marker just prior to surgery. It is imperative to mark the original IMF, and a good idea to mark the true midline of the anterior chest.

In addition to manual measurements, 3-D and 4-D systems are available to facilitate the measurement process in addition to enhancing the patients overall experience by increasing physician–patient interaction in selecting the appropriate implant.[32] The visual display of the implant selected increases the confidence of the patient in the results that will be achieved. The 4-D imaging system (Precision Light Inc., Los Gatos, CA) automatically measures and characterizes both the soft tissue and chest wall as this is an important step in surgical planning. There are times that minor chest wall or soft tissue asymmetries are missed by manual measurement and visualization. This new

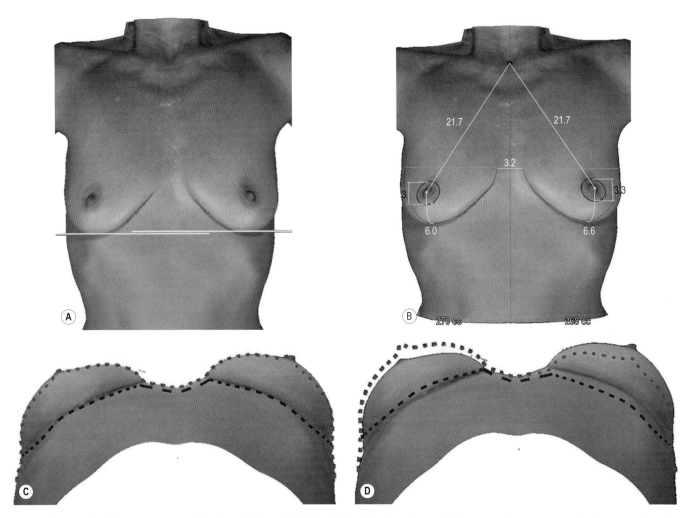

Fig. 2.2 Example of hard tissue asymmetry. **(A)** Patient's AP view. **(B)** Patients AP view following automated biodimensional measurements and volume characterization. **(C)** Bird's eye view of patient's chest. Red line delineating the soft tissue envelope, and blue line the chest wall. **(D)** Bird's eye view of patient's chest with superimposed soft tissue and chest wall outlines as mirror images with identification of chest wall asymmetry. Even though the volume is identical, the presenting anatomy is very different.

system captures all of the asymmetries preoperatively so that appropriate preoperative planning can be performed and the patient is advised with an accurate informed consent.[32] This system is based on the biodimensional principles as previously described. As we continue to pursue increased patient safety and satisfaction, while decreasing reoperation rates, this system will serve as another tool in our armamentarium to achieve these goals.

Informed consent

It is incumbent on the surgeon to evaluate the patient's emotional state, timing, and appropriateness of the desired outcome. It is the surgeon's responsibility to listen, educate, and evaluate; this process and the communication that takes place between patient and surgeon are documented in the medical record. Informed consent is not simply the signing of a paper or contract but refers to the entire process between patient and physician as well as physician extenders. To be "informed," the patient must be provided with adequate information about risks, benefits, and treatment alternatives to the proposed procedure. The authors recommend the use of official ASPS (American Society of Plastic Surgeons) informed consents. To "consent," the patient must be an adult (by age), be capable of rational communication, and be able to understand the information. The informed consent documentation must be thorough and specific

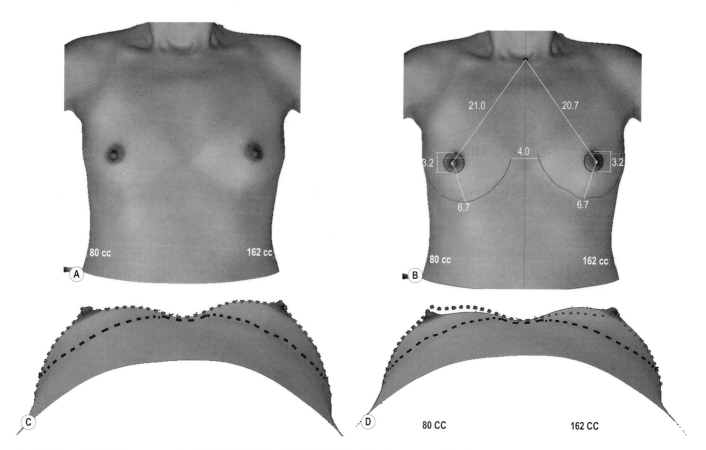

Fig. 2.3 Example of soft tissue asymmetry. **(A)** Patient's AP view. **(B)** Patients AP view following automated biodimensional measurements and volume characterization. Bird's eye view of patient's chest. Red line delineating the soft tissue envelope, and blue line the chest wall. **(C,D)** Bird's eye view of patient's chest with superimposed soft tissue and chest wall outlines as mirror images with identification of soft tissue asymmetry.

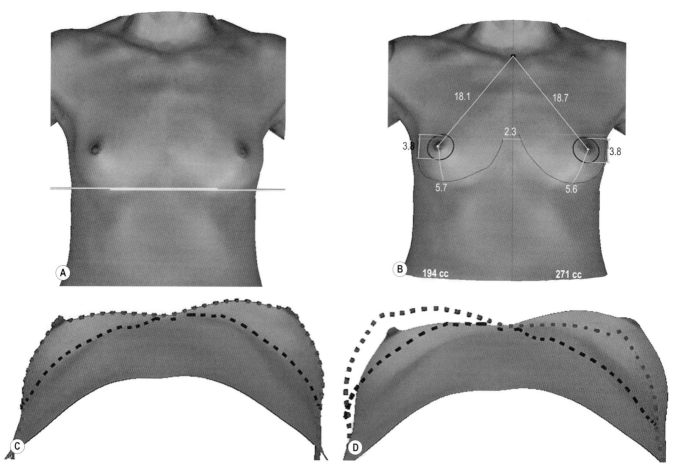

Fig. 2.4 Example of hard and soft tissue asymmetry. **(A)** Patient's AP view. **(B)** Patients AP view following automated biodimensional measurements and volume characterization. **(C,D)** Bird's eye view.

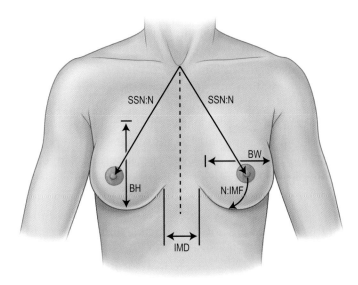

Fig. 2.5 Preoperative measures (taken before breast augmentation) include SSN : N (suprasternal notch to nipple); N : IMF (nipple to inframammary fold); BW (breast width); BH (breast height), and IMD (intermammary distance).

to the operation and preferably the surgeon. A checklist of specifics (which must be initialed by the patient) is considered advisable. "Before and after" photographs may be shown but should be realistic. Photographs of the patient are a necessary form of documentation, requiring appropriate permission. Their confidentiality is essential unless permission is given for any use other than medical review documentation. A male surgeon should be accompanied by a female chaperone during all breast photography and examinations. Because of the multiple options in breast augmentation surgery, a second office visit is advisable. There must be a clear understanding (which is documented in the medical record) between patient and surgeon of the specific desired outcome (size, shape), the alternative ways by which this can be achieved, and the risk-to-benefit ratio of the chosen "pathway."

Operative planning

Incision length and placement

Four types of incision are commonly employed in breast augmentation: transaxillary, inframammary, periareolar, and transumbilical. After implant selection, the decision as to which type of incision is to be used should be made by the patient and surgeon after the options, risks, and benefits of each have been thoroughly explained. Surgeons should offer only the techniques that they are comfortable performing. The final choice should allow the surgeon optimal control and visualization to deliver the desired outcome for the specific patient and the specific implant.

The *inframammary* incision permits complete visualization of either the prepectoral or subglandular pocket and allows precise placement of virtually all implants. The technique does leave a visible scar within the inframammary fold. Smaller incisions (<3 cm) can be used for saline-filled implants, but silicone gel implants often require incisions up to 5.0 cm in length. The incision should be placed in the projected inframammary fold rather than in the existing fold to avoid visibility and widening of the subsequent scar.

The *periareolar* incision is placed at the areolar-cutaneous juncture and generally heals inconspicuously in light pigmented patients. The dissection allows easy adjustment of the inframammary fold and direct access to the lower parenchyma for scoring and release when a constricted lower pole is present. Disadvantages include limited exposure of the surgical field, transection of the parenchymal ducts (which are often colonized with *Staphylococcus epidermidis*), potentially increased risk of nipple sensitivity changes, and visible scarring on the breast mound. This technique should not routinely be used on patients with an areola diameter <40 mm and may not allow introduction of larger gel or enhanced cohesive gel implants.

The *transaxillary* approach can be performed either bluntly or with the aid of an endoscope. The endoscope allows precise dissection and release of the inferior musculofascial attachments of the pectoralis major as well as direct visualization for hemostasis. This approach avoids any scarring on the breast mound and can be used with both saline and gel implants in either a subpectoral or subglandular pocket. Disadvantages include difficulty with parenchymal alterations and the probable need for a second incision on the breast mound for revisionary surgery. Precise implant placement can be more difficult with this incision, and enhanced cohesive gel and anatomic implants may be precluded.

Transumbilical breast augmentation has the obvious advantage of a single, well-hidden, remote incision. It can be used only with saline implants, however, and precise pocket dissection requires experience. The pocket is dissected bluntly, and hemostasis can be difficult from the remote access port. *As with the transaxillary approach, revisions often necessitate a second incision on the breast mound.*

Pocket position

The decision of subglandular/subfascial or subpectoral implant placement depends on implant selection (fill and texture) and tissue thickness *(Fig. 2.6)*. In theory, the best position for a mammary implant is in the subglandular plane. This is the most anatomically correct position to maintain natural shape and form. The authors, however, no longer utilize the subglandular plane and instead prefer the subfascial plane. The reasons for placement of implants in the subpectoral plane are to minimize the risk implant visibility and palpability. Risks of capsular contracture in either plane, is dependent on surgical preparation and technique and not necessarily the pocket. With sound surgical techniques and appropriate postoperative management, capsular contracture can be minimized in either pocket. Our belief is

that the subfascial pocket is more superior to subglandular, as this provides an additional durable layer between the implant and the gland.

The *subfascial* implant position has been advocated for augmentation mammaplasty in certain patients *(Fig. 2.7)*.[33–37] Theoretically, placement of the implant in the subfascial position between the anterior fascia of the pectoralis major and the muscle itself may provide additional support to the overlying soft tissue envelope, causing less distortion of the breast form and decreasing mobility of the implant within the pocket. The long-term outcome studies of breast augmentation employing this position are not yet available, but the procedure is gaining popularity worldwide.[34]

In patients with a pinch test result of >2 cm, the implant can safely be placed in the subfascial plane. Textured implants are the preferred implant for subfascial placement. If one chooses smooth gel implants for the subfascial plane, additional measures to prevent capsular contracture must be taken. These include larger pocket dissections with displacement exercises or possible dilute steroid pocket irrigation. Anatomic-shaped textured implants are placed in the appropriate pocket as determined by soft tissue thickness. Pockets for these

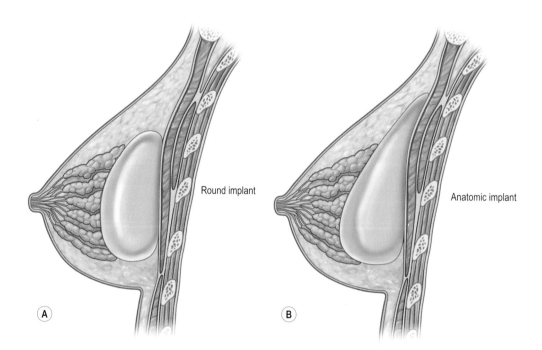

Round implant

Anatomic implant

(A)   **(B)**

Fig. 2.6 (A,B) When ample soft tissue is present, implants may be placed in the subglandular position or subfascial position. When there is soft tissue inadequacy, the subpectoral position is generally preferable.

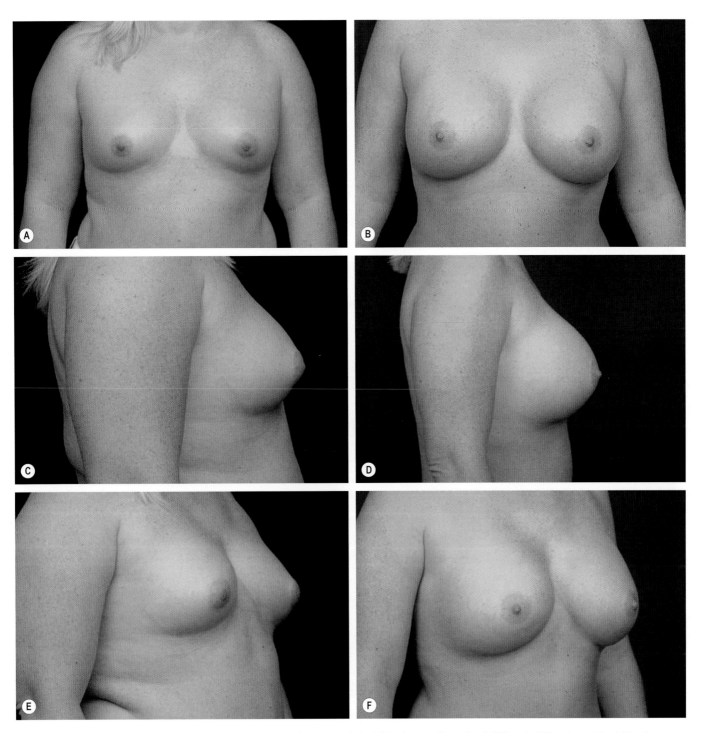

Fig. 2.7 (A–F) Preoperative and postoperative views of a 39-year-old female with Style 110 implants at 12 months: R, 360 cc; L, 360 cc in a subfascial location.

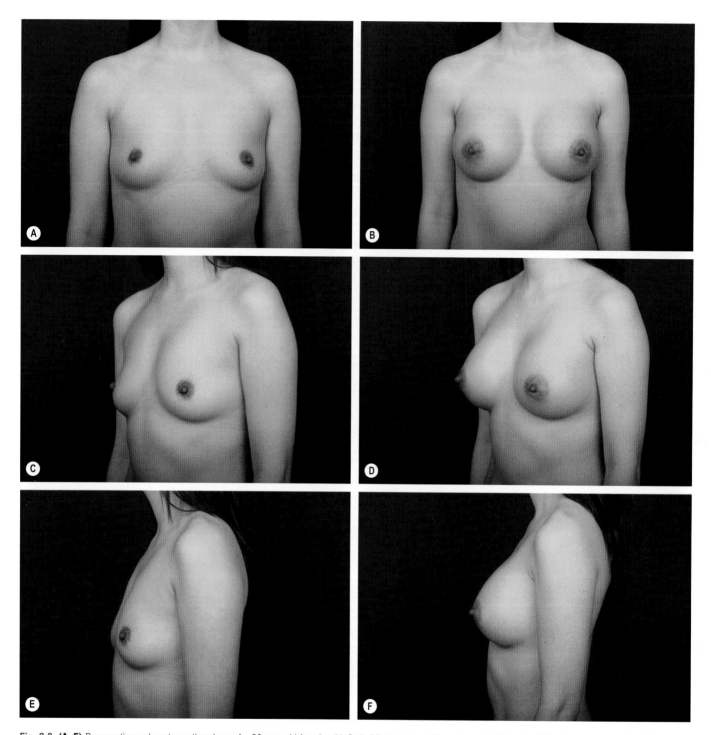

Fig. 2.8 (A–F) Preoperative and postoperative views of a 36-year-old female with Style 20 implants at 12 months: R, 400 cc; L, 400 cc in a subpectoral position.

implants are made only minimally larger than the footprint of the device to minimize displacement or malrotation.

When subpectoral pockets are selected, one generally divides the origin of the pectoralis major muscle just above the inframammary fold to allow better projection in the lower pole of the augmented breast and to maintain a natural inframammary fold *(Fig. 2.8)*. This places the superior portion of the implant in a subpectoral position while the inferior portion is subglandularly

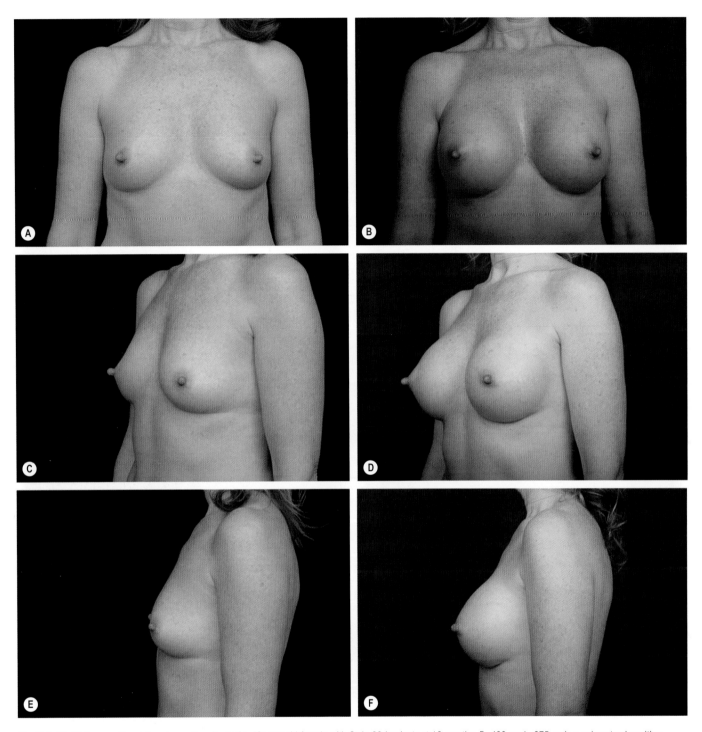

Fig. 2.9 (A–F) Preoperative and postoperative views of a 40-year-old female with Style 20 implants at 12 months: R, 400 cc; L, 375 cc in a subpectoral position.

located. In constricted breasts (tuberous breasts) or ptotic breasts, for which more parenchymal surgical manipulation is necessary, or when there is a greater need for the implant to fill out the lower soft tissue envelope, more dissection between parenchyma and muscle will allow the muscle to cover less of the implant with a resultant greater subglandular implant coverage. Alternatively, the pectoral muscle can be divided at a higher level to give a similar result *(Fig. 2.9)*. These pocket manipulations have been described

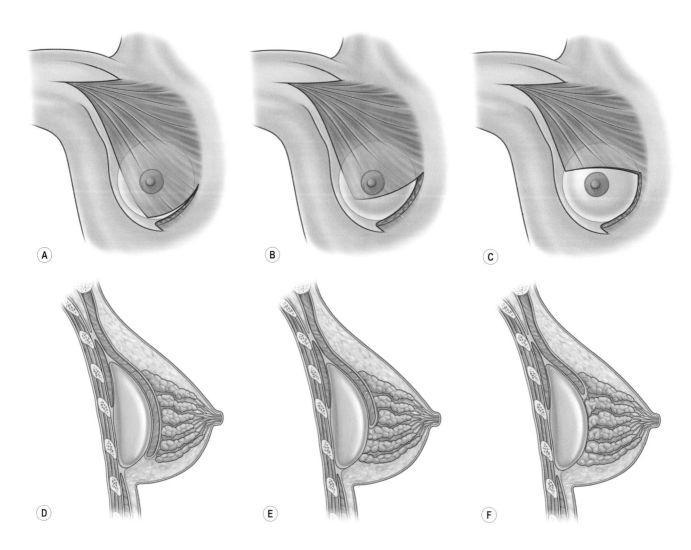

Fig. 2.10 Subpectoral implant placement generally involves release or division of the pectoralis major muscle, resulting in varying coverage relationships of muscles and parenchyma to implant. **(A)** For most routine breasts: *Muscle division* near the inframammary fold results in muscle coverage of most of the implant. **(B)** Breasts with mobile parenchyma muscle interface: *Muscle division* (or muscle-parenchymal detachment) to the lower areolar level results in muscle coverage of the upper half of the implant. **(C)** Breasts with glandular ptosis or lower pole constriction: *Muscle division* (or muscle-parenchymal detachment) to the upper areolar level results in muscle coverage of the upper third of the implant. **(D–F)** Lateral schematic views.

as dual-plane maneuvers to allow varying degrees of subpectoral to subglandular implant coverage.[31] This *dual-plane* dissection allows the pectoralis muscle to retract superiorly or *window-shade* upward, while the breast parenchyma is redraped over the inferior portion of the implant avoiding deformity of the resulting augmented breast *(Fig. 2.10)*.

Implant selection

Filling material

In the USA, there are two implant materials from which to choose: saline- and silicone-filled implants.

The decision between a saline-filled prosthesis and a silicone gel implant is one of the patient's preferences after the surgeon's conveyance of information. Experience has shown the results of silicone gel implants in primary breast augmentation to be generally soft and to have a natural feel and appearance, assuming capsular contracture is not present. Although the authors prefer silicone gel implants, saline implants placed in the subpectoral position can produce good results with a low incidence of capsular contracture. The thicker the soft tissue under which a saline implant is placed, the better it performs. Despite our preference for silicone gel, some patients will undoubtedly continue to have concerns about silicone-filled devices, and subpectoral saline implants have proved to be a reasonable alternative. Ultimately, the patient must feel comfortable with the implant device, so the final decision rests with the patient.

Implant size

The selection of the implant size is initiated during the preoperative consultation period based on both the patient's goals and the surgeon's assessment. In general, the critical factors in selecting a specific implant size are the dimensions of the nascent breast, the compliance and characteristics of the soft tissue envelope, and the desired volume for the resulting augmented breast. The base width of the breast is related to the width of the patient's chest and is proportional to the overall body habitus. It is imperative that this dimension is respected during augmentation in order to maintain the normal anatomical landmarks such as the lateral breast fold in the anterior axillary line and the intermammary distance (IMD). The same is true for breast height, but to a lesser degree than breast width. Violation of these landmarks may yield an unnatural and deformed appearance. Generally, the surgeon should select an implant that is slightly less wide than the existing breast. Implant manufacturers are now producing implants with varying degrees of projection for a given base width. In this way, the surgeon should be able to attain the desired amount of projection while preserving the normal aesthetic proportions of the breast *(Fig. 2.11)*.

The patient's request for a particular breast size and shape will largely determine the dimensions of the breast implant used. In addition to a thorough discussion with the patient as to her desire for the resultant form and size, the 4-D imaging system can be utilized to show the patient the outcomes based on the selection of a particular implant *(Figs 2.2–2.4)*.

Implant surface texture

The decision between textured and smooth-walled implants is only applicable for round implants. Anatomic implants are all textured by design to minimize malrotation *(Fig. 2.12)*. With round implants, the choice between textured and smooth-walled implants is based primarily on minimizing capsular contracture.

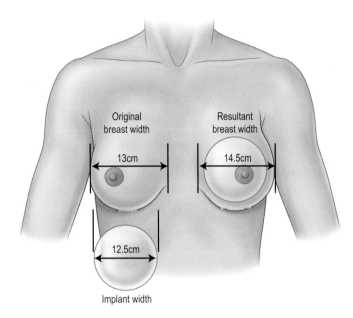

Fig. 2.11 After the width of the existing breast is measured and the desired resultant breast form is formulated, an implant is selected (generally just narrower than the original breast, shown on the patient's right) that in combination with the preoperative breast tissue will achieve the desired postoperative dimensions and form (shown on the patient's left).

For subpectoral augmentation, either implant can probably be used with comparable results. When the device is placed in the subfascial pocket, a textured implant is preferred to minimize capsular contracture. If a smooth walled implant is chosen, then the dissected pocket should be large enough to accommodate the implant displacement exercises *(Fig. 2.13)*.

Implant shape

It is important to reiterate the principle that the shape of the natural female breast is not a semicircle or a hemisphere. Dimensional analysis of the aesthetically pleasing breast form reveals a gently sloping upper pole and a curved lower pole with the nipple-areola complex at the point of maximum projection. The typical round shaped breast implant has its greatest projection centrally with the remainder of the volume distributed evenly along the base of the implant. In contrast, anatomically shaped breast implants have a flatter upper pole with the majority of the volume and projection in the lower pole *(Fig. 2.14)*. Thus, the anatomically shaped implant of a given base width and volume will produce less upper pole convexity than a round implant of the

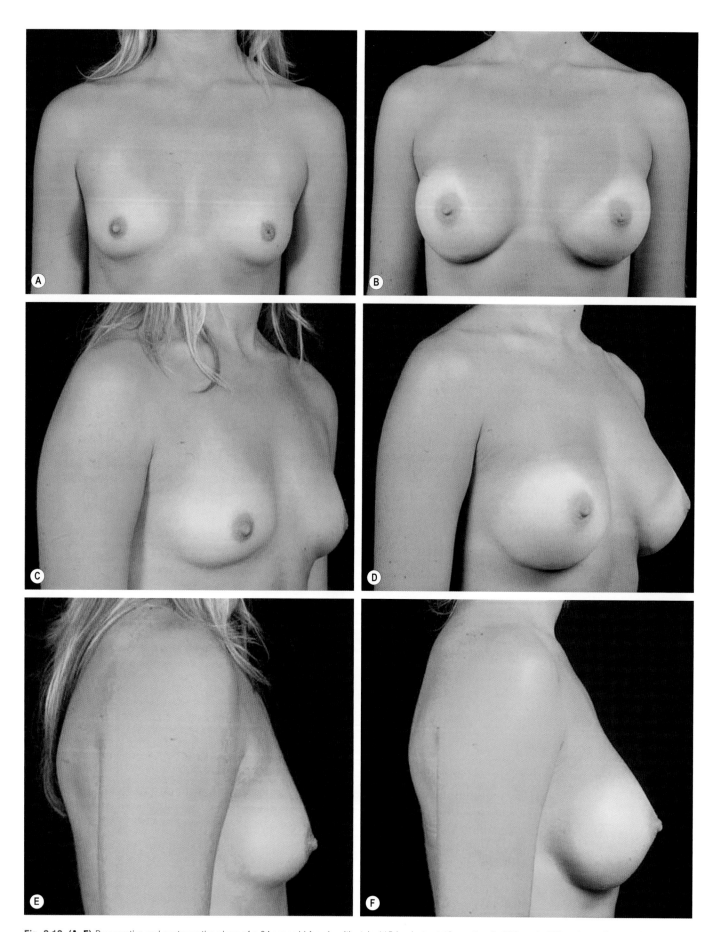

Fig. 2.12 (A–F) Preoperative and postoperative views of a 34-year-old female with style 115 implants at 12 months: R, 290 cc; L, 272 cc in a subpectoral position.

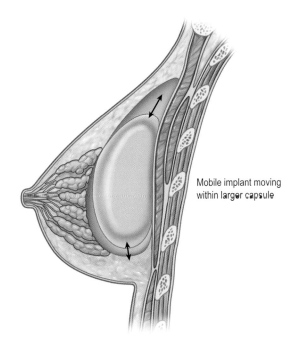

Mobile implant moving
within larger capsule

Fig. 2.13 Large pocket for smooth-surfaced implants to allow tissue redraping and encourage implant mobility, which is different than for textured devices (including anatomic), where a precise pocket is created that is either the same or slightly larger than the base and height of the implant to help maintain implant position.

same base width and volume *(Fig. 2.15)*. This characteristic of anatomically shaped implants can be extremely useful when the patient desires a significant volume augmentation but has a relatively narrow breast width.[19]

Treatment and surgical technique

Preoperative markings are made with the patient in the upright position and are useful as a reference point during the actual procedure. The surgeon should mark the chest midline in the frontal view from the suprasternal notch to the xiphoid process, the existing inframammary folds, and the likely position of the new inframammary folds as the proposed limits of the dissection. The patient is then asked to place her arms behind her head to visualize the displacement of the nipple and the true inframammary fold. The "yoga" type stretching exercises are also reviewed with the patient at this point. Following review of the consent and the plan, the patient is taken to the operating room. The patient is then placed in the supine position, centered on the operating table with the pelvis directly over

the flexion point of the bed. The arms must be well secured to the arm boards which are placed at 90° angles to the torso. These preparations are required so that the patient may be placed in the upright seated position as often as needed during the procedure. The sterile preparation and draping of the anterior chest must provide visualization of the patient's shoulders as an important anatomical reference point. Triple antibiotic solution irrigation will be used for all implant cases regardless of the incision type.

> **Hints and tips**
>
> It is imperative that dimensions are respected during augmentation in order to maintain the normal anatomical landmarks such as the lateral breast fold in the anterior axillary line and the intermammary distance (IMD).

> **Hints and tips**
>
> The patient's request for a particular breast size and shape will largely determine the dimensions of the breast implant used.

> **Hints and tips**
>
> Immediate stretching exercises are utilized postoperatively.

> **Hints and tips**
>
> Implant pocket is irrigated with an antibiotic solution containing 50 000 units of bacitracin, 1 g of cefazolin, and 80 mg of gentamicin per 500 mL of saline.

Inframammary incision

The inframammary approach permits complete visualization of the implant pocket with either subglandular, subfascial or subpectoral placement. The incision should be placed in the predicted location of the new inframammary fold which has been determined and marked preoperatively. Smaller incisions (<3 cm) may be used for inflatable saline-filled implants, but prefilled implants (silicone gel or saline) often require

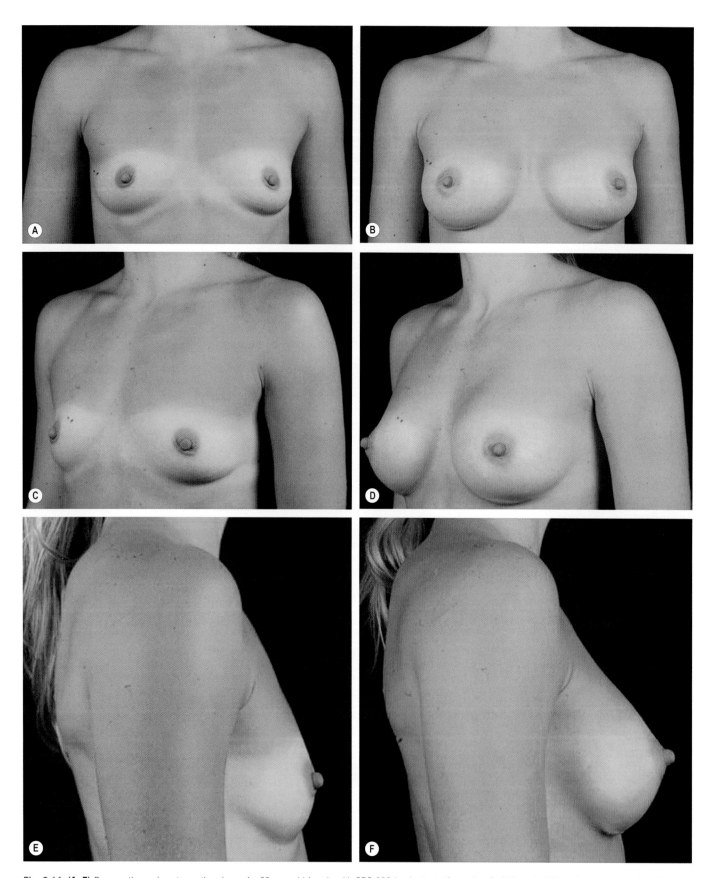

Fig. 2.14 (A–F) Preoperative and postoperative views of a 29-year-old female with CPG 332 implants at 12 months: R, 350 cc; L, 350 cc in a subpectoral position.

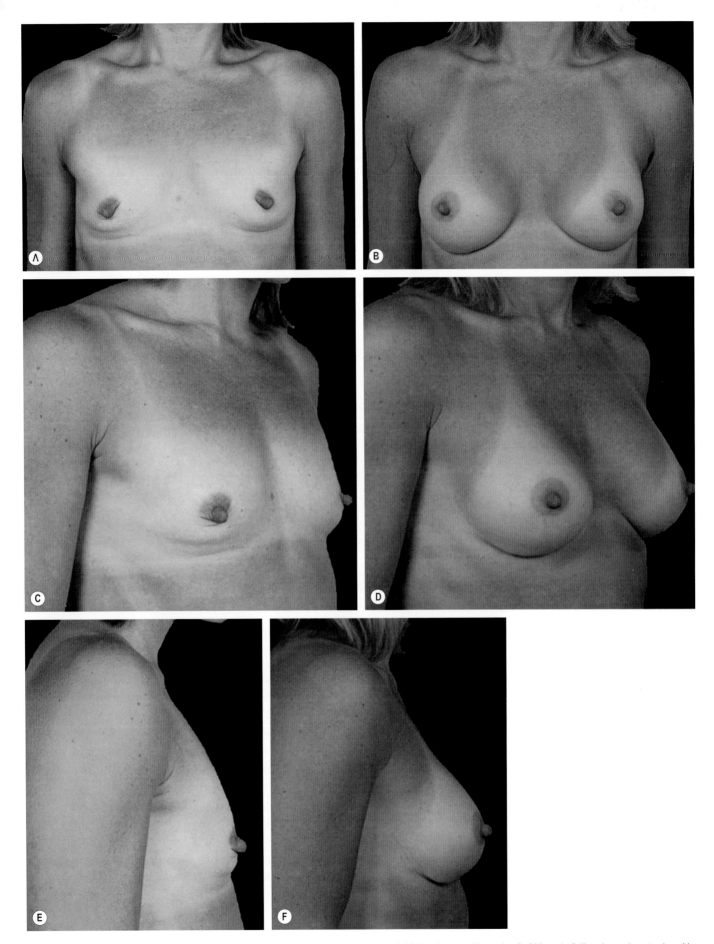

Fig. 2.15 (A–F) Preoperative and postoperative views of a 33-year-old female with Style 410 MM implants at 12 months: R, 280 cc; L, 245 cc in a subpectoral position.

incisions up to 5.0 cm in length. The incision should be designed with the majority of the incision lateral to the breast midline as this will place the resulting scar in the deepest portion of the new IMF.

The incision is made along the proposed markings, and the dissection is continued with an insulated electrocautery instrument through Scarpa fascia. A fiberoptic headlight is worn throughout the procedure, or a variety of lighted fiberoptic retractors are available to aid illumination and direct visualization within the pocket. If the implant is to be placed in the subfascial pocket, the dissection proceeds below the pectoralis fascia but above the pectoralis major fascia. Once the fascia is identified, it will be thicker as dissection proceeds more cephalad. Several medial intercostal perforating vessels may be encountered. These should be avoided or coagulated with insulated forceps if need be. For smooth-walled implants, a larger pocket is dissected to allow mobility of the implant. For anatomic implants, the pocket is precisely dissected to snugly accommodate the implant. Care should be taken to preserve the lateral intercostal cutaneous nerves, especially the fourth intercostal, which contains the primary sensory innervations of the nipple-areola complex.

If a subpectoral pocket is chosen, the dissection is initially carried out laterally to identify the lateral border of the pectoralis major muscle. The muscle edge can be lifted by forceps to allow easy entry into the submusculofascial plane. This plane is readily identified by the wispy areolar connective tissue and ease of dissection. An extended electrocautery instrument is used to complete the dissection. The inferior origin of the pectoralis major is released from lateral to medial at the level of the inframammary fold. Various slips of origin of the pectoralis major muscle are generally encountered and divided. Division of the pectoralis continues medially to the sternal border. Partial deep division may selectively be carried out 1–3 cm above the xiphoid, depending on which implant is to be used. Lateral dissection can be done bluntly with a finger to avoid injury to the lateral neurovascular bundles. The nerves can be stretched to accommodate the implant but should be preserved to minimize postoperative sensory changes. When the pectoralis major muscle is elevated, care must be taken to leave the pectoralis minor down on the chest wall. This will minimize bleeding and allow proper placement of the implant. At times, one may encounter several muscle interdigitations between the pectoralis minor and major and these are carefully dissected to prepare the pocket. In addition, if a dual plane pocket is planned preoperatively, further dissection over the muscle is carried out pending the level of the desired dual plane followed by release of the pectoralis major at the inframammary fold.

Exact implant "sizers" (gel or saline) are used when available to evaluate the pockets and resultant breast form. After the sizers are in place, the patient is placed in a 90° upright position and evaluated from various perspectives. Any asymmetry or underdissected areas are marked, and the patient is placed back in the supine position. Once adequate hemostasis is obtained and pocket dimensions are finalized, the pocket is irrigated with an antibiotic-containing solution,[38] and the implants are carefully placed by a minimal-touch technique.[38] The final results are assessed, again with the patient in a sitting position, and a multilayer closure is performed with absorbable suture. It is important to close off the implant pocket with a separate layer of suture before closing the skin. Once closure is complete, Steri-Strips are applied along the direction of the incisions.

Hints and tips

Exact implant "sizers" (gel or saline) are used when available to evaluate the pockets and resultant breast form.

Periareolar incision

The periareolar approach for augmentation mammaplasty was described by Jenny in 1972, and currently enjoys widespread use by plastic surgeons.[7] The periareolar incision is placed along the inferior portion of the areolar-cutaneous juncture. The principle advantage of this incision is that the resulting scar is usually well-camouflaged and quite inconspicuous. The periareolar approach allows easy adjustment of the IMF and direct access to the parenchyma for scoring and release when the lower pole of the breast is constricted. However, visualization and the dissection are typically inadequate with the periareolar incision in patients with areolas <3 cm in diameter. Other disadvantages of this approach include the potential risk of contamination if the lactiferous ducts are transected, the increased risk of changes in nipple sensitivity, and the risk of a hypopigmented scar in patients with darkly pigmented areolas.

The markings for a periareolar approach are similar to those for an inframammary augmentation. The incision is marked along the junction of the areola and the breast skin. The limits of the incision are the 3-o'clock and 9-o'clock positions.

The positioning of the patient is identical to that for an inframammary approach. It is imperative that the patient be able to fully flex at the waist for evaluation of the intraoperative appearance of the implants.

The precise incision is made. Wound edges are elevated directly up from the chest wall with an opposing pair of small sharp retractors. An insulated electrocautery unit is used to dissect straight down through the breast parenchyma to the pectoralis major fascia. The dissection is the same as described through the inframammary incision. If the inferior pole of the breast is constricted, radial scoring of the gland in the inferior pole can allow proper redraping of the soft tissue over the implant to correct the deformity. Before final implant placement, the pocket is once again checked for hemostasis and irrigated with an antibiotic solution. The closure is particularly important with this technique. The gland must be precisely reapproximated and closed with several layers of interrupted absorbable sutures to prevent distortion of the nipple-areola complex. The skin is closed with deep everting dermal sutures and a running subcuticular absorbable monofilament. Steri-Strips are applied to the closed incision.

Transaxillary incision

The transaxillary approach was described by Hoehler in 1973 and popularized by Bostwick and others.[39] This procedure can be performed either bluntly using the Montgomery dissector, or using an endoscope for precise visualization, and dissection of the implant pocket. The transaxillary approach avoids incisional scarring directly on the breast and places the incision in the inferior and anterior area of the axilla. The transaxillary incision usually provides adequate access when placing an inflatable round breast implant, and while not precluding is more difficult for placement of a large pre-filled implant, or an anatomically shaped device.

The markings for transaxillary breast augmentation are also made with the patient in the sitting or upright position. The existing and resultant inframammary folds are marked, as are the boundaries of the proposed dissection. To locate and mark the incision, the patient's arm is placed in complete adduction and the most anterior aspect of the axilla is marked. The incision should not extend beyond this line. The arm is then abducted approximately 45°, and a prominent axillary crease is identified. Any fold may be used, but preference is given to one high in the axilla, which aids in instrumentation during the procedure. For saline-filled implants, the incision should generally be 2.5–3.5 cm. Silicone implants require larger incisions. The patient is placed on the operating table in the supine position with arms abducted 90° and secured to arm boards that allow 10–15° variations in abduction and adduction from 90°. She must be able to flex 90° at the waist during the procedure. The incision is made, and small sharp retractors are used to elevate the medial aspect of the incision. Superficial subcutaneous dissection to the lateral border of the pectoralis major prevents injury to the intercostobrachial nerve. Scissor dissection is employed with use of the electrocautery and insulated forceps to control any bleeding. The fascia of the pectoralis major muscle is visualized at the lateral edge of the muscle, and the dissection is carried deep to this for a subfascial placement or deep to the muscle for subpectoral placement. One must be certain the correct plane is entered before continuing the dissection further.

For an endoscopically assisted augmentation, the endoscope is passed into the transaxillary tunnel, and the subpectoral space is seen under direct vision. This allows a more controlled release of the pectoralis major origin with a long insulated electrocautery instrument. On completion of the dissection, implant sizers are used to evaluate the pocket and identify any areas that need final adjustment. This must be done with the patient in the sitting position. The pockets are then irrigated with an antibiotic solution,[38] and the final implants are inserted. Before closure, the patient is once again placed in the sitting position for a final check of the implant position. The pectoralis muscle fascia is repaired with a single absorbable suture, and the incision is closed in one or two layers. Steri-Strips are applied to the incision.

Transumbilical

The markings for transumbilical breast augmentation are similar to those for a standard inframammary fold approach. The patient is placed on the operating table in the same manner as for an inframammary augmentation. An additional mark is made with the patient supine: a line is drawn from the umbilicus to the medial border of the areola bilaterally. An incision is made within the umbilicus, large enough to easily accommodate an index finger. An endotube with a blunt obturator is passed just above the rectus fascia along the line from the umbilicus to the areola. Care is taken to constantly palpate the progress of the obturator with the surgeon's other hand, always keeping the force up and away from the abdominal and thoracic cavities. The endotube is advanced over the costal margin. For subglandular implant placement, the force applied to the endotube is directed upward at the inframammary fold to prevent the obturator from slipping beneath the pectoralis major. The tunnel ends just cephalad to the nipple. Subpectoral positioning is possible by careful technique with use of special instruments to enter the fascial plane high laterally. The obturator is then removed, and an endoscope may be used to verify correct pocket identification. Hemostasis is also ensured. Both the endotube and endoscope are removed from the tunnel, and an expander is rolled up and placed within the incision. The expander is "milked" up the tunnel by manual external pressure. The expander is filled with saline to 150% of the final volume of the implant. Pocket adjustments can be made manually during filling. When the expansion is complete, the expander is drained and removed from the pocket by traction on the fill tube. The implant is placed and filled in exactly the same manner as the expander. The endotube is then replaced, and an endoscope may be used to verify implant position, valve patency, and hemostasis. The incision is closed with a single layer of absorbable suture. An abdominal binder is used for compression on the abdominal tunnels.

Postoperative care

In the overwhelming majority of cases, augmentation mammaplasty is performed as an outpatient procedure. Patients are given prescriptions for oral analgesics and a 3-day course of prophylactic oral antibiotics. Patient is shown yoga type stretching exercises of the chest to be performed on the same day following her surgery. Patients are allowed to remove operative dressings and shower as desired starting on the first postoperative day. The first follow-up visit is scheduled for 1–3 days after the procedure. If smooth (nontextured) implants were used, initiation of implant mobility exercises is recommended at this time. If the patient is at risk for superior implant displacement, a circumferential elastic strap may be used to apply continuous downward pressure during the early postoperative period. Patients are usually able to return to work a few days after surgery, but are not permitted to resume rigorous exercise for 2–3 weeks. Additional follow-up visits are scheduled at 4–6 weeks, 3 months, and 1 year. The importance of postoperative photo-documentation and critical analysis of the operative outcomes cannot be overemphasized. It is the author's practice to place patients on vitamin E 400 IU once a day for 2 years to minimize capsular contracture. Although there are no evidence based studies in the augmentation population on the use of Vitamin E, there is encouraging evidence in the treatment of RIF (radiation induced fibrosis) in mastectomy patients with radiation induced morbidities related to scarring.[40]

Perioperative complications

Alterations of nipple sensitivity after augmentation mammaplasty may be manifested as either anesthesia or hyperesthesia and are thought to result from traction injury, bruising, or transection of the lateral intercostal cutaneous nerves. The incidence and severity of nipple sensation changes does not vary with the surgical approach employed.[41]

Periprosthetic seroma fluid is usually resorbed by the soft tissues within the first week of surgery, and use of topical antibiotics intraoperatively has been shown to decrease the rates.[42] The authors do not use drains for primary breast augmentation.

The development of a hematoma after breast augmentation has several deleterious effects in both the early and late postoperative period including pain, blood loss, disfigurement, and capsular contracture.[43] Preoperatively, patients should receive a list of prescription and over-the-counter medications that may contribute to excessive postoperative bleeding. It is imperative that the patient discontinue any medications and herbal supplements that impair clotting or platelet function at least 1 week prior to surgery *(Table 2.1)*.[44-46] If a hematoma does develop in the perioperative period, immediate evacuation of the hematoma and exploration of the pocket is recommended. Unfortunately, the source of the hematoma is only rarely identified at the time of the exploration. Patients may occasionally present with a delayed hematoma 1–2 weeks or even months to years after augmentation, and frequently a history of breast trauma is elicited. Expanding hematomas require exploration and drainage regardless of the length of time from the augmentation. Nonoperative management of small nonexpanding hematomas is one option, but places the patient at a higher risk of subsequent periprosthetic capsular contracture.

Table 2.1 Herbs, herbal teas, homeopathic medicines, and dietary supplements associated with an increased risk of bleeding

Supplement type	Supplement name(s)	Treatment uses	Other side-effects (in addition to intrinsic bleeding risks)	Perioperative recommendations
Herbs and herbal extracts	Garlic (*Allium sativum*; Ajo)	Hypertension, hypercholesterolemia, fungal infections, cancer, MI prevention, PVD	Nausea, vomiting, hypoglycemia, halitosis, potentiation of warfarin, increased INR, abdominal pain, diarrhea, oral ulcers, anaphylaxis (rare)	Discontinue 7 days before surgery.[9] Resume 7 days after surgery.
	Ginger (*Zingiber officinale*)	Nausea, vomiting, GI bloating, dyspepsia, OA, RA, migraine, homeostasis restoration, weight loss	Nausea, GI bloating, worsen cholecystitis, arrhythmia (possible), hypoglycemia	Discontinue 2–3 weeks before surgery. Resume 2 weeks after surgery.
	Ginseng (*Panax ginseng*)	Stimulant, nausea, cancer prevention, CAD, DM2, dyspepsia, colic, infections, aging, stress, homeostasis restoration	Nausea, diarrhea, headaches, hypotension, hypertension, breast tenderness, hypoglycemia, insomnia (possible), interaction with warfarin	Discontinue 7 days before surgery.[9,30] Resume 2 weeks after surgery.
	Ginkgo (*Ginkgo biloba*) (Maidenhair tree)	Circulatory stimulant, dementia (Alzheimer's, multi-infarct), memory enhancement, PVD, ED	Nausea, vomiting, diarrhea, GI discomfort, headaches, palpitations, potentiates warfarin	Discontinue 36 h or more before surgery.[9] Resume 7 days after surgery.
	Feverfew (*Tanacetum parthenium*)	Fever, migraine, OA, GI upset, infertility	Oral ulcers, allergic reactions, GI discomfort and bloating	Taper and discontinue by 2–3 weeks before surgery to avoid withdrawal syndrome with abrupt cessation.[53] Resume 2 weeks after surgery.
	Bromelain	Inflammation, OA, autoimmune disorders, menstrual pain, digestion, gout	GI discomfort, diarrhea, tachycardia, menorrhagia (possible)	Discontinue 2–3 weeks before surgery. Resume 2 weeks after surgery.
	Liquorice/licorice (*Glycyrrhiza glabra*)	Aphthous ulcers, peptic ulcers, cancer, OA, adrenal insufficiency,	Hypokalemic paralysis, hypertension, weight loss/gain, infertility, temporary vision loss	Discontinue 2–3 weeks before surgery. Resume 2 weeks after surgery.
	Red chili pepper (*Capsaicin*)	Analgesic, chronic neuropathy, OA, uremic pruritis, psoriasis	Burning and stinging on contact, hypoglycemia, cough	Discontinue 2–3 weeks before surgery. Resume 2 weeks after surgery.

Table 2.1 Herbs, herbal teas, homeopathic medicines, and dietary supplements associated with an increased risk of bleeding—Cont'd

Supplement type	Supplement name(s)	Treatment uses	Other side-effects (in addition to intrinsic bleeding risks)	Perioperative recommendations
	Saw palmetto (*Serenoa repens*)	BPH, urinary tract infections	Nausea, vomiting, diarrhea, rhinitis, decreased libido, headache	Discontinue 2–3 weeks before surgery. Resume 2 weeks after surgery.
	Oil of Wintergreen (Methyl salicylate)	OA, joint discomfort, hypertension, inflammation, cellulite, flavoring agent	Displaces warfarin, nausea, vomiting, dizziness, increased INR	Discontinue 2–3 weeks before surgery. Resume 2 weeks after surgery.
	Devil's Claw (*Harpagophytum procumbens*)	Analgesic, fever, digestion aid, OA, appetite stimulant	Diarrhea, GI discomfort, tinnitus, headache, hypoglycemia, arrhythmia (possible)	Discontinue 2–3 weeks before surgery. Resume 2 weeks after surgery.
	Chinese Agrimony (*Agrimonia Pilosa*)	Analgesic, bacterial infection, helminthic infection, diarrhea, inflammation, cough, sore throat		Discontinue 2–3 weeks before surgery. Resume 2 weeks after surgery.
	Danshen (*Salvia miltiorrhiza*)	Atherosclerosis, stroke, angina pectoris, hypercholesterolemia, cancer, HIV, menstrual disorders, OA, insomnia, prostatitis	Hypotension, GI discomfort, reduced appetite, pruritis, seizures (possible), potentiates warfarin	Discontinue 2–3 weeks before surgery. Resume 2 weeks after surgery.
	Baical Skullcap Root (*Scutellaria baicalensis*)	Anxiety, inflammation, cancer, seizures, infections, insomnia, dysentery, diarrhea, rabies, menstrual disorders	Hepatotoxicity, pneumonitis	Discontinue 2–3 weeks before surgery. Resume 2 weeks after surgery.
	Geum japonicum	Diuretic, astringent, CAD, hypercholesterolemia		Discontinue 2–3 weeks before surgery. Resume 2 weeks after surgery.
	Chinese peony (*Paeoniae rubra*)	Inflammation, GI discomfort, spasm		Discontinue 2–3 weeks before surgery. Resume 2 weeks after surgery.
	Poncitrin (*Poncirus trifoliate*)	Constipation, diarrhea, spasm, expectorant		Discontinue 2–3 weeks before surgery. Resume 2 weeks after surgery.
	Fritillaria bulbs (*Fritillaria cirrhosa*)	Spasm, expectorant, hypertension, cough, asthma, opium toxicity		Discontinue 2–3 weeks before surgery. Resume 2 weeks after surgery.
	Japanese Honeysuckle (*Lonicera japonica*)	Fever, headache, cough, sore throat, bacterial infection, inflammation, ulcers		Discontinue 2–3 weeks before surgery. Resume 2 weeks after surgery.
Herbal formulas	Kangen-karyu	Hypertension, arteriosclerosis, memory impairment, headache		Discontinue 2–3 weeks before surgery. Resume 2 weeks after surgery.
	Bak Foong Pill	GI disturbances, cardiovascular disturbances, gynecological dysfunction		Discontinue 2–3 weeks before surgery. Resume 2 weeks after surgery.

Table 2.1 Herbs, herbal teas, homeopathic medicines, and dietary supplements associated with an increased risk of bleeding—Cont'd

Supplement type	Supplement name(s)	Treatment uses	Other side-effects (in addition to intrinsic bleeding risks)	Perioperative recommendations
Herbal teas	Te Gastronol	GI ulcers, intestinal inflammation, colitis, gastritis, flatulence		Discontinue 2–3 weeks before surgery. Resume 2 weeks after surgery.
	Seasonal tonic	Appetite suppressant		Discontinue 2–3 weeks before surgery. Resume 2 weeks after surgery.
Homeopathic medicines and other dietary supplements	Guīlinggāo (Tortoise jelly)	Fever, acne, enhancing circulation, improve intestinal function, constipation	None documented	Discontinue 2–3 weeks before surgery Resume 2 weeks after surgery.
	Vitamin E	Peyronie's disease, bladder cancer prevention, RA, Alzheimer's disease, PMS, movement disorders	Allergic reaction, fatigue, weakness, headache, nausea, diarrhea, vision disturbance, congenital heart defects in utero, heart failure	Discontinue 2–3 weeks before surgery. Resume when healing is complete.[3]
	Arnica Montana (Leopard's bane) (Wolf's bane)	OA, sprains, joint pain, inflammation	Gastroenteritis	Discontinue 2–3 weeks before surgery. Resume 2 weeks after surgery.
	Fish oil (Eicosapentaenoic acid)	Hypertension, hypertriglyceridemia, RA, angina pectoris, atherosclerosis	Hemorrhagic stroke, GI disturbances and bloating, diarrhea, hyperglycemia (possible)	Discontinue 2–3 weeks before surgery. Resume 2 weeks after surgery.
	Chondroitin	OA	Nausea, diarrhea, constipation, GI disturbances	Discontinue 2–3 weeks before surgery. Resume 2 weeks after surgery.
	Glucosamine	OA	Hypoglycemia, nausea, diarrhea, headache, insomnia, GI disturbances	Discontinue 2–3 weeks before surgery. Resume 2 weeks after surgery.

MI, myocardial infarction; PVD, peripheral vascular disease; INR, international normalized ratio; GI, gastrointestinal; OA, osteoarthritis; RA, rheumatoid arthritis; CAD, coronary artery disease; DM2, diabetes mellitus type II; ED, erectile dysfunction; HIV, human immunodeficiency virus.[44]

Postoperative wound infection may present with a spectrum of severity ranging from a mild cellulitis of the breast skin to a purulent periprosthetic space infection. The organism *Staphylococcus epidermidis* is part of the normal skin flora and is the most frequently identified pathogen in postoperative wound infections. Patients are given prophylactic antibiotics intra-operatively and postoperatively to reduce the risk of infection. Sterile technique is maintained during the procedure and the implant pocket is irrigated with an antibiotic solution containing 50 000 units of bacitracin, 1 g of cefazolin, and 80 mg of gentamicin per 500 mL of saline.[38] Further reduction of risk for bacterial contamination may be achieved by employing the *no-touch* technique in which only the surgeon handles the implant with fresh, powder free gloves. The implant is then inserted through a sterile sleeve to minimize contact with the patient's skin and inflated using a sterile closed filling system. A significant number of postoperative wound infections will respond to oral or intravenous antibiotics if therapy is initiated very early in the course of the infection. If the infection persists or progresses, then the implant should be removed and the wound should be allowed to heal over a drain or in severe cases by secondary intention. Once the infection has totally cleared, a secondary augmentation and scar revision should be planned in 6–12 months.

Mondor's disease is a superficial thrombophlebitis of the breast that may occur in up to 1–2% of augmentation patients.[47,48] This process usually affects the veins along the inferior aspect of the breast and occurs most frequently with the inframammary approach. Fortunately, this is a self-limiting process that usually resolves with warm compresses over a period of several weeks.

Delayed complications of augmentation mammaplasty

Periprosthetic capsular contracture

One of the most common delayed complications of augmentation mammaplasty is the development of a palpable and deforming periprosthetic capsular contracture. All surgical implants undergo some degree of encapsulation due to the natural foreign body reaction by the surrounding tissues. Clinically significant periprosthetic capsular contracture is characterized by excessive scar formation that leads to firmness, distortion, and displacement of the breast implant. Histological examination of these contractures reveals circumferential linear fibrosis, which is especially severe when formed in response to smooth shell implants. In 1975, Baker proposed a clinical classification system of capsular contracture after augmentation that is still commonly used to describe periprosthetic contractures *(Table 2.2)*.[49]

Table 2.2 **The grades of capsular contracture are divided into the following four types**

Grade	Description
I	Capsular contracture of the augmented breast feels as soft as an unoperated breast
II	Capsular contracture is minimal. The breast is less soft than an unoperated breast. The implant can be palpated but is not visible.
III	Capsular contracture is moderate. The breast is firmer. The implant can be palpated easily and may be distorted or visible
IV	Capsular contracture is severe. The breast is hard, tender, and painful, with significant distortion present. The capsule thickness is not directly proportional to palpable firmness, although some relationship may exist

(Reproduced with permission from Spear SL, Baker JL Jr. Classification of capsular contracture after prosthetic breast reconstruction. Plast Reconstr Surg 1995; 96(5):1119–1124.)

While several factors have been identified which contribute to capsular contracture, the precise etiology remains unknown. The hypertrophic, circumferential linear scar probably involves stimulation of myofibroblasts that are known to be present within the periprosthetic capsule. Irritation caused by periprosthetic hematoma, seroma, or silicone gel bleed may incite the capsular contracture. Other foreign body particles such as glove powder, lint, or dust may also contribute to the process.[50] Infectious etiologies have also been studied and are thought to play a role.[50] This theory describes a chronic subclinical infection located immediately adjacent to the implant shell within a microscopic biofilm that is relatively inaccessible to cellular and humoral immune function. Many strategies have been employed to prevent periprosthetic capsular contracture. One strategy has been the creation of a large implant pocket, and maintenance of this oversized pocket with implant displacement exercises. The use of implants with textured surfaces has been described above, and has been shown to reduce the rate of capsular contracture in breast augmentation. Other efforts have focused on minimizing operative trauma in order to reduce the risk of seroma or hematoma formation. Seromas, hematomas, and even blood staining of the periprosthetic tissues may incite capsular contracture. Any bleeding that does occur during the dissection needs to be controlled and the staining of the tissues with blood should be diluted with copious irrigation fluid.

Leukotriene receptor antagonists which are used to treat asthma, were studies in capsular contracture but are recommended to be used cautiously due to their side-effects.[51,52] Specifically zafirlukast (Accolate) and montelukast (Singulair) have been shown to reverse clinical signs of capsular contracture in patients taking the medication for asthma.[51,52] Treatment of established capsular contractures usually requires operative intervention. (This is discussed more completely in Chapter 3.) Open capsulotomy involves scoring the capsule circumferentially, and anteriorly to adequately release and expand the soft tissue envelope. With very thick fibrous capsules, or with calcified capsules containing silicone granulomas, it is often necessary to perform either a partial or complete capsulectomy to correct the deformity. This is often extremely effective in treating advanced grade IV capsular contractures, especially when the implant is replaced with a saline-filled or a no-bleed silicone gel-filled implant. Implant site change surgery has become popular for treating established or recurrent capsular contracture.[53–55] (Revisionary surgery will be discussed in the Chapter 3, in detail.)

Implant rupture and deflation

Any defect in the silicone elastomer shell of a saline-filled breast implant will ultimately result in *deflation* of the implant. The saline filling material leaks out of the implant and is harmlessly absorbed by the surrounding tissues. Clinical recognition of deflation is usually made by the patient and virtually always requires surgical explantation and replacement of the implant. A history of recent trauma is frequently elicited with deflation, and true *spontaneous* failure of the implant shell is relatively rare.

Magnetic resonance imaging (MRI) of the breast is considered the state-of-the-art technique for evaluating breast implant integrity. Modern fourth generation silicone gel is substantially more cohesive than the second and third-generation gel, and less likely to leak into the surrounding tissues, even when the implant shell is ruptured.

Recently, questions have been raised regarding case reports of suspected anaplastic large cell lymphoma (ALCL) in patients with breast implants. Since this initial report, the FDA has communicated up to 34 cases of ALCL in patients with breast implant which also occurs in patients without implants 12 total literature reports ($n=20$ cases) of ALCL in patients without breast implants.[56] ALCL is a rare peripheral T-cell lymphoma and prognosis varies by site, by age and by oncogene anaplastic lymphocyte kinase (ALK) expression. The 5-year survival ranges from 15% for ALCL-nodal, ALK-neg to 90% with the cutaneous form of ALCL.[57] In women with breast implants, it generally has been reported to behave in an indolent manner, which is inconsistent with the clinical course of ALCL in women without breast implants.[58,59] The clinical presentation has included patients with prior implant surgery who have developed late periprosthetic fluid collection which is an infrequently reported late occurrence. With our current knowledge about ALCL, for patients presenting with late fluid collection, at a minimum, image-guided aspiration of fluid, with appropriate fluid evaluation, including culture, cell count, and cytologic testing should be performed.[60] Further investigation will be necessary for refractory periprosthetic fluid collection. Even though the most common cause for such late fluid collections is idiopathic, in the absence of a diagnosed infectious or neoplastic cause, these collections will require capsulectomy, with or without implant replacement. It is important for plastic surgeons to consider such a process for all late seroma cases and even for late representing capsular contractures and formation of distinct masses. Clinical judgment is important and appropriate radiographic and laboratory tests (especially cytology) should be undertaken.[61]

Secondary procedures

Revisionary breast surgery (secondary or tertiary), often performed for the late complications of breast augmentation, pose a continual challenge to plastic surgeons. These procedures are complex, challenging, and unpredictable. Over the years, we have been dealing with thinned breast tissues from large implants that have been placed either in subglandular or subpectoral space leading to some long-term complications, such as implant extrusion, gel bleed, rupture with extravasation of gel, saline implant deflation, capsular contracture, palpability, rippling, "double bubble", "snoopy breast", symmastia, and implant malposition.

Historically, our options for revision and improvement have included, replacing saline implants with gel implants, using capsular flaps to gain additional stability and coverage, or performing a site change operation. None of these procedures have resulted in complete resolution of the described complaints. (The detailed management of revisionary procedures is discussed in Chapter 4.)

Access the complete references list online at **http://www.expertconsult.com**

15. Cunningham B. The Mentor study on contour profile gel silicone MemoryGel breast implants. *Plast Reconstr Surg.* 2007;120(7 Suppl 1):33S–39S.

17. Cunningham B, McCue J. Safety and effectiveness of Mentor's MemoryGel implants at 6 years. *Aesthet Plast Surg.* 2009;33(3):440–444.

    The authors update on the post-approval study for the Mentor Corporation. The study shows that Mentor MemoryGel silicone breast implants represent a safe and effective choice for women seeking breast augmentation or breast reconstruction following mastectomy.

19. Bengtson BP, Van Natta BW, Murphy DK, et al. Style 410 highly cohesive silicone breast implant core study results at 3 years. *Plast Reconstr Surg.* 2007;120 (7 Suppl 1):40S–48S.

25. Gabriel SE, O'Fallon WM, Kurland LT, et al. Risk of connective-tissue diseases and other disorders after breast implantation. *N Engl J Med.* 1994;330(24): 1697–1702.

    The authors conducted a population-based, retrospective study to examine the risk of a variety of connective-tissue diseases and other disorders after breast implantation. No association between breast implants and the connective-tissue diseases and other disorders that were studied was found.

27. Nelson N. Institute of Medicine finds no link between breast implants and disease. *J Natl Cancer Inst.* 1999;91(14):1191.

31. Tebbetts JB. Dual plane breast augmentation: optimizing implant-soft-tissue relationships in a wide range of breast types. *Plast Reconstr Surg.* 2001;107(5):1255–1272.

    This article describes specific indications and techniques for a dual plane approach to breast augmentation. Indications, operative techniques, results, and complications for this series of patients are presented. Dual plane augmentation mammaplasty adjusts implant and tissue relationships to ensure adequate soft-tissue coverage, while optimizing implant-soft-tissue dynamics to offer increased benefits and fewer tradeoffs compared with a single pocket location in a wide range of breast types.

38. Adams WP Jr, Rios JL, Smith SJ. Enhancing patient outcomes in aesthetic and reconstructive breast surgery using triple antibiotic breast irrigation: six-year prospective clinical study. *Plast Reconstr Surg.* 2006;117(1):30–36.

    The authors show the clinical importance of the use of triple antibiotic breast irrigation. This study shows the lower low incidence of capsular contracture compared with other published reports, and its clinical efficacy supports previously published in vitro studies. Application of triple antibiotic irrigation is recommended for all aesthetic and reconstructive breast procedures and is cost-effective.

40. Magnusson M, Hoglund P, Johansson K, et al. Pentoxifylline and vitamin E treatment for prevention of radiation-induced side-effects in women with breast cancer: a phase two, double-blind, placebo-controlled randomised clinical trial (Ptx-5). *Eur J Cancer.* 2009;45(14):2488–2495.

49. Spear SL, Baker JL Jr. Classification of capsular contracture after prosthetic breast reconstruction. *Plast Reconstr Surg.* 1995;96(5):1119–1124.

56. Spear SL, Murphy DK, Slicton A, et al. Inamed silicone breast implant core study results at 6 years. *Plast Reconstr Surg.* 2007;120(7 Suppl 1):8S–18S.

    The authors update on the post-approval study for Allergan Corporation. The study demonstrates the safety and effectiveness of Natrelle (formerly Inamed) silicone-filled breast implants through 6 years, including a low rupture rate and high satisfaction rate.

3

Secondary breast augmentation

Mitchell H. Brown

SYNOPSIS

- A defined process that encompasses careful patient selection, preoperative planning and education, precise surgical technique and standardized postoperative care will help to prevent the need for secondary augmentation surgery. It is never as easy to obtain an excellent result as it is at the time of initial implant insertion.
- A thorough understanding of the problems as they relate to patient expectations, soft tissue changes, implant characteristics and implant/pocket relationships are necessary before proceeding with revision surgery.
- Patients must clearly understand the risk/benefit equation for any revision procedure. Minor revisions should be performed with caution, as there is always a possibility of leaving the patient with a more significant problem.
- The treatment of capsular contracture should recognize the likely etiologic factors of subclinical infection and biofilm formation. Consideration should be made for exchange to a new implant and insertion of the implant in a new soft tissue environment, either through capsulectomy or site change.
- Implant malposition is a problem of the implant pocket. Treatment requires either an adjustment to the existing pocket or a site change to a new pocket.
- Rippling or implant edge palpability can be minimized by selecting an implant size that matches the dimensions of the patient's soft tissues and by ensuring adequate soft tissue coverage through proper pocket selection.

Introduction

Breast augmentation has been performed using breast implants since the early 1960s. Since then, millions of women worldwide have undergone breast augmentation. As the technique, surgical approach and implants have improved, results have become more predictable and stable. Given the sheer numbers of women who have breast implants in place, the number of women presenting for reoperative breast surgery continues to increase. In fact, many plastic surgeons who focus on breast aesthetics are seeing their practices evolve into specialty centers for revision breast surgery.

A consistent theme in this chapter will be prevention. The need to perform revisionary surgery has several consequences. It places the patient at an unnecessary risk. The best way to avoid risk is to avoid surgery. Revision surgery is costly to the patient. It is also costly to the surgeon and to the surgical practice. Most importantly, it is never as easy to get as good and as predictable a result as it is the very first time that the breast is operated on.

Revision breast augmentation can be a very difficult and challenging undertaking. The normal anatomy that exists in a primary procedure is no longer present. The surgeon must deal with a variety of factors, some predictable and some not predictable. These include: external and internal scarring, previously dissected tissue planes, alteration to the deep and superficial blood supply to the breast, alteration to the pectoralis major muscle (PMM), thinning and stretching of the overlying soft tissues and secondary effects related to the presence of a capsule around the pre-existing implant.

There are many reasons why a woman presents for secondary implant surgery, however the most common reason is for the management of capsular contracture.[1] Implant malposition is another common presentation and can be categorized into malpositions that are superior, inferior, lateral or medial. Other common indications include the management of rippling or implant edge palpability, size change, device failure and finally the correction of soft tissue changes secondary to hematoma, infection, radiation or previous surgery. Regardless of the presentation, the management of the secondary implant patient requires a systematic approach to identify the underlying problems, recognize the limitations, and develop a plan that is safe and maximizes the chances for a predictable outcome.

Basic science/disease process

When any implant is placed into the human body, a biologic response occurs. This response can take the form of regeneration, resorption or encapsulation. Regeneration occurs when the body recognizes the implant as self. This is seen with some types of acellular dermal matrices and the result is revascularization of the tissue and repopulation of the implant with the patient's own cells. Resorption occurs when the implant is recognized as foreign. The body attacks the material to break it down and eliminate it, depositing scar tissue in its place. This is seen with some types of resorbable mesh. Encapsulation typically occurs with cross linked materials such as synthetic mesh, Gore-Tex® or breast implants. This process involves an attempt by the body to wall off or encapsulate the device.

There are multiple factors that have been implicated in the formation of capsules. These include implant factors such as fill material and surface, patient factors such as local infection or previous radiation and technical factors such as bleeding or under-dissection of the pocket. A capsule is a normal and often desirable response by the body. It helps to stabilize the implant in the desired position. When the capsule is too thick or excessive, the result is deformity, pain and often further surgery. These concepts will be expanded upon in the section below on capsular contracture.

Diagnosis/patient presentation

The first step in evaluating the revision patient is to develop a clear understanding of their concerns and expectations. This may be easier to explain for some patients than others. Often, patients are abstract in the discussion of their concerns. Phrases such as, "this isn't what I wanted"; "I am very unhappy with my breasts"; "My friends tell me this can't be right, it should be fixed", demonstrate displeasure with the outcome but are hardly specific. To correct a problem, one must understand what the problem is, why it occurred and have a reasonable plan as to how to fix it. There is not a solution for every concern, nor is it reasonable to try to correct every outcome that is felt to be less than perfect.

A detailed history should include patient goals and expectations, general health and an assessment of risk factors for compromised healing including smoking history, systemic illness or previous radiation to the breast. The patient's breast health should be reviewed including the presence of past breast disease, family history of breast cancer and the timing of previous breast imaging. All prior breast surgeries should be well documented and operative notes obtained, if available. It is impossible to plan for a successful revision procedure without having a clear understanding as to what was done in the past. *Table 3.1* lists the key points of information that should be known about previous breast procedures.

Physical examination should focus on three components: the implant, the soft tissues, and the musculoskeletal framework. These three variables will completely define the dynamics of the presenting problem. The implant must be examined for position under the breast tissue and stability within the implant pocket. Malposition should be classified into medial (symmastia), lateral, inferior (double bubble) or superior. Implant stability within the pocket should be assessed with the patient in multiple positions including standing with arms at side, arms over head, lying supine and leaning forward. The presence of capsular contracture should be noted along with any areas of rippling or palpable implant edges.

Examination of the soft tissues is very important not only to determine a surgical plan but to inform the

Table 3.1 Previous breast surgery

Previous photographs (especially initial preoperative photographs)
  Pre-existing asymmetry
Timing
  How many procedures
  When performed
  Interval between procedures
  Time since most recent procedure
Implants
  Symmetric or asymmetric use of implants
  Implant size
  Implant fill
  Implant surface
  Implant shape and projection
Procedure
  Pocket selection
  Incision selection
  Management of skin envelope (previous mastopexy)
Complications
  Infection, hematoma, contracture, malposition, rupture
  Method of treatment
    Closed capsulotomy
    Open capsulotomy
    Pocket change
    Capsule repair
    Implant removal

patient what is realistically achievable with surgical correction. Any asymmetries should be recorded and discussed. Measurements include sternal notch to nipple distance, nipple to IMF distance and breast width. An attempt should be made to compare the width of the breast to the dimensions of the underlying implant. Nipple position on the breast mound should be noted, along with degree of ptosis or glandular ptosis. The quality and quantity of breast tissue in all four quadrants should be assessed to determine adequacy of soft tissue coverage. This may be done by subjective assessment or by more objective measures such as the pinch test. The breast and axilla is examined for abnormal masses and finally all scars are recorded for both location and quality.

As breast implants require a stable foundation to sit on, examination of the musculoskeletal anatomy is important. Pre-existing scoliosis or chest wall asymmetries should be recorded. Abnormal contour of the sternum either concave or convex will affect medial positioning of implants. Similarly, patients with asymmetric contour of the rib cage either superiorly or inferiorly will affect the upper pole fullness or the stability of the implant at the level of the IMF. The pectoralis muscle should be examined as it may have been damaged or excessively released with previous surgeries. In cases of Poland syndrome, the muscle may be absent or rudimentary.

Investigations should be patient specific. Implants can be imaged with a combination of ultrasound, mammography or MRI. The soft tissues should be imaged as necessary for abnormal masses or calcifications. In general, ultrasound and mammography are used to image the breast tissue and assess for actual breast pathology. The author routinely requires a screening mammogram within one year prior to any elective breast surgery for all women over the age of 40. MRI is indicated for assessment of integrity of the breast implant and specifics of soft tissue or skeletal asymmetries. It is also useful in identifying the exact plane of the implant and its relation to the pectoral muscle. In patients who have undergone multiple procedures, the exact implant location and the status of the pectoral muscle can often be difficult to determine. The value of any radiologic investigation should be weighed against the cost including actual financial cost of the test, radiation exposure and patient time. Concerns within the breast tissue or axilla may require a referral and opinion from a breast oncologic surgeon.

Classification

Revision breast augmentation surgery can be classified into three categories: related to the previous surgery, related to the soft tissues, related to the implant. Problems related to the previous surgery are most common. There are many decisions that go into planning any breast surgery. Improper pocket selection, improper implant selection, over or under dissection of the pocket, infection and postoperative bleeding can all affect the final outcome. Patients who would benefit from a skin tightening procedure but instead undergo the insertion of a large implant will likely have a short term gain with unacceptable results in the longer term. *Figure 3.1* shows a woman who underwent bilateral subpectoral augmentation and presented with concerns of breast asymmetry. Upon surgical exploration, it was determined that the right pectoral muscle had been released along the IMF to the level of the sternum, but

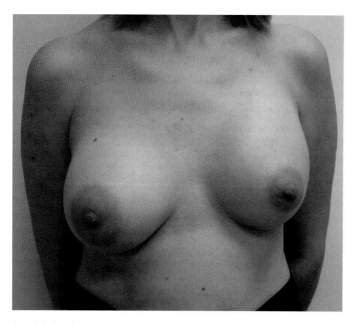

Fig. 3.1 Post-breast augmentation breast asymmetry. This patient underwent a subpectoral breast augmentation. Revision surgery demonstrated inferior release of the PMM on the right and no release of the PMM on the left.

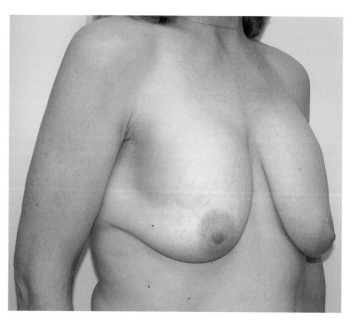

Fig. 3.2 Subpectoral breast augmentation. Implant is soft and in a normal position. There is overlying ptosis of the soft tissues causing a "waterfall" deformity.

the left muscle had not been released at all, resulting in a unilateral high riding implant.

The second category includes issues related to the soft tissues. Breast tissue will undergo normal physiologic changes throughout a woman's lifetime. These changes may include atrophy, hypertrophy, thinning or stretching. Changes are exaggerated by events such as pregnancy, breast-feeding or fluctuations in weight. The presence of an implant may hasten some of these changes, especially thinning of the skin, the development of striae and stretch marks or the development of ptosis and pseudoptosis. Even if the implant itself remains in a normal position, without complications, the development of soft tissue changes on their own can be enough to drive the need for revision surgery. *Figure 3.2* shows a woman with normal, soft implants and overlying breast ptosis. This "waterfall" deformity requires a mastopexy to bring the breast tissue back up to where the implant sits.

The final category includes issues related to the implant itself. This would include capsular contracture, implant malposition, implant deflation, rupture or implant palpability and rippling. The remainder of this chapter will focus on how to prevent and treat these causes of revision breast surgery.

Patient selection/indications

The decision to proceed with a revision breast augmentation should only be made after careful consideration of the patient's concerns and a thorough discussion regarding goals and expectations. As the primary surgeon, it is possible to decrease revision rates by committing to basic core principles that include; patient education, informed consent, preoperative planning, proper implant selection using tissue based planning, precise surgical technique and structured postoperative care. Each indication for a revision can find its roots embedded in one or more of these principles. For example, a patient whose implant was improperly matched to their soft tissue envelope will likely develop implant malposition, rotation or rippling. A patient who is concerned about an ongoing asymmetry but did not understand that this asymmetry existed preoperatively will not be prepared to accept the continued difference in her two breasts. Surgery that uses imprecise technique increases the likelihood of infection, contracture, hematoma and implant malposition. A device placed through too small an incision will be more likely to fail.

The best way to manage a revision is to have avoided it in the first place. Having said that, errors do occur, soft tissues do not always behave as planned, well intentioned decisions are not always born out to be correct, patient's bodies continue to change and the principles of gravity continue to exist. For these reasons, the need for revision augmentation surgery will persist.

The surgeon and patient should spend time performing a risk/benefit analysis. On one side of the equation are the reasons why the patient wishes a revision. The patient may have symptoms such as pain from a capsular contracture or a tight, poorly healed scar. She may have restriction of movement that affects her ability to do common activities. Other concerns may relate to the effect on quality of life. Asymmetry, improper sizing, malposition or contracture may limit the wearing of certain clothing styles and this may impact on the patients self image, self-esteem and confidence, all reasons for having the augmentation done in the first place. These concerns must be balanced against the inherent risks and complications of the revision as well as the likelihood for being able to meet the patients stated goals. The commonly used phrase; "the enemy of good is better" should be carefully considered and discussed with the patient. There is nothing worse than performing surgery to correct a relatively minor problem only to be left with a major one.

Not all revisions of previous breast augmentations require the use of an implant. Patients who have had multiple previous procedures, painful contractures, implant ruptures or complex malposition problems may be best served by implant removal with or without capsulectomy. Often, breast reshaping in the form of a mastopexy can be performed simultaneously or at a later date. For patients with saline implants, consideration can be given to preoperative deflation of the implant. This can be done in the office using a sterile prep-tray, needle and suction. Patients must sign a consent committing to the plan for definitive surgery. This short procedure allows both the patient and surgeon to assess the quantity and quality of breast tissue as well as visualize any existing asymmetries. On several occasions, the author has had patients decide to accept the breast as is (other than removal of the deflated device) or to perform a lift only.

As with any procedure, patients undergoing revision breast augmentation must have realistic expectations. There is not a solution for every problem and in some circumstances, it is best not to offer a surgical option.

Any implant can be used in reoperative breast surgery, however there are certain circumstances where a particular implant may offer a unique benefit. The surface of an implant may affect issues of rippling, palpability and capsule formation. Patients with rippling may gain benefit from the use of a smooth device whereas patients with repeated contractures may have less chance of a recurrence with a textured implant. In situations of implant malposition and capsular contracture, the author prefers using textured surface devices. This decision is not absolute and requires a new pocket for the implant and adequate soft tissue cover to minimize the risk of traction rippling. In most cases of secondary implant surgery, it is the author's view that everything possible should be done to attempt to correct the presenting problem. This usually requires the selection of a new device. The cost of new implants as well as surgical costs, are the responsibility of the patient. In primary implant surgery, the author discusses financial implications of subsequent surgery as part of the consent process. Patients are made aware that they may be responsible for the costs of any revision procedure and for the cost of new implants, if indicated. The author reserves the right to determine his surgical fee based upon the reason for revision and time since primary surgery. In Canada, the treatment of conditions such as symptomatic capsular contracture, infection or hematoma are considered insured services.

In situations where an implant is too wide for the breast, higher profile devices can be selected and in cases of breast asymmetry, the surgeon may select implants of different projection. Round implants produce a shape that is very different from anatomic devices and do not carry the added risk of implant rotation. Shaped implants however, have the potential to correct various asymmetries, produce a natural upper breast contour and have a low rate of capsular contracture.[2–4]

Specific contraindications exist when using shaped gel implants in revision surgery. Of course, a patient must be willing to accept the use of a gel device. Outside of North America, this is rarely an issue, but there are a number of women within Canada and the United States who continue to have a greater comfort level with saline implants. Understanding a woman's goals is key to selecting the best implant. Patients who would like a full looking upper pole are not good candidates for a shaped implant. The form stable nature of the gel results in a breast that is slightly firmer than what is seen with more responsive gel devices. Patients who are unwilling to accept this will do better with a softer round gel or saline implant.

The location and length of the surgical scar is an important consideration for most implant patients. In revision surgery, there will be a pre-existing scar. Surgery should always be performed through an incision that allows for direct access and precise correction of the underlying problem. If that cannot be done through the previous scar, then a new incision should be selected. When using a gel implant, it is critical to have a long enough incision to allow for implant insertion without damaging the device. This is generally in the range of 4 cm for a round implant and 5 cm for a form stable shaped device. This incision length limits the choice for scar location. Most commonly, the incision will be placed in the inframammary fold or through a large periareolar incision. If an axillary approach is selected, it is imperative that the incision be of adequate length. Patients who are not willing to accept the required scar length and location are not candidates for gel implants.

Treatment/surgical technique

Hints and tips

- Obtain all previous operative records, if available.
- For patients with saline implants, consider preoperative deflation to allow assessment of the soft tissues and asymmetry.
- Consider implant removal without replacement as an option in all revision procedures.
- Whenever possible, treatment of capsular contracture should include replacement of the implant, and insertion of the implant into a new soft tissue environment, either through capsulectomy or site change.
- Implant malposition is a problem of the implant pocket. Treatment requires adjusting the existing pocket or switching to a new pocket.
- Shaped implants in revision surgery require a new pocket where the dimensions of the pocket can be matched to the dimensions of the implant.
- When surgery is required on both the implant and the soft tissues, revise the implant first and then tailor the soft tissues around the new device.

Careful preoperative planning is a cornerstone of any successful breast augmentation. This statement is especially true in revision surgery. It is absolutely imperative to have a detailed understanding of all previous breast surgeries. Whenever possible, surgical records should be obtained and reviewed. Often, women presenting with breast implant problems have had multiple procedures. These may have included mastopexies, reductions, biopsies or lumpectomies. Each of these surgeries will have left scars and have caused an alteration to the normal blood flow within the breast and to the nipple areola complex. For each previous breast implant procedure, it is important to know the implant fill, surface, size, pocket and incision used. Any complications such as infection, contracture or malposition should be recorded, including the methods by which these complications were treated.

The exact surgical plan will be determined by the specifics of the patient. Revision procedures may involve implant removal with or without a mastopexy. When the plan calls for insertion of a new implant, there are several fundamental decisions that need to be made. Pocket selection is a very important consideration. Options for the implant pocket are summarized in **Table 3.2**.

When the capsule around the implant is normal, there is adequate soft tissue coverage and the implant/soft tissue relationships are acceptable then the same pocket can be utilized. This is most common with revisions for size change or minor malpositions. In the case of minor contractures, an open capsulotomy or partial capsulectomy may be indicated. With Baker III/IV contractures, implant malposition, rippling or edge palpability a site change is usually indicated. When revision surgery calls for the use of a shaped gel implant, a pocket change is mandatory to allow for a precise pocket to implant fit. Site change can take the form of a

Table 3.2 **Options for implant pocket**

Same pocket
Open capsulotomy
Partial capsulectomy
Same location with complete capsulectomy
Subglandular to subpectoral
Subpectoral to subglandular
Neo-subpectoral
Convert to dual plane

capsulectomy, subglandular to subpectoral conversion, subpectoral to subglandular conversion or the creation of a new subpectoral pocket on top of a previous subpectoral capsule.[5] A variation on site change is the conversion to a dual plane pocket as described by Spear.[6] This approach is helpful in many cases of contracture or superior implant malposition.

A second critical consideration is the implant type, shape and size. There is no single formula that can be applied to all cases of revision augmentation but certain principles can be followed. In cases of contracture, consider the use of a textured surface implant. Several studies suggest that there is a lower capsule contracture rate with textured implants, especially when the implant is placed in the subglandular space.[7,8,9] Consider the use of smaller implant sizes. Many problems following breast augmentation are as a result of soft tissue changes secondary to a large implant. It is usually better to use a smaller implant size with a skin tightening procedure rather than filling a skin envelope with larger volume devices. Shaped gel implants have a central role to play in implant selection for revision augmentation. Although they usually require a new pocket for insertion, they have many benefits including a lower contracture rate, less rippling, and shape stability. The variety of sizes allows for correction of asymmetries and the form

stable nature of the gel allows the implant to shape the breast rather than the breast shaping the implant. Selection of the implant size must be based on defined measurements of implant height, width and projection to insure stability of the implant under the soft tissues.[2,10]

The final preoperative decision relates to the soft tissues. In cases of ptosis, glandular ptosis, skin stretch, asymmetry or nipple malposition, an alteration to the soft tissue envelope may be necessary *(Fig. 3.3)*. Combining a mastopexy with revision of an augmentation is a complex procedure with many variables, some unpredictable. It should be undertaken with caution and only in patients with few risk factors for delayed wound healing. The soft tissues should be handled with extreme care and all skin undermining should be kept to a minimum to decrease the likelihood of skin flap or nipple loss.

The technical steps required to perform a successful breast augmentation are beyond the scope of this chapter, however many of the principles are shared when performing revision breast augmentation. Preoperative markings are done with the patient in a standing or sitting position. When using shaped implants, these markings are critical, as the implant pocket must be dissected just large enough to allow the implant to be inserted. The surgical steps will vary

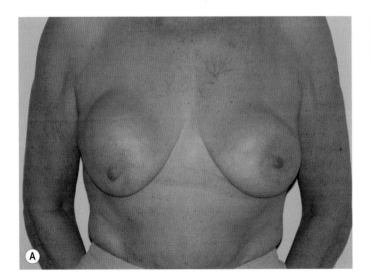
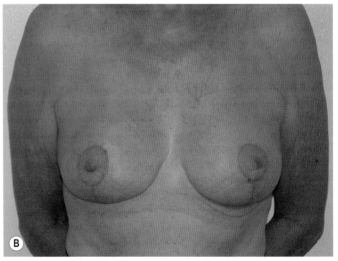

Fig. 3.3 **(A)** A patient with capsular contracture around a subglandular implant. **(B)** 6 weeks after explantation, capsulectomy, subpectoral implant replacement and mastopexy.

depending upon the individual case but usually follow a similar pattern; removal of the old implant; management of the existing capsule; creation or preparation of a pocket for the new implant; insertion of the new implant, and then contouring of the soft tissues. It is always advisable to use precise dissection techniques under direct vision. In primary augmentation, the use of sizers is rarely indicated but in revision cases, sizers may be used more frequently. When using a shaped implant, it is important to use a sizer slightly smaller then the anticipated implant size. Too large a sizer, will result in over-dissection of the pocket and increase the likelihood of rotational problems with the final implant.

Implant insertion is performed using a no touch or minimal touch technique. This is done to decrease the risk of implant contamination and eventual biofilm formation or infection. Minimal digital palpation is used to insure that the implant is sitting flush with the chest wall and in the desired location. Closed suction drains are usually necessary in revision procedures, especially when performing a capsulectomy or pocket change. In thin patients with minimal breast tissue, it is important to place the drain in such a way that there is a lengthy subcutaneous tunnel. This will minimize the likelihood of bacterial tracking especially following drain removal.

Contracture

Capsular contracture is classified according to the classification proposed by Baker. The Baker Classification is still used today and is very simple. The original Baker classification defines four classes[11,12]:

- Class I: Breast absolutely natural; no one could tell breast was augmented
- Class II: Minimal contracture: I can tell surgery was performed but patient has no complaint
- Class III: Moderate contracture: patient feels some firmness
- Class IV: Severe contracture: obvious just from observation.

Capsular contracture represents the most common reason for secondary breast implant surgery.[1] The treatment of capsular contracture begins with prevention. Multiple factors have been implicated in the development of contracted capsules and they are listed in *Table 3.3*.

Table 3.3 Etiology of capsular contracture

Infection
Pocket contamination
Hematoma/blood in implant pocket
Seroma
Silicone gel bleed
Foreign material in pocket (talc, gauze)
Implant surface
Excessive implant size relative to soft tissues
Trauma
Failure of postoperative massage
Delayed contamination – local, systemic
Pocket location
Implant type

Many of these factors can be controlled through precise surgical technique, proper patient and implant selection, patient education and defined post surgical protocols. Maintaining a clean, non contaminated pocket is critical in preventing contractures. The author places an OpSite shield over the nipple at the start of surgery to minimize contamination from the lactiferous ducts. After creation of the pocket, irrigation is performed with an antiseptic solution. Many recommendations have been made as to the ideal solution for irrigation and include betadine, bacitracin and antibiotic solutions. Adams has published extensively on this area and recommends a triple antibiotic mixture that includes 50 mL of povidone-iodine, 1 g of cefazolin and 80 mg of gentamicin in 500 mL normal saline.[13] This author has used a 50/50 mixture of povidone-iodine and normal saline for 15 years with good success. Following preparation of the pocket, the surgical gloves are changed prior to opening the implants. The implants are bathed in the irrigation solution and then inserted. Various techniques have been reported for implant insertion. These range from cleaning the skin around the incision to a complete no touch technique.[14] Other options include using an insertion sleeve or a lubricated funnel. Prophylactic antibiotics are given prior to surgery and for several days after surgery.

Our present understanding of the entire etiology of capsular contracture is lacking. It is necessary for us to develop a better understanding of the physiologic and biochemical processes responsible for capsular contracture if we expect to completely eradicate this problem. Until then, a certain percentage of implant patients will continue to present for treatment.

The decision to treat a contracture is usually based upon the aesthetic consequences of the contracture and the presence of patient symptoms. For minor degrees of contracture (Baker class II), it may be best to take an expectant approach. Given that there is no treatment that can guarantee success, the risks of treating low grade contractures often outweigh the potential benefits.

There are very few nonsurgical options for the treatment of established capsular contractures. In 2002, Schlesinger et al. reported on the use of Zafirlukast (Accolate) for the nonsurgical treatment of capsules.[15] Zafirlukast is a leukotriene receptor antagonist commonly used in the treatment of asthma. Its method of action is to inhibit eosinophilic influx and contractile activity of smooth muscle. Schlesinger noted the incidental improvement of a patient with capsular contracture while taking the medication for a separate indication. The authors report on a series of patients who had improvement in the softness of their capsules while taking zafirlukast. Not only was the treatment used for established capsules, but the authors suggested a potential preventative use in patients who were predisposed to capsule formation. Another medication, montelukast (Singulair) was also described. It is a pharmacologically similar drug that requires only once daily dosage. Risks of both of these drugs include drowsiness and hepatic toxicity. Other studies have also shown clinical improvement in capsule firmness with the use of Accolate.[16,17] The author of this chapter has used both Accolate and Singulair in several patients with established contractures. Treatment times have generally been for 3 months. Very little clinical improvement has been noted and at present, the author is not recommending it for either treatment or prevention of contracture.

When contracture is more significant (Baker III or IV), surgical correction is indicated. There are many surgical approaches for treating capsular contracture and they are summarized in *Table 3.4*.

Table 3.4 Surgical options for treating capsular contracture
Explantation
Open capsulotomy
Capsulectomy
Partial
Total
Pocket site change
Addition or interposition of ADM

Any treatment for capsular contracture has the potential to fail. With this information, some patients choose to have their implants removed with no reinsertion. This approach may be indicated for more elderly women, those who have had multiple previous procedures or those who are not willing to accept the possibility of recurrence and still further treatment. At the time of implant removal, a decision must be made with regards to the capsule. Indications for a capsulectomy include rupture of a gel filled device, or calcification within the capsule. If the capsule is thin and soft, then it may be left in situ, however it is often best to remove at least a portion of the capsule to allow the space to close and minimize the likelihood of a post-surgical fluid collection. Once the implant has been removed, a decision is required as to management of the soft tissues. Although the breast tissue can be left as is, consideration is made to performing a mastopexy and reshaping of the remaining gland. This option works well when there is adequate volume of tissue *(Fig. 3.4)*. When performing a simultaneous mastopexy, it is very important to minimize deep dissection around the areola. Because of the loss of the deep blood supply due to the implant pocket, the only blood supply to the areola is through the cutaneous circulation. The surgeon should minimize undermining and bevel acutely around the areola to preserve a layer of blood flow between the skin and the old implant capsule *(Fig. 3.5)*.

Closed and open capsulotomies have both been used to treat capsular contractures. The concept of a closed capsulotomy was first described by Baker in 1976.[18] Following this report, the use of closed capsulotomies became widespread. Over the next several years, surgeons began to report an association between implant rupture and closed capsulotomy. In addition, closed capsulotomy rarely provided more than temporary relief of capsular contracture. This technique is no longer recommended and in fact the FDA has stated that this procedure is contraindicated.

Open capsulotomy has been used for years to treat established contracture. This technique involves open scoring of the capsule, usually circumferentially. Several studies have demonstrated a low success rate with this technique.[19,20] The failure rate is even higher with successive attempts, approaching 75% after three capsulotomies.[20] This high rate of recurrence should not be surprising as nothing is being done to alter or change

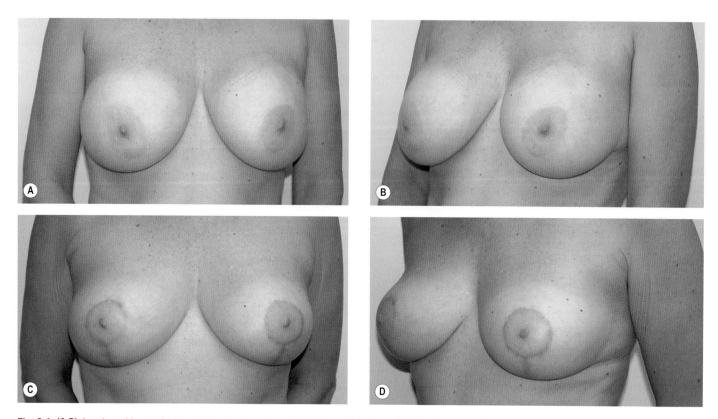

Fig. 3.4 (A,B) A patient with capsular contracture around a subglandular implant. **(C,D)** 3 months following explantation, capsulectomy and mastopexy.

the local environment in which the breast implant is sitting. Based upon much of what we know about the etiology of capsular contracture, it is the authors approach to always remove the implant from its previous pocket. This can be performed with either a capsulectomy or a site change.

When treating a patient with an established contracture, it is recommended to replace the actual implant. Not only do the implant package inserts suggest that implants are for single use only, but there is concern about either contamination or biofilm formation on the surface of the device. Biofilm is a proteinaceous layer that is produced by bacteria and coats the outer surface of an implant. The bacteria are able to hide within this layer making them resistant to systemic antibiotics. Occasionally, one can feel a slime-like substance on the surface of the device but often it is not possible to determine whether a biofilm layer is actually present. Although more work is required to fully understand the mechanism and treatment of biofilm, the best way to mange these patients is to have a high index of suspicion and a low threshold for implant replacement.

Consideration should be given for the use of a textured surface implant *(Fig. 3.6)*. Several studies have demonstrated a lower rate of capsular contracture with textured surface devices, especially when the implants are placed in a subglandular position.[7,8,9] If a textured device is used, it is important to carefully dissect the new pocket to the dimensions of the implant to promote stability within the pocket. For this reason, textured implants are less often used in association with a capsulectomy as the eventual pocket tends to be larger than the planned device. This is especially true when using an anatomic shaped implant where the unique potential for implant rotation exists.

Capsulectomy is one of the most effective ways to treat a contracture. It allows for the removal of the capsule and replacement of the implant into a fresh space. The potential for ongoing contamination of the space around the implant is minimized. Capsulectomy can either be partial or total. There are very few studies comparing the efficacy of these two approaches. Collis and Sharpe compared anterior capsulectomy and total capsulectomy. They replaced all implants with

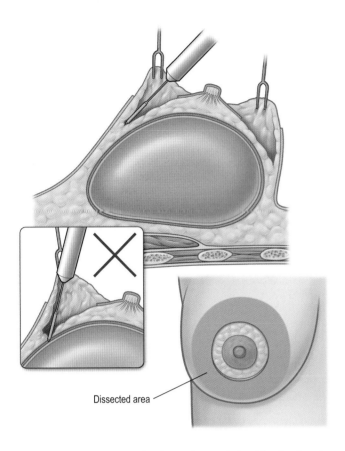

Fig. 3.5 Illustration demonstrating the need to acutely bevel the direction of dissection around the areola in order to maintain a layer of blood supply to the nipple areola complex.

Dissected area

a textured surface device. Contractures recurred in 46% of partial capsulectomies and only 10% of total capsulectomies.[21]

Any capsule with a Baker grade III or IV contracture should be removed, if technically possible. These capsules are generally thick and if not removed, can produce a palpable mass or a mammographic abnormality *(Fig. 3.7)*. They may be colonized by bacteria, and their removal will minimize the local bacterial load. Usually these capsules are calcified which is another indication for their complete removal. In some instances, a partial capsulectomy may be indicated. Subglandular capsules with minimal overlying tissue may be very difficult to remove without causing distortion of the overlying skin or compromise to the cutaneous blood supply. In these cases, a posterior capsulectomy may be more appropriate. For subpectoral implants, a total capsulectomy may be very difficult, especially when the capsule is stuck to the chest wall. The potential exists for bleeding, muscle injury or pneumothorax. Unless the capsule is calcified or grossly contaminated, consideration should be made for an anterior capsulectomy leaving the posterior capsule on the chest wall.

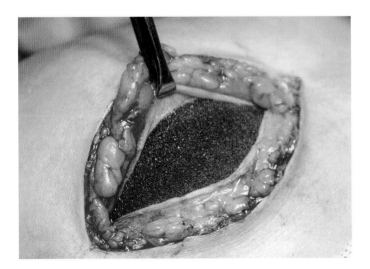

Fig. 3.6 Interface between the capsule and a textured surface implant. Note the tissue integration and the presence of a thin, pliable capsule.

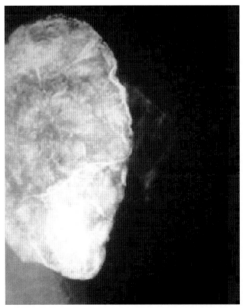

Fig. 3.7 Mammogram of a patient after explanation of a subglandular silicone gel implant without capsulectomy. The retained capsule is heavily calcified and produces both a palpable mass and this type of mammographic artifact, which makes visualization of the breast tissue nearly impossible. (Courtesy of Dr Leroy Young.)

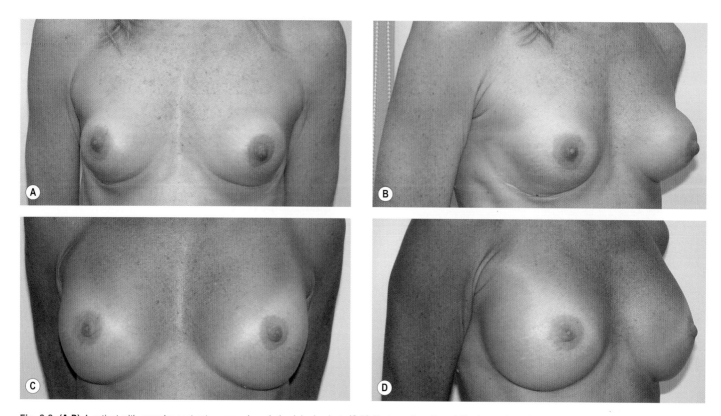

Fig. 3.8 (A,B) A patient with capsular contracture around a subglandular implant. **(C,D)** Postoperative views following explantation, capsulectomy and placement of subpectoral implants. Marionette sutures were used to stabilize the new implants under the PMM.

There are other situations when a complete capsulectomy is contraindicated. Occasionally, a capsule extends far superior towards or into the axilla. If excision jeopardizes the axillary structures then that portion of the capsule should be left in situ. Alternatively, a separate axillary incision may be made to provide safer and more direct access for excision. When moving an implant from a subglandular to a subpectoral position, capsular flaps may be helpful in supporting the implant in its new location. If the capsule is soft and noncalcified, a portion of the capsule may be left and used for support. Capsular flaps may also be used in cases of implant malposition to modify the existing pocket and support structures such as the inframammary fold or the medial breast border.

A powerful tool in treating capsular contracture is a site change, with or without a capsulectomy. Changing the site of the implant pocket allows for a new space that hopefully has minimal or no bacterial contamination, and optimal local blood flow. It also allows the surgeon to maximize the soft tissue coverage over the new device. Implants that were placed in a subglandular space years earlier often have minimal coverage due to natural atrophy and thinning of the tissues. *Figure 3.8* shows a patient with a Baker IV contracture in a subglandular position. Due to the minimal amount of remaining tissue, she underwent a total capsulectomy and replacement with an implant in the subpectoral plane. Percutaneous marionette sutures were used at the inferior edge of the PMM to secure the implant under the muscle in the early stages of healing. A wider implant was selected based upon measurements of the patient's breast width to better fill out the soft tissue envelope. *Figure 3.9* shows another subglandular to subpectoral conversion. In this case, the ptotic breast tissue necessitated a simultaneous lift.

Subpectoral implants can occasionally be moved to a subglandular position. Most often, there is inadequate overlying tissue and this site change is contraindicated. These patients are often treated with a conversion to a neo subpectoral pocket. *Figure 3.10* shows a patient with a unilateral Baker IV contracture. Her opposite breast

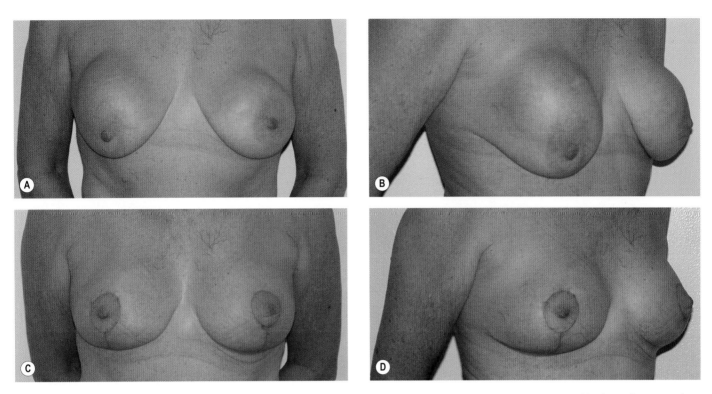

Fig. 3.9 (A,B) A patient with capsular contracture around a subglandular implant. **(C,D)** 6 weeks after explantation, capsulectomy, subpectoral implant replacement and mastopexy.

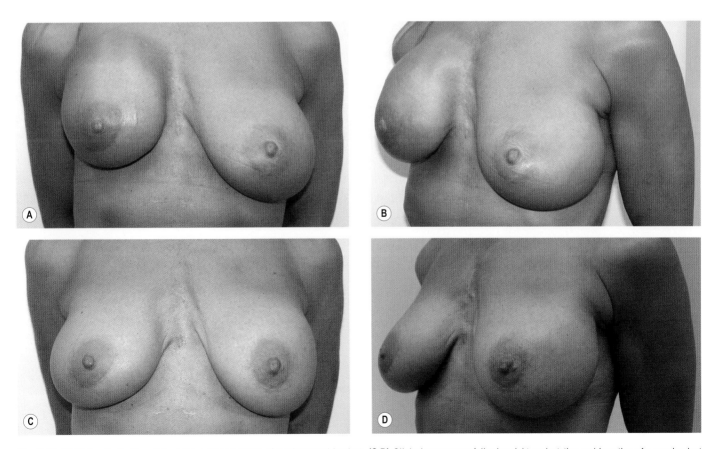

Fig. 3.10 (A,B) A patient with unilateral Baker IV contracture of a subpectoral implant. **(C,D)** Clinical appearance following right explantation and insertion of a new implant in a neo-subpectoral pocket. The left breast was left alone.

was soft and she did not wish to have it revised or changed. Surgery was performed on the affected side only with explantation and replacement of the implant in a neo subpectoral pocket. This allowed the implant

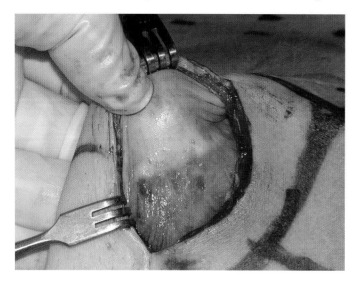

Fig. 3.11 Second stage of an expander/implant reconstruction. The normal capsule can be seen superiorly. Inferiorly, where the Alloderm has been placed, no capsule has formed.

to be covered by the muscle in the superior breast where soft tissue coverage was lacking. Although a capsulectomy and replacement under the muscle would have been an option, this approach was much less traumatic, easier for the patient and easier for the surgeon. In the event of a calcified capsule or a grossly contaminated pocket, preservation of the capsule is contraindicated and a complete capsulectomy should be performed.

Recently, an exciting new possible treatment for capsular contracture has been discussed. This involves the use of acellular dermal matrix (ADM). Although many types of ADM exist on the market, several induce a biologic response that promotes regeneration rather than resorption or encapsulation.[22–24] It has been observed that with these tissue substitutes, a capsule fails to form around the material *(Fig. 3.11)*. This may be due to the fact that the ADM is recognized as self rather than as a foreign material. The author has had anecdotal experience using ADM to assist in the treatment of an established contracture. *Figure 3.12* shows a patient who had previously undergone bilateral subpectoral saline implant augmentation. Subsequent

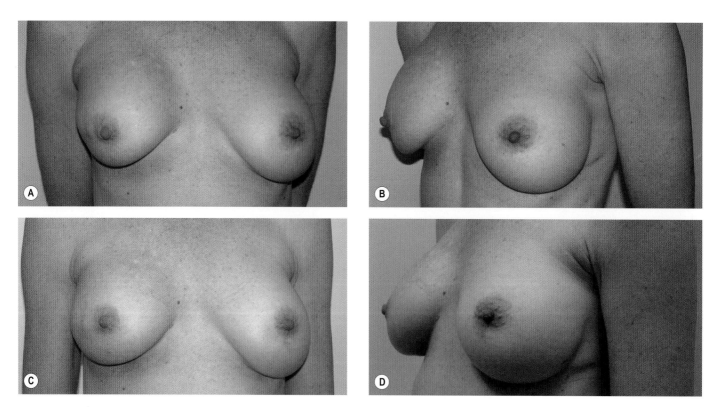

Fig. 3.12 (A,B) A patient with prior subpectoral saline implants. Developed right Baker IV contracture following lumpectomy and radiation. **(C,D)** 18 months following right inferior capsulectomy, circumferential capsulotomy, replacement of implant and Alloderm insertion inferiorly. Breast remains soft with no recurrence of contracture.

to this, she developed right breast cancer treated with lumpectomy, axillary node dissection and radiation therapy. She developed a unilateral Baker IV contracture. She wished to maintain her implants and was happy with the softness and appearance of her left breast. She was treated with right inferior capsulectomy, implant exchange and insertion of Alloderm (Lifecell Corporation, Brandenberg, NJ) to replace the inferior capsule. She is shown 18 months postoperatively with a soft breast and no recurrence of contracture. Further scientific study is necessary to better understand the mechanism of this response and the potential long term benefit of this material.

Malposition

Implant malposition is one of the most common reasons for revision surgery. It is important to carefully diagnose a malposition. In many instances, it may appear as if a malposition exists, when in fact the deformity is related to changes of the soft tissues *(Fig. 3.13)*. This is seen particularly with breast tissue ptosis. The ptosis makes the implant appear as if it is superiorly malpositioned when in fact the implant is in a normal position. Alternatively, in cases of lower pole stretch, the implant may look as if it is displaced inferiorly when the true problem relates to lengthening of the nipple to inframammary fold distance. It is best to identify where the ideal

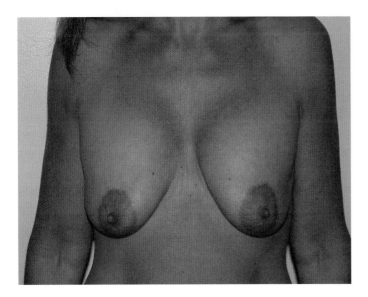

Fig. 3.13 Subpectoral implant. With age, overlying ptosis has developed requiring a mastopexy.

location of the nipple areola complex is and then determine whether or not the implant is sitting in the correct position on the chest wall. Capsular contracture is another common problem that can masquerade as a malposition. If contracture is severe, the deforming forces can cause the implant to shift into an abnormal location. Although this may be thought of as a malposition, the underlying problem requiring correction is the contracture of the capsule.

Implant malposition can be classified by the direction of the malposition. This may be superior (high riding implant), inferior (double bubble), medial (symmastia) or lateral *(Fig. 3.14)*. Occasionally, the malposition may be multidirectional.

Etiology

The etiology of a malposition is varied. Postoperative fluid collections such as hematoma or seroma can cause unexpected over-dissection of the implant pocket *(Fig. 3.15)*. It is important to avoid these collections by utilizing precise surgical technique, minimizing blunt dissection and ensuring complete hemostasis prior to closure. Although the author does not routinely use drains in primary breast augmentation, consideration is given to using drains in cases where the dissection is unusually difficult or when a textured device is being inserted. Drains are always used in secondary surgery. If a postoperative fluid collection does occur, early detection and drainage is mandatory to minimize the formation of a mature pocket that is too large for the implant.

Technical considerations such as under- or over-dissection of the pocket may result in a malposition. Pocket dissection should be done with care and under direct vision. Distant approaches for breast augmentation such as a transumbilical approach are at particular risk for asymmetry and malposition due to the blunt nature of the dissection. This is also true for the axillary approach when performed blind and without endoscopic assist. The author uses no blunt dissection when creating an implant pocket. Some surgeons advocate blunt dissection especially laterally, in an attempt to avoid injury to the lateral intercostal nerves. If this is done, then the amount of blunt dissection should be kept minimal and confined to this area only. The margins of the pocket dissection should be planned preoperatively and followed exactly at the time of surgery.

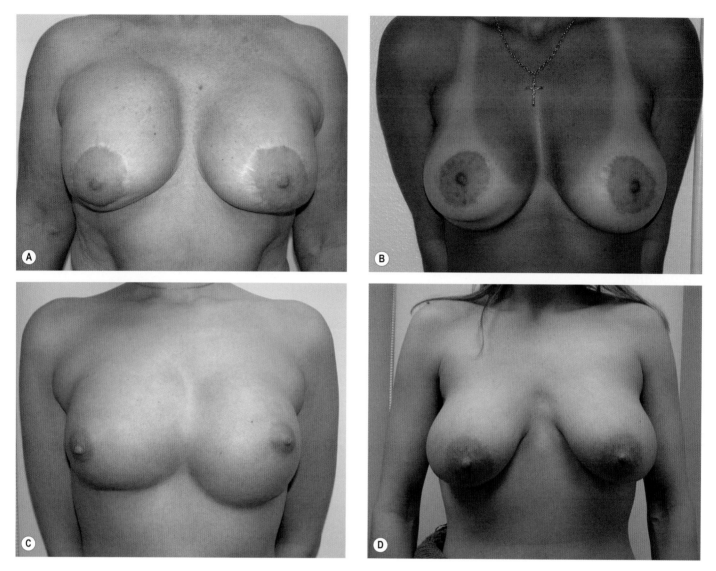

Fig. 3.14 The four directions of implant malposition. **(A)** superior, **(B)** inferior, **(C)** medial, **(D)** lateral.

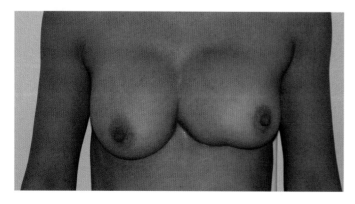

Fig. 3.15 Symmastia caused by an untreated postoperative hematoma.

The selection of an implant that is too wide or large for the soft tissue envelope will predispose to malposition. This is one of the most common causes of symmastia and lateral tissue stretch. The use of defined dimensional planning principles for implant selection is critical in order to avoid this problem. The patient who demands an implant too large for her soft tissues is a patient who should expect the need for further revision surgery.

Other technical factors that may result in implant malposition include inadequate release of the pectoralis major muscle (PMM), excessive release of the medial

PMM and excessive release or lowering of the inframammary fold. This last cause can be most difficult to avoid in certain patients. Women with tight inframammary folds or tuberous breast constrictions have a short nipple to fold distance. It is necessary to lower the fold in order to release the constricted lower pole and bring the nipple into a more central position on the eventual breast mound. Although precise planning can determine where to position the new fold, the old fold often remains tight and can give the appearance of a double crease. This possibility must be discussed with patients prior to surgery. Aggressive release of the constricted base and the use of form stable gel devices can help to minimize this problem.[25] One other patient group that is predisposed to implant malposition are those women with abnormalities of their chest wall. Patients with Poland syndrome or pectus excavatum are at high risk for medial displacement. It is important to recognize this in advance and adjust the surgical plan accordingly. Narrower implants should be considered and great care should be taken not to overly release the medial PMM, when it exists.

Treatment

Implant malpositions can be thought of as a problem of the implant pocket. Treatment either requires adjustment of the pocket or the creation of a new pocket. The options for treating an implant malposition are summarized in *Table 3.5*.

It is the author's preference to treat malpositions by moving the implant into a new, freshly created space whose boundaries can be very precisely defined. In

Table 3.5 **Treatment options for implant malposition**

Adjust the existing pocket
  Capsulodesis
  Capsulorrhaphy
  Partial capsulectomy and closure
  Capsular flap repair
  Repair with ADM/mesh/fascia
  Remove implant, repair pocket, delayed implant reinsertion
Change the pocket
  Subglandular to subpectoral
  Subpectoral to subglandular
  Subpectoral to neo subpectoral
  Conversion to dual plane pocket

some instances however, adjustment of the existing pocket is a very reasonable option. In order to adjust the pocket, the capsule must have enough thickness and substance to support the planned repair. There should be no evidence of calcification within the capsule and the pocket should be in the ideal location for the patient based upon overlying soft tissue characteristics. Options for adjusting the pocket include; suture capsulodesis, capsulorrhaphy, strip capsulectomy and suture repair or a variety of capsular flaps (*Fig. 3.16*). The use of acellular dermal matrix, mesh or fascia to act as an internal support has gained increasing popularity in the past several years. Not only does this tissue support the repair, but it can also provide added coverage in cases of implant palpability and rippling (*Fig. 3.17*). Acellular dermal matrix is used for the correction of a variety of malpositions. Most commonly, correction can be performed in a single stage however in complex cases involving multi-location malpositions a two-stage approach may be advocated. This involves adjusting the pocket to the desired dimensions, removing the implant and then letting the repair heal without the forces of an implant. Reinsertion of the device is then carried out several months later. A temporary, minimally inflated device can be used at the first stage to maintain integrity of the pocket. This approach has particular use in cases of recurrent symmastia.

A second approach to treating malpositions is to remove the implant from the abnormal pocket and replace into a new location. If the implant is subglandular then it can be placed in a new subpectoral pocket. If the implant is subpectoral then consideration can be made for moving to a subglandular position. Often, there is inadequate tissue to allow this site change and in this situation a new subpectoral pocket can be created.[5] This approach has great versatility. It allows for the implant to remain in a partial subpectoral position but be placed in a completely new pocket. Dissection is carried out on top of the old capsule inferiorly and when proceeding superiorly, the plane of dissection moves between the anterior wall of the capsule and the posterior surface of the pectoral muscle. Sutures are placed in the old capsule to close the potential space and the new implant is then placed on top of the old capsule. This neo-subpectoral approach has potential benefit in cases of inferior, medial and lateral malposition (*Fig. 3.18*). Superior malposition can certainly be treated with a

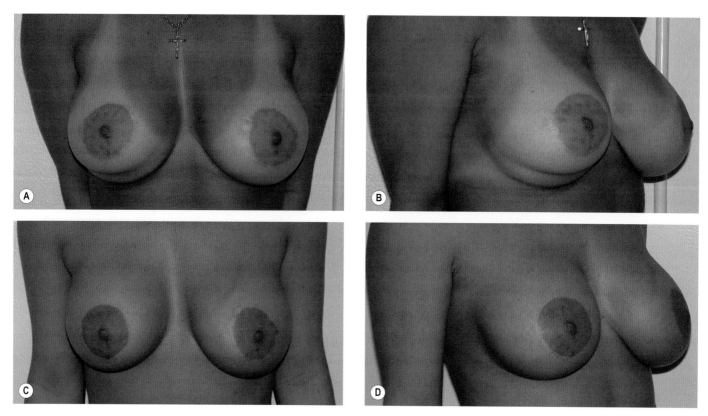

Fig. 3.16 (A,B) Patient with subpectoral implants and areola lift demonstrating inferior malposition of the right breast. **(C,D)** Clinical appearance following right inferior strip capsulectomy and suture repair of IMF.

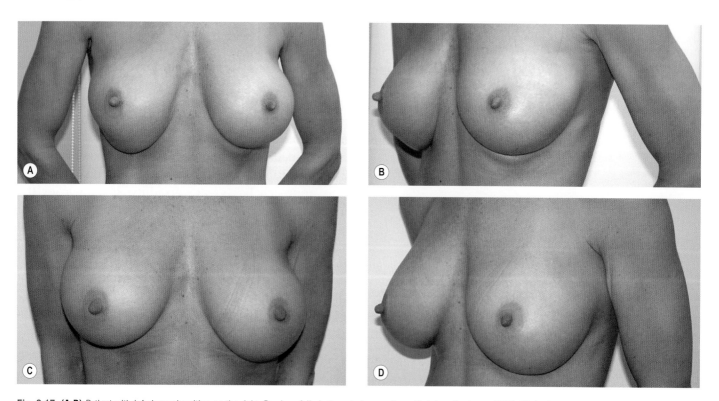

Fig. 3.17 (A,B) Patient with inferior malposition on the right. Previous failed attempt at correction with internal sutures. **(C,D)** Clinical appearance following correction of right inframammary fold position with Alloderm.

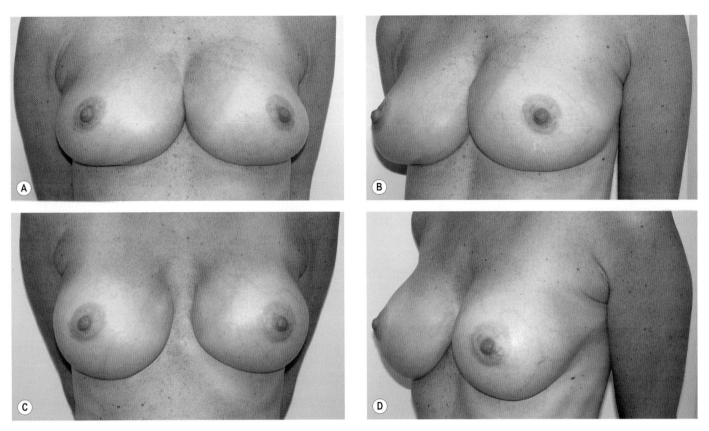

Fig. 3.18 (A,B) Patient with medial malposition following subpectoral augmentation. **(C,D)** Clinical appearance following implant removal, bilateral neosubpectoral pockets and insertion of new textured surface gel implants.

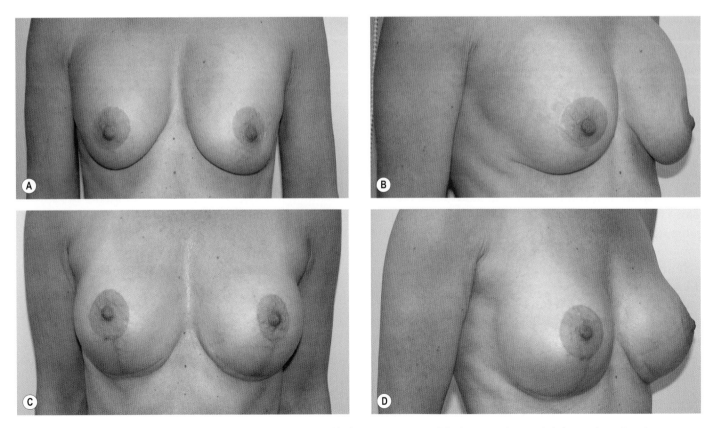

Fig. 3.19 (A,B) Patient with superior malposition and overlying breast ptosis. **(C,D)** Clinical appearance following conversion to a dual plane pocket and mastopexy.

pocket change but in cases where the capsule is soft and noncalcified a conversion to a dual plane pocket can be considered.[6] Dissection is carried out on top of the capsule from the IMF to the inferior border of the PMM. At this point, the anterior wall of the capsule is opened and the implant is allowed to drop down into the new subglandular space. The upper portion of the implant remains in the superior portion of the old capsule. When indicated, this lowering of the implant can be combined with a lift of the overlying tissues (*Fig. 3.19*).

Implant selection depends upon the type of malposition repair. When placing an implant into a mature pre-existing capsule, the author prefers a smooth surface device. When a new pocket is selected, a texture surface implant is selected in an attempt to stabilize the implant position and minimize the risk for recurrence of implant displacement. Postoperative care includes the use of a supportive sports bra for one month. Depending upon the type of repair, specialized bandaging may be used. For example with superior malpositions, a bandeau is applied and for symmastia correction a medial, presternal buttress bra is worn for the first month.

Implant failure

Prior to the breast implant controversy of the early 1990s, implant failure was felt to be a rare problem. As patients grew concerned about the safety of their implants they presented to plastic surgeons for further evaluation. It became apparent that implant rupture was more of a common problem then initially recognized. The lack of information about the failure rates and lifespan of breast implants stimulated many surgeons to assess rupture rates and cause of rupture in their own patients. Rupture seems to be time-dependent and specific to the particular generation of implant. Device failure is a complex issue to study, as there are many factors that can influence failure. These include: generation of implant; fill material; number of lumens; implant surface; normal variability in manufacturing technique; design modification; a history of closed capsulotomy or trauma to the breast; surgical technique, and method used for implant insertion or removal. Because of the compressive load placed on the implant, mammography has also been implicated in implant rupture. Other possible causes of device failure include needle biopsies as well as revision surgery without implant exchange. Although more information is known today about the incidence of implant failure, its exact incidence remains unknown and surgery to correct implant failure remains one of the most common reasons for reoperative breast surgery.

The etiology, diagnosis and treatment of implant failure varies considerably, depending upon the fill material of the implant. Although saline implants are subject to all of the issues listed above, surgeons have recognized that use of proper fill volume can minimize the deflation frequency of the implants. Underfilled implants may develop folding of the shell and subject the shell to unnatural strain that may lead to abrasions and fatigue fracture. Gutowski et al. studied 995 saline implants and determined that devices underfilled by more than 25 mL below the recommended range, were 3.3 times more likely to fail than were implants filled within 25 mL of the recommended range, or those that were overfilled.[26] When a saline implant fails, it is usually easy to detect clinically. Occasionally there may be a slow deflation, but typically, the device completely deflates. Treatment includes implant removal and replacement with a new device. If treatment is delayed, then an open capsulotomy may be necessary to re-establish desired pocket dimensions. In patients where there is an associated capsular contracture, capsulectomy may be indicated.

The exact incidence of gel-filled implant rupture remains unknown. Multiple studies have looked at incidence of device failure in relation to type of implant or length of time since initial surgery. Peters et al. reported on 352 explanted devices.[27] They found no ruptured generation one devices; a 77% rupture rate for generation two devices; and a 3.6% rate for generation three implants. Heden et al. evaluated fourth generation form stable gel implants with MRI.[28] He looked at 300 implants and found that five devices showed evidence of rupture, yielding a rupture prevalence of 1.7% at a median implant age of 8 years. Young and Watson studied 653 implants and stratified them by length of time *in situ*.[29] The overall rupture rate was 28.8% and the rate rose from 7% at 0–4 years, to 55% when implanted for over 20 years.

Physical features suggestive of a ruptured gel implant include a palpable mass adjacent to the implant representing gel herniation or a localized silicone granuloma, a change in shape of the breast, or unexplained pain or discomfort within the breast. Of course, ruptured implants may also be silent in their presentation. Patients should be questioned for any history of recent trauma, biopsies or mammograms. Imaging may be performed with ultrasound or mammography but the most reliable method for detecting a gel implant rupture is magnetic resonance imaging. MRI has been shown to have a high degree of both sensitivity and specificity, however the only way to diagnose an implant rupture with certainty is by surgical exploration. The most common positive finding on MRI is the "linguine sign," which represents disrupted fragments of the ruptured implant shell. MRI is also useful for detecting silicone granulomas, regional migration of gel and any evidence of residual silicone. In general, the T2-weighted sequence is considered the most helpful in evaluating silicone implants.

Implant ruptures are classified as either intracapsular or extracapsular. Ruptures that remain intracapsular are frequently silent. It should be noted that even with intracapsular ruptures, it is common to find silicone present within the implant capsule. Most surgeons recommend removal of ruptured silicone gel breast implants, especially if they are extracapsular. Asymptomatic intracapsular ruptures are more controversial, especially since it is much harder to definitively diagnose the rupture prior to surgery. Although some surgeons recommend leaving ruptured implants that have stayed confined within the capsule, it is the authors approach to remove all implants where there is clinical or radiographic evidence of rupture. A ruptured implant is no longer in the physical state that it was meant to be by the manufacturer who sold the device. Intracapsular ruptures have the potential of converting to extracapsular ruptures, a situation that is much more difficult to treat. Patients should be informed that the removal of a ruptured implant is not an emergency and can be planned around patient and surgeon convenience.

Surgical treatment includes implant removal with or without a capsulectomy. Ease of removal varies with the generation of the device. Generation two implants with their thin noncohesive gel are very difficult to remove, whereas newer third and fourth generation devices tend to come out more as a cohesive unit. Incision length should be adequate to allow for exposure of the implant, the capsule and any extracapsular gel. In cases where the capsule is thin and noncalcified, consideration may be given to implant removal only. Patients must be told that the remaining capsule may very well contain silicone gel particles. Today, this is less of a concern to women, but during the implant controversy of the early 1990s, *en bloc* resection, including the implant and capsule was done routinely. For all extracapsular ruptures and most intracapsular ruptures, implant removal and complete capsulectomy is recommended. This provides the best chance for total or near total removal of the gel. In patients who are having a new implant inserted, a total capsulectomy allows for a clean, fresh pocket for the new device. Of course, based on the soft tissue characteristics, a pocket change to a new location may be a more appropriate choice.

Rippling and palpability

Rippling or implant edge palpability is one of the more common concerns for patients following breast augmentation. Skin wrinkling and implant palpability arise from folding of the implant shell, inadequate soft tissue cover and stiffness of the shell of the implant. Rippling can be seen anywhere on the breast but is most frequently seen superiorly in the cleavage line or laterally. The causes of skin wrinkling and implant palpability are multifactorial, however the quality and quantity of the overlying soft tissues are the most critical factors.

All patients should be told that rippling can occur in any augmentation, however steps can be taken to minimize the likelihood or extent of rippling and palpability. This begins with prevention. Decisions such as pocket selection, implant size and dimensions of the pocket dissection are all selected to maximize the ratio of soft tissue to implant coverage. Patients must be educated as to why a certain pocket location is best. Tebbets described a method for assessing the amount of coverage in the upper portion of the breast.[30] The measured pinch thickness must be at least 2 cm to allow for a subglandular placement, otherwise a subpectoral or dual plane pocket is indicated. Attention should also be paid to the expected soft tissue changes that occur over time. A breast that has adequate soft tissues to cover a subglandular device, may atrophy and change over subsequent years, resulting in an implant with inadequate coverage and noticeable rippling. This is much more likely to happen with subglandular versus subpectoral positioning.

Initial implant size selection is critical and care should be taken to avoid selecting implants with a base diameter greater than the measured breast width. If greater volume is desired, the surgeon should consider higher profile devices rather than selecting an implant that is too wide for the soft tissue envelope. Exceptions to this include the severely hypoplastic breast or patients with a tuberous breast constriction. In these women it will be necessary to select a wider implant but patients should be told in advance that rippling, especially laterally, will likely occur.

The increased use of saline filled devices in the 1990s made rippling a much more common problem then seen previously. It is generally agreed that rippling is more common with a saline filled device, however it can certainly occur with gel filled implants. Rippling is more likely with implants that are not filled to ideal volumes. The percentage fill volume of a device describes the ratio of actual fill volume to maximum fill volume. As the fill volume increases, the chance of rippling decreases, however the implant assumes a more rounded shape and becomes firmer to the touch. With saline implants, surgeons should try to fill the implant to the upper limit that is recommended by the manufacturer, Underfilling should be avoided. With gel implants, there are various options with different fill volumes for a given size and base diameter. The surgeon must choose a device that will provide a low risk for rippling but at the same time, provide a pleasing feel and shape of the breast.

The stiffness of the elastomer shell also contributes to implant folding and palpability. Texturing the surface of an implant adds thickness and makes the shell stiffer. This explains why rippling is seen more commonly with textured surface implants. There are also some textured surfaces that promote tissue integration with the surrounding capsule. Although this may have a beneficial effect on preventing capsular contracture, the tissue adherence may lead to traction rippling, especially in the upper pole of the breast. For these reasons, it is very important to ensure that there is adequate soft tissue coverage when using a textured device.

The treatment of a patient with rippling or implant palpability begins with managing expectations. Unless the implant is removed, there can be no guarantee that the problem will be gone. The patient should understand that rippling and palpability can be minimized, not eliminated. All contributing factors must be considered when planning revision. The principles include: selecting an implant that matches the dimensions of the overlying breast tissue; maximizing soft tissue coverage over the implant; and selecting an implant that is least likely to result in rippling and palpable edges. This may mean a change of the implant fill material, surface, size or fill volume. *Figure 3.20* shows a patient with subglandular textured saline implants that have resulted in a palpable implant with visible rippling, most noticeable on the superior aspect of the left breast. She was treated with a pocket conversion to a subpectoral position to maximize upper pole coverage. A circumareolar lift was performed to tighten the skin envelope and the implant was changed to a smooth round gel device. The base width of the breast was measured at 13.5 cm. Accordingly, an implant was selected that did not extend past the lateral border of the breast.

Patients with superior or lateral rippling can also be improved by tightening the pocket that the implant sits in. This can be achieved by a combination of increasing implant volume and supporting the implant pocket. The use of capsular flaps or acellular dermal matrix (ADM) inferiorly can act as a sling and push the implant into a more superior position. Although this maneuver does not increase coverage over the implant, the added support has been shown to decrease traction rippling. The use of ADM to add soft tissue coverage has also been described. The material can be layered in the area of palpability or rippling. This technique, combined with pocket support inferiorly, is a very effective method of treatment when a pocket change is not indicated or possible.

One other option to consider is the use of micro fat injection. Fat has been used for years as a soft tissue filler. More recently, it has been described for use in the breast.[31,32] Fat injecting is an important tool in breast reconstruction and has been used to treat contour irregularities, palpable implant edges and lumpectomy or radiation induced deformities. The adipocyte derived stem cells would seem to have an effect on the local tissues inducing both a qualitative change and an increase in soft tissue volume. Fat injection for primary breast augmentation has been described, however at the time of writing this chapter, the use of large volume fat

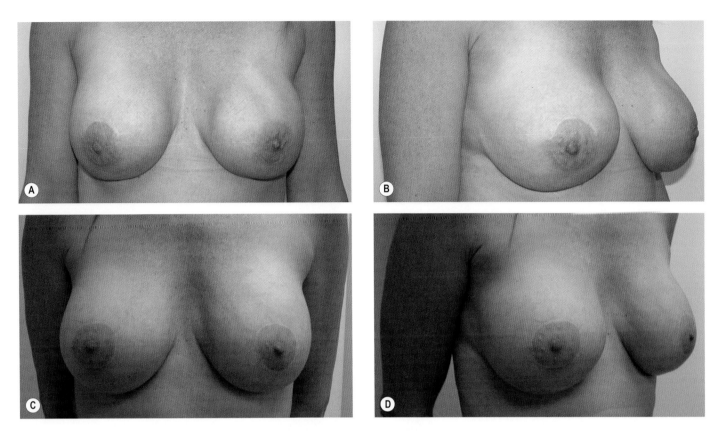

Fig. 3.20 **(A,B)** Patient with subglandular implants and visible rippling, especially on the left. **(C,D)** Clinical appearance after replacing the implants under the muscle and revising the areola lift. Visible rippling and implant edge palpability has been improved.

injection for breast enlargement is considered experimental and requires longer term follow-up. The author has had success using small volumes of fat, injecting superficially around the edges of implants where there has been clinical rippling. Injections must be superficial to the capsule. Small amounts of fat are deposited with each pass to minimize the risk of fat necrosis or irregular contour. Risks of this procedure include infection, intracapsular injection, damage to the implant, contour irregularities and resorption. The procedure is very technique dependent and patients are told that if complications occur, it may result in the need to remove the implant.

Breast asymmetry

All consultations or preoperative assessments for breast augmentation should include the statement that every woman's breasts are naturally asymmetric. Differences in the two breasts may include a difference in size, shape, areola position and diameter, and position of the IMF. The underlying chest wall or pectoral muscles may also be different. The chest wall acts as a foundation for the breast, and the breast implants to sit on. Asymmetries related to kyphosis, scoliosis or sternal abnormalities are probably under appreciated. *Figure 3.21* shows a woman with noticeable asymmetry in size and IMF position. It is important to note preoperatively that she has a scoliosis resulting in a concavity in the right upper chest and a convexity in the left upper chest. Although the use of different size and projection of implants may help to camouflage this asymmetry, complete correction is not possible. One common clinical scenario that merits attention is the patient presenting with asymmetric inframammary folds. There is a natural tendency to lower the fold on the higher side to match the fold on the opposite breast. Although correction of this problem will produce symmetric folds, the result is that the nipple on the corrected side will rotate superiorly on the breast mound more so than on the opposite side. This

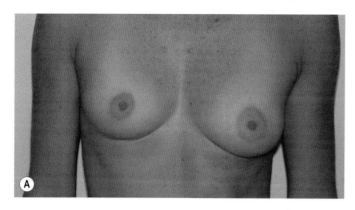 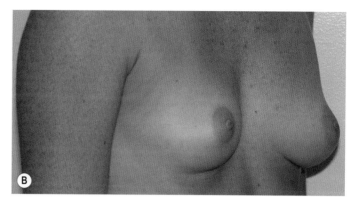

Fig. 3.21 Significant breast asymmetry largely related to abnormalities of the underlying muscle and chest wall. Although the breasts can be made to look more symmetric, noticeable asymmetry will certainly exist following breast augmentation.

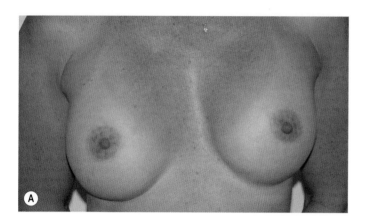 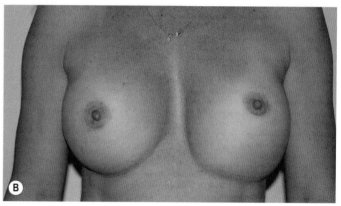

Fig. 3.22 (A) Patient following breast augmentation with asymmetric inframammary folds. **(B)** Clinical appearance following revision and lowering of the left inframammary fold. Although the folds are now more symmetric, the result has been to produce a high-riding nipple on the left.

may result in a high riding nipple on the treated side which becomes readily apparent when the patient wears a bra or bathing suit *(Fig. 3.22)*. In cases of minor fold asymmetries, it is often best to inform the patient that the folds should be left alone and that this minor degree of asymmetry will persist after surgery. In situations where asymmetry is either significant or is a major concern for the patient, steps can be taken surgically to try to minimize the asymmetry. Such steps may include using different implant sizes or projections, removing tissue or performing an asymmetric lift. Regardless of the surgical plan, some degree of asymmetry will remain following surgery.

Patients that are properly educated preoperatively will be prepared to accept minor asymmetries. At the time of consultation, measurements and photographs are taken to both document and illustrate asymmetry.

The author asks all his patients to stand in front of a full length mirror and clearly demonstrate where the asymmetries exist and which asymmetries can be corrected. Consent forms include a statement explaining that every attempt will be made to correct pre-existing asymmetries but the patient should expect that some degree of asymmetry will continue to be present following surgery.

After breast augmentation, some women do present with significant degrees of asymmetry. A full assessment is necessary to identify exactly what the causes of the asymmetry are. This should include a review of preoperative photographs or measurements (if available); a review of the operative report and implants selected; and a careful assessment of the breast tissue, implants and chest wall. Asymmetry may be due to many factors, including contracture, malposition or

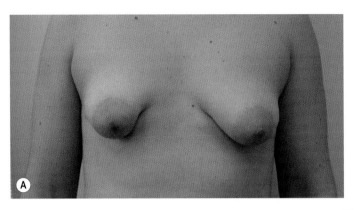 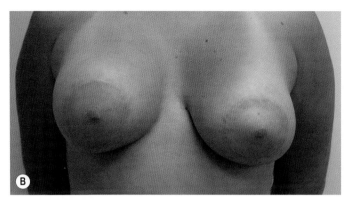

Fig 3.23 (A) A young woman with asymmetric type IV tuberous breast deformity. **(B)** Clinical appearance following a one-stage correction with areola lift and insertion of asymmetric shaped form-stable gel implants. She has ongoing asymmetry of her inframammary folds and nipple position as well as large areolas.

implant deflation. It may also be related to technical factors, such as incomplete muscle release or asymmetric pocket dissection.

Treatment is dependent upon the exact nature of the asymmetry. As with all secondary breast procedures, a full risk benefit analysis must be discussed with the patient. Minor asymmetries should be accepted, as the risks of complications and ongoing asymmetry outweigh the potential improvements. Existing contractures or implant malpositions can be treated as discussed previously. Differences in breast size can be corrected with reaugmentation using different implants or by adjusting the overlying soft tissues. The use of shaped gel implants can play an important role in managing the asymmetry patient. These implants allow surgeons to select devices based on width, height and projection. The added benefit of being able to individually adjust one of three dimensions provides great flexibility in balancing the two breasts.

Differences in shape can involve the breast mound, the areola or the nipple. Soft tissue asymmetry can be adjusted with asymmetric removal of tissue. Breasts of different width can be adjusted with pocket modification, implant size change or narrowing procedures such as a vertical scar mastopexy. Residual deformities following correction of a tuberous breast deformity can be particularly challenging. *Figure 3.23* shows a young woman with type 4 bilateral asymmetric tuberous breasts. She was treated in a single stage with a circumareolar correction of the herniated tissue, lowering of the inframammary folds, release of the constricted base and insertion of asymmetric shaped form stable gel

implants. She is shown 6 months later with ongoing asymmetry of her IMF and large areolas. She was advised to accept the difference in fold position, however her nipple height asymmetry and large areola diameter could be improved with an asymmetric areola lift and reduction using a permanent purse-string suture.

Breast asymmetry following augmentation is a very real concern for many patients, largely because augmentation can make pre-existing differences more noticeable. A detailed and thorough preoperative process that includes patient education will help patients to understand what is reasonable in terms of expectations and decrease the number of reoperations for residual asymmetry. If treatment is necessary, it must be based on a detailed assessment of the problem, an accurate diagnosis and a carefully executed surgical plan.

Soft tissue changes

Secondary breast surgery may be performed for indications other than problems related to the implant itself. The overlying breast tissue will undergo changes that are related to normal physiologic processes. Factors such as pregnancy, breast-feeding, weight gain and gravitational changes will result in ptosis of the overlying breast tissue. If the implant is subglandular, then it may descend into the lower pole of the breast, along with the glandular tissue. This will result in stretching and thinning of the lower pole and possibly lead to implant palpability and rippling. This problem would be exacerbated by insertion of implants that are too large or too heavy for the initial skin envelope

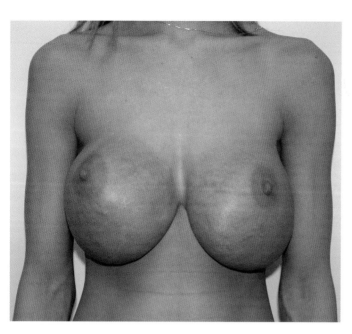

Fig. 3.24 Clinical appearance of a woman several years following subglandular breast augmentation. The soft tissue changes are as a result of poor tissue quality and the use of an excessively large implant.

(Fig. 3.24). Treatment of this problem can be challenging. One option is to remove the implant but this will leave a loose and empty skin envelope. Certainly a mastopexy may be performed but there needs to be adequate volume of tissue to allow the surgeon to shape a breast of adequate size. Care should be taken to minimize skin undermining, especially around the areola, in order to decrease the likelihood of vascular compromise. The most definitive treatment of a large, thinned out skin envelope is to remove the subglandular implant, place a smaller implant under the muscle and perform a lift of the lower pole tissues.

For subpectoral implants, the device will tend to remain high with the breast tissue falling off the implant in what has been described as a "waterfall deformity". If the implant is soft and felt to be in a normal position, then treatment would involve performing a mastopexy of the ptotic tissues. Otherwise, the implant may need to be removed and placed in a slightly lower position, or converted to a dual plane location.

Size change

In some surgical practices, a patient's request for a change in the size of her implants is a common reason

for reoperative surgery. A size change is not a complication in the truest sense of the word. It does however, require the patient to undergo further surgery, risk and expense. It is also a burden to the surgeon in terms of cost and time. When size change is requested within the first few years after surgery, it represents a miscommunication between the initial surgeon and the patient. A request for size change years after surgery may be more understandable as the patient's body and soft tissues may have undergone changes related to aging, weight fluctuations or pregnancy.

The steps required to minimize the number of requests for size change are several, however the underlying principle is patient education. For years, women have been under the impression that they were able to select any implant size that matches their perception of ideal. This was the era of volume. This approach resulted in a very high rate of secondary surgery. Implants that were too large for the patient's anatomy caused thinning and stretching of the soft tissues, rippling and palpability, and a high rate of implant malposition. Implants that were too small or narrow for the breast either failed to provide a pleasing aesthetic shape or resulted in implants with excessive mobility under the breast. This often leads to collapse of the implant pocket in certain positions and a very unnatural appearance.

The present era of implant selection could be called the dimensional era. Patients are encouraged to select implants that complement the measurements of their breasts and their underlying musculoskeletal anatomy. This requires a strong dedication to education. Key measurements such as breast width, nipple to inframammary fold distance and soft tissue thickness determine what dimensions of an implant will adequately fill out a breast envelope without stretching past the natural boundaries of the breast.[2,4,10] Of course certain exceptions exist such as in the tuberous breast or severely hypoplastic breast, but this approach will apply to the vast majority of patients. It has been the author's experience that a well educated patient will quite readily accept this approach to implant sizing. This commitment may result in the loss of certain patients who are only prepared to think in terms of volume, but it will certainly allow the surgeon to maintain a low rate of revision for problems related to improper size selection.

Once the proper size is selected preoperatively, there are several steps that can be taken to illustrate for the patient what they can reasonably expect. Sizers can be tried on in the office; photographs of patients with similar body proportions are viewed; and newer 3D programs can simulate the anticipated result. Patients who bring in representative photographs that deviate significantly from what is being shown are unlikely to be happy with their surgical result.

In the few situations where a size change is indicated, the surgical procedure is generally straightforward. Most often, a capsulotomy is performed to allow for adequate space for the new device. Drains are used in all reoperative cases. Patients undergoing a delayed size change require a more thorough analysis. Changes to the soft tissues may dictate the need for a skin tightening procedure and perhaps a smaller implant. It is important to resist the temptation of filling a looser skin envelope with larger implants. This slippery slope will eventually result in a situation that can be very difficult to manage.

Postoperative care

A routine process for managing patients in the postoperative period is important in all surgeries but especially with revision procedures. Surgery may be more complex involving work on the soft tissues, the implants or both. The specific care will depend upon the exact procedure performed. In most secondary cases, drains are used. Patients are given instructions on how to care for the drains and ensure that they do not fill with clots. A sterile dressing is placed around the drain site and patients must be instructed how to care for the dressing to minimize the likelihood of drain site infection. Patients are maintained on oral antibiotics until the drains are removed.

When correcting implant malposition, bandaging may be desirable to support the implant in a certain position. For example, when correcting symmastia, bandages or a bolster are often placed over the sternum to support the medial repair. Many surgeons place patients in a supportive bra for the first 4–6 weeks to encourage implant stability within the implant pocket. Postoperative activity should be tailored to the procedure. If a malposition is corrected and the implant is in a subpectoral position, the patient will be required to minimize pectoral activity until the new capsule has formed around the implant. Often, patients need to be given very clear instructions as to what it means to minimize pectoral contraction.

Displacement massage techniques are routinely used with smooth surface devices. This is started within a few days of surgery and is recommended to be performed several times a day. Patients must be shown exactly how to perform displacement massage, as most women are very cautious and tend to be too gentle. Postoperative massage with shaped implants or textured round devices is contraindicated.

Outcomes, prognosis, and complications

The expected outcomes in reoperative breast surgery are dependent upon the individual case and particularly, the complexity of the procedure performed. Patients should expect it to take longer for the tissues to heal then it would with primary surgery. In routine primary breast augmentation, patients are often instructed that it may take 6 months to a year for them to see the actual final result of their surgery. Scars must heal, tissue must redrape and soften and implants must stabilize in position. With secondary surgery, it will take even longer before the result reaches a plateau. It is probably best to wait at least a year before considering any revision surgery to be successful. Of course with capsular contracture, recurrence can occur at any time, even years after surgery.

As with primary surgery, the perception of the results is often based on preoperative expectations. It is imperative that the patient have realistic expectations as to what is possible. Setting these expectations early will assist in how patients assess their outcomes. This is especially true with reoperative cases.

The complications from reoperative breast surgery are similar to those in primary cases. These are summarized in *Table 3.6*. One specific risk in revision procedures that warrants special comment is potential compromise of the blood supply to the NAC. This risk rises with increased complexity of previous surgery and planned surgery. The surgeon must take into consideration previous sites of implant pocket(s) and previous

Table 3.6 **Risks associated with revision breast augmentation**	
Infection	Implant rupture
Hematoma	Contracture
Seroma	Interference with mammography
Decrease sensation	Rotation
Possible effect on breast-feeding	Malposition
Poor scarring	Asymmetry
Necrosis of tissue	Reoperations for replacement
Skin	Rippling
Nipple/areola	Implant edge palpability
Fat	Failure to meet patient expectations
Secondary changes to the soft tissues	

pedicle elevation. In cases where both implant revision and soft tissue reshaping is required, a staged approach should be considered. The likelihood for further revision surgery is greater in secondary cases than in primary augmentation. It is important to have a discussion with your patient in advance as to who will bear the financial responsibility for further surgery. Every practice will have their own approach, but setting the ground rules in advance will assist in limiting confusion and frustration after the fact.

All potential risks are more likely to occur in secondary procedures. Careful patient selection, intelligent surgical planning, meticulous technique and follow-up care will help to keep these complications to a minimum.

 Access the complete reference list online at **http://www.expertconsult.com**

1. Spear SL, Murphy DK, Slicton A, et al. Inamed silicone breast implant core study results at 6 years. *Plast Reconstr Surg*. 2007;120(Suppl):8S–16S.

   The FDA core study of silicone gel breast implants is one of the best available references for implant related complications and reoperation rates. This article reports on 6-year data with Inamed (Allergan) silicone gel breast implants and has been a stimulus for educational initiatives to decrease complications and reoperations in breast implant surgery.

5. Maxwell GP, Gabriel A. The neopectoral pocket in revisionary breast surgery. *Aesthetic Surg J*. 2008; 28:463–467.

   One of the most important tools in revision breast surgery is the ability to perform a site change. When implants are subpectoral and there is inadequate tissue for a subglandular location, the neosubpectoral pocket is often indicated. This excellent article discusses the indications and technique for this procedure.

6. Spear SL, Carter ME, Ganz JC. The correction of capsular contracture by conversion to "dual plane" positioning: Technique and outcomes. *Plast Reconstr Surg*. 2006;(Suppl):S118.

7. Barnsley GP, Sigurdson LJ, Barnsley SE. Textured surface breast implants in the prevention of capsular contracture among breast augmentation patients: A meta-analysis of randomized controlled trials. *Plast Reconstr Surg*. 2006;117:2182–2190.

   This meta-analysis is regularly quoted when discussing the effect of implant surface on the development of capsular contracture. Statistically low rates of contracture are found with textured devices in a subglandular pocket. This effect is lost for subpectoral implants.

10. Heden P, Jernbeck J, Hober M. Breast augmentation with anatomical cohesive gel implants. *Clin Plast Surg*. 2001;28:531–552.

    This paper describes the largest published experience with shaped form stable gel implants. It is an important reference that reviews patient selection, implant selection, outcomes and how to minimize complications.

13. Adams WP, Rios JL, Smith SJ. Enhancing patient outcomes in aesthetic and reconstructive breast surgery using triple antibiotic breast irrigation: six year prospective clinical study. *Plast Reconstr Surg*. 2006; 118(Suppl):S46–S52.

    The senior author of this paper has published extensively on biofilm and managing the microbial environment around breast implants. This prospective trial illustrates the use of a triple antibiotic solution in association with a defined stepwise approach to implant insertion in order to maintain low rates of infection and capsular contracture.

22. Breuing KH, Warren SM. Immediate bilateral breast reconstruction with implants and inferolateral Alloderm slings. *Ann Plast Surg*. 2005;55:232–239.

29. Young VL, Watson ME. Breast implant research: where we have been, where we are, where we need to go. *Clin Plast Surg*. 2001;28:451–483.

30. Tebbets JB. Alternatives and trade-offs in breast augmentation. *Clin Plast Surg*. 2001;28:485–500.

32. Rigotti G, Marchi A, Galiè M, et al. Clinical treatment of radiotherapy tissue damage by lipoaspirate transplant: A healing process mediated by adipocyte-derived adult stem cells. *Plast Reconstr Surg*. 2007;119:1409–1421.

4

Current concepts in revisionary breast surgery

G. Patrick Maxwell and Allen Gabriel

SYNOPSIS

- Breast augmentation is the most common aesthetic procedure performed in the United States.
- Revisionary breast surgeries are complex, challenging, and unpredictable.
- Four main drivers for revisionary surgery: capsular contracture, implant malposition, ptosis, and implant visibility or palpability.
- Authors introduce revisionary surgery techniques, utilizing a site change operation with the use of acellular dermal matrix (ADM).

 Access the Historical Perspective section online at
http://www.expertconsult.com

Introduction

It is estimated that over 300 000 primary breast augmentations were performed in the United States in 2009, and therefore there are now over 3 million women with augmented breasts in this country.[1-3] Based on current data, between 15% and 30% of these women, will have a reoperation within 5 years of their initial procedure.[1-3] Unfortunately, this rate climbs to 35% in patients with a prior history of revisionary breast augmentation.[4] As procedures become more complex in nature and number, new techniques and solutions are required of surgeons who perform these challenging operations to improve long-term patient outcomes.

Capsular contracture has historically been the most common complication of aesthetic and reconstructive breast surgery and remains the primary reason for most revisionary surgeries.[2,3,5,6] While increasing data suggests capsular contracture can be minimized in primary augmentation by technical detail including precise, atraumatic, bloodless dissection; appropriate antibiotic breast pocket irrigation; and minimizing any points of contamination during the procedure,[4,7] treatment of an established capsule remains even more challenging than the application of these techniques alone.

The enforcement of the US FDA restrictions on silicone gel implants in the early 1990s led American surgeons to use saline implants.[1] While prior to the 1992 "moratorium", the majority of silicone gel implants were placed in the subglandular position, saline implants (due to their palpability) began to be placed under the muscle in an effort to conceal the untoward contour irregularities of these implants.[8] As a number of these implants were of larger volumes, many patients experienced thinning of breast parenchyma and the overlying soft tissue, whether the implants were in subglandular or subpectoral positions. The thinned tissues, in turn, can lead to long-term complications, which had led to some key drivers of revisionary breast surgery.

The four primary reasons (or "Drivers") for aesthetic revision surgery in the Pre-Market Approval (PMA) studies were as follows:[9] (1) capsular contracture, (2) implant malposition, (3) ptosis, and (4) implant visibility or palpability. Frequently, these indications were not singularly distinct, but were combined with two or more being present in a given patient.

Hints and tips

- There are four key drivers to revisionary breast surgery: (1) capsular contracture; (2) implant malposition; (3) ptosis, and (4) implant visibility or palpability. Frequently, these indications are not singularly distinct, but were combined with two or more being present in a given patient.
- Capsular contracture is the most common driver for revisionary breast surgery.
- Site change and acellular dermal matrix are key for successful outcomes in revisionary breast surgery.

Basic science and disease process

Acellular dermal materials, biologically derived from allograft and xenograft, when placed in the human body, are thought to serve as a regenerative scaffold, promoting the organization of the healing process. These materials have become popular in breast cancer reconstruction, where they are said to serve as a tissue extension or tissue replacement ("soft-tissue patch") following cancer extirpation of the breast (so-called "sling technique").[22,23,27]

Our work with acellular dermal matrix (ADM) began in revisionary aesthetic breast surgery, attempting to prevent capsular contracture, rather than as a tissue replacement in breast reconstruction. Having previously employed "host-compatible" implant surfaces,[28] here we have utilized a similar concept in our clinical approach to breast revision: a dermal regenerative interface engaging the surface geometric contour of a breast implant.

Understanding the changes that occur in the breast tissue is part of management of the problem at hand. Following breast surgery, many factors play a role in the changes that are observed in the breast form and at times are considered late complications of breast augmentation. Patients lose or gain weight which contributes directly to the breast shape. In addition, some patients may undergo surgical or nonsurgical menopause which has deleterious effects on the wellbeing of the skin, causing thinning of the breast skin, decreased elasticity, and increased ptosis. There are other physiological factors that a play a big role in the pathophysiology of the changing breast forms. Patients present with any of the following complaints: *capsular contracture, implant malposition, ptosis*, and *implant visibility or palpability*. Interestingly, patients with capsular contracture do not realize the primary reason for the deformity of their breast and present to the office for other complaints as stated above.

Capsular contracture has plagued plastic surgery as the most common complication of aesthetic and reconstructive breast surgery for many years.[2,5] The majority of revisionary breast surgeries are performed to correct capsular contracture.[2,6] Many etiologies have been proposed for this process, and it is clear that prevention of it in primary cases includes sound techniques – including precise, atraumatic, bloodless dissection; appropriate triple antibiotic breast pocket irrigation; and minimizing any points of contamination during the procedure.[4,7] Treatment of an established capsule can be more challenging, and multiple techniques have been utilized for this. The bottom line for any pathophysiological process is to understand the disease at the cellular level. In this case, it is perspicuous that at the cellular level, capsular contracture is most likely caused by any process that will produce increased inflammation, leading to formation of deleterious cytokines within the periprosthetic pocket. Consequently, in addition to all of the techniques for treating and preventing capsular contracture described by many of our colleagues,[4,5,8,29–35] we believe that the addition of ADM is another modality in fighting the evolution of the capsule. ADM can counteract the inflammatory process, adding additional availability of tissue in-growth and controlling the interface of the pocket.

Acellular dermal matrix

Use of acellular dermal matrices have been popularized in both breast and abdominal wall reconstructions and has been reported in a range of clinical settings.[13–23] In reconstructive cases, it has been used to replace tissue, extend existing tissue, or act as a supplement. In aesthetic cases, it has been used to correct implant rippling and displacement, including symmastia.[25,26,36]

Immediate breast reconstruction using tissue expanders or implants has become one of the most commonly used surgical techniques, which has made visible rippling and contour deformity a more frequently encountered problem.[27] The recent use of allogeneic tissue supplements avoids the problems of autologous tissue coverage and provides camouflage, thus decreasing rippling, and increasing soft tissue padding.[27]

Rising demand has spurred a tremendous growth in the number of available ADMs. Published research regarding the use and efficacy of acellular dermal matrices in immediate breast reconstruction is growing but has not kept pace with the market explosion. The many features and indications of all ADMs can confound the decision making process for surgeons who want to incorporate ADMs in their treatment armamentarium.

Acellular dermal matrices can be categorized under either xenograft or allograft in origin. All are produced with a similar objective of removing cellular and antigenic components that can cause rejection and infection. The lack of immunogenic epitopes enables the evasion of rejection, absorption, and extrusion.[14,15,23] Production processes allow the basement membrane and cellular matrix to remain intact. This scaffold is left in place to allow in-growth of host fibroblasts and capillaries to eventually incorporate as its own. Much of this scaffold matrix consists of intact collagen fibers and bundles to support tissue in-growth, proteins, intact elastin, hyaluronic acid, fibronectin, fibrillar collagen, collagen VI, vascular channels and proteoglycan – all of which allow the body to mount its own tissue regeneration process.[14,15,22,23]

All ADMs are FDA cleared for homologous use only. Although features and processing may vary between ADMs, the success of the product will ultimately depend on its ability to meet the desired characteristics of a model ADM for revisionary breast surgery. A list of ADMs that are available on the market for a variety of applications are included in *Table 4.1*.

Published literature

AlloDerm is clearly in the forefront regarding published literature concerning ADMs for immediate breast reconstruction. A PubMed search using specific brand names and breast reconstruction reveals the majority of the publications involving AlloDerm. Ten of these papers relate directly to adjunctive ADM treatment of immediate breast reconstruction using AlloDerm,[14,15,22,23,27,37–39] Dermamatrix,[40] and Neoform.[41] All of these papers are recent publications, the oldest dating from 2005.[14] All are noncontrolled, retrospective case series. PubMed searches were also performed matching each name of all other human and xenograft ADMs – FlexHD, Allomax, Surgimend, Enduragen, Synovis, Permacol, and Strattice – with *breast reconstruction* and revealed no listings. It is likely that studies are underway and not yet completed.

As new products are introduced to the market place, it is always crucial to understand the science behind each technology. The device industry should be evaluated as critically as the pharmaceutical industry, questioning the science and understanding the mechanism of action.

When evaluating ADMs critically, it is important that we understand the differences on how the body responds to the different materials. Not all soft tissue materials elicit the same biological response. There are three unique processes that can take place with any tissue material that is placed into the body, whether it's a biologic or synthetic material. All products placed into a body elicit an inflammatory response with involvement of multiple cytoprotective and cytotoxic cytokines. The continuum of this reaction is controlled by the intrinsic mechanism unique to each scaffold.

Regeneration

With this process, the product is accepted by the body where the intact tissue matrix integrates and becomes part of the host through rapid revascularization and cellular repopulation. This is the process that is most beneficial and important to obtain good outcomes in breast surgery and perhaps the reason why we see less peri-prosthetic capsular contracture.

Resorption

This is the process where the human body attacks the replaced tissue and breaks it down by completely eliminating it, while depositing scar in its place. This is commonly seen with absorbable mesh products.

Table 4.1 Comparison of different commercially available acellular dermal matrices

Product name	Manufacturer	Origin	Method of preservation	Year introduced	Time to hydrate	Shelf-life	Refrigeration required
AlloDerm	LifeCell	Human dermis	Lyophilized; patented freeze-drying process prevents damaging ice crystals from forming	1994	10–40 min, depending on thickness, with warmed saline solution in two-step bath with light agitation	2 years	No
DermaMatrix	Processed by Musculoskeletal Transplant Foundation (MTF) for Synthes CMF	Human dermis	Aseptic processing method; lyophilized	2005	3 min	3 years	No
FlexHD	Processed by Musculoskeletal Transplant Foundation (MTF) for Ethicon	Human dermis	Aseptic processing method; packaged in an ethanol solution	2007	None	18 months	No
SurgiMend	TEI Biosciences	Fetal bovine dermal collagen	Terminally sterilized with ethylene oxide	2007	60 s with room temperature saline	3 years	No
Strattice	LifeCell	Porcine dermal collagen	Terminally sterilized via low dose e-beam; retains critical biochemical components; significantly reduces the key component believed to play a major role in the xenogeneic rejection response	2008	Minimum of 2 min in sterile saline	2 years	No
Veritas	Synovis Surgical Innovations	Bovine pericardium collagen	Terminally sterilized; sodium hydroxide treatment for purification and microbiological security	2008	None	2 years	No
Surgisis	Cook Biotech	Porcine Small Intestinal Submucosa	Sterilized with ethylene oxide	2004	3–10 min	1 year	No
AlloMax	Manufactured by Regeneration Technologies/ Tutogen Medical, Inc. for Bard Davol	Human dermis	Terminally sterilized	2007	Hydrates rapidly	5 years	No
MatriStem	Acell/Medline	Porcine bladder	Unavailable	2009	None	2 years	No

Encapsulation

During this process, the product is encapsulated through an inflammatory response which is unable to break down the product due to its synthetic nature. Therefore the product is encapsulated and walled off from the host. This process is not unique to synthetic products, but applies to any foreign body (e.g., pacemaker, implants) that is placed into the host.

The goal of regenerating tissue is to recapitulate in adult wounded tissue the intrinsic regenerative processes that are involved in normal adult tissue maintenance.[42] Scar does not have the native structure, function, and physiology of the original normal tissue. When a wound exceeds a critical deficit, it requires a scaffold to organize tissue replacement. Depending on the type of scaffold that is in place, different processes as described earlier will respond. At this point, the intrinsic factors of the ADM will be important to aid in each specific regenerative or reparative process. While regenerative healing is characterized by the restoration of the structure, function, and physiology of damaged or absent tissue, reparative healing is characterized by wound closure through scar formation.[42] All biologic scaffolds are not the same because of differences in the methods used to process them – materials that encapsulate and scar do not offer the benefits of regenerative healing but lead to suboptimal results.

Diagnosis and patient presentation

Acellular dermal matrix is utilized as an adjunct to the sound surgical principles necessary to diagnose and treat the underlying cause(s) necessitating revisionary aesthetic breast surgery. Clinical data shows the four main indications (drivers) for revisionary surgery are capsular contracture, implant malposition, ptosis, and implant visibility or palpability.[24–26] Each patient must be individually evaluated regarding concerns, goals, knowledge of previous surgical and implant specifics, and careful evaluation of her breasts – dimensions, quality/quantity of overlying soft tissue, and scarring (critical in planning surgery and maintaining necessary vascularity to manipulated tissues).

Despite the apparent complexity of a given clinical presentation, there are five underlying basic components which may be the cause, or contribute to the cause, of the problem: the skin, soft tissue, capsule, implant and chest wall. These underlying components must be carefully and systematically analyzed from *outside in*, or *inside out*, until all layers involved are evaluated.

Patient selection

The main drivers for reoperative surgery mentioned above should always be kept in mind as these five components are evaluated. We have learned from our revisionary and reconstructive breast experience that one or more of these components and layers may need to be addressed, in addition to the use of ADM. Such surgical manipulations may include skin envelope reduction, fat injection, lamellar separation, capsulectomy, capsulotomy, and site change of the replacement implant. In order to help plan for the surgery some general principles can be followed.

For patients whose original implants were subglandular, a pocket change to a subpectoral plane and lower pole coverage with acellular dermal matrix is generally performed. For those patients whose original implants were subpectoral, a neopectoral pocket with the addition of acellular dermal matrix is generally performed. Patients who did have adequate breast tissue, a subfascial pocket may be utilized with ADM coverage or support as indicated. As always, appropriate candidate selection is important for achieving a successful outcome, and high risk patients (e.g., smoker and those with BMI >35) should be discouraged from having elective surgery. The core principles for aesthetic breast revisions are summarized in *Table 4.2*.

Treatment and surgical technique

The use of ADM can be categorized into four distinct indications based upon the underlying clinical presentation: (1) Coverage of implant lower pole (usually for revision mastopexy); (2) implant stabilizer (usually for malposition correction); (3) tissue thickener (usually superomedially or inferiorly), and (4) treatment of capsular contracture (which may be technically similar to lower pole cover or superomedial thickening.) *(Fig. 4.1)*.

Video 1

Table 4.2 **The process of aesthetic breast revision core principles**

Patient–physician education: Patient evaluation	Preoperative planning
1. Listen to the patient	1. Dimensional and tissue evaluation (asymmetry)
2. Obtain accurate history	2. Implant evaluation
3. Interactive assessment	3. Periprosthetic pocket evaluation
4. Define *problem*(s)	4. Define *operative strategy*
5. Craft *solution*(s)	5. Implant selection
6. Educate/expectations	6. Pocket selection
Surgical technique	7. Soft tissue management
1. Access: incision location/length	8. Adjunctive techniques
2. Implant removal/evaluation	**Postoperative management**
3. Pocket alteration (location/size/capsule/technique)	1. Comprehensive patient experience
4. Implant selection (intraoperative information) (Sizers(?), upright evaluation)	2. Commitment to surgical excellence
5. Implant handling/irrigation/positioning	3. Short-term postoperative care (movement, drains, dressings, sutures)
6. Soft tissue alterations (tailor tac)	4. Long-term postoperative care
7. Additional maneuvers (ADM, fat injection)	5. Management of revisions
8. Placement of drains	

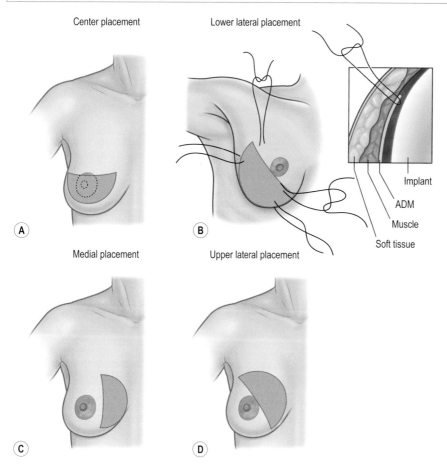

Fig. 4.1 Placement of ADM at various anatomical locations during revisionary surgery.

Hints and tips

- A careful history is imperative in understanding how a problem came to exist. This includes all previous operations, what was done, and what implants were used. Previous operative notes and documentation of detail specifics of existing implants are highly desirable. A careful analysis of the patient's existing "form", asymmetries, dimensional measurements, and tissue characterization is mandatory, in addition to documentation of current implant type, volume, location, and "status". Any previous or current pathological concerns should be known, as well as any diagnostic imaging of the breasts or implants, in addition to the patient's overall health, surgeries, and medications.
- Site change to *dual plane* if original implant in subglandular pocket.
- Site change to *neopectoral pocket* if original implant in subpectoral pocket.
- ADM should be handled in the same manner as the silicone implant. The surgeon should only be handling the implantable materials, and both the prosthetic device and ADM are bathed in a solution consisting of 50 000 U of bacitracin, 1 g of cephazolin, 80 mg of gentamicin, in 500 mL of normal saline.
- ADM contour shapes, with a geometric contour to engage the geometry of the implant surface, are exclusively selected for the lower pole indications (capsular contracture and ptosis correction).
- Extra thick ADMs, which are hand shaped intraoperatively for its geometry to conform to that of the superomedial implant geometric contour for superior "tissue thickener" are selected.
- Key decisions regarding implant (type, volume, dimensions, filler, shape, and surface) are made, as well as treatment of existing capsule, overlying parenchyma, soft tissue, and skin envelope (mastopexy). We have a preference for the creation of "site-changed" pockets, silicone gel implants (generally having a "Biocell texture"), ADMs selected by their biomechanical properties, "design", indications for use, documented outcomes, as well as considerations of cost.

Coverage of the lower pole

This important concept and technique, which is our most frequently utilized ADM placement, is employed when performing soft tissue and skin envelope alterations in redo surgery (revision mastopexy with augmentation). As many patients with previously placed implants develop laxity, sag, or tissue thinning over time, mastopexy or revision mastopexy over the

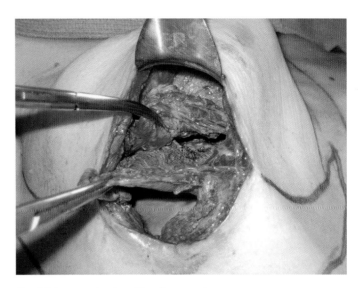

Fig. 4.2 Intraoperative view of lamellar separation.

replacement implant is required to achieve the aesthetic breast form. If the existing implant is subglandular, a subpectoral (subpectoral-fascial) pocket is created (after capsule treatment), the new implant inserted in the newly created subpectoral pocket, and the lower portion of the implant covered with ADM. This allows a "circumvertical" or "inverted T" mastopexy to be safely performed without underlying muscle, as the ADM separates the skin closure from the implant. If the existing implant is already subpectoral, a neopectoral site change is carried out, and the ADM utilized similarly. If there has been a previous implant in both the subglandular and subpectoral pockets, "lamellar" separation (dissecting the pectoralis muscle from its superficial and deep scarred attachments) may be necessary *(Fig. 4.2)*. ADM is considered to be the outer layer of the underlying implant (to which it is intimately engaged by proximity of placement), and may also require suture stabilization. Thus the ADM may be tacked to the inferior border of the pectoralis major above and to Scarpa's fascia or deep fascia below (at the level of the IMF). Parachute pull-out sutures may alternatively be used to redrape the ADM. When there is lamellar scarring requiring lamellar separation, the remaining pectoralis muscle may be "window shaded" up in the pocket, requiring lower muscle inferior pull following its release. This lower pole coverage situation is best achieved by suturing of the ADM along the entire length of the lower pectoral border, draping it over the implant inferiorly,

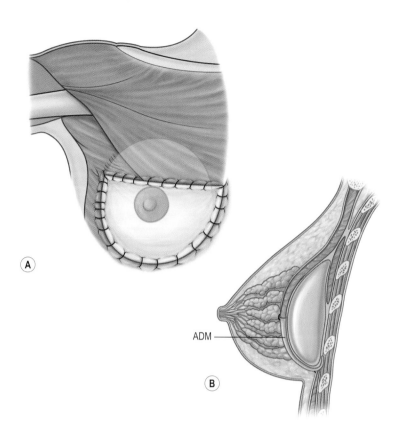

ADM

Fig. 4.3 Interposition of regenerative matrix between implant and skin closure. This is similar to the "reconstructive model".

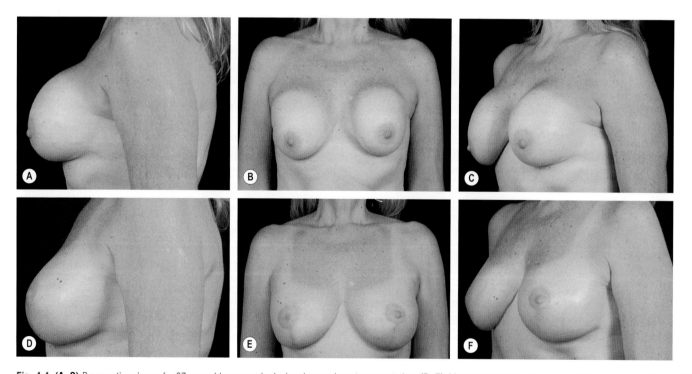

Fig. 4.4 (A–C) Preoperative views of a 37-year-old woman who had undergone breast augmentation; **(D–F)** 32 months after revision augmentation mastopexy (inverted-T), which included the development of neopectoral pocket, lower pole coverage with ADM and replacement of implants with form stable, highly cohesive gel anatomic implants.

and securing it (under more taughtness) at or near the IMF. This application is similar to the "reconstructive model', as a "pectoral muscle extension" *(Fig. 4.3)*. In all instances, an adequate environment, cover and stability over the non muscle covered portion of the implant (lower pole) by the ADM, allows the skin envelope to be safely lifted and tightened (Mastopexy), assuming adequate respect for the vascularity of the redraped tissue, as well as compliance with all sound surgical principles *(Figs 4.4–4.6)*.

Regarding the desired biomechanical properties of the desired ADM, rapid revascularization is required for conformability of the ADM to redrape over the surface of the implant (intimate engagement of surface contours). If the patient had capsular contracture, then a more compliant material may be desired. If the patient had more laxity or stretch deformity, a more taught material might be preferable.

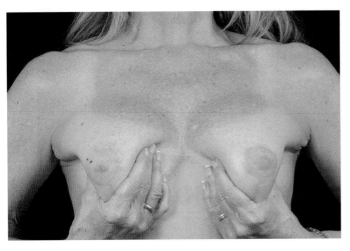

Fig. 4.5 Same patient as seen in *Fig. 4.4*, demonstrating the softness of implants 32 months following the treatment of her capsular contracture and ptosis.

Implant stabilizer

ADM allows the surgeon enhanced control in maintaining implant position in a newly created "neo" pocket or for re-enforcement after capsulorrhaphy in various forms of implant malposition correction. Inferior malposition (double bubble), medial malposition (symmastia), or lateral malposition are generally treated by capsulorrhaphy or site change (the author's preference and recommendation). In a certain percentage of patients, the tissue is strong enough to support this correction with a new pocket and appropriate suturing alone. A number of these patients, however, will have thin tissue, previous scar, or problematic bony contour slopes, such that re-enforcement of the site change (i.e.,

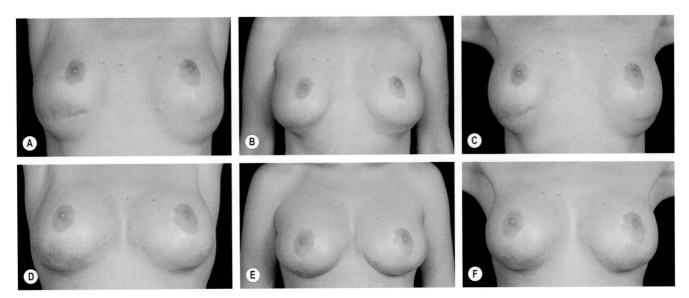

Fig. 4.6 (A–C) Preoperative views of a 49-year-old woman who had undergone augmentation mastopexy; **(D–F)** 30 months after revision augmentation mastopexy (inverted-T), which included the development of neopectoral pocket, lower pole coverage and reinforcement of inferior and lateral walls with ADM and replacement of implants form stable, highly cohesive gel anatomic implants. Successful correction of inferior and lateral malposition was achieved.

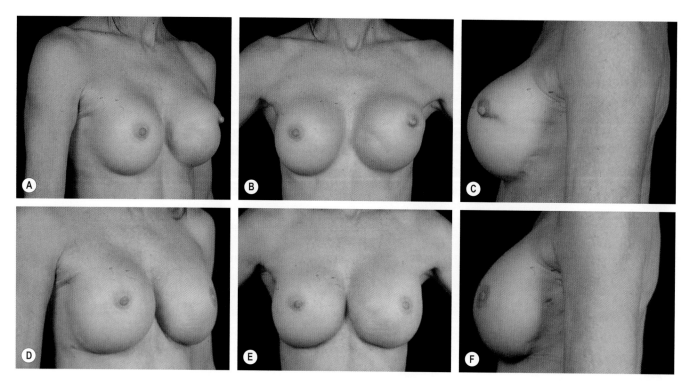

Fig. 4.7 (A–C) Preoperative views of a 38-year-old woman who had undergone multiple previous revision augmentations. **(D–F)** 26 months after revision augmentation through IMF incision, which included the development of neopectoral pocket, lamellar separation, lower pole coverage with ADM and replacement of implants with textured gel implants.

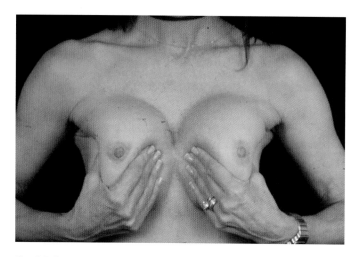

Fig. 4.8 Same patient as seen in **Fig. 4.7**, demonstrating the softness of implants 26 months following the treatment of her implant malposition, lamellar scarring and tissue thinning.

neopectoral pocket of appropriate dimensions in the correct location with old pocket obliteration) with ADM is highly advised to re-enforce or buttress the corrected implant position (*Figs 4.7, 4.8*). These materials are sutured in appropriate position with proper purchase to achieve support. The biomechanical properties of the ADM for this indication are strength and taughtness to maintain implant stabilization.

Tissue thickener

This concept is an extension of second stage breast reconstruction, where expander to implant conversion is facilitated by a superomedial placement of an extra-thick ADM, to enhance soft tissue cover of the implant and give a better visual and palpable confluence of chest to breast form.[43] In aesthetic revisions this is also most frequently applied to upper pole (or superomedial area) to thicken tissue, minimize visibility of traction rippling, camouflage implant edges, and enhance cleavage. An extra thick allograft material is generally utilized and appropriately trimmed. It is draped over the implant (intimate engagement on its deep surface) and in contact with existing capsule or new/neo pocket on its superficial surface. Parachute 2-0 Prolene sutures with Keith needles are utilized in the ADM corners, and interspersed on the medial side to facilitate placement and

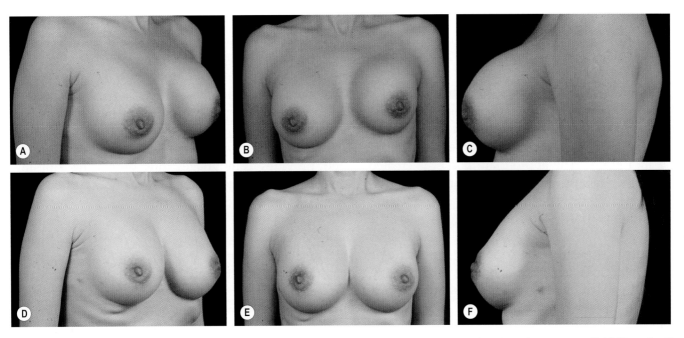

Fig. 4.9 (A–C) Preoperative views of a 45-year-old woman who had undergone multiple previous attempts at correction of capsular contracture; **(D–F)** 22 months after revision augmentation through IMF incision, which included the development of neopectoral pocket, lower pole coverage with ADM and replacement of implants with higher-profile, lower-volume textured gel implants.

redraping. The suture ends are tied to themselves externally, under no tension, and covered with a Tegaderm for 7–10 days. This same application is occasionally used laterally or inferolaterally for implant visibility or palpability, and inferiorly to "thicken" a very thin cutaneous cover *(Figs 4.7, 4.8)*. The key to success is proper pocket alteration with incorporation of the extra thick ADM providing bulk and ultimately revascularization and cellular repopulation.

Treatment of capsular contracture

Even though the presenting problem may be capsular contracture, additional deformities may be identified following detailed analysis from skin envelope to chest wall as noted above. This can include thinned tissue over an encapsulated implant, malposition of the encapsulated implant, or stretched deformity, snoopy, or ptosis over an encapsulated implant. If the encapsulation is in the subglandular position a total capsulectomy with site change to the subpectoral position is usually performed. If the encapsulation is in the subpectoral position, a neopectoral pocket with partial anterior capsule excision and residual capsule obliteration, or total (perhaps partial) capsulectomy is performed In

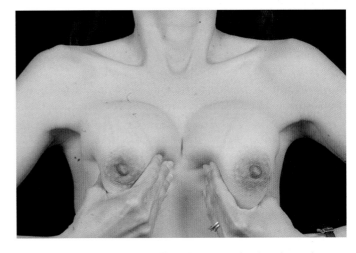

Fig. 4.10 Same patient as seen in *Fig. 4.9*, demonstrating the softness of implants 22 months following the treatment of her capsular contracture.

these cases the ADM is again selected for rapid revascularization, conformability to the implant, and performance. The technique is most frequently similar to the "lower pole cover" concept, but may be closer to a "medial thickener" or "malposition reinforce," depending upon the presenting problem *(Figs 4.9, 4.10)*. There is an increasing body of documentation that the coupling of the ADM to the implant will further reduce the incidence of capsular contracture.[12,24] If capsular contracture is the only clinical diagnosis, then we recommend placement of the ADM at the lower or middle poles.

The surgical techniques used are based on the preoperative findings and the indications as described above. The ADM should be conformed to, and in intimate contact with, the outer surface of the implant (like a hand in a glove). The appropriate pocket is created whether it's a neopectoral, subpectoral, or subfascial.[8,11] Three to five half-mattress stabilizing parachute sutures are placed between the skin and ADM to stabilize the tissue and place it in the desired location. Sizes selected are normally in the 6–8×10–16 cm range (depending on size of implant), rectangle or "contour" shapes, and trimmed as needed. Seroma formation should be prevented in all breast revisions to improve revascularization and cellular repopulation of the ADM, so drains are always recommended.

Outcomes, prognosis and complications

Breast augmentation is the most common aesthetic procedure performed in the United States and perhaps in the world.[44] As plastic surgeons, we strive to achieve perfection and continue to improve our surgical techniques to achieve the aesthetic breast form. Despite advances in implant technology and surgical techniques, undesired outcomes are encountered leading to revisionary surgeries. In preparing for a revisionary breast augmentation, one must understand patients' goals and expectations and evaluate the probability of their accomplishment, as well as the risk/benefit ratio. When the decision is made to move forward, the goal should be to plan and execute the most precise and efficient surgical correction as is possible. To achieve this goal, one must understand the problem(s) and variables involved, and then look for new solutions.

In the past, our options were limited to working with only native tissues that were available for these procedures. With the advent of ADM, the indications and the spectrum of correcting secondary deformities has improved.

Use of acellular dermal products has been popularized in both breast and abdominal wall reconstructions.[13–23] In reconstruction cases, ADMs have been used to replace tissue, extend existing tissue or act as a supplement. In aesthetic revisions, the ADM essentially becomes an outer conforming, regenerative layer around the implant. ADMs have been used to correct implant rippling and displacement, ptosis, and capsular contracture.[25,26,36] ADMs are used as an alternative to other autologous tissue methods of coverage and provides camouflage, thus decreasing rippling, and increasing soft tissue padding.[27] In addition to all the indications described previously, we have also used ADMs as a mode of treatment for capsular contracture.[24] Breast capsular contracture is similar to lamellar scarring in the eyelids. At the cellular level, capsular contracture is most likely caused by any process that produces increased inflammation, which in turn leads to the formation of deleterious cytokines within the periprosthetic pocket. Consequently, in addition to the many techniques described for treating and preventing capsular contracture,[4,5,8,29–35] we believe that the addition of acellular dermal matrix is another modality in fighting the evolution of the capsule. An ADM can counteract the inflammatory process, adding more tissue in-growth availability and controlling the interface of the pocket by providing a regenerative layer between device and native tissue.

The rising demand for the use of ADM, coupled with good outcomes in breast reconstructions, has spurred tremendous interest in its use for aesthetic breast surgery patients. In the past, revisionary surgeries were generally performed with a total capsulectomy, removal of the implant from the subglandular plane, and placement of a new implant in the subpectoral position.[5,8,10] This is a fairly simple procedure, involving a change in implant placement from over the muscle to under the muscle. More recently, it has become necessary to perform revisionary surgery on volume-depleted or severely scarred breasts. In correcting these deformities, as described above, in addition to the site change operation, ADMs can provide additional coverage where the repair is performed.

The recently published series of 78 consecutive patients who underwent revisionary breast augmentation/mastopexies with acellular dermal matrices was one of the largest series to date to address the use of ADM in revisionary aesthetic breast surgery.[12] Of the 78 patients, 56 had their original implants in the

Table 4.3 Complications

Complication	Patients (n)
Hematoma	1
Seroma	0
Implant malposition	1
Implant rupture	0
Infection	0
Total	2

Table 4.4 Presenting clinical signs

Clinical signs	Patients (n)
Capsular contracture	56
Implant exposure	2
Rippling	7
Implant malposition	5
Bottoming out	4
Symmastia	4
Total	78

Table 4.5 Augmentation versus augmentation mastopexy

	Patients (n)
Augmentation	49
Augmentation/mastopexy	29
Total	78

Table 4.6 Preoperative and postoperative Baker classification in all patients

	Patients (%)	
	Preoperative	Postoperative
Baker I	6.4	97.4
Baker II	20.5	2.6
Baker III	64.1	0
Baker IV	9.0	0

subpectoral position, and 22 had them in the subglandular position. Complications included two patients (2.5%) requiring reoperation, one for a hematoma and the other for an implant malposition *(Table 4.3)*.

Presenting clinical signs are listed in *Table 4.4* and the type of operation performed is listed in *Table 4.5*. As expected, the majority of complaints were due to "implant hardening."

Of 78 patients, 76 (97.4%) were assessed as having soft implants with a Baker I level of capsular contracture at final follow-up; two patients (2.6%) had a Baker II contracture. No patient had a Baker III or Baker IV classification postoperatively *(Table 4.6)*.

Currently, we have performed over 150 revisionary augmentations with ADM. As the results continue to be satisfactory both to surgeon and patient, we continue to explore new concepts and techniques to improve outcomes, minimize risks while enhancing patient safety, improve efficiency, and lower costs. We are now seeing product differentiation in outcome assessment. Thus, we are carefully documenting these findings to report in peer reviewed literature.

A challenge we continue to face in aesthetic revisionary surgery is the cost of these products and their affordability by the patient. On the other hand, the biggest possible cost of performing a revisionary surgical procedure (to patient and surgeon alike), is the need to perform another surgical revision due to failure of the planned procedure. Therefore as we continue to report our outcome data using ADMs in revisionary aesthetic breast surgery, and compare it with the outcomes without use of ADMs, a new picture may emerge. Undoubtedly, the coming years will be exciting as we further define the issues, advance the science, and improve our understanding via evidence-based medicine for the benefit of our patient population.

 Access the complete references list online at **http://www.expertconsult.com**

2. Spear SL, Murphy DK, Slicton A, et al. Inamed silicone breast implant core study results at 6 years. *Plast Reconstr Surg.* 2007;120(7 Suppl 1):8S–18S.

The authors update on the post-approval study for the Allergan Corporation. The study demonstrates the safety and effectiveness of Natrelle (formerly Inamed) silicone-filled breast implants through 6 years, including a low rupture rate and high satisfaction rate.

3. Cunningham B, McCue J. Safety and effectiveness of Mentor's MemoryGel implants at 6 years. *Aesthet Plast Surg.* 2009;33(3):440–444.

   The authors update on the post-approval study for the Mentor Corporation. The study shows that Mentor MemoryGel silicone breast implants represent a safe and effective choice for women seeking breast augmentation or breast reconstruction following mastectomy.

4. Adams WP Jr, Rios JL, Smith SJ. Enhancing patient outcomes in aesthetic and reconstructive breast surgery using triple antibiotic breast irrigation: six-year prospective clinical study. *Plast Reconstr Surg.* 2006;117(1):30–36.

   The authors show the clinical importance of the use of triple antibiotic breast irrigation. This study shows the lower incidence of capsular contracture compared with other published reports, and its clinical efficacy supports previously published in vitro studies. Application of triple antibiotic irrigation is recommended for all aesthetic and reconstructive breast procedures and is cost-effective.

8. Maxwell GP, Gabriel A. The neopectoral pocket in revisionary breast surgery. *Aesthet Surg J.* 2008;28(4):463–467.

12. Maxwell GP, Gabriel A. Use of the acellular dermal matrix in revisionary aesthetic breast surgery. *Aesthet Surg J.* 2009;29(6):485–493.

    The authors show the largest ADM-based revisionary surgeries, including both revisionary augmentation and revision of augmentation mastopexy. This series shows that the ADM can be used both safely and effectively in revisionary cases, resulting in decreased rates of capsular contracture and implant cushioning/stabilization.

13. Bindingnavele V, Gaon M, Ota KS, et al. Use of acellular cadaveric dermis and tissue expansion in postmastectomy breast reconstruction. *J Plast Reconstr Aesthet Surg.* 2007;60(11):1214–1218.

22. Salzberg CA. Nonexpansive immediate breast reconstruction using human acellular tissue matrix graft (AlloDerm). *Ann Plast Surg.* 2006;57(1):1–5.

23. Spear SL, Parikh PM, Reisin E, et al. Acellular dermis-assisted breast reconstruction. *Aesthetic Plast Surg.* 2008;32(3):418–425.

25. Duncan DI. Correction of implant rippling using allograft dermis. *Aesthet Surg J.* 2001;21(1):81–84.

42. Harper JR, McQuillan DJ. A novel regenerative tissue matrix (RTM) technology for connective tissue reconstruction. *Wounds.* 2007;2007(6):20–24.

5

Endoscopic approaches to the breast

Neil A. Fine and Clark F. Schierle

SYNOPSIS

- Applications for surgical endoscopes have been developed in both cosmetic and reconstructive breast surgery.
- As in other surgical applications, surgical endoscopes allow for the use of distant, more cosmetically acceptable incisions in performing cosmetic and reconstructive breast surgery.
- Use of surgical endoscopes in cosmetic breast surgery allow for dissection of an implant pocket from a remote incision, typically located in the axilla.
- In reconstructive breast surgery, the endoscope allows for a skin sparing technique in the harvest of the latissimus dorsi muscle for partial breast reconstruction.
- Techniques and approaches utilizing surgical endoscopy to optimize visualization while minimizing scarring continue to evolve.

 Access the Historical Perspective section online at
http://www.expertconsult.com

Introduction

Endoscopic approaches to conventional surgical problems have significantly enhanced treatment options since their introduction in the latter half of the 20th century (Berger 1996; Paige 1997).[6,15] Less traumatic tissue dissection in conjunction with smaller surgical incisions have enabled many patients to benefit from reduced postoperative pain, expedited recovery, and improved cosmesis (Cho 1997).[8] The surgical endoscope has been used by the senior author to perform over 200 endoscopic augmentation mammaplasties and over 50 endoscopic lumpectomy reconstructions. Unlike intra-abdominal or thoracic applications, plastic surgery frequently involves extensive soft tissue and neurovascular dissection within enclosed potential spaces. Limited surgical apertures and confined optical cavities have therefore inhibited the development and widespread usage of minimally invasive plastic surgical techniques. Widespread availability of endoscopic equipment and refinements in technique have improved the relevance and utilization of endoscopic approaches in a wide variety of plastic surgical applications in recent years. As endoscopic approaches to the breast and other areas of plastic surgery have gained acceptance, it is important to have a fundamental understanding of the basic concepts of surgical endoscopy. These include the principle of the optical cavity, support systems, illumination equipment, imaging technology, incision planning, and some basic technical considerations.

The optical cavity

The development and maintenance of an optical cavity is the primary technical challenge of endoscopic surgery. Optical cavities may be formed from preexisting, potential, or dissected spaces and can vary greatly with bony and soft tissue anatomy. Optical cavities are characterized by space, support, medium, and pressure. Space refers to the anatomic space which they occupy and may be existing, potential, or dissected. Support may be provided by existing bony or soft tissue anatomy, mechanical retraction, or through the infiltration of an optical medium. The optical medium refers to the gaseous or liquid contents of the cavity which allow for transmission of visible light. The pressure within the cavity can be modulated in closed endoscopic systems depending on the anatomic constraints of the space in which the surgeon is working. In plastic surgical approaches to the breast, be they cosmetic or reconstructive, the optical cavity is a mechanically maintained, dissected space with room air providing the optical transmission medium.

Support systems

Due to the fact that the optical cavity in both endoscopic flap harvest for breast reconstruction and endoscopic augmentation mammaplasty are continuous with the ambient air of the operating room, support cannot be provided by an optical fluid medium under pressure. Further, since the planes are ones which are dissected rather than preexisting, there is no inherent anatomic support for maintenance of the optical cavity. Therefore, the only option for creation and maintenance of the optical cavity is mechanical retraction. Internal mechanical retractors apply a centrifugally directed force on the roof of the optical cavity. This provides the lift necessary to deepen the space for optimal visualization and manipulation of the surgical field. The force applied must be sufficient to counteract the elastic and gravitational forces acting to collapse the optical cavity. Mechanical retraction for cosmetic and reconstructive breast surgery can be free or coaxial with the camera. A single, well designed coaxial retractor allows a single surgeon to control both the visual field and optical cavity with relative ease. If necessary, an assistant may use a free retractor to briefly enhance the optical cavity during a particularly challenging or distant portion of the operation.

Illumination and imaging

Several technological advances in illumination and imaging technology have proven instrumental in the development of surgical endoscopy. Glass fiber optic cables allow for the use of distant light sources bright enough to provide full spectrum illumination of the surgical field.

Fine and colleagues were the first to report a clinical experience with endoscopic latissimus dorsi flaps in 1994.[20] This harvesting technique utilized smaller incisions and was performed with the use of modified laparoscopic cholecystectomy instruments. Since this publication, the limiting factor for improving endoscopic harvest has been creation of an adequate optical cavity. Innovative ideas to optimize visualization within soft tissue planes have gradually emerged. Several authors have described external retraction with sutures, balloon dilation, CO_2 insufflation, and the use of additional ports. We have further refined our technique, namely the endoscopic assisted reconstruction with latissimus dorsi (EARLi) flap. This procedure, first performed by the senior author in 1998, for reconstruction after breast conserving therapy, only requires an axillary incision and is therefore cosmetically appealing. Seminal studies in the late 1990s, documenting the equivalence of BC with mastectomy for the treatment of small breast cancers resulted in many women requesting BCT. Unfortunately, adequate carcinoma excisions, especially excisions for relatively large T2 or T3 breast cancers, may lead to poor cosmetic results. The severity of the aesthetic defect is a direct relation between the size of the tumor resection with adequate margins, and the size of the affected breast. A recent report has shown that BCT combining radiation and immediate myosubcutaneous latissimus dorsi flap reconstruction is an oncologically safe treatment for larger breast cancers. Several authors have described a latissimus mini-flap, a procedure for filling in the breast defect which utilizes an incision running from the apex of the axilla along the lateral border of the breast towards the outer aspect of the inframammary fold. This innovative approach allows both wide local excision in women who would otherwise have required a mastectomy as well as a more cosmetically appealing outcome. At our institution, we perform the EARLi flap, a procedure with even less scarring, to achieve a favorable cosmetic outcome after BCT. The principle goals of the EARLi flap are to replace excised tissue volume and prevent breast deformity following lumpectomy. In addition, breast size and contour are maintained, and scar tissue contracture is minimized. Because of the small incision and limited soft tissue dissection, postoperative pain is reduced and recovery time is diminished.

Endoscopic augmentation mammaplasty

Basic science/disease process

The female breast covers the anterior chest wall from approximately the second rib superiorly to the fourth or fifth rib inferiorly. Its upper one half overlies the pectoralis major muscle, the serratus anterior its lower one half, and some of the axillary fascia laterally. The breast is essentially a skin organ. It is attached intimately to the skin by suspensory ligaments (Cooper ligaments). This is because developmentally it forms from the ectoderm of the anterolateral body wall, and epithelial proliferation from that site creates the gland. For this reason, opening the natural plane between the muscle and the breast is easy; an implant can be inserted into this space. The blood supply of the breast is derived from branches of the axillary artery, the intercostal arteries, and the internal mammary artery. Few if any vessels penetrate into the gland from the underlying central muscle. The nerve supply to the breast comes from the anterior and lateral cutaneous branches of the third, fourth, and fifth thoracic nerves. One of the larger lateral cutaneous branches often can be visualized and preserved during augmentation surgery.

Diagnosis/patient presentation

Micromastia or mammary hypoplasia is chief complaint in patients seeking an enlargement procedure. Significant breast asymmetry, ptosis, or tubular breast deformity are difficult if not impossible to address through the transaxillary approach and, as such, must be comprehensively assessed and ruled out. Absence of any significant abnormality must be ruled out clinically and, when appropriate, mammographically prior to any elective breast surgical procedure.

Patient selection

Indications for endoscopic breast augmentation include the patient's desire for a remote incision and the absence of a well-developed inframammary crease to hide a crease incision from view in the horizontal visual axis. Patients without significant ptosis are ideal candidates. This minimizes the need for excessive manipulation or dissection during creation of the implant pocket from a remote site. A constricted lower pole with a short distance from the inframammary crease to the areola is significantly more difficult and can require radial scoring of the breast parenchyma. The potential exists for inferior implant displacement from over-dissection (lowering) of the inframammary crease and superior implant displacement from under-dissection of the inframammary crease. Tubular breast deformities also present a contraindication to endoscopic transaxillary augmentation mammaplasty. The need for correction of the herniated areola and the scoring of the constricted lower-pole parenchyma makes the periareolar access incision ideal for tubular breast deformity. Some degree of ptosis can also represent a relative or absolute contraindication to the technique. Mild pseudoptosis and Regnault grade 1 ptosis may be addressed during a transaxillary, endoscopically assisted dissection, but this anatomy requires manipulation of the inframammary crease to control the vertical descent of the breast. Due to the need for control and accuracy in this dissection and concerns over the risk of under- or over-dissection, aggressive management of ptosis via this approach is not recommended for the inexperienced surgeon. While it is possible to place an implant into the subglandular plane from the axillary approach to improve moderate ptosis, the very fact that moderate (or greater) ptosis exists means that an inframammary crease incision will be well hidden and a periareolar incision may be hidden by or incorporated into a mastopexy incision, negating a primary benefit of the endoscopic transaxillary approach: a hidden scar in a breast that would show other incisions. Both silicone and saline devices may be introduced through the transaxillary approach, although due to the physical constraints of the transaxillary tunnel, introduction of silicone gel implants >300 cc may be challenging and require special care to avoid damage to the device or surrounding anatomic structures during insertion. This limitation is due to a desire to have a 'hidden' transaxillary scar. For the scar to blend into a high transverse axillary crease it can rarely be longer than 5 cm. As the scar becomes longer in runs the risk of being more visible if a woman's arm is raised. A saline implant

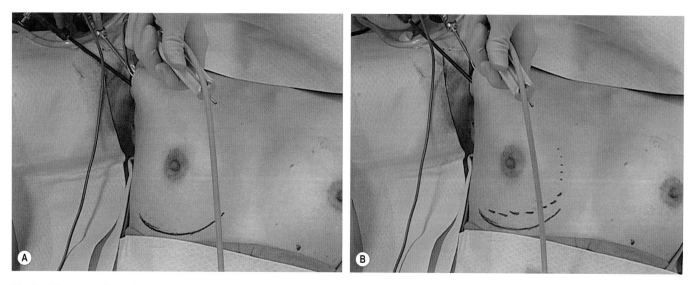

Fig. 5.1 **(A)** Preoperative markings demonstrating planned location of inframammary fold (solid line). **(B)** Preoperative markings demonstrating planned release of pectoralis muscle origin (dotted line).

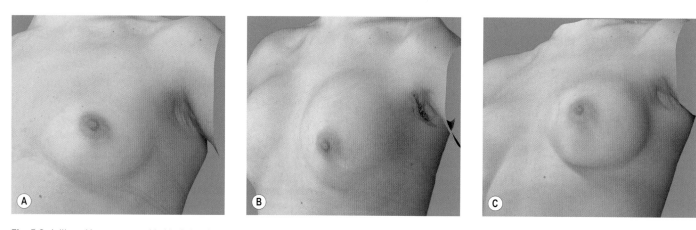

Fig. 5.2 Axillary skin creases provide ideal sites for incision placement. **(A)** Preoperative; **(B)** one week postoperative; and **(C)** three month postoperative appearance of axillary incision site.

of any size can be placed through an incision of 3 cm. Therefore, women who desire a hidden scar and an implant >300 ccs will need to consider the trade-off of a longer, more visible scar with a silicone implant vs a short, hidden scar with a saline device.

Treatment/surgical technique

Video 1

Preoperative considerations include accurate marking of the native and proposed placement of the inframammary crease, as well as anticipated areas of release of the pectoralis major muscle. The pectoralis muscle should be completely divided along its inferior origin from the rectus fascia *(Fig. 5.1)*. This complete myotomy is transitioned gradually to a partial thickness release as the dissection approaches the medial origins along the sternal border until the level of the nipple is reached. Mark the first axillary crease with an incision behind the anterior axillary line. The incision should measure 3 cm if a saline implant is planned, 4.5–5 cm if silicone is to be used. If concealed in a natural skin crease within the hair bearing portion of the axilla, the incision will typically be extremely favorable if not disappear almost completely when fully mature *(Fig. 5.2)*.

Endoscopic transaxillary breast augmentation is easily performed under conscious sedation, although

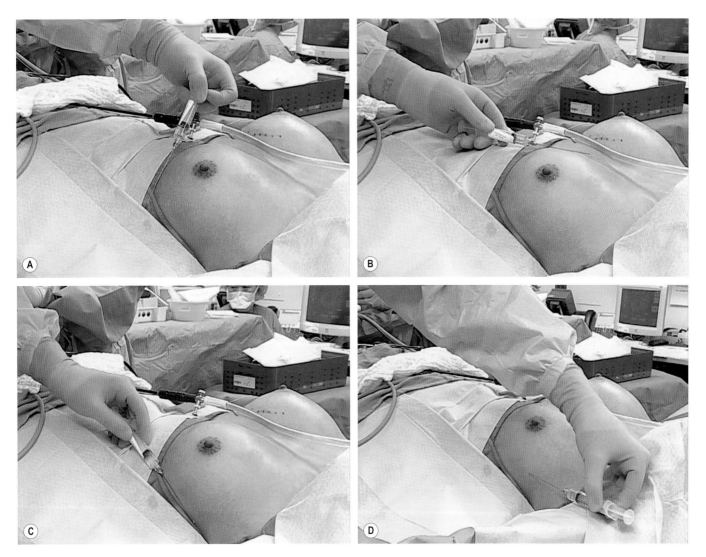

Fig. 5.3 A wetting solution of dilute local anesthetic containing epinephrine is infiltrated along the **(A)** Inferior pectoralis muscle border. **(B)** Medial pectoralis muscle border. **(C)** Lateral chest wall with special attention to the course of the intercostal nerves, and **(D)** Axillary tunnel along the course of the planned dissection with a bolus placed under the pectoralis muscle.

a general anesthetic may be considered based on patient preference, and in cases involving a larger silicone implant requiring more vigorous technique to introduce the implant through the tunnel. Regardless of anesthetic technique, a wetting solution is introduced into the site of the axillary tunnel extending to underneath the pectoralis major muscle as well as along the lateral, inferior, and medial boundaries of dissection *(Fig. 5.3)*. A spinal needle may be utilized to minimize sites of needle puncture. The needle is directed tangentially to the ribcage to prevent penetration of the chest wall. The epinephrine in the wetting solution will limit bleeding, either stopping small bleeding vessels or

slowing larger vessels that may be injured during the dissection. It is important to limit or avoid bleeding due to limitations on visualization that occur more easily within the optical cavity of an endoscopic procedure due to limited ability to simultaneously suction, apply pressure, clamp and visualize a vigorous, actively bleeding vessel. The best solution for dealing with bleeding is to avoid it by using epinephrine in a wetting solution and using careful coagulating cautery to perform the dissection.

Perform the incision in the preoperatively marked axillary crease with a No. 15 blade. Place two skin hooks and perform vertical spreading through the

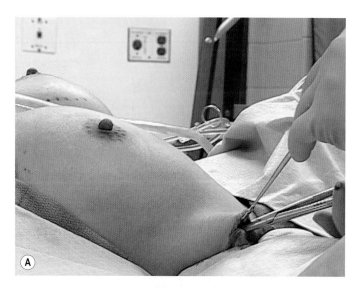

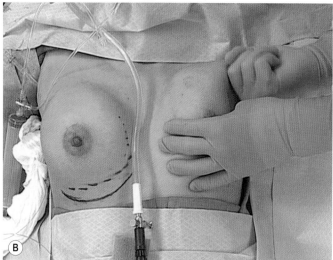

Fig. 5.4 (A) The axillary tunnel is created in a blunt fashion using scissors in a spreading motion. Care is taken to avoid injuring the intercostobrachial nerve or creating multiple tunnels. **(B)** The subpectoral space is entered bluntly with finger dissection.

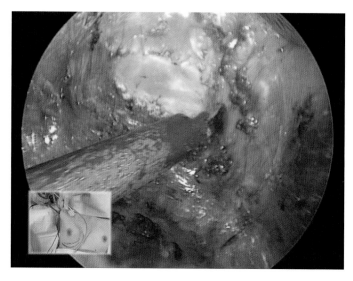

Fig. 5.5 Dissection with electrocautery is used to selectively release the pectoralis muscle origin.

subcutaneous tissues until the pectoral fascia is reached. Dissect in the subcutaneous plane, aiming the tunnel toward the nipple to avoid injury to the intercostal brachial nerve *(Fig. 5.4)*. Take extreme care during this initial tunnel dissection not to create more than one subcutaneous dissection plane, or tunnel. This will greatly facilitate insertion and reinsertion of retractors, instruments, and the implants later. Multiple tunnels, if created, will hinder insertion of all devices as they will tend to catch and trap the device in them and be a source of delay and frustration for the surgeon. Insert the index finger, identify the underside of the pectoralis,

and perforate the fascia bluntly to allow access to the submuscular plane.

An endoscopic retractor is then introduced, followed by the surgical endoscope. After establishing the optical cavity, a monopolar electrocautery dissector is utilized for both dissection and hemostasis. The retractor or dissector may be fitted with a port to allow attachment to low wall suction to assist in evacuation of smoke from the optical cavity during dissection. This suction will also help to keep the lens from fogging. Too much suction however, may collapse the pocket. It is best to be able to turn the suction on and off. An assistant may hold the retractor during dissection; however, the need for this assistance is diminished with experience. Dissection may then proceed in a sequential fashion lateral to medial to completely release the pectoralis major origin inferiorly and partially release the pectoralis major muscle origin inferomedially. Complete release is confirmed by the clear visualization of subcutaneous, yellow fat during the dissection *(Fig. 5.5)*. Partial thinning of the pectoralis muscle origin inferomedially is critical to improve cleavage, but care must be taken to avoid over dissection which can result in visible rippling or symnastia. The operating surgeon should constantly reassess the internal position of the retractor with relation to the breast external anatomy by looking at the scope's transillumination through the skin and by watching the tissues move through

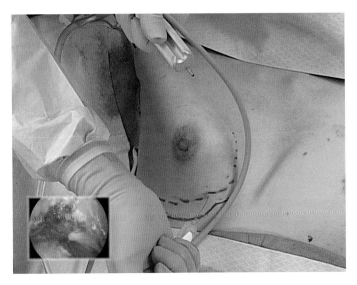

Fig. 5.6 Intraoperative supplementation with wetting solution aids in hemostasis of selected vessels under direct visualization.

the scope during manipulation of the external breast tissues. Transcutaneous supplementation of wetting solution under direct endoscopic vision helps minimize blood loss and improve visualization during dissection *(Fig. 5.6)*.

After meticulous hemostasis is confirmed, the endoscope is removed and the pocket irrigated with antibiotic irrigation. In our practice, a local anesthetic catheter is then introduced for postoperative pain control, taking care to tunnel the path of the catheter subcutaneously with the introducer needle. This prevents leakage of anesthetic fluid and translocation of skin flora into the implant cavity. The implant is then introduced through the axillary tunnel and position confirmed. Saline implants are then inflated with the use of a closed system. If using silicone implants you should open the tunnel wider in order to accommodate the introduction of a silicone implant. If there is trouble inserting, it is usually a problem with the tunnel being too small at some point rather than a problem with the external incision.

At this point, additional blunt dissection may be performed either with the surgeons finger or a large urethral dilator. The patient is flexed to ninety degrees upright to assess final implant positioning and symmetry. The patient is then laid back down and the axillary incision closed. Closure of the tunnel is typically not performed in the case of saline implants. If a silicone implant is used and the tunnel seems overly dissected, sutures may be used to close this space to avoid implant migration. The skin of the axillary incision is closed in standard fashion with absorbable deep dermal sutures followed by a permanent running intradermal monofilament suture.

Postoperative care

A light ACE wrap is applied for support and comfort Walking and daily living activities, including hair combing and teeth brushing, is encouraged immediately. Low impact aerobic activity may be resumed after 2 weeks. More strenuous physical activity, including lifting, is restricted for 4–6 weeks.

Outcomes, prognosis, and complications

Outcomes are shown in *Figure 5.7*. Complication rates for these procedures are comparable with other techniques for breast augmentation. Most implant malpositions are related to superior displacement; however, inferior displacement with bottoming out is more difficult to treat. This occasionally cannot be corrected remotely and requires an inframammary incision. Axillary banding across the axillary incision may be related to hypertrophic scarring, lymphatic channels or thrombophlebitis (Mondor disease). Although meticulous hemostasis is one of the benefits of the endoscopic approach, axillary hematoma has been described, although rarely. Published reports suggest rates of deflation and capsular contracture to be similar to those of any other technique. Reports of malposition are typically due to inadequate release of the pectoralis major muscle origin and relate to transaxillary augmentation that is not assisted with video endoscopy. In our experience, use of the video endoscope allows a precise, complete release, resulting in no significant increase in rates of malposition compared with other approaches. Similarly, we have not found any significant difference in rates of capsular contracture or infectious complications. Minor complications such as implant deflation, mild capsular contracture, or small hematomas may often be dealt with through the existing transaxillary approach with video endoscopic assistance. More significant complications may necessitate conversion to a

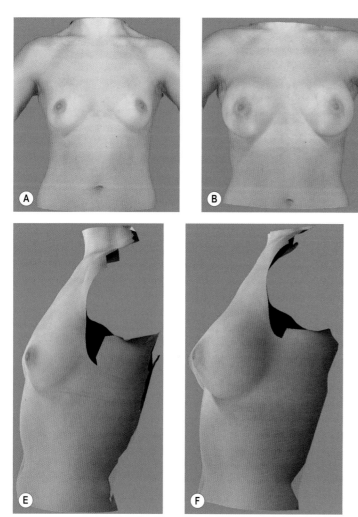

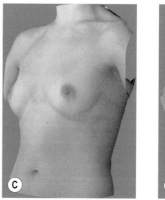

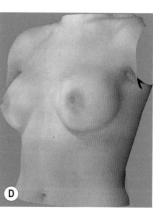

Fig. 5.7 **(A,B)** Anterior, **(C,D)** oblique, and **(E,F)** lateral pre- and postoperative photographs. A 275 cc smooth round saline filled device.

traditional open approach through an inframammary fold incision. Locating this incision in the revision patient is typically more straightforward, as the patient has typically developed a well-defined inframammary fold after the original augmentation (assuming the pectoralis release has been performed adequately).

Endoscopic breast reconstruction

Basic science/disease process

The latissimus dorsi muscle is broad and flat, with an origin arising from the spinous processes of the sacral, lumbar and caudal six thoracic vertebrae and inserting on the lesser tubercle and intertubercular groove of the humerus. It is adherent to the serratus anterior, lower four ribs, and teres major muscle at the level on the scapula. One of two Mathes and Nahai type five muscle flaps, the latissimus dorsi is served by a single dominant pedicle in the form of the thoracodorsal artery and its venae comitantes and several segmental intercostal and lumbar perforators near the posterior midline. Of important clinical significance are the one or multiple branches of the thoracodorsal artery that supply the serratus anterior muscle prior to its entry into the latissimus dorsi muscle. The neural innervation of the latissimus dorsi muscle is supplied by the thoracodorsal nerve which accompanies the path of its co-named artery and vein.

Diagnosis/patient presentation

It is important for the reconstructive breast surgeon to have a good understanding of the relative indications for BCT vs mastectomy. Approximately two-thirds of women with operable locoregional cancer, namely stage I/II breast carcinoma, are afforded the choice between BCT with lumpectomy, axillary lymph node sampling and breast irradiation, or mastectomy with sentinel lymph node biopsy. Both treatment options have been shown to be medically equivalent with regard to overall survival rates. BCT has focused on optimizing cosmetic goals and minimizing the psychological morbidity of a mastectomy, while maintaining low rates of local recurrence. Completeness of tumor excision using wide margins are important in reducing local recurrence, however cosmesis and patient satisfaction after BCT is dependent on the volume excised. Significant volume loss during BCT surgery can be anticipated in patients with large tumor to breast ratios and in women with large tumor burden, therefore breast reshaping or volume replacement should be considered to maintain breast shape in these patients.

Patient selection

The EARLi technique is best suited for women requiring resection of 20–30% of their breast volume. It is optimal for defects in the upper outer quadrant, the site of occurrence for approximately 75% of breast cancers. The EARLi flap is least suited for breast defects in the lower inner quadrant, where less than 6% of breast cancers reside. The procedure has been used in patients with significant breast defects that compromise cosmesis, including those requiring quadrantectomy for large unicentric breast tumors, benign disease, or recurrent infection. The EARLi flap is performed only after lesion excision and confirmation of final pathology reports. Therefore the procedure could be performed as early as 3 days after lumpectomy, but the procedure has been delayed for as long as three weeks to accommodate patient preference for timing of surgery.

The EARLi flap has similar contraindications as other latissimus muscle flaps. Pedicle compromise, division of the thoracodorsal vessels, is a contraindication to the EARLi flap. A previous thoracotomy or axillary incision should raise the concern of an injured or ligated pedicle. Because the latissimus muscle is transferred, muscle function may be compromised. However, muscle weakness is not usually seen except in women active in sports requiring extreme upper body strength such as mountain climbers and competitive swimmers. Defect location in the lower, inner quadrant is also a contraindication. A large cavity in this location cannot be adequately filled with a pedicled latissimus flap.

Treatment/surgical technique

Timing of the EARLi procedure is a critical component to success with this technique. The procedure is best performed in the early postoperative period (1–3 weeks); it is not performed immediately with the lumpectomy. Staging the two procedures in this manner avoids false negative pathology which may require a subsequent mastectomy. While a short interval between lumpectomy and EARLi flap reconstruction is important, it is advantageous to carry out the flap prior to the formation of scar contracture in order to obviate the need for a skin paddle to release contracted skin.

After the induction of general anesthesia, the patient is placed in a lateral decubitus position, with the operative side up *(Fig. 5.8)*. A vacuum molded pad or bean bag is placed beneath the patient in order to maintain position throughout the operation. The arm on the side of the defect is prepped into the operative field so that during the procedure it can be moved to allow optimal visualization. The primary surgeon stands facing the patient's anterior chest, while the assistant stands facing the patient's back. Proper preparation and function

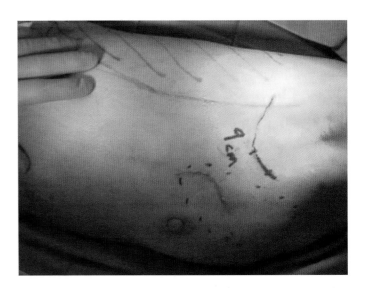

Fig. 5.8 Preoperative markings indicating planned incision (solid line), latissimus muscle (hash marks), and lumpectomy cavity (dotted circle).

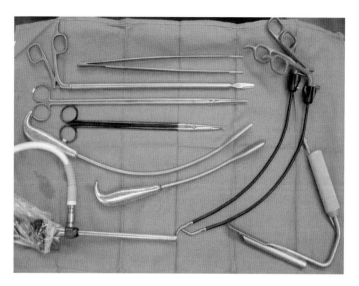

Fig. 5.9 Instrumentation used in endoscopically assisted harvest of the latissimus dorsi muscle.

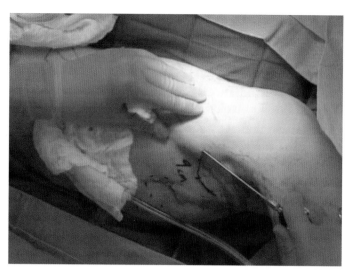

Fig. 5.10 Wetting solution consisting of dilute local anesthetic containing epinephrine is infiltrated in a superficial plane overlying the latissimus dorsi muscle.

of endoscopic camera and dissection equipment is confirmed *(Fig. 5.9)*

Wetting solution is infused into the subcutaneous tissue overlying the latissimus dorsi muscle in order to facilitate local hemostasis and atraumatic tissue plane dissection *(Fig. 5.10)*. It is generally not necessary to attempt infiltration of wetting solution under the latissimus muscle as the effects of the tumescent anesthesia will typically diffuse to affect the entire operative field. The existing lumpectomy incision is then opened and the extent of the soft tissue defect is appreciated. This allows time for the epinephrine in the tumescent fluid to take effect and also allows for estimation of the amount of latissimus needed to fill the defect. The extent of distal latissimus dissection is dependent upon the amount of tissue required to fill the breast defect. Ideally, the quantity of transferred latissimus muscle should be tailored to provide an aesthetically contoured breast mound. The approximate size and configuration of the sheet-like latissimus dorsi muscle is approximated with the use of a laparotomy sponge *(Fig. 5.11)*. The amount of additional sub-Scarpa's fatty tissue incorporated onto the superficial aspect of the latissimus flap is gauged to appropriately augment the reconstruction of a large defect. A curvilinear incision is then made in the axilla along the inferior hair line. The length of the incision is variable and is tailored to accommodate the size of the surgeon's hand. The typical incision length is approximately 9 cm. In patients who have previously undergone transaxillary sentinel lymph node sampling, the incision incorporates the existing scar line. If the lumpectomy incision is high in the upper outer quadrant, it may also be used for the latissimus dissection.

Initial dissection is focused on identification of the thoracodorsal pedicle, which is located along the lateral edge of the latissimus dorsi muscle. Once the thoracodorsal pedicle is unequivocally identified, arterial tributaries supplying the serratus anterior must be clip-ligated and divided. The serratus branch must be ligated to allow full latissimus elevation without risk of avulsion. Because of the high axillary incision, the thoracodorsal pedicle may be mistaken for the serratus branch, so care must be exercised at this point.

The deep surface of the latissimus dorsi muscle is then elevated off the chest wall using a combination of monopolar electrocautery, blunt and sharp dissection *(Fig. 5.12)*. The surgeons hand is inserted to assist with blunt dissection and to ensure proper plane of dissection by palpating the scapula below the plane of dissection. A retractor with an endoscope is then introduced into the operative field and utilized to facilitate mobilization of the latissimus dorsi from its myofascial attachments. Lumbar perforators may be visualized and clipped or cauterized using endoscopic guidance at this point. After completing the deep dissection plane, sharp

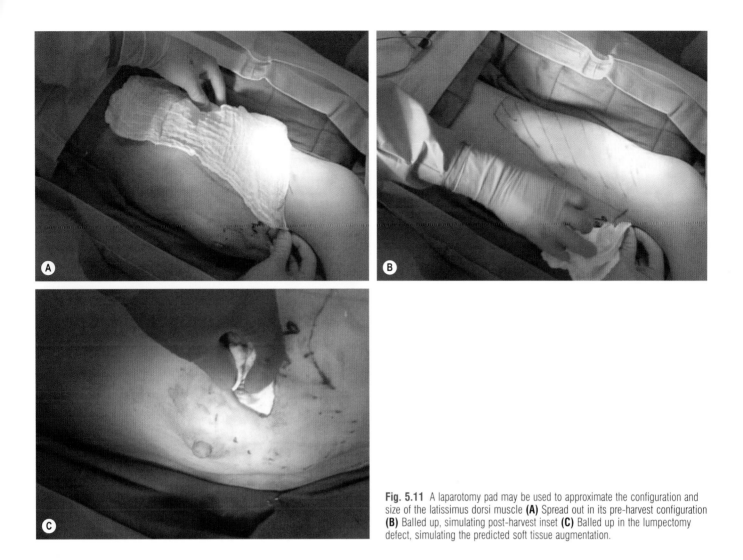

Fig. 5.11 A laparotomy pad may be used to approximate the configuration and size of the latissimus dorsi muscle **(A)** Spread out in its pre-harvest configuration **(B)** Balled up, simulating post-harvest inset **(C)** Balled up in the lumpectomy defect, simulating the predicted soft tissue augmentation.

Fig. 5.12 A blunt dissector which is part of the endoscopic latissimus harvest instrument set is used to assist in dissection of the muscle off of the posterior chest wall and the overlying skin flap. **(A)** View of the dissector instrument outside the operative cavity **(B)** Dissector in use within the operative cavity.

dissection with scissors is used to free the anterior and posterior border of the muscle. Initially, this is done via direct vision, then endoscopic visualization is used, followed by "blind" pushing of the scissors to get maximal length of the muscle. The scissors used are typically long Metzenbaum with some use of the endoscopic 10 mm scissors. The next step is to dissect the superficial surface. Initially, this is done right on the muscle. This tissue will end up in the axilla so extra bulk is not needed. After 5–6 cm on the muscle the plane of dissection transitions to the level of Scarpa's fascia. This adds a layer of fat to the muscle increasing the bulk and allowing larger defects to be adequately filled. The procedure for this dissection is the same as freeing the edges, first direct vision, then some endoscopic work and finally blind or externally visualized dissection with progressively longer Metzenbaum and endoscopic scissors.

At this point in the procedure, the latissimus is left adherent to only its distal origin along the thoracolumbar vertebral column and posterior iliac crest, and its insertion on the humerus. The distal extent of the muscular flap is sharply divided using tactile guidance and endoscopic scissors. The division of the distal muscular origin is the most challenging part of the procedure. The author has tried many methods and has found sharp division with tactile guidance to be the most efficient *(Fig. 5.13)*. Tactile guidance refers to the technique whereby the surgeon inserts one hand into the incision and grips the distal muscle between the thumb and fingers and then cuts just beyond the finger tips with endoscopic scissors. *(Fig. 5.14)* The surgeon's hand provides both guidance and traction and greatly facilitates this portion of the procedure. It is at this point that many surgeons may want to hesitate proceeding with sharp division of muscle due to concerns over bleeding. Active bleeding is not a problem with this, or any other part of the procedure due to the hemostatic effect of the epinephrine in the tumescent fluid instilled at the beginning of the procedure. After distal division is complete, the muscle is delivered into the axillary incision *(Fig. 5.15)*.

The muscle flap is carefully examined and hemostasis is achieved with the aid of bipolar electrocautery. Special attention is given to identify the number and location of lumbar and intercostal perforators severed during mobilization of the latissimus flap as this will play a role

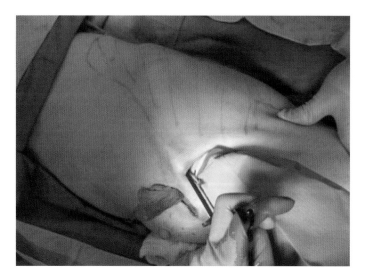

Fig. 5.13 Scissor dissection is used to release the inferior origin of the latissimus muscle.

in final hemostasis prior to closure *(Fig. 5.16)*. These vessels usually are not actively bleeding, due the tumescent fluid but they can be seen. The insertion of the muscle into the humerus is completely divided using monopolar electrocautery, which allows for further anterior arc rotation to reach defects in a more medial location. This also limits pulling on the arm and breast with subsequent muscle flexion. After complete mobilization of the latissimus dorsi, the flap is tethered only by its neurovascular pedicle. A subcutaneous tunnel is created from the axillary incision into the breast defect. The muscle is then passed through the tunnel and guided into the breast defect through the existing breast lumpectomy incision. Once the flap is adequately positioned to fill the breast defect, absorbable sutures are used to loosely tack the muscle in its final position.

Attention is now turned to the donor site. This is the portion of the operation that truly depends on the endoscope. Using the endoscope, perforators are identified and coagulated along the posterior midline. Curved, insulated endoscopic grasping forceps are used to coagulate the most posterior vessels. The number and location of bleeding sites should correspond to perforators identified on the muscle during flap hemostasis. Two 7 mm drains are placed into the donor site on the back, and one is placed into the breast. A local anesthetic catheter may be inserted into the axilla to assist with post operative pain management. The axillary and

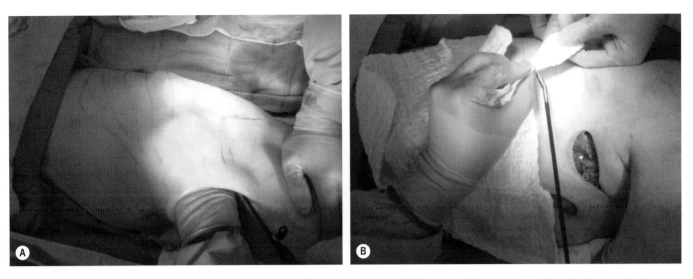

Fig. 5.14 (A) Scissor dissection is used to release the posterior origin of the latissimus muscle. **(B)** Simulation of the tactile scissor dissection technique is demonstrated using a laparotomy pad.

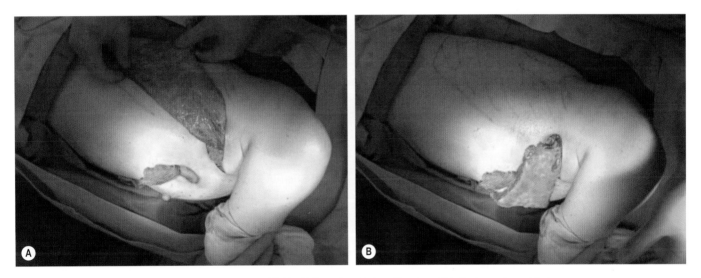

Fig. 5.15 (A) Completed dissection of the latissimus muscle **(B)** After delivery through the axillary tunnel into the lumpectomy defect.

breast incisions are then closed in standard fashion. Typical operative time is between 2 and 3 hours.

Postoperative care

Loosely applied dressings are removed after approximately 24 h. Patients' postoperative hospital course is typically 24–48 h. The suction drains are kept in place until the output is <30 mL in a 24 h period. Often, a more conservative approach is used to manage the back donor site drains secondary to high risk of post operative seroma formation. Walking and daily living activities, including hair combing and teeth brushing

are encouraged immediately. More strenuous physical activity, including lifting, is restricted for 4–6 weeks.

Outcomes, prognosis, and complications

The spectrum of postoperative complications after EARLi flap breast reconstruction is much the same as with a traditional open latissimus flap. Outcomes are shown in *Figure 5.17*. In our series, donor site seromas requiring office aspiration have occurred in approximately 10% of cases, all managed by office aspiration. There have been no postoperative hematomas in this series. In another study comparing donor site morbidity

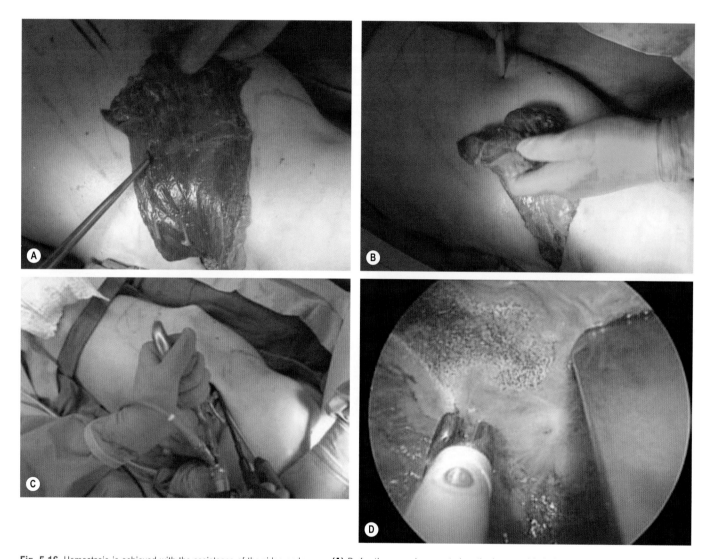

Fig. 5.16 Hemostasis is achieved with the assistance of the video endoscope **(A)** Perforating vessels are noted on the harvested latissimus muscle. **(B)** Locations of perforators are transposed onto the skin using surgical marking pen. **(C,D)** Perforators are located, identified, and cauterized using the marked perforator locations as a road map.

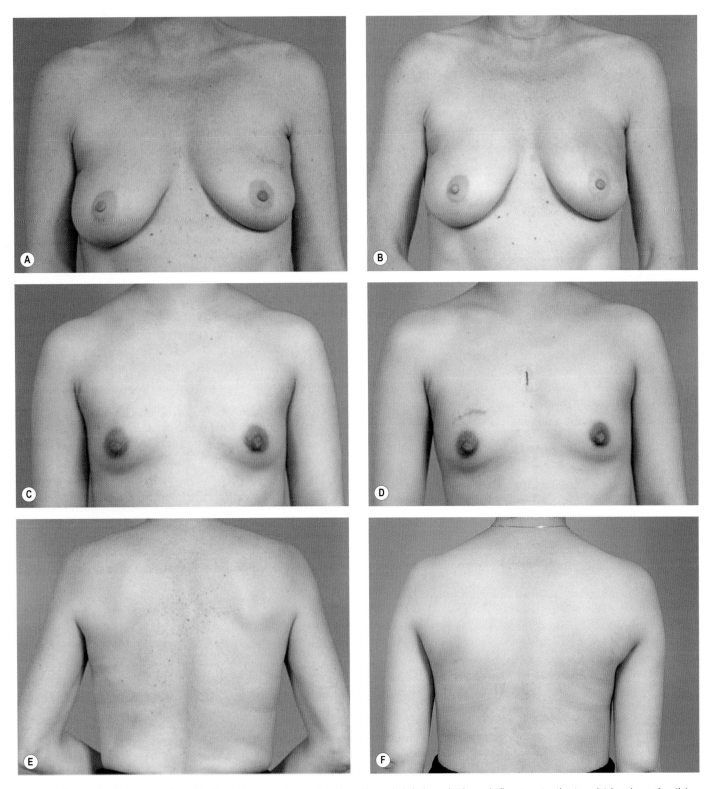

Fig. 5.17 Preoperative **(A,C)** and postoperative **(B,D)** views of patients undergoing endoscopic latissimus dorsi muscle flap reconstruction to maintain volume of partial mastectomy defects. Minimal donor site deformity is seen **(E,F)**.

between endoscopically assisted and traditional harvest of free latissimus dorsi muscle flaps, results revealed no statistically significant differences in hematomas or seromas. Importantly, patient based questionnaires have shown endoscopically assisted latissimus harvests to have less pain and allow for early upper extremity movement and overall improved cosmesis. Depressed back contour can occur if fat is taken superficial to Scarpa's fascia. Temporary paresis of deltoid function was seen in two patients in our series, presumably due to prolonged arm abduction during muscle harvest.

References

1. Nahai F, Eaves F. Fundamentals of endoscopic plastic surgery. In: Nahai F, Saltz R, eds. *Endoscopic plastic surgery*, 2nd ed. St Louis: Quality Medical; 2008.
   Good overview of endoscopic principles for plastic surgery.

2. Delmar H. Axillary approach for endoscopically assisted breast augmentation. In: Nahai F, Saltz R, eds. *Endoscopic plastic surgery*, 2nd ed. St Louis: Quality Medical; 2008.
   General discussion of endoscopic breast augmentation.

3. Nahai F, Eaves F. Submuscular breast augmentation. In: Nahai F, Saltz R, eds. *Endoscopic plastic surgery*, 2nd ed. St Louis: Quality Medical; 2008.
   Specific considerations for the submuscular approach.

4. Strock L. Transaxillary breast augmentation. In: Spear S, ed. *Surgery of the breast*, 3rd ed. Philadelphia: Wolters Kluwer Lippincott Williams & Wilkins; 2011.
   Well illustrated overview of the surgical technique.

5. Fine N, O'Shaughnessy K. Endoscopic delayed-immediate autologous reconstruction with latissimus muscle only flaps. In: Spear S, ed. *Surgery of the breast*, 3rd ed. Philadelphia: Wolters Kluwer Lippincott Williams & Wilkins; 2011.
   Comprehensive description of endoscopically assisted breast reconstruction using the latissimus muscle.

6. Berger A, Krause-Bergmann A. [Use of endoscopy in plastic surgery]. *Langenbecks Arch Chir*. 1996;381(2):114–122.

7. Benito-Ruiz J. Transaxillary subfascial breast augmentation. *Aesthetic Plast Surg*. 2003;23:480–483.

8. Cho BC, Lee JH, Ramasastry SS, et al. Free latissimus dorsi muscle transfer using an endoscopic technique. *Ann Plast Surg*. 1997;38(6):586–593.

9. Graf RM, Bernardes A, Auersvald A, et al. Subfascial endoscopic transaxillary augmentation mammaplasty. *Aesthetic Plast Surg*. 2000;24:216–220.

10. Ho LC. Endoscopic assisted transaxillary augmentation mammaplasty. *Br J Plast Surg*. 1993;46:332–336.

11. Howard PS, Oslin BD, Moore JR. Endoscopic transaxillary submuscular augmentation mammaplasty with textured saline breast implants. *Ann Plast Surg*. 1996;37:12–17.

12. Price CI, Eaves 3rd FF, Nahai F, et al. Endoscopic transaxillary subpectoral breast augmentation. *Plast Recon Surg*. 1994;94:612–619.

13. Eaves 3rd FF, Price CI, Bostwick J 3rd, et al. Subcutaneous endoscopic plastic surgery using a retractor-mounted endoscopic system. *Perspect Plast Surg*. 1993;7:1–22.

14. Johnson GW, Crhist JE. The endoscopic breast augmentation: the transumbilical insertion of saline-filled breast implants. *Plast Reconstr Surg*. 1993;92:801–808.

15. Paige KT, Eaves 3rd FF, Wood RJ. Endoscopically assisted plastic surgical procedures in the pediatric patient. *J Craniofac Surg*. 1997;8(3):164–169.

16. Vasconez LO. Expert commentary. *Perspect Plast Surg*. 1993;7:23–26.

17. Vasconez LO, Core GB, Oslin B. Endoscopy in plastic surgery. An overview. *Clin Plast Surg*. 1995;22(4):585–589.

18. Miller MJ, Robb GL. Endoscopic technique for free flap harvesting. *Clin Plast Surg*. 1995;22(4):755–773.

19. Friedlander L, Sundin J. Minimally invasive harvesting of the latissimus dorsi. *Plast Reconstr Surg*. 1994;94(6):881–884.

20. Fine NA, Orgill DP, Pribaz JJ. Early clinical experience in endoscopic-assisted muscle flap harvest. *Ann Plast Surg*. 1994;33(5):465–472.

21. Masuoka T, Fujikawa M, Yamamoto H, et al. Breast reconstruction after mastectomy without additional scarring: application of endoscopic latissimus dorsi muscle harvest. *Ann Plast Surg*. 1998;40(2):123–127.

22. Pomel C, Missana MC, Atallah D, et al. Endoscopic muscular latissimus dorsi flap harvesting for immediate breast reconstruction after skin sparing mastectomy. *Eur J Surg Oncol*. 2003;29(2):127–131.

23. Kronowitz SJ. Endoscopic subcutaneous surgery: a new surgical approach. *Ann Plast Surg*. 1999;42(4):357–364.

24. Van Buskirk ER, Rehnke RD, Montgomery RL, et al. Endoscopic harvest of the latissimus dorsi muscle using the balloon dissection technique. *Plast Reconstr Surg*. 1997;99(3):899–905.

25. Lin CH, Wei FC, Levin LS, et al. Donor-site morbidity comparison between endoscopically assisted and traditional harvest of free latissimus dorsi muscle flap. *Plast Reconstr Surg*. 1999;104(4):1070–1078.

6

Iatrogenic disorders following breast surgery

Walter Peters

SYNOPSIS

Iatrogenic deformity after breast augmentation can result from the following factors:

- Nature of the injected material
- Nature of the implant
- Surgical technique
- Treatment of previous complications.

Introduction

The word "iatrogenic" is defined as illness caused by medical examination or treatment. During the early years (1900–1950), breast augmentation was usually accomplished by the injection of foreign material, generally paraffin or liquid silicone. Iatrogenic disorders were very common during this period. They resulted primarily from the foreign material that was injected. Breast implants were introduced in the early 1950s. They resulted in a totally different group of iatrogenic disorders. Some of these were due to the implants. Others were due to untoward complications, surgical techniques, and patient anomalies. The purpose of this chapter is to review the iatrogenic disorders that can occur after breast augmentation.

Injection materials

The history of breast augmentation occupies the past 110 years. Fewer surgical procedures have a history as fascinating as breast augmentation. There have been four main eras of injectable materials for breast augmentation. Each of these eras has produced iatrogenic breast conditions of major proportions:

- Paraffin (1899–1914)
- A plethora of material (1915–1943)
- Liquid silicone (1944–1991)
- Polyacrylamide hydrogel (PAH) (1988–2009)

Paraffin (1899–1914)

Paraffin injections[1,2] were used extensively for breast augmentation from 1900 to 1914. Paraffin is a group of hydrocarbons, which is saturated with carbon to hydrogen bonds, making them relatively inert. The basic repeating unit in the polymers is: $-(CH_2)\,n-$. Paraffin exists as a hard form (wax) and a soft form (Vaseline). Paraffin was usually liquefied in a warming chamber prior to injection. The first published report of paraffin injections into a patient dates back to a report by Gersuny, of Vienna, in 1899. A young man had undergone a bilateral orchidectomy for tuberculous disease. Gersuny injected paraffin into his scrotum, so that the patient could pass the physical examination necessary to join the army. Paraffin injections were subsequently used extensively for breast augmentation in Europe, the Far East and North America, until about 1914, when its complications became known. However, in the Far East, the practice was continued into the 1950s and 1960s.

The early results of paraffin injections were often quite acceptable. The complications that followed frequently did not show up until 5 or 10 years later. The local complications included migration, ulceration, fistulae, infection and necrosis. A new term was coined – "paraffinomas" – to describe these changes, which involved both skin and underlying soft tissues. These complications would frequently lead to breast amputation. Ultimately, in his 1925 textbook, H. Lyons Hunt called an "inexcusable practice" and blamed "beauty doctors and other such imposters" for its continued use. The disastrous experience with paraffin was to live on in the collective memory of the plastic surgery profession.

Figure 6.1 shows the clinical status of a woman who received paraffin injections in the Far East 40 years earlier. She had undergone multiple debridement procedures and bilateral mastectomies over the years to treat multiple ulcers, infections and fistulae. She continued to suffer from these problems.

After the paraffin saga, there was a period of approximately 30 years during which a huge plethora of materials was used for breast augmentation. The list of these materials was limited only by the extent of man's imagination. During this time, the following materials

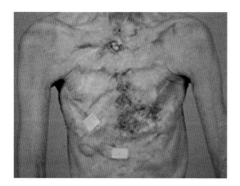

Fig. 6.1 Clinical status of a woman who had received paraffin injections in the Far East 40 years previously. She has had many operations over the years, including bilateral mastectomies, to treat ulcers and fistulae. She continues to suffer from these problems.

were used: ivory balls, glass balls, vegetable oils, mineral oil, lanolin, beeswax, shellac, silk fabric, epoxy resin, ground rubber, ox cartilage, sponges, sacs, rubber, goat's milk, Teflon, soybean and peanut oil, and glazier's putty. The outcome with each of these materials was similar – chronic inflammation, infection, and foreign body granulomas. Many of the materials had severe tissue reactions. Infections were common. Ultimately, none of the materials proved to be useful for breast augmentation.

Liquid silicone injections (1944–1991)

In 1943, the Dow Corning Corporation and Corning Glass formed a joint venture in the United States, to develop silicone products to be used for military purposes during the Second World War. Ultimately, these silicones were used for waterproofing, to prepare grease and oil products for aircraft, to insulate electrical transformers, and to prepare high-temperature-resistant rubbers. When the war came to an end, Dow Corning redirected their efforts to the formulation of medical-grade silicones. Medical grade refers to material that is pure in quality, sterile, and of constant viscosity. Medical-grade silicone was not available until 1960.

Near the end of the Second World War, prostitutes in Japan used industrial-grade liquid silicone extensively. United States' servicemen preferred women with larger breasts than those of Asian women. Barrels of industrial-grade silicone began to mysteriously disappear from Japanese docks, destined for injection into the breasts of these unfortunate women.

Many of the complications of paraffin injections were repeated – a half-century later – with silicone injections. Some of them were even worse, because of impurities and additives in the silicone preparations. Only industrial-grade silicone was available. This material was never meant for injection because of its impurities. In addition, in many of the preparations, contaminants were purposely added to the injected material. Their purpose was to cause a sclerosis reaction in the breasts, to contain the liquid silicone and to hopefully prevent it from migrating through the breast tissue to other sites. Common sclerosing agents included croton oil, cobra venom, olive oil and peanut oil. The adverse effects of injected liquid silicone were very similar to those of paraffin. These included: migration of silicone to other parts of the body, inflammation, discoloration, and the formation of granulomas, ulceration and fistulae.

During the late 1950s and 1960s, a number of physicians and lay clinics in North America turned to liquid silicone injections for augmenting women's breasts. Las Vegas became a "center" for silicone injections. In the entertainment business, these silicone injections were referred to as "Cleopatra's Needle". They were often injected into woman's breasts under great pressure, using equipment resembling a caulking gun. It has been estimated that in Las Vegas in the 1960s, liquid silicone was used to inject the breasts of over 10 000 women. Ultimately, in 1975, because of the horrendous complications from silicone injections into breasts in Las Vegas, the state of Nevada declared that it was a felony to inject silicone or to transport liquid silicone across the state line.

In 1966, the FDA authorized nine plastic surgeons and one dermatologist to investigate the cosmetic use of Dow Corning's highly purified medical-grade liquid silicone (Dow Corning 360) for certain specific problems in patients. The study was limited to only these particular physicians. However, over time, many other physicians used this medical-grade silicone, although they were not part of the official study. Subsequently, Dow Corning decided to discontinue efforts to gain FDA approval, because they could not prevent misuse of the product.

Figure 6.2 shows the clinical status of a woman who received silicone breast injections in San Francisco in 1972. Over the next 30 years, much of the silicone has migrated to her abdomen. Her breasts show chronic inflammation from silicone granulomas that have infiltrated the overlying skin. Mammography of breasts injected with silicone usually demonstrates multiple cystic masses, ranging from 0.2 cm to 2.0 cm in diameter, often with calcification *(Fig. 6.3)*. This can interfere with clinical and radiological breast evaluation.

Figure 6.4 shows the microscopic appearance of a silicone granuloma, which has been excised from silicone-injected breast tissue. This shows extensive destruction of the breast parenchyma. Silicone appears as empty spaces or vacuoles, where it has been washed out during tissue preparation. Histology also shows occasional giant cells, vascular obliteration, a chronic inflammatory response and destruction of the breast parenchyma.

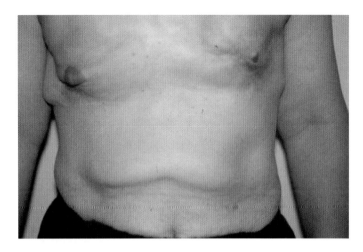

Fig. 6.2 Clinical status of a woman who received breast silicone injections in San Francisco in 1972. Over the following 30 years, much of the silicone has migrated to her abdomen. Her breasts show chronic inflammation from silicone granulomas that have infiltrated the overlying skin.

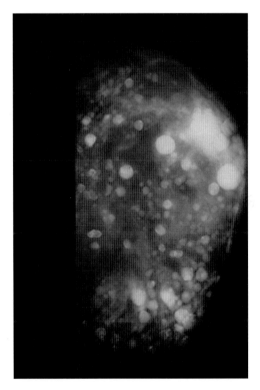

Fig. 6.3 Mammography following liquid silicone injections demonstrates multiple cystic masses ranging from 0.2 cm to 2.0 cm in diameter, often with calcification.

The reactions of liquid silicone injected into breasts vary considerably. Not all patients appear to be equally susceptible to the deleterious effects of silicone. Some patients do not develop significant symptoms at all. In

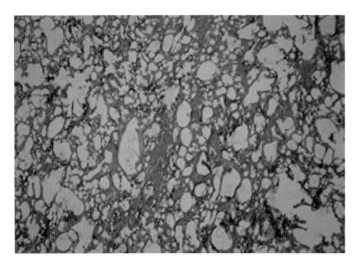

Fig. 6.4 Histology of breast tissue which was injected with liquid silicone. There is extensive destruction of breast parenchyma. Silicone shows up as empty spaces or vacuoles, where it been washed out during the tissue preparation. There are occasional multinucleated giant cells, areas of vascular obliterans, and chronic inflammation (H&E stain, magnification ×50).

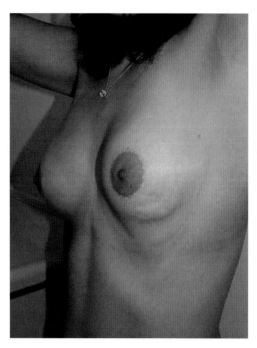

Fig. 6.5 Clinical status of a 29-year-old woman, 1 year after she received breast PAH injections in Iran. Visible and palpable tender masses are apparent in the inframammary and inferior-lateral aspect of both breasts.

general, the average time from injection of silicone to the development of complications is 9 years. There are two main types of clinical presentations. The first type of patient usually presents with multiple and/or painful lumps in their breasts. In some patients, these may occur within two to three years of injection. In other patients, they may not occur until 10 or 15 years after injection. Many patients have also had multiple injections of cortisone, in an attempt to decrease the inflammatory reaction. This can complicate the clinical picture.

The second type of patient presents with skin inflammation and impending breakdown (see *Fig. 6.2*). As the silicone invades the dermis and epidermis of the overlying skin, the breast may show varying stages of skin circulatory difficulties, from fine telangiectasia to necrosis. Skin capillary filling time is increased. Migration of the silicone is common.

Injectable liquid silicone has many qualities that could make it a suitable material for long-term soft-tissue augmentation. At the same time, there are still many unanswered questions pertaining to potential complications that need to be addressed before it can be considered for this purpose. A well conducted, controlled, long-term study is needed to answer these questions.

Polyacrylamide hydrogel (1988–2010)

During the past 20 years, a newer class of injectable material has been used, mainly in Ukraine, Russia, and China: polyacrylamide hydrogel (PAH).[3] It is an extensively cross-linked polymeric soft tissue filler substance that has been used extensively for breast augmentation. Initially, PAH appeared to be an ideal soft tissue filler material. However, several reports have subsequently appeared, demonstrating that numerous complications can occur after PAH injections. These can develop from several months to three years after injection. They include: migration, breast lumps, pain, infection, firmness and disfigurement. The use of PAH has now been banned in China and many other countries.

Figure 6.5 shows a 29-year-old woman who received PAH injections into both breasts in a plastic surgery clinic in Iran 1-year previously. Over the following year, she developed visible and palpable tender masses. A T1-weighted magnetic resonance imaging study of the left breast shows low signal intensity material, mostly superficial to the pectoral muscles, in the subglandular plane *(Fig. 6.6)*. The PAH was easily removed

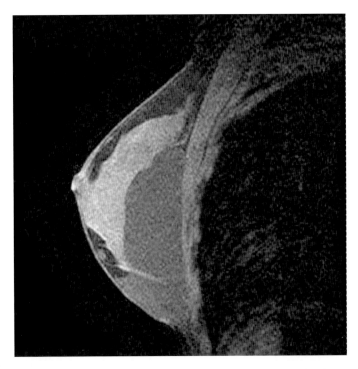

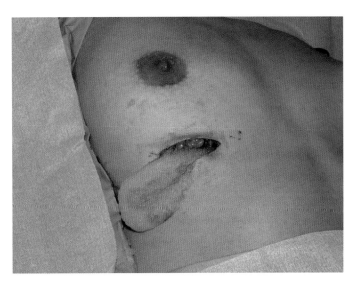

Fig. 6.7 The PAH was easily removed through bilateral inframammary incisions. It had the consistency of "Cream of Wheat".

Fig. 6.6 A T1-weighted image of the left breast *(Fig. 6.3)* showed low signal intensity material, mostly superficial to the pectoral muscles, in the subglandular plane.

through bilateral inframammary incisions. It had the consistency of "cream of wheat" *(Fig. 6.7)*. The patient underwent an uneventful subglandular breast augmentation with cohesive gel implants 2 years later.

This particular patient, who was injected with PAH in Iran, showed only minimal complications with migration and surface lumps in her breasts. However, we have seen other patients (e.g., from Russia), who have presented with major recurrent infections and multiple sinuses, and fistulae, many years after receiving PAH injections *(Fig. 6.8)*. There may be different chemical formulations and different purifications of PAH in certain areas of the world.

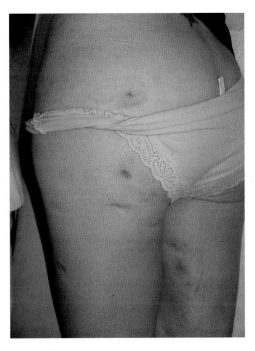

Fig. 6.8 This 32-year-old woman received PAH injections 6 years earlier in Russia. She has been plagued with recurrent infections and draining sinuses.

Breast implants

The sponges (1951–1962, the early years)

The initial breast implants were developed in 1951. This introduced a totally new concept. Solid devices were now inserted behind the breast tissue to augment the size and shape of the breast. Breast implants have evolved over the past 60 years. Ivalon (polyvinyl alcohol) (Beverly Hills Surgical Supply Company) sponge was the first significant implantation material used for breast augmentation. The original sponges were manufactured by Clay-Adams Company (USA) and the Poly-Plastic

Company (USA). Pangman and Wallace[4] published the first study on these implants in 1955. They surmised that the outer surface of these sponges could become infiltrated with vascularized tissue, to produce a "living sponge". Subsequent investigations showed that this process did not occur. Although the initial results were encouraging, within 1 year of augmentation, breasts became very firm and lost over 25% of their volume. Pangman introduced many modifications of his implant, including: a double-layered construction and wrapping the implant in a polyethylene sac. In spite of these modifications, all of these patients developed major firmness and shrinkage of their implants.

Figure 6.9 shows the breast appearance 19 years after augmentation with Ivalon double-layered sponge implants (*circa* 1958).[5] This patient presented with bilateral very painful capsular contractures. She was subsequently treated by explantation and capsulectomy.

From 1952 to 1962, other sponges were also used for breast augmentation. These included: polyethylene sponge, Etheron (a polyether sponge), and Polystan (fabric tapes that were cut by machine and then wound by hand into a ball). Another type of implant that was used from 1958 to 1962 consisted of shredded polyethylene strips, each about 2 mm wide, enclosed in a casing.[6]

All of the implant materials from this era had a similar outcome. Within a year of implantation, they developed major and painful breast firmness and a loss of breast volume. This was due to capsular contracture, a process that would lead to collapse of the sponge and which would continue to plague plastic surgeons and their patients for the next 50 years. Many of these sponges also developed infection. Because of this high complication rate, the popularity of breast augmentation surgery declined progressively until 1963, when the silicone gel implant was introduced.

Silicone gel implants

In 1963, Cronin and Gerow introduced silicone gel implants, as the new "natural feel" implants. This revolutionized breast augmentation surgery. Subsequently, newer types of silicone gel implants were introduced. From 1963 until 1992, silicone gel breast implants were far from being homogeneous. About 10 different companies manufactured many different types of silicone gel breast implants. They obtained their raw materials for gels and shells from a similar number of other companies, who entered and left the market at intervals. Many of the suppliers and manufactures changed their names and ownership over the years. Most of the companies no longer exist. No formal process of FDA premarket testing was in effect until 1988.

Silicone gel breast implants were originally implanted in small numbers, and these numbers slowly increased.[7] From 1962 to 1970, only about 50 000 women received gel implants in the United States. Subsequently, this number rose annually. In 1982, about 100 000 women received silicone gel implants. From 1983 to 1991, this number remained constant at 120 000–130 000 per year. Estimates indicate that, by 1992, over 2 million women had received breast implants globally, and that over 95% were silicone gel implants. Over half of these implants were inserted in North America.

As breast augmentation surgery continued to flourish, iatrogenic disorders from this procedure became more common. These disorders included: implant disruption, hematoma, infection, capsular contracture, capsular calcification, implant displacement, and other complications.

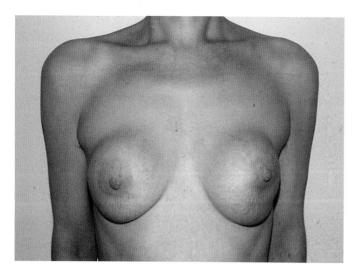

Fig. 6.9 Breast appearance 19 years after augmentation with Ivalon double-layered sponge implants (*circa* 1958). She presented with bilateral painful capsular contractures. All sponge implants tended to have this same outcome. This patient was treated by explantation and capsulectomy.

Implant disruption: silicone gel implants

Most of the implant disruption studies[6–9] were done in the 1990s. Before 1993, the incidence of implant disruption was thought to be very low. In January 1992, Dr David Kessler, the then Commissioner of the FDA, called for a moratorium on the use of silicone gel breast implants. Following this, hundreds of thousands of women with gel implants rushed to have their implants removed. They perceived that there was an association between their implants and medical disease. Why else would they have been banned? This huge number of women with gel implants provided very large numbers of implants for disruption assessment.

From 1963 to 1992, there have been three generations of gel implants, and a number of other lesser variations. First generation implants (1963–1972) had a thick gel and thick wall. They have generally remained intact over the years. Most first generation implants were "tear-drop shaped". They had woven Dacron (DuPont Co, DE) patches on their posterior surfaces *(Fig. 6.10)* to anchor them to the chest wall in an attempt to restrict ptosis. These patches adhered very tenaciously to adjacent tissues. Subsequently, when capsular contracture developed, these patches could cause major breast distortion. In addition, significant torsion could be placed at the site of this patch. This could lead to exposure with subsequent extrusion of the implant *(Fig. 6.11)*.

Most women with first generation implants developed very firm breasts, usually within a year of implantation. This was due to capsular contracture, a process that was not well understood at the time. It was surmised that this firmness was due to firmness of the implants. Softer implants (second generation) were therefore developed, with the hope that they would result in softer breasts.

Second generation implants (1973 to the mid-1980s) had a thin gel and thin wall. Studies have shown that these implants were much more prone to disruption than first generation implants. In addition, the watery nature of the second generation implants *(Fig. 6.12)* could result in gel migration, which had not been seen with first generation implants. Manufacturers ultimately addressed the implant disruption problem by developing the third generation implant. Third generation implants (mid-1980s to 1992) had a stronger and thicker shell and a much more cohesive gel *(Fig. 6.13)*. They also had a barrier layer to reduce the diffusion of silicone oil, which was thought to increase capsular contracture. They proved to be much more durable that second generation implants in general, but there were differences among manufacturers.[10]

The breast implant business was competitive and companies introduced changes such as softer gels, barrier low-bleed shells, greater or lesser shell thickness, surface texturing, different sizes, contours, shapes and multiple lumens in search of better aesthetics. Ultimately, over 240 styles and 8300 models of silicone gel breast implants were manufactured in the United States alone. After the moratorium, manufacturers developed the

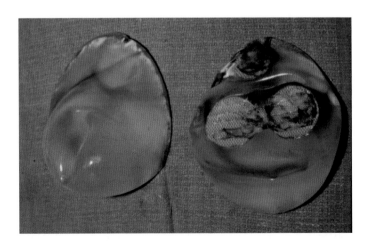

Fig. 6.10 Most first generation silicone gel implants were "tear-drop" shaped and had Dacron patches on their posterior surface. These were designed in an attempt to restrict ptosis of the implant.

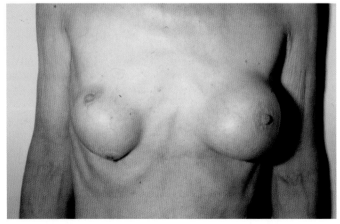

Fig. 6.11 Dacron patches of first generation implants adhered very tenaciously to adjacent tissues. This resulted in major distortion after capsular contracture developed. In this patient, torsion at the site of a Dacron patch has caused breakdown, with exposure of the implant and subsequent infection.

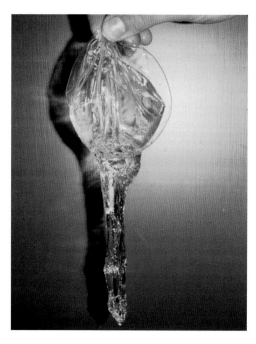

Fig. 6.12 Second generation silicone gel implants (1973 to the mid-1980s) had thin elastomeric shells and were filled with a watery gel. The watery nature of this get could result in gel migration. This had not been seen with first generation implants, which had a thick viscous gel.

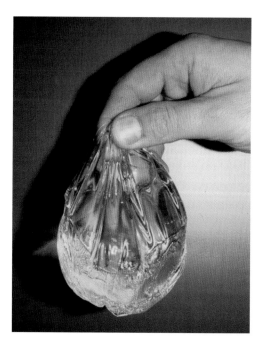

Fig. 6.13 Third generation implants had a stronger and thicker shell and a much more cohesive gel. They also had a barrier layer to reduce the diffusion of silicone oil.

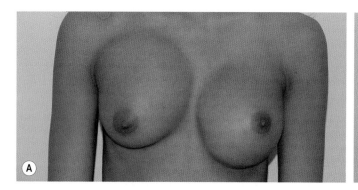

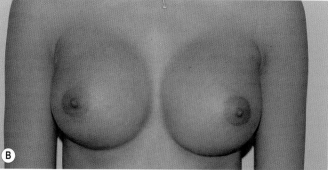

Fig. 6.14 (A) Breasts of a 26-year-old woman 10 months after a bilateral inframammary submuscular augmentation with 350 cc saline implants. She gave a history of bilateral hematomas that were "squeezed out" daily for 1 week after the surgery. She has a class IV contracture on the right side and a class III contracture on the left side. Hematology testing revealed a coagulopathy, with an elevated bleeding time. **(B)** Breast appearance of the patient one year after coagulopathy correction, open capsulotomy, partial capsulectomy, and insertion of new 420 cc submuscular silicone gel implants.

fourth and fifth generations of silicone gel implants, which had stronger shells and more cohesive gels.

Hematoma

The incidence of hematoma after breast augmentation is about 3%. The incidence of subclinical hematomas may be higher. Most hematomas develop *early*, within hours or days of surgery. Most require surgical removal. Some studies have shown a strong association between hematomas and the subsequent development of capsular contracture. Other studies have not found this association.

Figure 6.14A shows the breasts of a 26-year-old woman who presented 10 months after she had a bilateral inframammary submuscular augmentation with 350 cc saline implants. She gave a history of bilateral hematomas that were "squeezed out" on a daily basis for 1 week after the surgery. Ever since the surgery, her right breast remained much larger and higher than the left side. Currently, she presented with a class IV contracture on the right side and a class III contracture on the left side. Hematology testing indicated that her bleeding time was markedly elevated. Ultimately, she was proven to have a factor VIII deficiency. Once this factor was replaced, an uneventful bilateral open capsulotomy was performed and new 420 cc silicone gel implants were inserted in the submuscular plane. *Figure 6.14B* shows that 1 year later, she had excellent symmetry with a Baker class I result 1 year after surgery.

Late hematomas are much less common. Most studies are in the form of case reports.[11,12] *Figure 6.15* shows the

appearance of a 51-year-old woman who presented 12 years, after a bilateral breast augmentation with 250 cc silicone gel breast implants. She had a 1-year history of a progressive and painful doubling of her left breast size. At explantation, there was evidence of old hemorrhage and recent organizing blood clot. It has been suggested that a late hematoma can result from actual erosion of small- to medium-sized arteries in the breast capsule. This could develop from various causes, including normal wear and tear from friction of the implants against the capsule. Capsular contracture and trauma may also be factors.

Infection

Infection after breast augmentation is uncommon.[13] It is usually classified as early (within 4 weeks of augmentation) or late (from the second month onwards). The incidence of early infection is thought to be about 1%. Late infection is very rare and cases are largely anecdotal. Endogenous bacteria usually cause early infections, either from the skin or from the milk ducts. By contrast, the pathogenesis of late infections usually involves a bacteremia.

Figure 6.16A shows a 36-year-old woman who presented 3 weeks after undergoing a bilateral, periareolar, subglandular, breast augmentation using textured cohesive gel implants in a clinic in Mexico. She gave a history

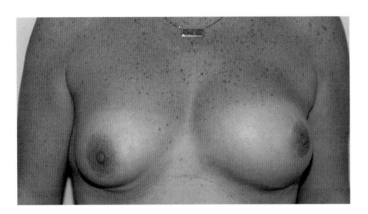

Fig. 6.15 This 51-year-old woman presented with a chronic hematoma 12 years after a bilateral inframammary submuscular breast augmentation with 250 cc silicone gel implants. Her left breast had slowly doubled in size over the preceding year. This may have resulted from an erosion of an artery in the breast capsule.

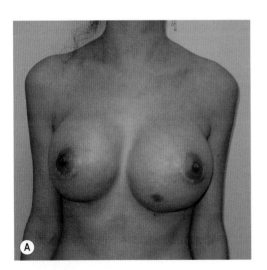
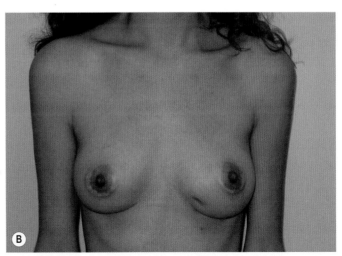

Fig. 6.16 **(A)** This 36-year-old woman presented 4 weeks after a bilateral periareolar subglandular breast augmentation in Mexico. She gave a history of bilateral hematomas which were "squeezed out" daily for many days postoperatively. Currently, she presented with an enlarged, painful left breast with an exposed implant and infection. **(B)** Three months after bilateral inframammary explantation. On the left side, a total capsulectomy was done. The pocket was then irrigated with antibiotic solution daily for 2 weeks.

of bilateral hematomas, which were "squeezed out" daily for many days postoperatively. She now presented with an enlarged, painful left breast with an exposed implant and drainage from the exposure site. Both implants were removed through inframammary incisions. On the left side, a total capsulectomy was done. A drain was left in place on the left side for daily antibiotic irrigations. Cultures from the left capsule demonstrated a heavy growth of *Serratia marcescens*, which was resistant to many antibiotics. She was treated with daily pocket irrigations with antibiotic solution for 2 weeks. Several months later, the breasts settled down (*Fig. 6.16B*). She subsequently decided to forego further implants. If new implants were inserted, then that would usually be done after 1 year. They would usually be inserted in a different (submuscular) plane, to avoid the scar tissue from her earlier infection.

Figure 6.17 shows the breasts of a 29-year-old woman who developed a painful late infection of her right breast, 9.5 years after a bilateral, inframammary, submuscular, 300 cc silicone gel breast implants. This was treated by bilateral explantation and capsulectomy on the right side. Cultures from the right capsule grew strains of *Bacillus* and *Staphylococcus* that were resistant to multiple antibiotics. This patient had a history of intravenous drug abuse, which may have led to a seeding of her capsule.

Capsular contracture

The incidence of capsular contracture from 1965 to 1990 was reported to range between 10% and 97%. During this time, many surgeons felt that capsular contracture was a "side effect" of breast augmentation, rather than a complication. With the development of newer 3rd, 4th, and 5th generation implants, the incidence of capsular contracture appears to have been reduced to single digit levels.[14] However, most of these studies have been done over relatively short time intervals. Some studies have shown that surface texturing of silicone gel implants reduces the incidence of capsular contracture.[15] Other studies have not supported this finding. Most of these studies have been done over relatively short time periods. Time will tell the ultimate incidence of capsular contracture over longer periods of time.

Capsular contracture can occur in many forms. *Figure 6.18* show the breasts of a 55-year-old woman, who had received bilateral first generation subglandular silicone gel implants 25 years earlier. She developed bilateral class IV contractures. They were distorted, firm and painful. Capsular contracture appears to be more common with subglandular implants than with submuscular implants. It also appears to be more common with silicone gel implants than with saline implants.

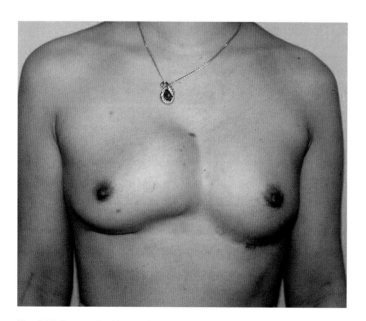

Fig. 6.17 Breasts of a 29-year-old woman who developed a painful late infection of her right breast, 9.5 years after a bilateral inframammary submuscular breast augmentation. This likely developed following a bacteremia.

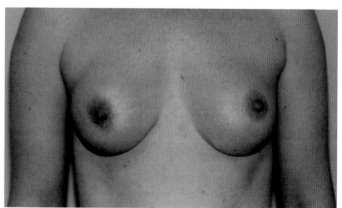

Fig. 6.18 A 55-year-old woman with bilateral class IV capsular contractures 25 years after a bilateral subglandular breast augmentation with first generation implants.

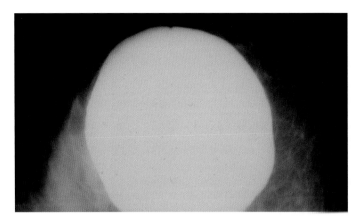

Fig. 6.19 Capsular contracture can interfere with mammographic imaging of a breast, particularly if there is minimal breast tissue, with a large implant in the subglandular plane. This silicone gel implant has been in place for 26 years.

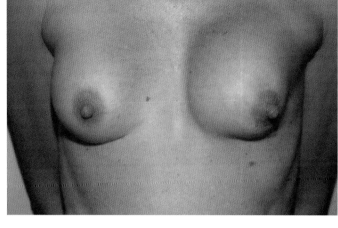

Fig. 6.20 Malposition of the left breast implant following a closed capsulotomy. The implant has moved upwards through a rent in the capsule.

Capsular contracture can limit the clinical and mammographic visualization of breast tissue, particularly if there is minimal breast tissue with a large implant in the subglandular position *(Fig. 6.19)*.

Closed capsulotomy

In the late 1970s and early 1980s, most patients with silicone gel implants developed capsular contractures. The classical treatment for this condition was open capsulotomy with or without capsular resection. However, at that point in time, closed capsulotomy became a popular method of dealing with capsular contracture.[16] Various techniques were developed to vigorously squeeze the breast, so that the scar tissue around the implant could be disrupted, in an attempt to restore softness to the augmented breast. This technique was used mainly for subglandular implants. Sufficient leverage was not usually possible to disrupt the capsule around submuscular implants. At that time, most implants had been placed in the subglandular plane. The pressures generated during closed capsulotomy were shown to be 10.6–15.2 pounds per square inch. Unfortunately, capsular contracture tended to recur after closed capsulotomy. In addition, the technique opened up a horrendous number of new iatrogenic complications. These included: implant displacement, hematoma, implant rupture, and even a gamekeeper's thumb in the surgeon!

Figure 6.20 shows malposition of the left breast implant following a closed capsulotomy. The implant has migrated upwards through a rent in the capsule. *Figure 6.21* shows a 53-year-old woman with second generation gel implants. She presented several months after a vigorous closed capsulotomy in another city. She had experienced immediate pain and swelling in her left axilla and antecubital area after the procedure. Excisional biopsy showed that silicone from the watery gel had migrated to her axilla and antecubital areas.

Figure 6.22 shows the radiological appearance of a breast with a second generation implant, after several vigorous closed capsulotomies at another center. The force of the procedures likely contributed to the current mammographic appearance, with dispersal of silicone globules throughout the breast. This pattern is similar to that seen after silicone injections *(Fig. 6.3)*.

By the mid-1980s, it was recognized that most capsular contractures recurred after closed capsulotomy, and that there was a very high complication rate with the procedure. Surgeons reverted back to open capsulotomy, with or without capsular resection.

Capsular calcification: silicone gel implants

Capsular calcification is a relatively common finding in patients who have received first and second generation subglandular silicone gel implants.[17] By contrast, capsular calcification is very rare with submuscular gel implants. Capsular calcification has not been studied

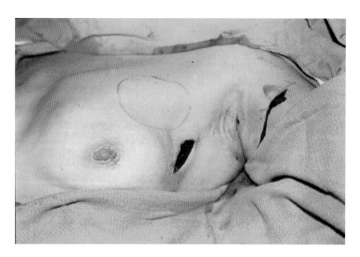

Fig. 6.21 Patient with silicone, which has extruded to her left axilla and antecubital fossa after a vigorous closed capsulotomy at another institution.

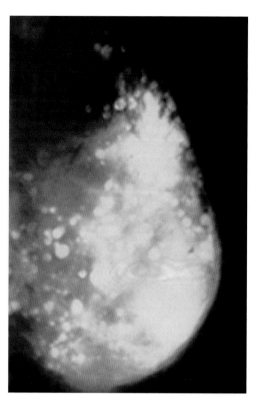

Fig. 6.22 Radiological appearance of a breast after multiple vigorous closed capsulotomy procedures.

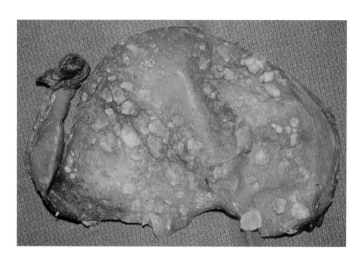

Fig. 6.23 Calcified capsules around silicone gel implants usually demonstrate clinically visible white or gray plaques on their inner surface, adjacent to the implant.

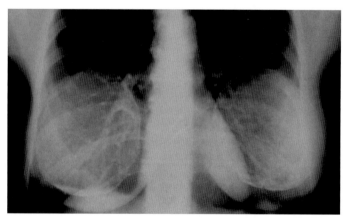

Fig. 6.24 Capsular calcification can show up on routine chest X-ray.

in women with third, fourth, or fifth generation gel implants. Clinically, subglandular calcified capsules from first and second generation gel implants demonstrate visible white or gray plaques on their inner surface, adjacent to the gel implant *(Fig. 6.23)*. This calcification can even show up on a routine chest X-ray *(Fig. 6.24)*. One patient showed extensive bilateral heterotopic calcification[18] 1.2–2.2 cm thick *(Fig. 6.25)*. Most patients with capsular calcification demonstrate class III or IV contractures with significant breast pain.

One study reported on the incidence and nature of capsular calcification in 404 capsules around silicone gel implants.[17] This study demonstrated that all first generation silicone gel implants demonstrated capsular calcification after a mean duration of 17.6 years (range, 14–28 years). By contrast, only 9.8% of second generation implants were associated with capsular calcification. Their mean duration *in situ* was 16.0 years (range, 13–22 years). No second generation implants developed clinical calcification until they had been in place for at least 11 years. In all capsules, calcification existed in two

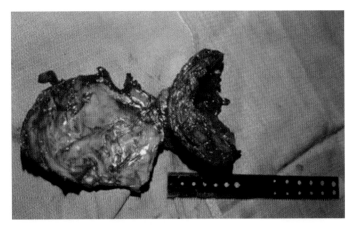

Fig. 6.25 This calcified capsule developed over 17 years in a 63-year-old woman with first generation implants. This represented heterotopic ossification with a thickness of 1.2–2.2 cm.

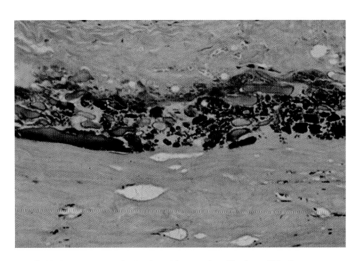

Fig. 6.26 Photomicrograph showing pink area of ossification within the capsule around a first generation gel implant that had been in place for 28 years (H&E stain, magnification ×200).

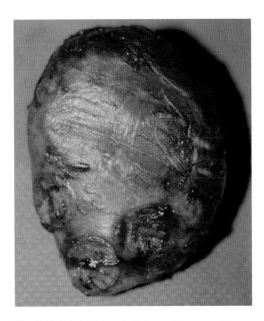

Fig. 6.27 Subglandular calcified capsules are usually removed en masse if implants are removed. This is a first generation gel implant with five Dacron patches on its posterior surface.

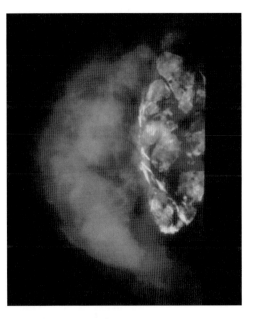

Fig. 6.28 Radiological appearance of a calcified capsule, 7 years after explantation of silicone gel implants. The capsule has persisted over time.

forms: globular aggregates on the surface of the capsule (adjacent to the implant) and actual bone formation within the fibrous tissue of the capsule *(Fig. 6.26)*. Ultrastructural analysis has confirmed two types of calcification, each with hydroxyapatite crystals.

If silicone gel implants are removed from patients with significant capsular calcification, then it is important to remove the calcified capsule as well.[19] This is usually done as an *en masse* procedure if the implants are in the subglandular plane. *Figure 6.27* shows the calcified capsule around a first generation gel implant with five Dacron patches on its posterior surface.

If calcified capsules are not removed at the time of explantation, then they will persist and can interfere with the subsequent clinical and radiological assessment of the breast. *Figure 6.28* shows a calcified capsule that was not removed at the time of explantation. It continues to persist 7 years later.

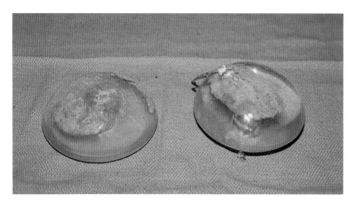

Fig. 6.29 With a saline implant, calcification is rare. When it occurs, it develops mainly on the surface of the implant as an ivory-colored tenaciously adherent deposit of calcium apatite.

Calcified capsules with saline implants

Calcification has also been reported following the insertion of saline implants.[20] Here, the calcification occurs mainly on the anterior surface of the implant as an ivory-colored, tenaciously adherent deposit *(Fig. 6.29)*. Ultrastructure analysis has shown individual crystals measuring approximately $40×10×10$ nm, in the form of calcium apatite. In these patients, capsular calcification was also observed, but it was seen only microscopically.

It has been postulated that capsular calcification with silicone gel and saline could result from abrasion of the implant surface, to release silica-rich sites, which could serve as a nidus for capsular calcification. With silicone gel implants, the lubricant effect of the silicone "bleed" may reduce movement between the capsule and the implant. Calcification would therefore tend to occur in the capsule, rather than on the surface of the implant. With saline-filled implants, there would be no such lubricant effect and nucleation would be expected to occur on the surface of the implant as well as the capsule.

Steroid atrophy

The high incidence of capsular contracture with first and second generation silicone gel implants stimulated some surgeons to instill cortisone solutions (usually Kenalog) into the breast pocket during breast augmentation.[21] Some surgeons also added steroid to the implant, hoping for slow diffusion into the implant pocket. In certain patients, this resulted in steroid

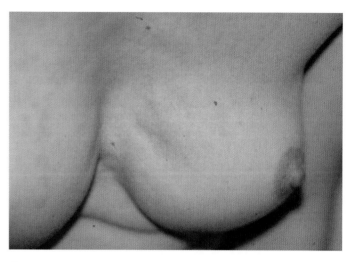

Fig. 6.30 Steroid atrophy after Kenalog was instilled into the pocket of a silicone gel breast implant. Over 9 years, the soft tissue on the medial breast has thinned out.

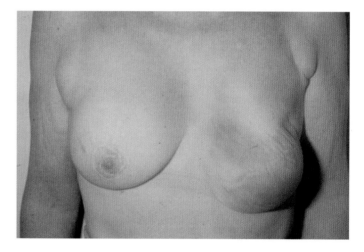

Fig. 6.31 Major steroid atrophy after Kenalog was instilled into the pocket around a silicone gel breast implant.

atrophy of the soft tissues. This could occur in localized areas *(Fig. 6.30)* or in large areas, resulting in impending implant extrusion *(Fig. 6.31)*.

Complications specific to saline implants

Deflation

Saline implants were introduced in 1965 with the Simaplast implant. Other companies followed over the next decade. Spontaneous deflation of early saline

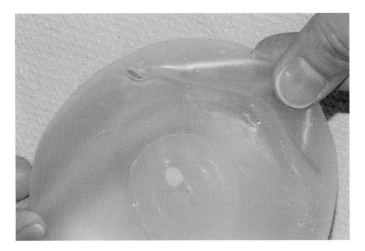

Fig. 6.32 Leakage of a saline implant tends to occur at the end of a fold in the implant shell, presumably from weakening of the shell at this area.

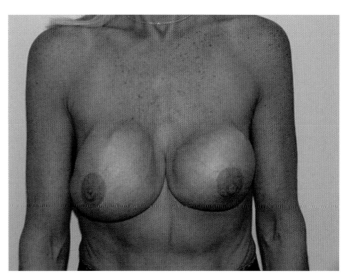

Fig. 6.33 Extensive rippling in a 45-year-old woman with subglandular saline implants.

implants was very common. By 1973, several types of saline implants had demonstrated spontaneous deflation rates of 76–88% over 3 years. Most leaks occurred at the seams and valves of the implants. With this incidence of deflation, most plastic surgeons stopped using saline implants for the next decade. Over the years, manufacturers have developed much stronger and more durable saline implants with much more effective valves. Currently, the incidence of deflation of saline implants is very low.[22] When leakage does occur, it tends to develop at the end of a fold in the implant shell, presumably from weakening of the shell in that area *(Fig. 6.32)*.

Ripples and folds

Ripples and folds are common after the insertion of saline implants if there is insufficient soft tissue (<2 cm) overlying the implant. This problem can occur if saline implants are in the subglandular or submuscular position. This can be quite devastating to the patient *(Fig. 6.33)*. Rippling can sometimes be reduced by overfilling the implant. Implant exchange with silicone gel implants can often improve this problem. However, in the rare patient with a major paucity of soft tissue overlying the implant, ripples and folds can develop even with modern cohesive gel implants *(Fig. 6.34)*.

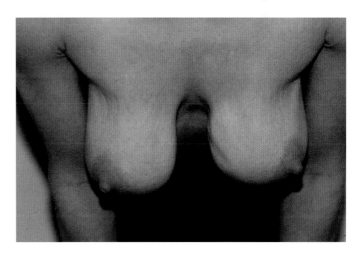

Fig. 6.34 Ripples and folds resulting after subglandular fourth generation cohesive gel implants. These have developed because this woman had very thin overlying soft tissue (0.6 cm).

Autoinflation

Spontaneous autoinflation of saline implants is a rare phenomenon, whereby patients develop spontaneous implant inflation over many years.[23,24] Several theories have been advocated to explain this phenomenon. Currently, however, there appear to be only two possible mechanisms: a hypertonic filling solution or alterations of the valve mechanism, which would allow fluid from the implant pocket to pass into the lumen of the

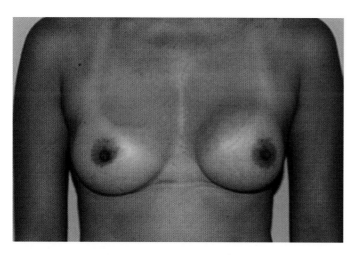

Fig. 6.35 Appearance of a patient 23 years after subglandular augmentation with Simaplast implants. The left breast is larger than the right side. There was a class II contracture of the right side and a class IV contracture on the left side.

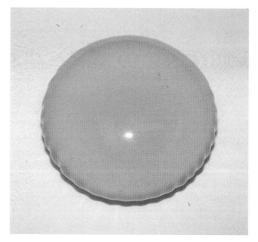

Fig. 6.37 This saline implant enlarged 88% from 330 cc to 620 cc during its 4 years *in situ*. The fluid in the implant had high levels of uric acid.

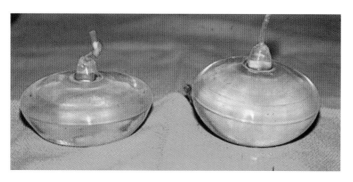

Fig. 6.36 Posterior surface of the Simaplast implants removed after 23 years *in situ*. The left implant had expanded 45% from 200 cc to 290 cc. The right implant was unchanged (220 cc). The left unilateral autoinflation probably resulted after hypertonic fluid was injected on that side.

implant. *Figure 6.35* shows the appearance of a 44-year-old woman who received Simaplast inflatable implants 23 years earlier. Over time, the left breast has progressively enlarged. At explantation, the left implant weighed 290 g, whereas the right side weighed only 220 g *(Fig. 6.36)*. The osmolality of the fluid in the right implant was 302 mmol/kg (isotonic) compared with 407 mmol/kg on the left side. Calculations showed that the most likely explanation for the autoinflation is that the original filling solution of the autoinflated implant had an osmolality that was twice than that of normal saline. Further expansion was likely constrained by the class IV capsular contracture on the left side.

Figure 6.37 shows a saline-filled implant that had enlarged from 330 cc to 620 cc during the 4-years that it was *in situ*. The solution in this implant demonstrated very high levels of uric acid. It was suggested that material from the implant pocket may have entered through the valve. It may have then been degraded to uric acid.

Implant malposition

Iatrogenic malposition of breast implants can result from a number of causes. Surgical technique is often a major factor. Developmental anomalies can also play a role.

Plane of insertion

Some iatrogenic developments are related to the plane of dissection. *Figure 6.38A* shows the breasts of a 21-year-old woman who presented for a left unilateral breast augmentation. She had a short distance (4 cm) from her nipple to the inframammary fold. On the right side, this distance was 6 cm. When a left, unilateral submuscular, 250 cc silicone gel implant was inserted, she developed a "snoopy" deformity (a configuration like "Snoopy's nose") *(Fig. 6.38B)*. This is also an example of a "double-bubble". This problem was easily addressed by changing the implant from the submuscular to the subglandular position *(Fig. 6.38C)*.

Figure 6.39 shows the breast of a 33-year-old woman who had 300 cc silicone gel implants inserted in the

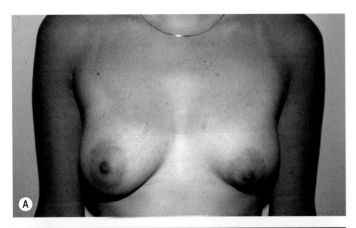

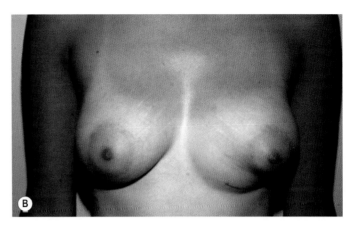

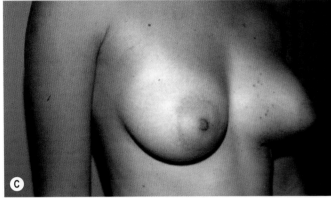

Fig. 6.38 (A) Breasts of a 21-year-old woman who presented for a left unilateral breast augmentation. She had a short distance (4 cm) from her nipple to the inframammary fold. On the other side, this distance was 6 cm. **(B)** When a 250 cc implant was inserted in the submuscular plane, the patient developed a "Snoopy" deformity or double-bubble, because of the short 4 cm distance from the nipple to the fold. **(C)** The "Snoopy" deformity was easily corrected by placing the implant in the subglandular plane.

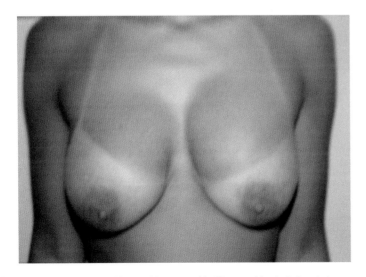

Fig. 6.39 Breasts of a 33-year-old woman with silicone gel implants inserted in the submuscular plane. Preoperatively, her nipples were about 2 cm below the inframammary fold. She would likely have had a better cosmetic result if the implants were placed in the subglandular plane. This would have lifted her nipples better.

submuscular plane. Preoperatively, her nipples were about 2 cm below the inframammary fold. She would probably have had a better cosmetic result if the implants were placed in the subglandular plane. This would have lifted her nipples more effectively.

Inadequate muscle release

The submuscular plane of insertion has advantages for certain patients, particularly if there is a marked paucity of breast tissue. *Figure 6.40A* shows the breasts of a 29-year-old woman with submuscular 300 cc silicone gel implants. At rest, she has a Baker class I result with excellent breast symmetry. However, when she contracts her pectoralis major muscles *(Fig. 6.40B)*, the contraction causes a major distortion of her breast. Better symmetry could have been obtained by more release of the origin of her pectoralis major muscle on the left side.

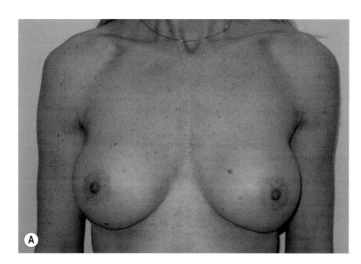
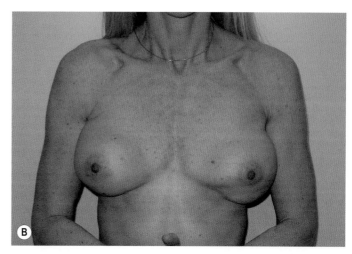

Fig. 6.40 (A) Breasts of a 29-year-old woman with submuscular 300 cc silicone gel implants. At rest, she has a Baker class I result with excellent breast symmetry. **(B)** When the patient contracts her pectoralis major muscles, the contraction causes a major distortion of her left breast. Better symmetry could have been obtained by more release of the origin of her left pectoralis major muscle.

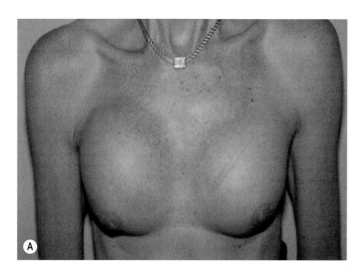
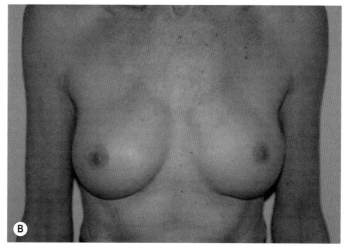

Fig. 6.41 (A) Breasts of a 54-year-old woman who had a submusculofascial insertion of silicone gel implants 20 years previously. Over 20 years, the implants have been lifted superiorly and laterally. **(B)** Breast appearance of the patient after closing the submuscular pockets, and then inserting new implants in the subglandular plane.

Submusculofascial plane

During the 1980s, implants were often inserted in the submusculofascial plane. It was generally accepted that placement in the deeper plane resulted in softer breasts. The implant was placed beneath the pectoralis major muscle and portions of the serratus anterior, rectus abdominis, and external oblique muscles. Subsequently, over time, many of these implants became displaced superior-laterally. *Figure 6.41A* shows the breasts of a

54-year-old woman who had a submusculofascial insertion of silicone gel implants 20 years previously. She developed the classical "up and out" appearance of implants that were inserted in this plane. This has resulted from the superior lateral force of the musculofascial tissues. This problem was addressed by removing her implants, closing the submuscular pockets, and then inserting new 300 cc silicone gel implants in the subglandular plane *(Fig. 6.41B)*.

In the late 1980s, many plastic surgeons changed from the submusculofascial plane to a purely submuscular

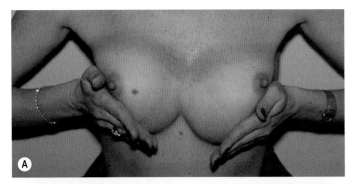
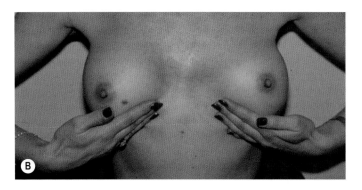
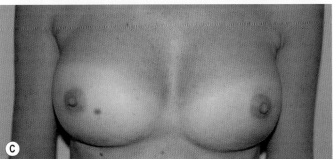

Fig. 6.42 **(A,B)** Breasts of a 25-year-old woman who underwent a transaxillary breast augmentation. A very aggressive pocket dissection was performed at another institution, resulting in pockets that were too large in all directions. **(C)** The patient after an inframammary incision to close the submusculofascial plane and then carefully insert new 300 cc silicone gel implants in the newly-dissected subglandular plane.

plane. Implants tended to be located quite high. In many cases, they would descend as the tissues settled. However, in some cases, they remained high. To address this problem Tebbetts introduced the concept of a dual plane insertion.[25] This allowed the upper part of the implant to be in the submuscular plane, while the lower part was located in the subglandular plane. This decreased the tendency of implants to be positioned too high.

Minor degrees of implant malposition can often be addressed by doing a capsulorraphy procedure. This generally works better if the implants are not overly large and if the affected area of the pocket is not large.

Transaxillary dissection

With the emergence of the transaxillary approach to breast augmentation, a whole new set of potential iatrogenic complications became available. This procedure has the advantage that the incision is hidden within the axillary fold. With this technique, a large urethral sound or similar type of dissector is used to partially detach the pectoral muscle bluntly from the sternum and from its lower costal origins. It is essential that the lower Pectoralis major fibers be divided and that a pocket is

created sufficiently low, beneath the musculofascial layer. Otherwise, the implant position will be too high. This led to significant problems with breast symmetry. If the procedure is done without an endoscope, then it must be performed quite "blindly". This resulted in some implants being situated too low. Others were located too far laterally or too far medially. Some of the problems were difficult to correct. In addition, many patients developed wrinkles and folds, because of inadequate soft tissues to cover the folds in their saline implants.

Figures 6.42A,B show the breasts of a 25-year-old woman who underwent a transaxillary breast augmentation at another institution. A very aggressive pocket dissection was performed, resulting in pockets that were too large in all directions. This problem was easily addressed by removing her implants, closing the submusculofascial pocket with sutures, and then inserting new silicone gel implants in the subglandular plane *(Fig. 6.42C)*.

Symmastia

Symmastia results from over-dissection of the implant pocket medially. Congenital anomalies can play a role.

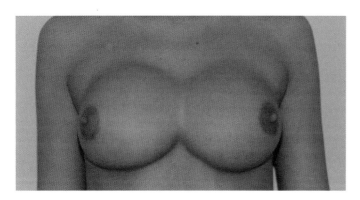

Fig. 6.43 Symmastia after 700 cc saline implants were inserted in the submuscular plane in another city. This problem is very difficult to correct.

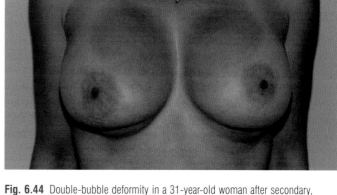

Fig. 6.44 Double-bubble deformity in a 31-year-old woman after secondary, periareolar, submuscular 600 cc saline implants were inserted at another center.

Symmastia is more common with large implants and with submuscular placement. Milder forms of the symmastia can be corrected by conversion of the implant from the submuscular to the subglandular plane. Major forms of symmastia are much more difficult to correct. *Figure 6.43* shows a woman with major symmastia after bilateral submuscular 700 cc saline implants were inserted in another city. Capsular flaps have been described to treat this problem. However, in most cases of major symmastia, the implants need to be removed, and the resulting tissues need to be sewn down to deeper tissues and underlying bone. Then, after a year or so, when the tissues have healed, a secondary augmentation can be attempted with smaller implants, usually in the subglandular plane. Even then, success is not guaranteed.

Double-bubble deformity

Figure 6.44 shows the breast appearance of a 29-year-old woman who has developed a "double-bubble" deformity after primary and secondary surgery at another center. She initially had 400 cc silicone gel implants inserted in the submuscular plane, through periareolar incisions. Subsequently, she requested larger implants. Her surgeon then inserted 650 cc silicone gel implants, again – in the submuscular plane through a periareolar incision. Her double-bubble deformity has resulted because the dissection was done too far inferiorly. There is one "bubble" from the implant that is located below the fold, and another "bubble" at the level of the fold.

This problem is more common with large implants that are inserted in the submuscular plane. It is also more common with secondary surgery that is done through a periareolar incision, because it is difficult to assess the lower limit of the dissection through that incision. The treatment of this condition is challenging. In this case, the implant would need to be removed through an inframammary incision, the lower part of the pocket would need to be sutured to adjacent soft tissue, and the implant would need to be left out for 6–12 months, to let the lower area of the pocket scar down. Then, a further implant could be inserted. If a large implant were inserted in the same stage, then it would likely pull through the repair site. As with many secondary breast implant procedures, the ultimate success of this revisionary surgery cannot be assured.

Ptosis of the augmented breast

Ptosis of the augmented breast can range from minor to severe. Minor ptosis can be addressed by performing an areolar "mastopexy". This can be done by via crescent-shaped excision of skin above the areola or a concentric circumferential (donut) excision of skin around the areola. Although neither procedure yields much nipple elevation, they can be useful with minor degrees of ptosis. The major concern with a circumferential mastopexy is that the surgeon must use a nonabsorbable purse-string suture in the dermis of the outer circle, in order to permanently reduce its diameter. Otherwise, the diameter of the new areola would become much larger. *Figure 6.45* shows the breasts of a 26-year-old

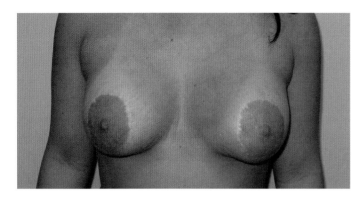

Fig. 6.45 This 26-year-old woman had a circumareolar mastopexy done at the same time as a periareolar breast augmentation at another institution. No purse-string suture was used. The procedure did not lift her nipple, but it did double the size of her areola.

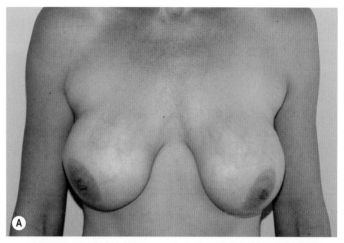

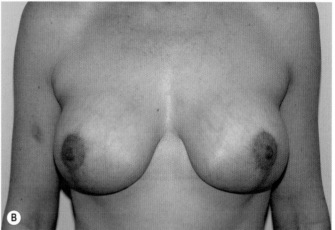

Fig. 6.46 (A) This 29-year-old woman had an inframammary subglandular breast augmentation done in Saudi Arabia 10 years earlier, with "an excellent result". Subsequently, she breast fed each of her two children for 2 years. She now presents with significant ptosis. **(B)** The patient after a very careful McKissock mastopexy procedure and insertion of new 300 cc cohesive gel implants in the subglandular plane.

woman who underwent a circumareolar mastopexy without using a purse-string suture. The procedure did not lift her nipple, but it did double the diameter of her areola.

Secondary ptosis after pregnancy

Figure 6.46A shows a 29-year-old woman who had a bilateral subglandular breast augmentation in Saudi Arabia 10 years earlier, with "a very satisfactory result". Subsequently, she had two children and breast-fed them each for 2 years. Following that time, she presented with major ptosis. This problem was addressed by removing her implants, performing a McKissock mastopexy procedure, and at the same time, inserting new subglandular 300 cc silicone gel implants. This resulted in a very satisfactory breast appearance *(Fig. 6.46B).* Simultaneous mastopexy/augmentation procedures can be fraught with complications. However, if the patient already has implants, then, with careful surgery, the risks can be minimized.

Breast augmentation surgery is considered by many to be a relatively simple type of operation. This can certainly be the case. However, when complications unfold, the outcome can be disastrous, even after multiple operations. Over the years, breast augmentation has produced a plethora of iatrogenic disorders.

Access the complete reference list online at **http://www.expertconsult.com**

2. Peters WJ, Fornasier V. Complications from injectable materials used for breast augmentation. *Can J Plast Surg.* 2009;17:89–96.

   A fantastic review of this topic.

5. Peters WJ, Smith DC. Ivalon breast prostheses: Evaluation 19 years after implantation. *Plast Reconstr Surg.* 1981;67: 514–518.

   An excellent review of this topic.

6. Peters WJ. The evolution of breast implants. *Can J Plast Surg.* 2002;10:223–236.

   An excellent review of this topic.

7. Bondurant S, Ernster V, Herdman R, eds. *Safety of Silicone Breast Implants.* Washington DC: National Academy Press; 2000.

   A fantastic review of this topic.

7

Mastopexy

Kent K. Higdon and James C. Grotting

SYNOPSIS

- Breast ptosis is a common problem caused by several different factors: pregnancy, weight changes, aging, delayed effect of breast implants and developmental deformities.
- Mastopexy and augmentation-mastopexy techniques are varied and can be applied to different breast shape deformities.
- Mastopexy techniques can be periareolar, vertical or based on the inverted-T techniques, as well as being performed in some instances by liposuction alone.
- Preoperative deflation prior to mastopexy or augmentation-mastopexy is a safe and effective technique that offers the patient and surgeon many benefits.

 Access the Historical Perspective section online at
http://www.expertconsult.com

Introduction

The desire for the aesthetic breast has long been captivating to humankind, and its allure permeates many feminine descriptions in classic literature. In the 'Reeve's Tale', from his novel *The Canterbury Tales*, Geoffrey Chaucer describes Malyne, the young and lusty daughter of the miller Symkyn, as follows:

This wenche thikke and wel ygrowen was, with camus nose and yen greye as glas, with buttokes brode, and brestes rounde and hye, but right fair was hir heer, I wol nat lie.

(Chaucer G, Donaldson ET. Chaucer's poetry: an anthology for the modern reader. New York: Ronald Press; 1958:133.)

Though written in Middle English and dating back to *c*1387–1400, this excerpt from the Reeve's Tale clearly conveys that Chaucer's youthful character Malyne, with her "rounde and hye" breasts, is particularly attractive to her suitors. In their pursuit of the aesthetic breast, plastic surgeons have relied heavily on the mastopexy, an operation often referred to by the lay public as the "breast lift." In performing mastopexies, plastic surgeons address breast *ptosis*, a word whose etymologic root is Greek for "falling." What was true in Chaucer's time still holds today: that the "falling" or sagging breast is not the aesthetic ideal. Techniques for addressing the ptotic breast were borne from reduction mammaplasty procedures, essentially exchanging significant parenchymal resections for parenchymal reshaping and redraping the skin envelope. It is not surprising to note the confusion among patients between what is a breast reduction and what is truly a mastopexy. In fact, even among plastic surgeons there are gray areas between the two operations. For example, the patient with primarily breast skin excess and a much more minor component of glandular excess would likely benefit from a small parenchymal reduction in addition to skin resection and parenchymal redistribution. But does that constitute reduction mammoplasty? Mastopexy is a parenchymal reshaping that may or may not require a small parenchymal reduction. Reduction mammaplasties always require parenchymal reduction. What defines the difference between mastopexy and reduction mammoplasty, is whether the patient truly exhibits symptoms of macromastia – the affirmative being the case of a reduction mammoplasty. The issue is further confused from a general standpoint when you consider that some plastic surgeons treat breast ptosis with augmentation alone or in combination with mastopexy in certain instances. Plastic surgeons must be clear that ptosis as a separate entity from macromastia and gigantomastia is treated differently from cases of macromastia or gigantomastia that happen to have ptosis. Typically, the ptotic breast has a paucity of breast parenchyma in relation to a lax, excessive skin envelope. Contrarily, the cardinal finding of the hypertrophic breasts seen in cases of macromastia, gigantomastia, etc., is a predominance of parenchyma without skin excess. The vast majority of patients undergoing surgical intervention to treat ptosis of the breast are treated with skin resection and redraping over a repositioned breast mound – the operation that is the mastopexy.

Basic science/disease process

The pathophysiology of breast ptosis is multifaceted – but can be conceptualized as being the result of the combination of expansion and aging, or separately as a result of a congenital deformity. In its classic description, breast ptosis is the result of inadequate parenchyma or parenchymal maldistribution in the face of excess, lax skin and connective tissues. The ligaments described by Sir Astley Cooper run from the pectoralis muscular fascia, through breast parenchyma, and insert into the dermis *(Fig. 7.1)*. Parenchymal changes with aging (accentuated by the case of the patient with an implant), weight changes in the obese, and pregnancy, are also accompanied by specific alterations in the integrity of Cooper's ligaments, the breast's fascial components, and the overlying skin. These processes essentially function as tissue expansion, as the parenchyma ebbs and flows with the tides of hormonal fluctuations in

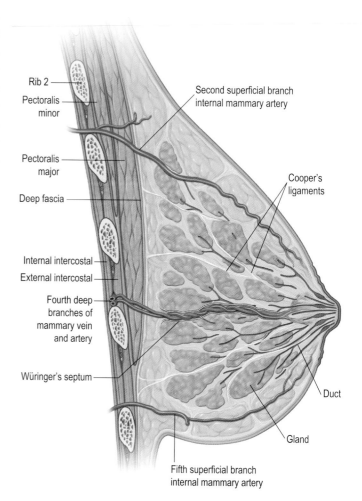

Fig. 7.1 Profile anatomic view of the hemisected human breast. The ligaments described by Sir Astley Cooper are clearly demonstrated to run from the posterior, or deep, breast fascia, which is intimately associated with the pectoralis major muscle fascia, to the anterior, or superficial, breast fascia, and insert into the dermis. The parenchyma, which is encapsulated within these fascial borders, changes with aging, implants, weight changes, and pregnancy. These types of parenchymal changes result in alterations to the integrity of Cooper's ligaments, the breast's fascial components, and the overlying skin and fat.

pregnancy or menopause, or with the weight fluctuations in the obese having lost massive amounts of weight, or with the expanded breast that is created with a breast implant. The skin becomes thin and stretched, and supporting structures, such as Cooper's ligaments and the superficial and deep layers of the superficial breast fascia, lose their inherent elasticity. The breast parenchyma, once held in place on the chest wall by and within these structures, becomes mobile and descends with the constant pull of gravity. Adding the effects of time with aging only exacerbates these

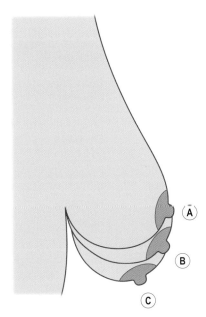

Fig. 7.2 Breast ptosis classification as described by Regnault. **(A)** Minimal ptosis: the nipple is at the level of or just inferior to the inframammary crease. **(B)** Moderate ptosis: the nipple is 1–3 cm below the inframammary crease. **(C)** Severe ptosis: the nipple is >3 cm below the inframammary crease. (Redrawn from: Georgiade GS, Georgiade NG, Riefkohl R. Esthetic breast surgery: In: McCarthy JG, ed. Plastic surgery. Philadelphia: WB Saunders; 1991:3839.)

pathophysiologic changes. The loss of elastic recoil of the skin and connective tissue, coupled with involutional atrophy of the parenchymal mound, results in an unshapely, falling, and unaesthetic breast.

Breast ptosis in its various degrees is defined by its anatomic relationship to the inframammary fold. The original classification scheme for breast ptosis was set forth by Regnault,[11] who in 1976 described the degrees of breast ptosis *(Fig. 7.2)*. Grade I ptosis, or mild ptosis, was defined as having the nipple within 1 cm of the inframammary fold and being above the lower pole of the breast. Grade II, or moderate, breast ptosis exists when the nipple is 1–3 cm below the inframammary fold but still is above the lower pole of the breast. In grade III (severe) ptosis, the nipple is more than 3 cm below the inframammary fold and is situated below the lower breast contour. There is a fourth category of breast ptosis, commonly known as glandular or pseudoptosis, in which the nipple rests above the inframammary fold but the majority of breast tissue rests below and gives the appearance of ptosis.

An additional caveat to the Regnault classification was submitted by Brink, which takes into account other causes of the ptotic breast, such as parenchymal maldistribution, and posits an algorithm by which they can be surgically addressed *(Table 7.1, Fig. 7.3)*. One example of such parenchymal maldistribution is the tuberous breast deformity, also known as the tubular breast or constricted breast, which manifests as a high inframammary fold, hypoplastic lower pole, and nipple-areolar complex resting on the inferior-most aspect of the breast.[12] Other classic features of the tuberous breast include herniation of the nipple-areolar complex as well as a constriction of the base of the breast.[13] The tuberous breast deformity consists of a spectrum of different presentations to include some or all of these findings, the more severe cases representing the more challenging cases to correct *(Fig. 7.4)*. Tuberous breasts can occur unilaterally, with the contralateral breast being unaffected, or can present to similar or vastly different degrees in bilateral cases. There are three classes of tuberous breast as described by Grolleau *(Fig. 7.5)*. Type I deformities manifest as deficiency only in the lower medial quadrant, leaving the inferomedial shaped like an italic S and the inferolateral aspect comparably oversized. Both the inferomedial and inferolateral quadrants are deficient in the type II anomaly, leaving a paucity of skin in the infraareolar segment, which causes the areola to point downward. Finally, in a type III deformity, all four quadrants are deficient, and the breast base is constricted both horizontally and vertically.[14] Von Heimburg describes a second classification scheme for the tuberous breast deformity *(Table 7.2)*. In von Heimburg class I tuberous breasts, there is parenchymal hypoplasia of the inferomedial breast quadrant, similar to that described by Grolleau. The von Heimburg class II tuberous breast is also similar in description to Grolleau's classification, with hypoplasia of the inferomedial and inferolateral breast parenchyma, and an adequate amount of periareolar skin. The third class of tuberous breast described by von Heimburg manifests as hypoplastic parenchyma inferomedially and inferolaterally, but with limited or inadequate periareolar skin. The fourth and final class of tuberous breast deformity described by von Heimburg is presents with hypoplastic parenchyma in all four breast quadrants.[15] Various techniques, such as periareolar nipple-areolar reduction, radial scoring, dermoglandular flaps, autologous and alloplastic augmentation, and tissue expansion, among others, have been used for the correction of this deformity.

Table 7.1 Procedural specifics for forms of breast ptosis

	Inframammary fold position	Parenchymal position	Nipple–areola position	Nipple to fold distance	Clavicle to nipple distance	Clavicle to fold distance
True ptosis	Fixed normal	Fixed rotated	Low downward pointing	Unchanged normal	Elongated	Unchanged normal
Glandular ptosis						
Common	Mobile descended	Mobile descended	Low forward pointing	Elongated	Elongated	Elongated
Uncommon	Fixed normal / Normal	Mobile descended	Low relative to fold	Elongated	Normal to elongated	Unchanged / Normal
Parenchymal maldistribution	Fixed high	Fixed high	Normal downward pointing	Short	Normal	Short
Pseudoptosis[a]	Variable, usually low[a]	Mobile re-descended	Surgically fixed	Elongated	Surgically fixed	Variable, usually elongated[a]

[a]Pseudoptosis is most common after corrective procedures for glandular ptosis where the fold has descended preoperatively. (From: Brink RR. Management of true ptosis of the breast. Plast Reconstr Surg 1993; 91:657–662.)

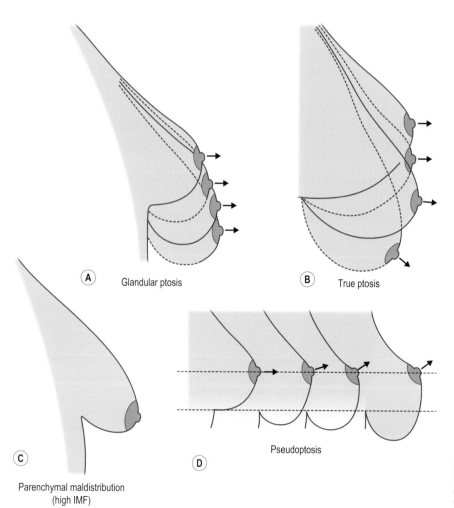

(A) Glandular ptosis

(B) True ptosis

(C) Parenchymal maldistribution (high IMF)

(D) Pseudoptosis

Fig. 7.3 (A–D) Different types of breast ptosis. IMF, inframammary fold. (Redrawn after: Brink RR. Management of true ptosis of the breast. Plast Reconstr Surg 1993; 91:657–662.)

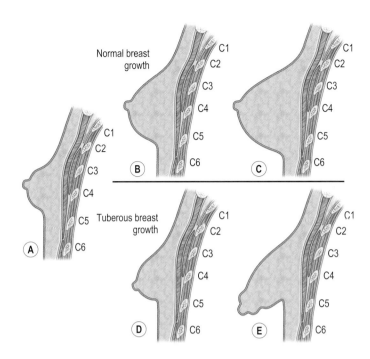

Fig. 7.4 (Top) Normal breast development with forward and peripheral expansion. (Bottom) Development of a tuberous breast, with limited peripheral expansion and exaggerated forward expansion. (Redrawn from: Grolleau JL, Lanfrey E, Lavigne B, et al. Breast base anomalies: treatment strategy for tuberous breasts, minor deformities, and asymmetry. Plast Reconstr Surg 1999; 104(7):2040–2048.)

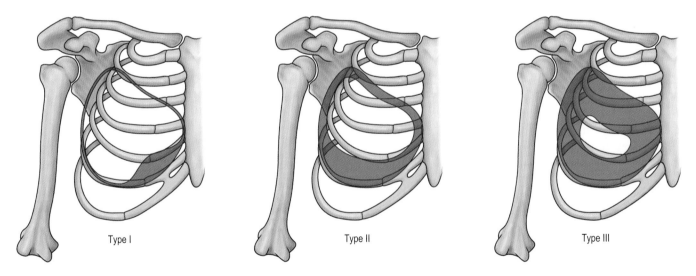

Fig. 7.5 Classification system for breast base anomalies. Type I breasts have hypoplasia of the lower medial quadrant. Type II breasts have hypoplasia of both lower quadrants. Type III breasts have hypoplasia of all four quadrants. (Redrawn from: Grolleau JL, Lanfrey E, Lavigne B, et al. Breast base anomalies: treatment strategy for tuberous breasts, minor deformities, and asymmetry. Plast Reconstr Surg 1999; 104(7):2040–2048.)

Table 7.2 von Heimburg's tuberous breast classification

Class	Anatomic features
von Heimburg class I	Hypoplasia of lower medial quadrant
von Heimburg class II	Hypoplasia of both lower quadrants with adequate areolar skin
von Heimburg class III	Hypoplasia of both lower quadrants with limited areolar skin
von Heimburg class IV	Hypoplasia of all quadrants

(From von Heimburg D, Exner K, Kruft S, et al. The tuberous breast deformity: classification and treatment. Br J Plast Surg 1996; 49:339–345. Reprinted with permission from the British Association of Plastic Surgeons.)

Diagnosis and patient presentation

Patient evaluation

Most patients present for consultations with certain notions as to what they should expect from the operation itself. These predetermined ideas often come from surfing the internet and perusing before-and-after photographic images, in addition to talking to other people who have undergone mastopexy. Analysis by the patient can take into account how pretty or aesthetic the breast is postoperatively, as well as some or all of the aspects a plastic surgeon might evaluate, such as the breast shape, position on the chest wall, nipple areolar complex position on the breast mound, and scarring. Often, this can be helpful during the patient evaluation, answering some preliminary questions and setting a conceptual basis upon which the surgeon can explain the rationale for the technique to be implemented. In cases where patient expectations are out of line with a reasonable outcome, the predetermined notions must be addressed and misunderstandings must be resolved preoperatively. For example, the patient with very large, ptotic breasts desiring to maintain her large breast size in addition to having the breasts be replaced to a more uplifted position will be uniformly disappointed. Without a reduction, the results in this type of patient will not only likely be inadequate with regard to the degree of lift but also with regard to the longevity of the lifted result. So patient expectations are a key component of the patient analysis, and questions to assess these predetermined notions during the evaluation can be helpful to the patient and the surgeon.

Many patients are initially seen requesting implants, thinking that the implants lift the breast. Implants never lift the breasts in and of themselves, and this part of the consultation can be confusing to patients because this counters their preconceived notions. On the contrary, other patients present desiring a breast lift but are advised to get implants by surgeons who may not be confident in their ability to achieve a long-lasting and well-shaped mastopexy. The end result can be an implant breast construct that is too large for the patient's frame and fails to satisfy the patient's goals.

We find that one of the most helpful questions that can be posed to a patient is "can you make your breasts look the way you want them to in a bra?" If the answer is yes, then perhaps a mastopexy alone is the best recommendation. If the answer is no, and the patient relies on adding volume by stuffing or padding, then adding an implant may be necessary. Of course, combinations of small reductions and implants – the "Addition/ Subtraction Concept" – can be a very satisfactory approach.

Discussing the typical pattern of the incisions and the expected scars is important. Patients will often have in mind a smaller scar pattern, hoping for a "lollipop" or "doughnut" lift, instead of the "anchor" scar. These patients may even accept a suboptimal mastopexy in order to avoid additional scar placement. However, if you as a surgeon agree to meet these types of demands, then you should also be aware that if the patient is unhappy later with the result of this trade-off, they may forget about the conversation about shorter scars for a more limited result! The plastic surgeon must take into account the degree of skin laxity, the excess amount of skin in relation to the parenchyma, the position or malposition of the parenchyma, and degree of nipple-areolar complex elevation anticipated – and then incorporate that physical examination information with the patient's history of chest or breast surgery, the patient's history of scarring, including hypertrophic scarring or keloid formation, the patient's desires with regard to scar placement, and the surgeon's experience and technical ability to achieve the most aesthetic and durable result.

Measurements are another key component to the diagnosis and treatment of the patient with breast ptosis. Such marks, such as the sternal notch to nipple distance, define current nipple position on the breast and chest wall and can help define symmetry. The nipple to inframammary fold distance quantitates the skin of the lower breast pole, as well as assisting in defining symmetry. The breast base diameter gives a width of the breast on the chest wall, allowing for implant selection in the case where mastopexy is to be performed in conjunction with augmentation. These measurements, in addition to the classification of the degree of ptosis, can be quite useful in planning, as well as achieving an aesthetic result.

Preoperative breast imaging, in the form of high-resolution digital color photography is another important tool for documentation to demonstrate the degree of preoperative ptosis, as well as the degree of improvement postoperatively. The advent of three-dimensional imaging and computerized image-enhancing software has diversified the options for plastic surgeons to demonstrate to patients the implant sizes, asymmetries, and expected outcomes during consultations, as well as their postoperative improvement. Some of these concepts are covered in greater detail in Chapter 2.

A careful conversation describing the rationale of the pattern to be used and the expected scars can go a long way toward warding off disappointment in the postoperative period. Further, specific counseling as far as the risks, benefits, and alternatives to the proposed surgical intervention should be documented as part of the informed consent. It is often useful to have the patient come back for a second visit prior to surgery, especially in cases where the operation may be delayed for any reason. At that time, the details of the previous evaluation, having been documented in detail, can be easily covered again and any new concerns can be raised and addressed. We use an interactive computerized consultation system that allows the patient to revisit the consultation as well as teaching materials online using any internet connection as often as they wish.

Patient selection

The majority of patients presenting for mastopexy procedures typically fall into three categories: those who indeed would benefit from mastopexy, those who need an augmentation with mastopexy, and those who need a formal reduction mammaplasty. The analysis of the quality and amount of skin in relation to the mass and anatomic distribution of the breast parenchyma usually dictates which procedure is necessary. The ideal mastopexy patient has a normal volume of breast parenchyma and a minimal-to-moderate excess of skin that is of good quality. When patients present with minimal glandular mass and breast ptosis, consideration must be given to the skin amount and quality – as this patient will likely need a mastopexy in addition to an augmentation with an implant, either as combined or staged operations. Conversely, the patient who presents with an overabundance of parenchyma and ptosis will need a breast reduction.

Part of the informed consent process and patient evaluation is a determination of the patient's surgical risk. Risk factors for surgery, such as age, history of recent weight loss, cardiopulmonary health, medications and recent changes to medication regimen, history of stroke, hepatic or renal insufficiency, abnormal bleeding or clotting tendencies, and possibilities the patient is or may become pregnant, etc., must be thoroughly completed and documented. The patient's breast history is important to acquire and completely document and discuss. Any history of breast changes/masses, nipple-areolar changes or discharge, mammography, previous breast surgery, pregnancies and breast-feeding, radiation therapy to the chest or breast, and personal or family history of breast cancer must be explored with the patient in detail. It is the practice of the authors to have patients over 35 years of age obtain a recent mammogram, unless a normal one has been documented in the year prior, before proceeding with surgery.

Treatment/surgical technique

The vast array of surgical options and approaches for mastopexy is best condensed into a classification scheme based on scar pattern. Generally, mastopexy techniques are described by the scar pattern from the skin reduction. There are four basic scar patterns for mastopexy techniques: periareolar, vertical, J or L, and inverted-T. More specifically, however, each of these broad categories of scar pattern has techniques within them that cross the boundaries of this basic classification scheme. This comes as a direct result of the multiple modifications of each technique that surgeons have developed in an attempt to reduce scarring, yet still address the degree of glandular ptosis in relation to the degree of skin quality and excess. The basic tenets for implementation and application of each of the mastopexy techniques, as well as their inherent risk-benefit analysis, are detailed in the following sections, in which the specifics of the techniques are also discussed.

Periareolar techniques

Generally, the periareolar technique is best-suited for patients with mild to moderate breast ptosis and in whom the parenchyma is adequate from a volume standpoint. Firmer parenchyma is preferable to softer tissues in implementing this technique. The incisions for this technique range from a superior crescent of excised skin to a complete donut. Patients who present with mild to moderate breast ptosis but with inadequate parenchymal volume can be treated with an implant via the periareolar technique. The obvious advantage of the periareolar technique, be it for mastopexy, augmentation, or augmentation-mastopexy, which is described later in the chapter, is that the incision is camouflaged in the aesthetic transition from breast skin to the skin of the nipple-areola. Disadvantages of periareolar techniques relate to precise skin excision and ultimately a limited degree of cephalic nipple-areolar complex movement. Other disadvantages include possible scar widening and decreased breast projection. Removal of too much skin leads to an unaesthetic widening of the areola. Widened scars are multifactorial in nature and can be the result of excessive tension on the closure, which can result from the weight of the implant or aggressive skin excision. The patient's skin quality, such as its thickness, elasticity, and degree of aging/damage, can also contribute to widened periareolar scars. Achieving a well-hidden scar and appropriate nipple areolar elevation at the expense of creating an aesthetically-flat, misshapen breast is also not ideal and should be avoided or corrected when possible. Loss of projection with the periareolar techniques, however, can be used to achieve goal the aesthetic in some cases, such as the tuberous breast deformity, but caution must be taken to avoid flattening of the breast.

Small, mildly ptotic breasts with adequate parenchyma respond best to these techniques. Modifications can be made, however, to accommodate moderate degrees of breast ptosis as well as inadequate parenchymal volume using periareolar mastopexy approaches. Typically, the modification required is the addition of a small implant to replace the lacking parenchyma, simultaneously filling the skin envelope. This results in an aesthetic breast mound, though it often can also result in a low-set nipple-areolar complex on the breast. Excising skin around the nipple-areola at the same operative setting elevates the nipple-areolar complex to a more aesthetic location and completes the periareolar mastopexy. Usually, the amount of lift obtained is limited to 1–2 cm.

In an effort to limit complications associated with periareolar mastopexy techniques, Spear et al. designed a series of rules to follow.[16,17]

Rule 1: $D_{outside} \leq D_{original} + (D_{original} - D_{inside})$. The amount of nonpigmented skin excised should be less than the amount of pigmented skin excised. In doing so, there will be no undue tension on the new areola that could cause subsequent widening. This should prevent a postoperative areola larger than the original. The distance from the edge of the areola to the outer diameter located on the normal breast skin should roughly equal the distance to the inner diameter, which should be located within the areola.

Rule 2: $D_{outside} < 2 \times D_{inside}$. The design of the outside diameter should be no more than two times the inside diameter in order to minimize the discrepancy in circle sizes, thereby reducing tension on the closure. This should prevent against an overly-ambitious plan to remove skin, and, as a result, limit the risk of poor scars and overly-flattened breasts. Keep in mind, however, that some leeway exists in the case of skin envelope laxity, the degree of which is ultimately a judgment call.

Rule 3: D_{final} = Rule 3: $D_{final} = \frac{1}{2}(D_{outside} + D_{inside})$. This final rule helps predict the final areolar size, which is particularly useful in asymmetry cases, as well as those in whom no round block suture is employed **(Fig. 7.6)**.

Concentric mastopexy without parenchymal reshaping

The amount of skin to be excised is determined by the position of the nipple-areola complex. One must take care to excise only the amount of skin necessary to raise the nipple-areola complex to the proper level for

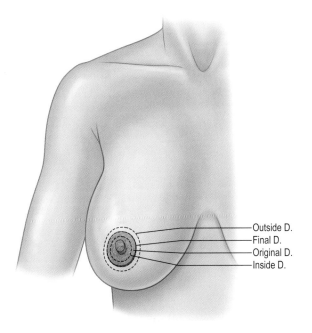

Outside D.
Final D.
Original D.
Inside D.

Fig. 7.6 Periareolar design guides as described by Spear et al. D, diameter. (Modified from: Michelow BJ, Nahai F. Mastopexy. In: Achauer BM, Erikson E, Guyuron B, et al., eds. Plastic surgery: indications, operations and outcomes, Vol. 5. St Louis: Mosby; 2000.)

Periareolar Benelli mastopexy

The Benelli mastopexy technique is an extension of the donut mastopexy that was borne from dissatisfaction with the limitations of the simpler periareolar methods of mastopexy.[18,19] The Benelli modifications allow the periareolar technique to be used to treat larger breasts with increasing degrees of ptosis. This technique can be combined with reduction techniques when necessary to ensure the best possible result while remaining true to the idea of a minimal scar. The fundamental concept behind the Benelli mastopexy is treatment of the skin and the gland as two separate components. The glandular tissue of the breast is accessed through the periareolar incision and separated from the overlying skin component. Superior, medial, and lateral dermoglandular flaps are created, with resection of intervening tissues and thinning of the flaps as is indicated for cases of macromastia. Glandular reassembly consists of reducing the glandular width, tightening the lower pole, and coning the breast construct by crisscrossing the medial and lateral dermoglandular flaps. The skin envelope is redraped over this newly formed glandular scaffold. A round block cerclage stitch is used as in the donut mastopexy to help control tension at the areola-skin junction. As can be seen, this technique allows precise shaping of the breast by the inverted T type of incision through the gland, while requiring no additional incisions in the skin.

Because this technique affords access to the gland, and thus more flexibility in reshaping the gland, the indications for this procedure can be broadened to include patients with larger breasts or greater degrees of ptosis while still satisfying the requirement of minimal scars. It can be used on breasts with minimal glandular tissue by forgoing the glandular incision in favor of plication while simultaneously adding an implant. It can be used as described for larger breasts requiring a modest degree of reduction. This technique, however, is not recommended for breasts that are mainly fat or have a large amount of skin excess, especially if skin is of poor quality. Also, this technique is not indicated in large breasts for which a formal reduction may be the more appropriate procedure. The main advantages are the improved ability to shape the gland and recontour the breast and the commitment to minimizing the scar. The disadvantages of this technique include those of the donut and

correction of the ptosis. Consideration must be given to any excess areola that is to be removed. The lines of excision are marked on the breast with the patient in a sitting or standing position in the preoperative area. Symmetry is checked by comparing sternal notch to nipple distance and sternum to nipple distance. In the operating room, the amount of the areola that is to remain is marked on the stretched breast with an areolar marker. The skin between these two marks is infiltrated with 0.5% lidocaine with 1:200 000 epinephrine to facilitate de-epithelialization. Once the skin is removed, the edge of the dermis can be elevated. At the same time, the remaining skin around the exposed dermis can be elevated off the gland for a short distance superiorly. The freed dermis can then be tacked to the gland under the elevated skin, giving additional support to the breast. A purse-string suture of 4-0 Gore-Tex® or Mersilene is then placed in the deep dermis of the skin edge. This is then cinched to the approximate size of the areola and tied. The areola is then approximated to the skin with half-buried horizontal mattress sutures, followed by a running, subcuticular 4-0 Monocryl or polydioxanone closure.

crescent mastopexies. In addition, care must be taken on incision and reconstruction of the gland to avoid damage to the vascular supply of the gland and overlying skin. There is a significant learning curve associated with Benelli's technique. If there is an over-resection of skin or inadequate glandular support, the breast has a marked tendency toward a flattened appearance along with widening of the nipple-areola complex.

Technique

Preoperative marking is initiated by marking the midline and the estimated meridian of the newly shaped breast with the patient in the upright position. The new meridian is often medial to the breast meridian approximately 6 cm from the midline. The future superior border of the areola, point A, is marked on the meridian approximately 2 cm above the anterior projection of the inframammary fold. The future inferior border of the areola, point B, is marked with the patient supine approximately 5–12 cm above the inframammary fold on the basis of the estimated final breast volume and the expected skin retraction. The medial and lateral limits of the new areola, points C and D, are marked on the basis of estimates of the final breast volume. These limits are equidistant from the previously-marked meridian, and point C averages 8–12 cm from the midline *(Fig. 7.7)*. The opposite breast is marked with reference to the already marked breast. The preoperative markings are verified by pinching together the superior and inferior points and then the medial and lateral points, ensuring that enough skin will remain to adequately cover the breast tissue without tension.

Infiltration with dilute saline (1000 mL), epinephrine (0.25 mg) and lidocaine 2% (20 mL) is performed subcutaneously in the area that will be detached. The ellipse and surrounding 3 cm is not infiltrated to preserve vascularity of the skin edges. The prepectoral area is also infiltrated. The desired areolar diameter is marked, and the periareolar ellipse is de-epithelialized. The de-epithelialized dermis is incised from the 2-o'clock to the 10-o'clock position. The dissection is extended toward the inframammary fold in the subcutaneous plane *(Fig. 7.8)*. The dissection continues to the upper outer quadrant of the breast and becomes more superficial to preserve the vessels coming from the lateral thoracic artery.

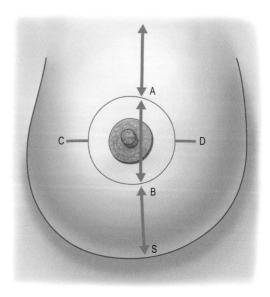

Fig. 7.7 Markings for Benelli mastopexy. **(A)** Future superior point of the nipple; **(B)** future inferior point of the nipple; **(C)** medial limit of the nipple; **(D)** lateral limit of the nipple. Point C averages 8–12 cm from the midline. S is the point where the breast meridian intersects the inframammary fold. (Redrawn after: Benelli L. A new periareolar mammaplasty: the "round block" technique. Aesthetic Plast Surg 1990; 14:93–100.)

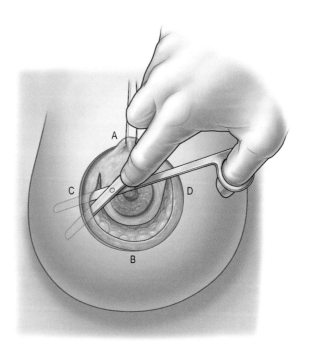

Fig. 7.8 Dissection of the breast during Benelli mastopexy. Incision of dermis from the 2-o'clock to the 10-o'clock position with dissection to the inframammary fold subcutaneously. (Redrawn after Benelli LC. Periareolar Benelli mastopexy and reduction. In: Spear SL, ed. Surgery of the breast: principles and art. Philadelphia: Lippincott-Raven; 1998:685.)

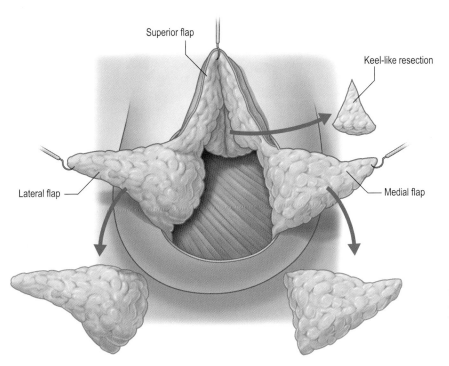

Superior flap

Keel-like resection

Lateral flap

Medial flap

Fig. 7.9 Four flaps of the Benelli mastopexy: superior dermoglandular flap supporting glandular medial and lateral flaps, and detached skin flap. (Redrawn after Benelli LC. Periareolar Benelli mastopexy and reduction. In: Spear SL, ed. Surgery of the breast: principles and art. Philadelphia: Lippincott-Raven; 1998:685.)

Glandular dissection is then initiated with a semicircular incision approximately 3 cm from the inferior areola edge to preserve innervation and blood supply to the areola. Dissection is continued to the prepectoral space in the avascular central space, preserving the peripheral blood supply. The inferior glandular flap is then cut vertically beyond the breast meridian up to the fascia. Four flaps will have thus been created: a superior dermoglandular flap supporting the areola, a glandular medial flap, a glandular lateral flap, and the detached skin flap *(Fig. 7.9)*. These glandular flaps will be reassembled and repositioned to decrease the base of the breast, thus promoting the lifted appearance. If necessary, these flaps can be trimmed to reduce unwanted fullness. Volume reduction should be performed at the distal ends of the flaps to limit their length.

Once the appropriate resection is complete, the gland is initially lifted by placing a stitch in the glandular tissue of the superior flap and fixating this to the pectoralis fascia *(Fig. 7.10)*. This should elevate the areola and cause an exaggerated convexity in the superior pole of the breast *(Fig. 7.11)*. This exaggerated convexity will disappear within a few weeks secondary to gravity and the weight of the breast. Next, the medial and lateral flaps are folded over one another and sutured in place.

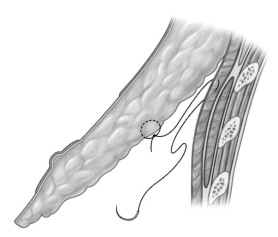

Fig. 7.10 Benelli mastopexy. Attachment of the superior flap to the chest wall by the pectoralis fascia. (Redrawn after Benelli LC. Periareolar Benelli mastopexy and reduction. In: Spear SL, ed. Surgery of the breast: principles and art. Philadelphia: Lippincott-Raven; 1998:685.)

Because most ptosis involves a lateral migration of the breast, the goal here is to medialize the breast. Therefore, the crisscross mastopexy is begun by rotating and folding the medial flap behind the areola, fixing its distal portion to the pectoralis muscle with superficial stitches *(Fig. 7.12)*. The lateral flap is then crossed over and fixed to the medial flap *(Fig. 7.13)*. The movement

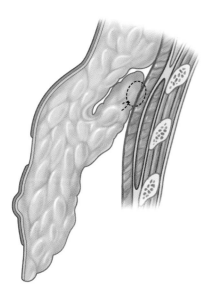

Fig. 7.11 Benelli mastopexy. Superior flap attached to the chest wall demonstrating areolar elevation and exaggerated convexity of superior pole. (Redrawn after Benelli LC. Periareolar Benelli mastopexy and reduction. In: Spear SL, ed. Surgery of the breast: principles and art. Philadelphia: Lippincott-Raven; 1998:685.)

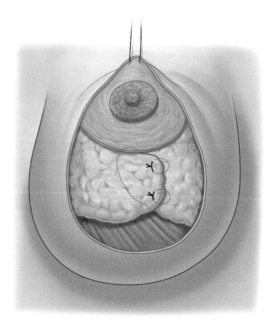

Fig. 7.13 Benelli mastopexy. Lateral flap is affixed to the medial flap. (Redrawn after Benelli LC. Periareolar Benelli mastopexy and reduction. In: Spear SL, ed. Surgery of the breast: principles and art. Philadelphia: Lippincott-Raven; 1998:685.

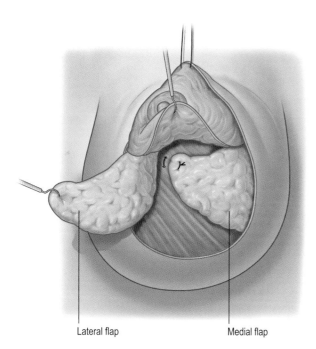

Lateral flap   Medial flap

Fig. 7.12 Benelli mastopexy. Medial glandular flap affixed to the underlying pectoralis muscle. (Redrawn after Benelli LC. Periareolar Benelli mastopexy and reduction. In: Spear SL, ed. Surgery of the breast: principles and art. Philadelphia: Lippincott-Raven; 1998:685.)

of these flaps reduces the base of the breast, forming a glandular cone on which to place the areola. If the gland requires no resection, a plication invagination can be performed to achieve an elevated conical breast shape *(Fig. 7.14)*. The areola is fixated to the superior border of the ellipse through a 1-cm dermal incision made near the superior skin edge. This allows the knot to be buried and the areola to be supported without tension on the skin *(Fig. 7.15)*. Support for the breast shape is achieved by full-breast lacing. Braided polyester suture on a long straight needle is used for the large inverted sutures along the underside of the gland. The superior stitch should pass through the superior dermoglandular flap, allowing control of the anterior projection of the nipple-areola complex. These full-breast lacing sutures should be applied without tension, their goal being to provide passive support of the newly formed conical breast. Tying these lacing sutures overly tight can result in glandular necrosis. The skin is redraped over the breast, and a round block cerclage stitch is passed in the deep dermis in purse-string fashion *(Fig. 7.16)*. It is then cinched around a tube of the desired diameter, ensuring even distribution of the skin pleats. The block stitch is then tied, burying the knot in the previously formed

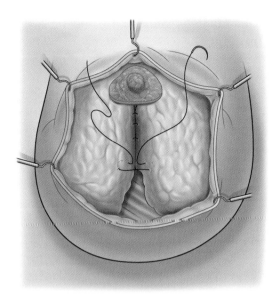

Fig. 7.14 Benelli mastopexy. Plication invagination of the gland to form a conical shape. (Redrawn after Benelli LC. Periareolar Benelli mastopexy and reduction. In: Spear SL, ed. Surgery of the breast: principles and art. Philadelphia: Lippincott-Raven; 1998:685.)

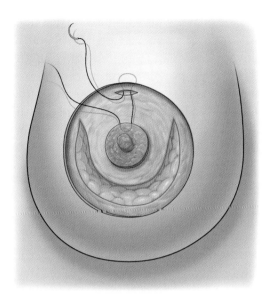

Fig. 7.15 Benelli mastopexy. Fixation of areola to the superior border of the ellipse. (Redrawn after Benelli LC. Periareolar Benelli mastopexy and reduction. In: Spear SL, ed. Surgery of the breast: principles and art. Philadelphia: Lippincott-Raven; 1998:685.)

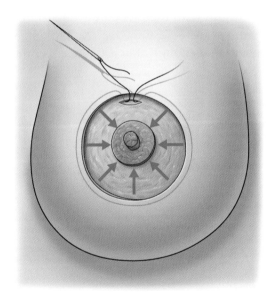

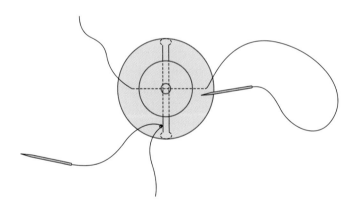

Fig. 7.17 U stitches to help prevent areolar herniation and aid in producing a round shape in the Benelli mastopexy. (Redrawn after Benelli LC. Periareolar Benelli mastopexy and reduction. In: Spear SL, ed. Surgery of the breast: principles and art. Philadelphia: Lippincott-Raven; 1998:685.)

Fig. 7.16 Benelli mastopexy round block suture. (Redrawn after Benelli LC. Periareolar Benelli mastopexy and reduction. In: Spear SL, ed. Surgery of the breast: principles and art. Philadelphia: Lippincott-Raven; 1998:685.)

dermal window. Further regulation of the projection of the areola is accomplished by an inverted dermoarcolar stitch that takes a large vertical bite in the areola and a large horizontal bite in the dermal ellipse. This helps distribute any remaining deep pleats evenly around the areola. A diametrical transareolar U suture is placed to serve as a barrier and help prevent areola protrusion (*Fig. 7.17*). It can also be used to give a circular shape to the areola in those patients in whom it tends to be ovoid. A 4-0 Vicryl intradermal suture around the areola completes the procedure.

Dressings consist of wet compresses on the areola and dry compresses on the detached skin, held in place by an adhesive bandage of moderate compression to reduce hematoma risk. These are removed on postoperative day 2, along with any drains and replaced with a sterile, ultrathin, semi-occlusive polyurethane foam adhesive pad. This dressing covers the areola and scar and maintains all the detached skin in place. This pad will be changed weekly. The patient wears a mammary support bra for 2 months, day and night.

Góes periareolar technique with mesh support

Further expanding the indications for the periareolar technique is Joao Carlos Sampaio Góes of Brazil.[20,21] He introduced the "double skin" technique, in which the basic principle involves formation of a resistant lining of the breast by the use of a layer of prosthetic mesh. This mesh provides increased support of the new breast shape during the healing and skin contraction processes. Like Benelli, Góes treats the glandular unit separately from the cutaneous lining. This method forms an internal brassiere, making use of the anterior pectoral fascia, the intramammary connective ligaments, a periareolar dermal flap (used as internal skin lining), an absorbable mixed mesh, and the external skin lining. Recently, Góes described a variation in his technique, employing the use of a biologic mesh, trilaminate purified porcine collagen matrix, in lieu of woven polypropylene/polyglactin or polyglactin/ Dacron meshes. The rationale for using an alternative mesh is the prolonged duration of the result using the biologic mesh, demonstrating lasting shape and projection for the majority of patients for >5 years postoperatively.[22]

The primary indication for this method is the correction of ptosis or a slight reduction of hypertrophy with or without ptosis. Reductions from each breast ideally should be no more than 500 g. Better aesthetic results can be obtained in younger patients with firmer tissue, more elastic skin, and little fatty tissue. Obesity, as in all periareolar techniques, can be regarded as a contraindication. The main advantages of this technique have much to do with the addition of a mesh layer. The mesh causes a fibrotic reaction that serves to support the breast for a longer time during the healing and cicatrization process. Whereas this goal necessitates a more rigid postoperative breast, which can last for up to 2 months, the gland ultimately does regain its elastic

consistency and normal movement. By the time the mesh is absorbed (in the case of mixed or woven meshes) or integrated (in the case of biologic meshes), the cicatrization that has occurred is strong enough to enable the breast to maintain its new shape against its own weight and the effects of gravity. Breast palpation is normal, and no mesh can be felt by either patient or physician after healing is complete. The main disadvantages of this procedure are the increased technical difficulty and the steep learning curve, in addition to mesh-related complications, such as infection, palpability, retraction, skin necrosis, or extrusion. Although Góes indicates minimal rates of mesh-related complications, there are many opportunities for the inexperienced surgeon to get into trouble. Extreme vigilance in excising the skin flaps and optimal retraction with meticulous placement and securing of the mesh are imperative to prevent suboptimal results and potentially disastrous outcomes.

Technique

The technique is begun with the preoperative marking. Four cardinal points are determined *(Fig. 7.18)*. It is important to ensure that enough skin is left to cover the

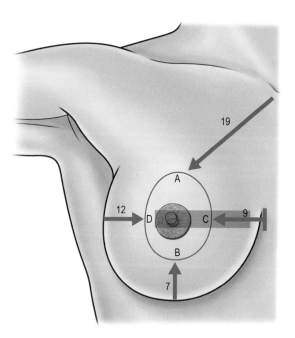

Fig. 7.18 Four cardinal points for the Góes mammaplasty. (Redrawn after Góes JC. Periareolar mastopexy and reduction with mesh support. In: Spear SL, ed. Surgery of the breast: principles and art. Philadelphia: Lippincott-Raven; 1998:697.)

newly formed breast mound. Point A is the level of the top of the new areola. Point B marks the distance from the inframammary fold to the bottom of the new areola (average 7 cm). Point C is the distance from the medial breast border to the medial aspect of the new areola at the level of the nipple (average 9 cm). Point D is the distance from the anterior axillary line to the lateral aspect of the new areola at the level of the nipple (average 12 cm). The area between the areolar and the skin marking is de-epithelialized. An incision is made along the outer ellipse, and the skin flap is developed. The superior dissection proceeds along the base; the thickness of the subcutaneous fat tissue is progressively increased as one gets closer to the base of the breast. Undermining continues over the pectoral fascia for approximately 5 cm superiorly and then inferiorly under the gland approximately one third of the way into the retromammary space. Care should be taken to identify and preserve all perforating vessels *(Fig. 7.19)*. Once the skin and the gland are separated, wedges of tissue can be removed superiorly and inferiorly to accomplish any needed reduction of breast tissue. The base of the mammary gland should not be disturbed. To reassemble the gland, any superior excisional defect is closed, and the gland is fixed to the thorax in a way that fills and elevates the upper pole of the breast *(Fig. 7.20)*. The lower hemisphere excisional defect is then closed and secured to the intramammary connective ligaments and the anterior pectoral fascia. The dermal flap, which has been undermined to the areola, is gently stretched over the gland; it is attached inferiorly to the anterior pectoral fascia when possible and superiorly to the connective ligaments. This dermal component is the so-called internal skin lining *(Fig. 7.21)*. Next, the mixed mesh (polyglactin mesh with Dacron filaments), woven mesh (polyglactin/polypropylene), or biologic mesh is applied over the dermal flap as a brassiere. It is used to give an ideal shape to the parenchymal cone and to elevate the breast slightly. It is sutured to the anterior pectoral fascia. Overcorrection of the breast mound is not necessary and in fact is detrimental because there is no postoperative settling of the breast tissue. The external skin lining is brought up over the breast mound and closed around the areola with a circular continuous deep intradermal suture of Mersilene 2-0 on a straight needle. A continuous, intradermal Monocryl 4-0 suture is used to fix the areola skin to the external skin lining.

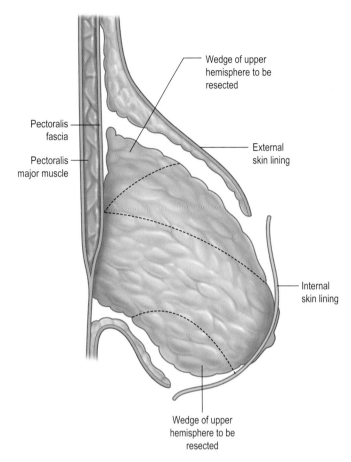

Fig. 7.19 Góes technique. Dissection of the gland to separate it from the skin along with lines of excision of the gland. Note the formation of the internal skin lining. (Redrawn after Góes JC. Periareolar mastopexy and reduction with mesh support. In: Spear SL, ed. Surgery of the breast: principles and art. Philadelphia: Lippincott-Raven; 1998:697.)

Dressings consist of triangular pieces of Micropore tape covering the whole gland, which is left in place for 20 days. Tegaderm also works well for this purpose. Suction drains are removed after approximately 5 days.

Vertical/short scar techniques

As the degree of the breast ptosis increases, so does the total length of the incision necessary to correct it. The logical extension of the periareolar scar is the addition of a vertical component. We believe that some type of parenchymal reconstruction is necessary to create a long-lasting result in mastopexy. There are specific cases where a surgeon may elect not to perform parenchymal remodeling, such as in a contralateral mastopexy for symmetry in breast reconstruction, where follow-up

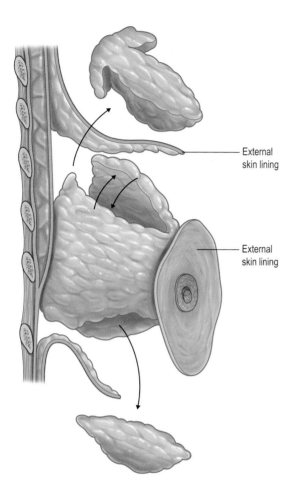

Fig. 7.20 Góes technique. Lines of resection from the superior and inferior hemispheres to narrow the base. Note that mastopexy alone, these regions can simply be imbricated rather than resected. (Redrawn after Góes JC. Periareolar mastopexy and reduction with mesh support. In: Spear SL, ed. Surgery of the breast: principles and art. Philadelphia: Lippincott-Raven; 1998:697.)

imaging may be a concern. In such cases, the surgeon may elect to perform a skin tightening procedure alone by de-epithelializing in the pattern of Wise or in a vertical pattern.

Lassus vertical scar technique

Claude Lassus developed a technique for reduction and mastopexy combining four principles: a central wedge resection to reduce the size of the breast, if needed; transposition of the areola on a superiorly-based flap; no undermining of the skin; and addition of a vertical scar component.[23–26]

The best candidate for this procedure is a young woman with good skin elasticity, a firm, glandular

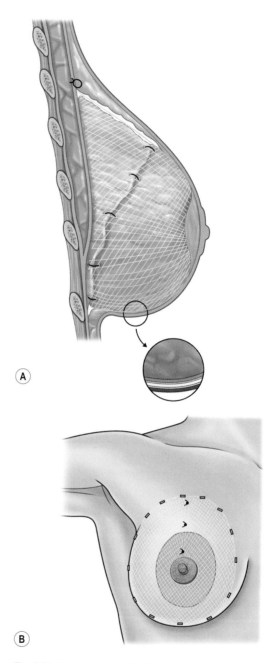

Fig. 7.21 Góes technique. **(A)** The breast projects anteriorly and superiorly after formation of the cone and reinforcement of the breast with mesh. **(B)** Schematic for the placement of mesh. The polyglactin-Dacron composite mesh of Góes' original description is replaced with a Vicryl-Prolene composite. (Redrawn after Góes JC. Periareolar mastopexy and reduction with mesh support. In: Spear SL, ed. Surgery of the breast: principles and art. Philadelphia: Lippincott-Raven; 1998:697.)

breast, and breasts that are not excessively large or ptotic. Lassus cites numerous advantages of this technique. First, the central vertical wedge resection, when necessary, does not impair the blood supply to the gland. Because there is no undermining of the skin from the gland or the gland from the muscle, the vascular perforators are not disturbed, theoretically eliminating the possibility of skin or glandular necrosis. In addition, the use of a superiorly based pedicle to transpose the nipple-areola complex preserves most of the neurovascular supply of the areola, thereby reducing the occurrence of necrosis or decreased nipple sensation. If, however, the nipple-areola complex has to be elevated more than 10 cm, a lateral pedicle as advocated by Skoog is used.[27] A superior pedicle flap would necessarily have to be folded over onto itself, increasing the risk for venous congestion and possible areolar necrosis. Because no undermining is performed, the risk for necrosis of skin and areola is decreased. By joining composite blocks of skin, fat, and gland to shape the breast, subsequent healing produces a solid, fibrous band the thickness of the breast. This becomes the main breast support, ensuring projection helping maintain long-lasting results. Also, because there is no undermining, drains are usually not necessary. A disadvantage of the procedure is the visible vertical scar. Although some would argue that a vertical scar in the standing position may be hidden, and that most of the time it vanishes over the years – it is still a scar on the breast and many woman are not willing to accept this. The patient must also be made aware that the early postoperative breast shape will be less than aesthetically-pleasing and that it may take several months for the breasts to obtain their final shape. Some women may not psychologically be able to wait 3 months or more to obtain a result they can accept. In addition, an important aspect of the procedure is an "adjust as you go" philosophy. Thus, there is an inherent need to remove sutures and revise the breast shape using multiple excisions. Some surgeons may find this removal and replacement of suture lines frustrating. Also, one must be careful not to handle the tissue too aggressively while making these fine adjustments, which can result in problems with wound healing.

Lejour vertical scar technique

Madeleine Lejour derived her variation of the vertical scar technique by modifying concepts from Lassus, Marchac, Arie and Pitanguy.[5,23,24,28–32] This technique uses adjustable markings, a superior pedicle for the areola, and central pedicle reduction where necessary, with lower pole skin undermining. Lejour's modifications can be described by the following three principles: wide lower pole skin undermining to promote skin retraction and to reduce the amount of scarring; overcorrection of the deformity to promote better late results; and liposuction of the breast to facilitate molding and to remove unnecessary fat tissue, which has a tendency to resorb if the patient loses weight and thereby contribute to recurrent ptosis.

The Lejour technique can be used either as a reduction technique or as a mastopexy technique; therefore, it is applicable to many breast sizes and skin qualities. The author points to many advantages of this technique.[33] First, by detachment of the skin from the lower portion of the breast and use of strong subglandular sutures to reshape the gland, postoperative stability is enhanced. Also, the redraped skin can retract over the gland without pressure from the weight of the gland acting against the contraction forces. By performing minimal skin excision, one can avoid over-resection, which can lead to widening of scars and wound complications. The remaining skin is gathered into fine wrinkles to reduce the length of the closure. These wrinkles flatten within a few weeks to months. The resulting scar is limited to the periareolar region with a vertical limb that does not cross the inframammary fold. Nipple sensitivity is preserved by superior pedicle techniques, especially when the base of the upper pedicle is large (as with this technique). Liposuction, which is used when volume reduction of the breast is necessary, is considered by Lejour to be advantageous because it helps make the breast softer, more pliable, and easier to shape. It protects nerves, vessels, parenchyma, and connective tissue while removing breast volume. Suction can be used at the end of the procedure to decrease any tension on the closure. Any noted asymmetry can be corrected before leaving the operating room. Finally, because liposuction removes more fat than other tissue, the resulting breast is less susceptible to recurrent ptosis in cases when the patient experiences subsequent weight loss. This contributes to the stability of the final breast shape. As with the Lassus technique, the major drawback is the amount of time postoperatively before the final result can be realized and appreciated. Both the surgeon and the patient must have patience while the skin retracts, the wrinkles flatten, and the overcorrected breast, with its superior bulge and inferior flatness, evolves to an aesthetically pleasing breast. The author notes that some skin redundancy occasionally remains, which necessitates excision by a horizontal approach. Although this horizontal incision is small, it does add a horizontal component to the resulting scar.

Grotting sculpted vertical pillar mastopexy

With increasingly better results being shown with the vertical techniques of mastopexy and reduction, the authors developed a modification of the vertical technique to produce a beautiful shape with short scars that also minimized complications. The current preferred method has the latitude to allow resection of glandular tissue, if desired, and also the insertion of an implant in either the subglandular or the subpectoral plane if more volume is required. The markings are performed with the patient in the standing position with the arms hanging at the sides. The inframammary fold is marked on both sides. Next, the future nipple position is determined using a combination of reference points. The inframammary fold in transposed onto the anterior surface of the breast. Typically, this point is about 2 cm lower than the point chosen for inverted T techniques. Then, the lower pole breast tissue is gathered to simulate the mastopexy in order to determine if the nipple seems to elevate to the marked point of transposition. Next, the point is cross-checked against the mid-humeral line. The sternal notch to new nipple position is measured, and this typically is 20–23 cm (*Fig. 7.22*). Symmetry between the sides is checked, and, if any measurements are significantly disparate, then appropriate adjustments are made. An important consideration is parenchymal volume asymmetry. In cases where this exists, it is often necessary to mark the A point a centimeter or so lower on the larger side than the smaller side, in order to account for skin recoil after tissue resection. Final nipple position is usually determined intraoperatively after completing the vertical closure.

Hints and tips

Multiple reference points should be used preoperatively to estimate the final placement of the nipple areolar complex. However, it is the intraoperative assessment after closure of the vertical pillars where the final position of the nipple areolar complex is determined.

The next mark is the breast meridian, marked on its anterior surface. The midpoint of the inframammary fold is measured and will be the reference point for creating the marks for the medial and lateral pillars that will approximate at this point after completing the vertical closure. It is preferable to use the standard superior pedicle for the nipple-areolar complex, but if the density of the gland or distance of elevation appears restrictive, the superomedial pedicle recommended by Elizabeth Hall-Findlay is used.[6,7] The medial and lateral pillar lines are drawn by manually distracting the breast tissue medially and laterally. These marks are joined inferiorly by a parabolic line whose lowest-point of the curve is approximately 2–3 cm above the inframammary fold (*Fig. 7.23*). Superiorly, the vertical lines are curved up to the new nipple point. Small inflections of the lines to create a mosque-dome effect can be used to accentuate the future 6-o'clock position on the areolar closure if desired. The top of the vertical closure at this point is pinched approximated to ensure adequate skin will remain for closure. From the top of the vertical closure, one measures down 5–6 cm and makes another mark that will represent the approximate position of the new inframammary fold. The breast tissue below that point will comprise the bottom of the future superiorly-based dermoglandular flap (if the intention of the surgeon is to autologously-augment the patient) or be resected (as in small reductions, with or without an implant). Preaxillary fullnesses and lateral chest rolls may need liposuction to contour and should be marked.

Hints and tips

Contouring the preaxillary fullness and lateral chest rolls with liposuction is an option to further improve breast aesthetics when fatty excess exists in these areas at the same time as the mastopexy procedure. The results are improved and patients appreciate it.

Flap design depends on the need to augment the upper pole of the breast. As mentioned, though, in cases where a small amount of parenchymal reduction is required, this flap represents a readily available source for removal. The volume to be left behind is again approximated, and the resulting shape is visualized (*Fig. 7.24*). If tissue is to be removed (small reduction),

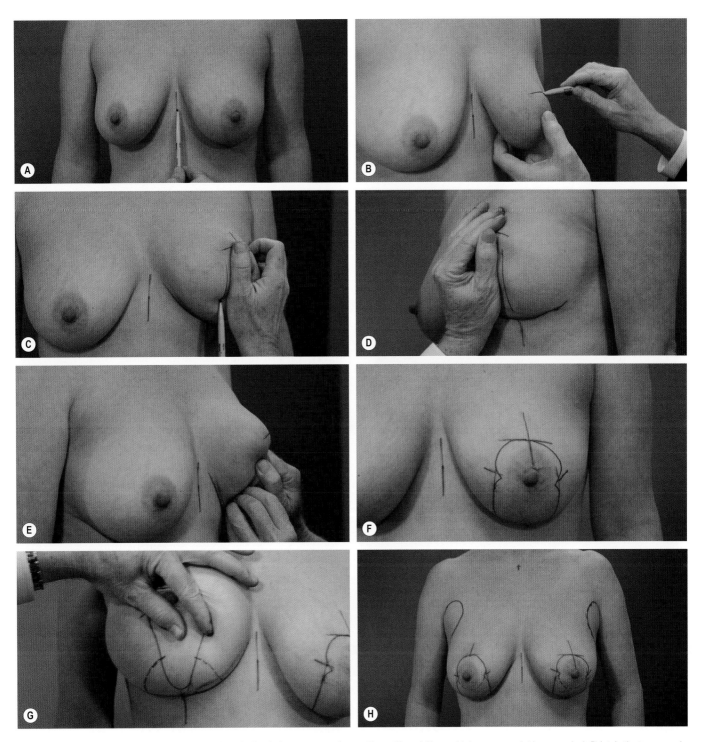

Fig. 7.22 (A–H) Authors' preferred modification of vertical technique, preoperative markings. The midline and inframammary folds are marked. Point A, the transposed location of the inframammary fold, is marked on the breast anteriorly, as is the breast meridian. The breast is then manually distracted laterally and then medially to estimate and mark the medial and lateral vertical limbs, respectively. Points C and D are the cephalic extents of these vertical limbs and will become the bottom of the new areola. Often the vertical limbs can be manually approximated to simulate the mastopexy. The upper curved line represents the new areola boundary and is usually 12–14 cm in length.

the lines should anticipate that, but similarly, if an implant is to be added, the final tension on the closure is a critical factor. The lines are adjusted in or out on the basis of those factors. It is also preferable to mark on the skin surface any inferior glandular tissue that will be resected, much the same way as one would mark this in an inverted-T reduction.

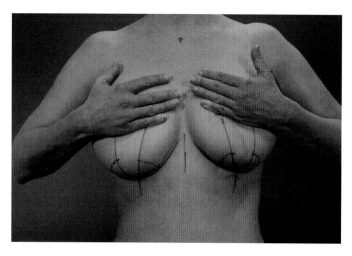

Fig. 7.23 Note the bottom of the incision line coming to a V approximately 2 cm above the inframammary fold (point B). The hatched lines show the location of the glandular resection at the bases of the medial and lateral pillars. A superiorly-based flap can be created from the tissues between the marked medial and lateral pillars, rotated retro-areolarly, and then sutured to the pectoralis fascia to improve upper pole fill.

Technique

Once general anesthesia is satisfactorily induced, we ensure proper positioning on the operating room table. The patient's body should be centered on the operating room table, and the arms should be properly secured and padded to allow the patient to be sat up and the surgeon assess the result intraoperatively. After the patient is prepped and draped, pendulum sutures are placed at the sternal notch and xiphoid areas to enable symmetry later in the operation. Simulated mastopexies using skin staples or Adair clamps can be performed at this point to ensure adequate tissue will remain for vertical pillar closure. The nipple areola is marked with an appropriate sized nipple marker, and then lidocaine 0.5% with epinephrine 1:200000 is infiltrated in the intended lines of incision, areas to be de-epithelialized, as well as beneath the gland. In a straightforward mastopexy, the superiorly-based inferior flap will be completely de-epithelialized and folded underneath the nipple-areola complex to fill the upper pole. It is often necessary to resect the base of the pillars at a level that measures approximately 6 cm from the top of the vertical limb down to the pectoral muscle beneath it. Appropriate projection of the gland left behind prevents recurrence of ptosis. After de-epithelialization of the periareolar skin and that between the medial and lateral pillar marks, the lower pole of the breast is undermined in the subcutaneous plane over that portion of the breast

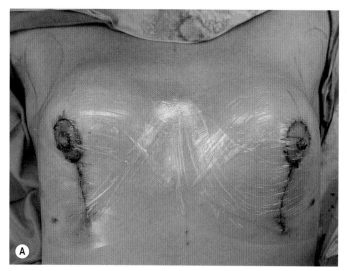
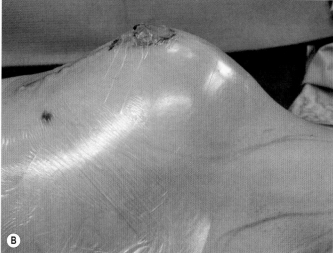

Fig. 7.24 (A,B) Authors' preferred technique. Rounded superior pole, flat lower pole, and slightly downward pointing nipple.

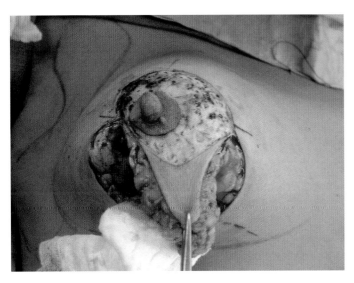

Fig. 7.25 The lower pole of the breast has been detached. The resulting flap may be transposed into the retro-areolar location to augment the upper pole or resected in cases such as a small reduction or when an implant is to be added (addition-subtraction concept).

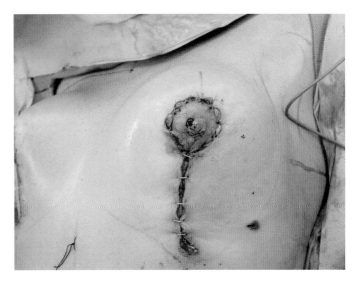

Fig. 7.26 Temporary closure of the breast.

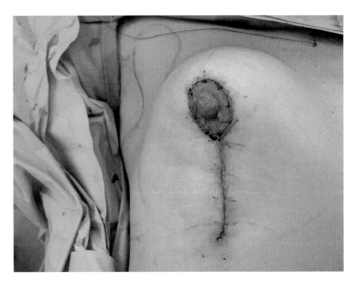

Fig. 7.27 Authors' preferred technique. Rounded superior pole, flat lower pole, and slightly downward pointing nipple.

to be resected inferiorly, if any *(Fig. 7.25)*. The gland is then undermined at the level of the pectoralis fascia from the inframammary fold inferiorly to the superior pole to establish space into which to fold the superiorly based inferior flap. At this point, the bases of the pillars can be trimmed if needed. If this is not the case, then not much medial or lateral undermining is necessary. The flap is sutured into an appropriate position. If no flap is used and the tissue is resected between the medial and lateral pillars, then a suture is used from the undersurface of the gland beneath the nipple-areola complex to the pectoral fascia as high up in the upper pole as possible. This imparts roundness and fullness to the upper pole. In cases where no implant is planned, a "lateral shaping suture" is used to bring the lateral parenchyma at the anterior axillary fold toward the midline of the breast to form an aesthetic curve to the lateral portion of the breast. The medial and lateral pillars are then simply reapproximated with 2-0 Vicryl sutures in the parenchyma and 3-0 polydioxanone as a layered and running skin closure. The nipple-areola complex is exteriorized in its virtual position with the patient sitting up in the operating room *(Fig. 7.26)*. The "on the table" shape is usually one of a flattened lower pole and a rounded upper pole with the nipple pointing slightly inferiorly, creating the so-called "upside-down breast" *(Fig. 7.27)*. The use of Tegaderm to support the

final shape is an important aspect of postoperative care *(Fig. 7.28)*. It should be left on for up to 2 weeks, at which point a bra should be used day and night for 6–8 weeks *(Figs 7.29, 7.30)*.

Authors' preferred technique for augmentation mastopexy

Augmentation mastopexy is the combination of augmentation techniques with mastopexy techniques for the correction of ptosis. Because ptosis is the result of

Video 1

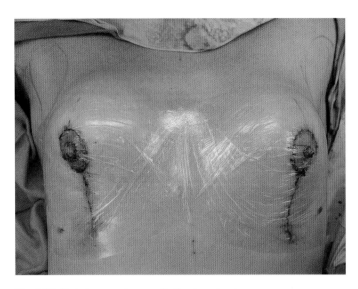

Fig. 7.28 Final closure and cover with Tegaderm dressing.

deficient glandular tissue, excess skin with nipple malposition, or more commonly a combination of both, it makes sense that correction of this deformity would combine a technique that increases breast volume (augmentation) with a technique that decreases the skin envelope and allows repositioning of the nipple-areolar complex (mastopexy). These techniques are by no means for everyone, but they should be included in the plastic surgeon's choice of techniques for the correction of breast ptosis. Many patients want the lift but also prefer the shape created by the breast implant.

Any of the previously discussed mastopexy techniques can be combined with augmentation. The chosen combination will depend on the patient's presenting complaints and anatomy. In general, this technique is most useful for those women with a deficit of glandular

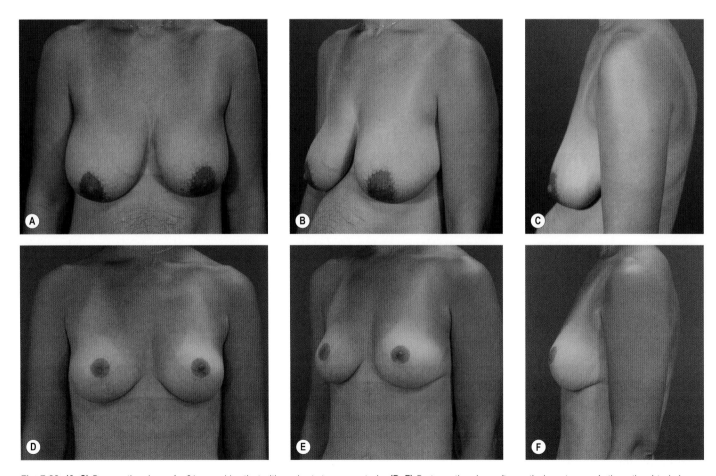

Fig. 7.29 (A–C) Preoperative views of a 31-year-old patient with moderate to severe ptosis. **(D–F)** Postoperative views after vertical mastopexy via the authors' technique.

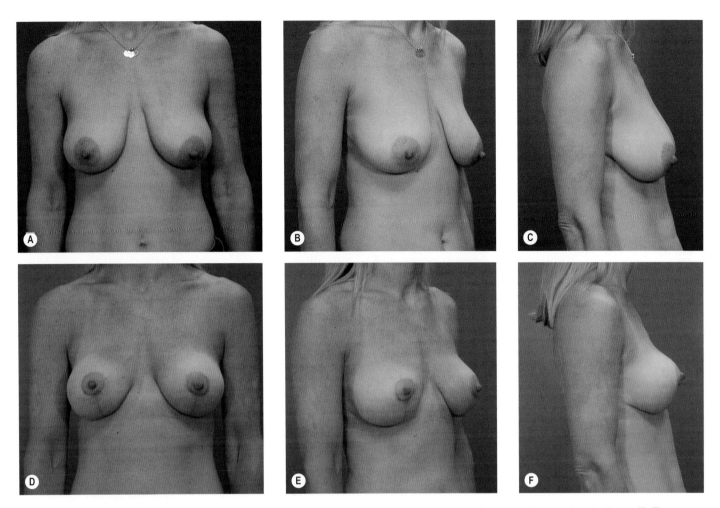

Fig. 7.30 (A–C) Preoperative views of a 37-year-old female with bilateral breast ptosis with asymmetric nipple position but similar parenchymal volumes. **(D–F)** Postoperative views after bilateral vertical mastopexy via the authors' technique.

tissue regardless of the size of the skin envelope. Another good indication is asymmetry when one breast is hypoplastic and the other is ptotic.

The advantages and disadvantages of the mastopexy techniques remain the same, as already noted. However, the added benefits and risks of augmentation mammaplasty must now be considered. Advantages include improved fill of the skin envelope by virtue of the implant, particularly in the superior and superomedial aspects of the breasts. The risks include an increased chance of wound problems and dehiscence because of the added weight of the implant. This creates increased tension on the suture lines, especially in the face of over resection of the skin flaps by the surgeon's incorrectly estimating the final breast volume in light of the implant. The increased risk for wound problems and

dehiscence can be lessened if the surgeon is vigilant and keeps skin resection to a minimum at the beginning of the procedure. Additional skin resection can always be performed at the end of the procedure on the basis of the final volume of the breast with the implant in place. There are also the inherent risks of the implants (malpositioning, leakage, rupture, capsular contracture) and the patient's perceived risks of silicone.[34] The patient has the choice of silicone gel or saline implants if concurrent mastopexy is to be performed. Implant selection for augmentation-mastopexy is different than in augmentation without mastopexy. In general, we scale down the base diameter and projection of implants chosen for augmentation-mastopexy. Selecting a textured surface device may assist in avoiding malposition, especially when the subglandular plane is chosen. If the parenchymal volume is deficient in the upper pole (<3 cm pinch thickness), then we prefer a subpectoral placement. The augmentation-mastopexy is also an excellent situation to improve breast shape, especially in cases of asymmetry. Usually, the ptotic breast has excess lower pole volume and is deficient in the superior pole. Often the asymmetry exists in the lower pole of the breast. A technique we have found quite helpful in cases such as these is to reduce the lower pole parenchyma and augment the breast with an implant – what we call the "Addition–Subtraction Concept." This concept can be applied to several areas of aesthetic and reconstructive plastic surgery and is particularly apropos in the setting of breast ptosis and asymmetry. We find it useful in asymmetry cases to perform a differential lower pole parenchymal resection, followed by placement of an implant to improve upper pole fill and elevate the upper breast border. Even in the symmetric patient, it is often necessary to reduce the lower pole and add an implant to improve breast shape and upper pole fill.

> ### Hints and tips
>
> Lower pole excess and upper pole deficiency are typical findings in breast ptosis. Often asymmetries exist as well, with asymmetry existing in the lower pole tissues. Lower pole parenchymal resections (asymmetric resections in asymmetry cases, symmetric resections in cases of symmetry) combined with implant augmentations, the "Addition–Subtraction Concept'" can be employed to achieve beautiful breast shape and treat these areas of excess and deficiency simultaneously.

Again, the implant is placed in the subglandular or subpectoral position based on the adequacy of the available parenchyma as determined by skin pinch thickness of >3 cm. A further variation on this technique is to use autologous fat grafts in the upper pole to improve upper pole fill in cases where the patient does not desire an implant.

Technique

Augmentation mammaplasty proceeds with marking and incisions according to the mastopexy technique chosen. Once the breast tissue or muscle is exposed, the pocket for the implant, either submuscular or subglandular, can be formed and the implant inserted. The mastopexy can then be completed.

There is one final point that should be carefully considered before augmentation mastopexy, especially in women with severe ptosis in whom a formal Wise-pattern mastopexy is planned – the blood and nerve supply to the nipple-areolar complex and the skin flaps. Surgeons must remain cognizant of the perfusion and innervation in relation to the incisions made for both the augmentation and the mastopexy portions of the procedure. Whereas the neurovascular supply is usually not compromised by formal mastopexy alone, the addition of the augmentation procedure may cause significant alteration in blood supply. Any mastopexy technique that requires wide undermining of skin flaps (e.g., Góes or Benelli techniques) should not be combined with subglandular augmentation because this would almost certainly result in glandular necrosis. With the combination of these two procedures, there is the possibility of a denervated or devascularized nipple-areola complex, breast tissue, or skin flap.

> ### Hints and tips
>
> Careful attention must always be paid to the perfusion and innervation of the breast in mastopexy and augmentation-mastopexy procedures. Whereas the neurovascular supply is usually not compromised by formal mastopexy alone, the addition of the augmentation procedure may cause significant alteration in blood supply. However, mastopexy techniques that require extensive undermining can jeopardize perfusion and should be implemented carefully.

One should undermine judiciously and carefully evaluate the mastopexy technique as it is being performed to help avoid these potential complications. Should there be a suggestion of nipple or skin flap compromise at the conclusion of the procedure, then there are steps that can be taken in an attempt to reverse this process. These include removing the periareolar skin sutures to allow relaxation of the tissues and increased blood supply to the nipple-areola complex. Removal of the implant may be necessary to reduce tension on both the skin flaps and the nipple-areolar complex. This too can sometimes allow increased blood flow to the tissues. Loss of the nipple is a devastating complication for both the patient and the surgeon, and aggressive measures must be undertaken when there is concern about its viability. Nerve damage is difficult to assess immediately postoperatively. Therefore, one must perform careful and well thought out dissection in an attempt to minimize damage to these structures. In one's enthusiasm to treat severe degrees of ptosis, one should not lose sight of the main goal, which is the formation of a well-shaped, well-proportioned, viable breast with intact sensation. Most of the time, this goal can be achieved with proper selection of patients and careful planning and execution of the surgical technique, much to the delight of the patient and the satisfaction of the surgeon *(Fig. 7.31)*.

Mastopexy post-explantation

A woman may request explantation of her breast implants for many reasons.[35] Some women have concerns about the safety of silicone; some have implants that have ruptured or leaked; some have disfiguring or painful capsular contractures; some have malpositioned implants that have not responded to subsequent attempts at correction, and some have implants that have become infected. Other women may present with unaesthetic implant visibility, whereas some may complain of palpability and desire explantation. Finally, there are those women

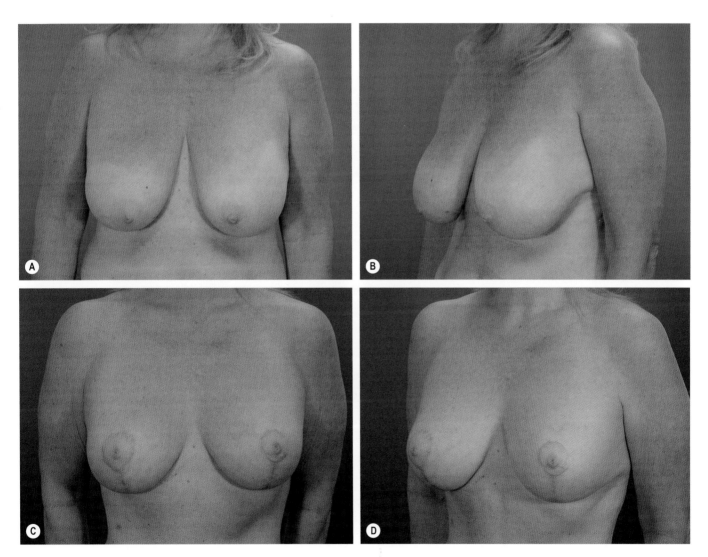

Fig. 7.31 (A,B) Preoperative views of a 44-year-old female post-lapband and a 60 lb weight loss. She had previously-placed oversized subpectoral implants. **(C,D)** Postoperative views after bilateral removal of implants and replacement with subglandularly-placed silicone gel implants in combination with parenchymal resection (Addition–Subtraction Concept).

who after many years no longer wish to be as large as they are.

When an implant is removed, the breast may assume an excessively lax and ptotic position. Often, there will also be a maldistribution of glandular tissue with inferior pole deformities. The potential for this post-explantation result should be included when the explantation procedure is discussed with a patient. The surgeon should also be prepared to discuss procedures that are available to help reshape the remaining breast tissue. This discussion should include realistic expectations of what can be accomplished along with the possibility of needing additional scars to achieve an optimal breast shape. If additional scarring is not acceptable, the patient must be made aware of the probability of a suboptimal result. The surgeon should ascertain the patient's motivation for removal and post-removal expectations. If a woman has had an implant rupture, whether it is silicone or saline, she may merely wish to have it replaced with the same type of implant; if she had silicone implants, she may wish to have both implants removed and replaced with saline, or vice versa. Those women with capsular contractures may opt for replacement, but there are those patients who just want the implants removed. This is similar to those women with malpositioned implants that have not responded to secondary or even tertiary procedures. Then there are those

women who for one reason or another, mostly because of changes in body image, decide after many years to have their implants removed. These women all have the option of explantation alone, explantation with replacement, or explantation with some type of concurrent mastopexy procedure. The women with only one option are those with an infected implant. These women require explantation, irrigation, and drainage. Implant replacement or mastopexy procedures must be postponed until the infection has resolved and the tissues have healed. One other group of women needs to be mentioned here, and these are women who have had implants placed secondary to reconstruction after mastectomy. These women have one other option on explantation, that being reconstruction with autologous tissue (e.g., latissimus dorsi flap, TRAM flap). This subject is beyond the scope of this chapter and is not discussed. The reader is referred to the chapters on breast reconstruction in this book. Our discussion here focuses on those women who wish to have explantation with mastopexy.

A particularly useful technique in the case where mastopexy is planned post-explantation of saline-filled implants is the intentional deflation of the implants preoperatively. We perform this technique in the office under sterile conditions after first placing local anesthetic, which is 1% lidocaine with epinephrine 1:200 000, in the lower pole of the breast *(Fig. 7.32)*. A sterile

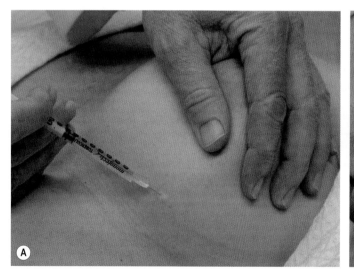
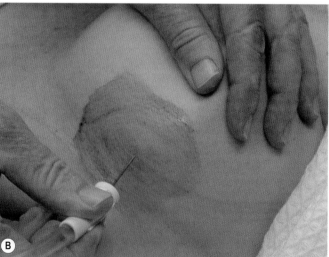

Fig. 7.32 (A,B) Preoperative saline implant deflation. Local anesthetic (1% lidocaine with epinephrine 1:200 000) is infiltrated into the lower pole of the breast, and then the area is prepped with Betadine solution. A sterile 18-gauge needle is attached to sterile suction tubing, and, after allowing analgesia to take effect, the needle is placed through the anesthetized skin, subcutaneous tissue, and parenchyma, into the implant.

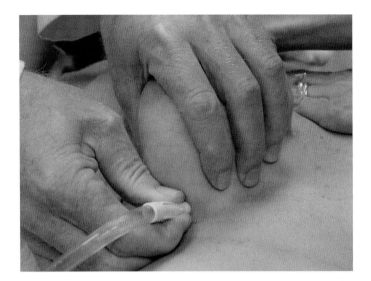

Fig. 7.33 Preoperative saline implant deflation. The right hand guides the needle, holding it in place within the implant cavity, while the left hand compresses the implant and displaces it inferiorly.

18-gauge needle is then attached to sterile suction tubing, and, after allowing analgesia to take effect, the needle is placed through the anesthetized skin, subcutaneous tissue, and parenchyma, into the implant. The right hand guides the needle, holding it in place within the implant cavity, while the left hand compresses the implant and displaces it inferiorly *(Fig. 7.33)*. There are several benefits that this technique affords the patient and surgeon. First, the actual volumes within each implant can be directly measured, thereby giving the patient and surgeon a true reference for implant size selection in cases where implant removal and replacement, with or without mastopexy, is being considered. This is particularly helpful in cases where the patient is not sure of the volumes or when autoinflation of the implants is suspected. Additionally, the preoperative deflation allows the patient to assess how much residual parenchymal volume she has without the implant fill. We recommend deflation approximately one month ahead of the planned surgery to allow the tissues to recoil from the burgeoning and stretch caused by the implant. During this time, we also have the patients evaluate their deflated breasts in a bra to see if they are happy with how much tissue remains. If they are dissatisfied, then an implant will most likely be required in addition to the mastopexy. Often, however, women are very satisfied and frequently happy to be relieved of the volume of the implants.

As with mastopexy procedures in general, the most important component in determining the ability to reshape the gland is the amount of glandular tissue available. In those women with minimal glandular tissue, explantation followed by mastopexy procedures alone will produce a suboptimal result. These women may best be served by some type of augmentation mastopexy procedure. Another option for patients with silicone gel implants would be just to perform the explantation and then allow the skin envelope to contract, a concept similar to that for the preoperative saline implant deflation technique described above. Some of these women may obtain significant improvement after contraction is allowed to take place. For them, a simple nipple-areola complex repositioning procedure may be all that is required to achieve a satisfactory result. Whichever procedure is chosen for reshaping, the neurovascular supply for the nipple-areolar complex must always be considered. The mastopexy procedure chosen must always take into consideration possible alterations to the nerves and vessels secondary to the original augmentation. In some patients, especially when there is little native breast tissue, it may be prudent to perform mastopexy as a delayed operation.

The next issue that needs to be addressed is whether to perform capsulectomy or capsulotomy. Although there are many differing opinions among surgeons and many special situations, in general, capsulectomy should be performed in patients with ruptured silicone gel implants, in patients with severe capsular contracture, or when the capsule contains large amounts of calcium deposits. Otherwise, the capsule, with or without additional capsulotomy incisions, may be left in place to add bulk to the glandular reconstruction.

Technique

Before removal of the implant, the new areolar border is marked. De-epithelialization is performed on the basis of the mastopexy technique. Any of the previously discussed mastopexy procedures may be used. It is usually easier to perform the initial mastopexy maneuvers with the implant in place, and this is the method we prefer. An incision is usually made in the inframammary fold, but a periareolar incision can occasionally be used to gain access to the implant or capsule. If the implant to be removed is silicone and there is suspected leakage of the implant, the capsule is left intact. Dissection proceeds on its anterior surface followed by posterior release from the pectoralis muscle or chest wall, depending on where the implant was originally placed. Dissection is with a combination of cautery and blunt technique. In dissecting anteriorly over the capsule in a submuscularly placed implant, one should take care to avoid the thoracoacromial artery because cautery-induced muscle contraction brings the artery close to the dissection plane. Once the capsule is freed, it is removed totally and intact. The pocket is then visualized and palpated. Any lumps or irregularities are excised for biopsy. The pocket is then irrigated, and the mastopexy portion of the procedure is begun. If the implant to be removed is silicone without evidence of leakage or if it is a saline implant, a total capsulectomy is usually not necessary. An exception to this is the silicone implant that is subsequently found to be ruptured. In addition, if the capsule is calcified to such an extent that leaving it in place would distort the subsequent breast reshaping, a partial capsulectomy is in order. If the capsule is to be left in place, dissection should proceed through the tissues to the capsule. The capsule can be opened and the implant delivered. The capsule should be palpated for calcifications and irregularities, and, if these are found, a partial capsulectomy can be performed. Reshaping of the gland can then be accomplished. Drains are placed, and the skin envelope is closed. The nipple is repositioned and sutured in place.

When sufficient glandular tissue is available, mastopexy after explantation often yields an aesthetically pleasing breast shape. This is most often accomplished by use of a superiorly based dermoglandular flap that is folded back on itself to establish projection and upper pole fill.

Inverted-T technique

The inverted-T or keyhole closure is the technique most-familiar to plastic surgeons trained in the USA.[31,36] The Wise pattern vertical scar with long horizontal scar is based on the reduction technique of the same name.[8,37,38] Regardless of the name, the long horizontal component allows adequate resection of the skin envelope in extremely ptotic breasts.

The inverted T-scar technique is reserved for those women with moderate to severe breast ptosis with a large excess of skin and a moderate amount of glandular tissue. This technique uses the same markings as traditional reduction techniques. However, a reduction procedure is usually not required for mastopexy in these patients. The advantages of this technique are the ability to excise all excess skin and the ability to see the final shape of the breast while the patient is still on the operating table. This allows final adjustments to shape and symmetry to be made before the end of the procedure and decreases the chance that a subsequent revision will be necessary.

The major disadvantage of this procedure is the increased length of the incisions, which increases the length of subsequent scars. The horizontal component usually runs from the most medial aspect of the breast to the most lateral aspect. In no patient should the medial incisions meet or be within 1–2 cm of midline. The risk for hypertrophic scarring is greatly increased in this area, and lengthening the medial extent of these incisions should be avoided. Another potential disadvantage is that the shape of the new breast is supported mainly by the skin envelope. There are no pillars or intraglandular sutures to help support the newly formed breast shape. This lack of internal support increases the chance of recurrent ptosis during the subsequent months and years.

Technique

Markings proceed with the standard Wise pattern. First, the meridian line of the breast is marked. The new position of the nipple is marked along this line at the anterior projection of the inframammary fold. A wire keyhole pattern is spread to allow it to just encompass the original areola. The superior aspect of the pattern is placed approximately 2 cm above the location of the projected nipple position. These markings can be checked by bringing these points together with infolding of the central and inferior skin and assessing tension. Some tension is necessary to com-

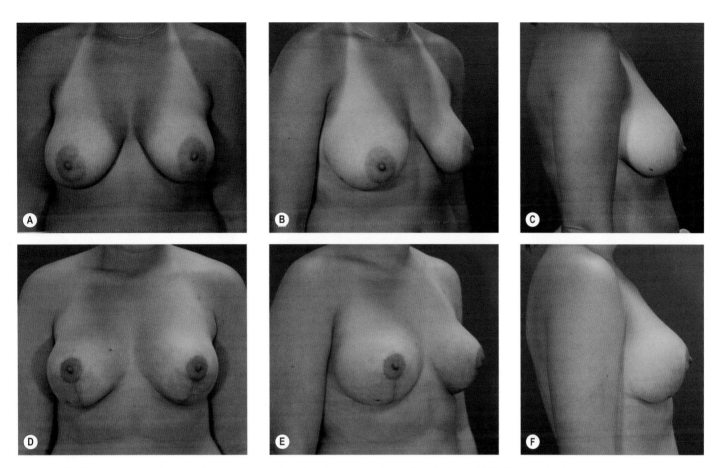

Fig. 7.34 (A–C) A 35-year-old patient with bilateral breast pseudoptosis and asymmetry of parenchymal volume. **(D–F)**, Postoperative views after inverted-T technique mastopexy and asymmetric small reduction of the inferior pole parenchyma.

pensate for the inevitable postoperative relaxation of skin support; however, it should not be so great as to risk ischemia or wound problems or to cause an unnatural tightness to the base of the breast. These vertically-oriented markings are extended laterally and medially on the breast to converge with the inframammary fold.

In the operating room, the portion of the areola to be preserved is marked with an areolar marking device of the appropriate diameter. The area within the marks is de-epithelialized. Transdermal incisions are made along the upper portion of what would be the vertical bipedicle flap of a reduction mammoplasty on either side of the nipple-areola complex. If there is an abundance of de-epithelialized breast tissue below the inframammary fold, dissection of the gland off the pectoralis muscle is undertaken starting from the inframammary fold and

proceeding upward to establish a superiorly based dermoglandular pedicle. The dissection continues until the pocket can accept the excess inferior glandular tissue. This tissue is folded behind the breast and attached to the pectoralis fascia high enough to eliminate gross glandular redundancy. Skin closure is accomplished in standard fashion with little or no further undermining. The nipple-areola complex is positioned and sutured into place *(Fig. 7.34)*.

Postoperative care

Management of the post-mastopexy in the perioperative period has many facets, ranging from medication administration to dressing and drain use to activity limitations and even what type of bra to use. It is typical in the practice of these authors not to continue antibiotic prophylaxis postoperatively after routine mastopexy. Perioperative intravenous antibiotics covering skin flora, such as the first generation cephalosporin cefazolin or alternative in the case of allergy, are given less than an hour prior to incision and are typically all that is required. Postoperative narcotic analgesics are typically used as needed within the first week or two after surgery, counseling the patients on side-effects such as sedation and constipation, among others, and recommendations for care in those circumstances are given in a preoperative packet. Antiemetics, such as the selective 5-HT3 receptor antagonist ondansetron or the phenothiazine H-1 receptor antagonist promethazine, are usually used for postoperative nausea and vomiting. It is the practice of the authors to dress the breasts in Tegaderms applied without stretch to decrease shear forces and blistering. The Tegaderms have aperture at the nipples that allows oozing to drain out onto gauze pads held in place by a postoperative brassiere. These Tegaderms are left in place for 2 weeks after surgery. Scar care is begun at 3 weeks after surgery, with over-the-counter scar treatments that are then transitioned to silicone sheeting, which is continued for up to a year or more as indicated. Drains are rarely used in typical mastopexy cases. Postoperative brassieres are used for at least 8 weeks after surgery, in an effort to support the new breast as the postoperative edema begins to egress. Exercise by the patient is minimal in the first week or so after surgery, which is typical while postoperative pain begins to improve. During the second week, mild activities such as walking can be initiated. During the third week, elliptical trainers or stationary bicycles can be used without the adjunctive use of the upper body lever arms that are available at some gymnasiums. Full-on running or activities that tend to cause vigorous up and down motion of the new breasts are restricted until 8 weeks postoperatively. Though exceptions can sometimes be made in certain circumstances, rigorous adherence to minimizing pectoralis muscle activity in augmentation mastopexy patients, especially reoperative cases, must be maintained to protect the integrity of the internal sutures against the weight of the implant. Capsular displacement or massage exercises are not recommended in cases where textured devices are used or reoperative cases.

Outcomes, prognosis, complications

Although most mastopexy procedures produce a higher-positioned and shapely breast that pleases most patients, there are complications that may require revisional procedures. These include nipple loss, unacceptable scars, flap necrosis, nipple malposition, and cosmetic disappointments. In the event of any of these complications, secondary procedures to correct any shortcomings should be made available to the patient. The primary goal, however, is to avoid any of these adverse sequelae.

Nipple loss

Nipple loss is one of the most devastating complications that can happen to both patient and surgeon. The incidence of nipple loss by various techniques is reported to be less than 10%, usually in the range of 0–5%. In addition to technical errors, nipple loss can be predicted by a variety of patient factors including smoking, diabetes, obesity, and hypertension. Minimizing risk for this complication begins with proper selection of patients and technique. In high-risk patients (smokers, patients with diabetes or obesity, or those with severe ptosis), a free nipple graft technique is an option that can be considered. This is also a possibility intraoperatively or postoperatively if the viability of the transposed nipple appears compromised. Until approximately 12 h postoperatively, the compromised nipple-areolar complex may be converted to a free nipple graft. This, of course, assumes that a satisfactory dermal bed can be found to accept the nipple graft. After 12 h, conservative treatment of any nipple necrosis should be undertaken, including release of sutures, topical nitropaste or leeches, greasy dressings, hyperbaric oxygen therapy (if available), and appropriate antibiotic therapy. Many times, conservative treatment and closure by secondary intention produce a satisfactory result. Whereas the usual rule with ischemic tissues is early sharp débridement, in nipple necrosis, debridement should be delayed as long as possible. If healing does not produce a satisfactory result, the nipple-areola complex can be reconstructed by standard reconstruction techniques ranging from simple tattooing of the areola to flap reconstructions of the nipple itself.

Scars

Although scars are an inherent part of any surgical procedure, their final quality cannot be predicted. Ironically, those who are the least concerned with scarring (i.e., elderly women with thin skin) tend to have scars of the best quality, whereas those who are most concerned with their scars (i.e., young women 16–25 years of age, especially those with darker, thick, acne-prone skin) tend to have the worst scarring results. Obviously, the best way to minimize the occurrence of poor quality scars is to minimize the incision. The surgeon can help with this by choosing the proper mastopexy technique, by proper execution with gentle skin handling, by minimal or no tension on the wound, and by minimizing the incisions where appropriate. Once healed, prominent scars may first receive a trial of vitamin E, compression with tape or silicone sheeting, laser treatment, or intralesional triamcinolone (Kenalog) injections. In some situations, particularly bad scars can be resected, followed by a precise and careful closure. It is preferable to assess patients for scar revision after 1 year.

Flap necrosis

Flap necrosis can occur by virtue of the flaps used, especially when the inverted-T or Wise-pattern mastopexy technique is used. The lateral flap is most commonly affected secondary to the substantial undermining required in this region to allow proper shaping of the breast. Although excessive tension is thought occasionally to play a small role, most flap loss is primarily ischemic. Treatment is similar to that of the ischemic nipple: greasy dressings, hyperbaric oxygen, or antibiotics. Débridement of large areas of flap necrosis should be undertaken when they are clearly demarcated. Delayed closure can be performed, thereby avoiding weeks or months of caring for an open breast wound. Small areas of skin necrosis (1–2 cm) may be treated conservatively, especially along the inframammary fold.

Nipple malposition

Although there are many formulas and methods to determine nipple position (i.e., sternal notch to nipple distance, inframammary fold to nipple distance, nipple to sternal distance, and mid-humeral position), none is perfect and nipple malposition may occur. This type of result can cause a patient's disappointment with the procedure no matter how well shaped the newly constructed breast is or how well the incisions have healed. The nipple should be properly situated on the breast, at or near the point of greatest projection, with ample but not an excessive amount of tissue underneath it.

When malposition of the nipple occurs, one can attempt to reposition it; however, one should wait at least several months to allow complete healing of the breast and nipple-areolar complex. The tissues should be soft and supple. It is easier to raise the nipple-areolar complex than to lower it. If the nipple-areola complex is too low, then a small crescent of skin can be removed above it that will result in an elevated nipple-areolar complex. More often, all the incisions must be reopened and the skin envelope tightened.

Nipples that appear too high can be caused by one of two situations. The breast may have bottomed-out – and if this has occurred, a simple tissue resection can be performed inferiorly with use of the already present vertical and horizontal incision sites. If a high-riding nipple is the result of incorrect positioning, this is a more complex problem. One can attempt to lower the nipple by one of a series of maneuvers including V-Y advancement inferiorly, transposition as a flap, or transfer as a graft. Regardless of the method used, a scar superior to the areola will be produced. This scar will be subject to the same potential problems as are other breast scars. In addition, a scar above the nipple-areolar complex, regardless of how well it heals, is not particularly aesthetic and will not be well accepted by the patient.

Cosmetic disappointments

Regardless of the technique, the goal of mastopexy is to produce attractive, symmetric, higher-positioned, fuller breasts. In some instances, this goal is not reached. Over-resection, under-resection, and healing complications can contribute to cosmetic disappointments. Under-resection can easily be corrected by additional tissue excision. Over-resection, however, presents a more disturbing problem that may require placement of an implant for correction. Residual tissue deformities secondary to infection, hematoma, or fat necrosis may require additional surgery for excision of resultant lumps and bumps to produce a breast with a soft, smooth contour.

Cosmetic problems may be apparent immediately postoperatively, or they may take weeks and even months to become evident. Although it is not always possible to avoid these cosmetic disappointments, one should do everything one can to keep them from occurring. In the majority of patients, mastopexy is a useful and rewarding procedure for both the patient and the surgeon.

Other complications

Complications such as infection and hematoma also may occur, though their incidence is uncommon. The main point for decreasing their incidence is minimizing risk for their occurrence. In the case of hemorrhage, stopping anticoagulants and antiplatelet medications prior to surgery in a timeframe appropriate to the specific medication is helpful in minimizing risk. Often, these medications are held for a week or so postoperatively. Controlling hypertension intraoperatively and postoperatively is also important, as is meticulous hemostasis intraoperatively, in reducing complications from hemorrhage in mastopexy. Should significant hemorrhage occur, early surgical intervention is warranted, with evacuation of hematoma and ensuring hemostasis. Infection is also a relatively infrequent complication due to vigilance in administration of perioperative antibiotics, which is typically one intravenous dose given prior to incision but no longer than one hour prior to incision.[39] Early recognition and appropriate management, whether oral antibiotics or incision and drainage with intravenous antibiotics based on sound surgical principles, represent classic management of infectious complications.

Secondary procedures

Secondary procedures are sometimes necessary after mastopexy and related operations, and they may be indicated in cases of infection, hematoma, scarring, or an unacceptable cosmetic result, to name a few. Each complication has its own particular method of management, which have been detailed in their dedicated segments in the preceding section of this chapter. The unifying theme, however, in addressing complications in mastopexy and procedures related to mastopexy, is minimizing risk. Understanding and adhering to sound anatomic and surgical principles is paramount. Thorough history and physicals, and holding or continuing medications that may portend bleeding, wound healing, or other risks, are important in reducing the occurrence of these complications. Discussing with anesthesia providers any concerns, such as controlling blood pressure and redosing antibiotics in a specific timeframe, may reduce risk in certain circumstances. Ultimately, secondary procedures are necessary, but our primary objective is to prevent their occurrence.

Access the complete references list online at **http://www.expertconsult.com**

5. Lejour M. Vertical mammaplasty and liposuction of the breast. *Plast Reconstr Surg*. 1994;94:100–114.
   From 1989 to 1994, the author has used vertical mammaplasty without a submammary scar for all breast reductions. Using a technique relying on adjustable markings, an upper pedicle for the areola, and a central breast reduction with limited skin undermining, the author achieves a breast whose shape is created by suturing the gland and does not rely on the skin. A personal series of 100 consecutive patients (192 breasts) operated on from 1990 through 1992 is reviewed, and mastopexy was performed in 39 breasts. Among the 153 breasts that required reduction, liposuction was attempted as a complementary procedure before the surgical reduction in the 120 fattest breasts. Between 100 and 1000 cc of fat (mean 300 cc) was suctioned in 86 breasts. This figure represents 50% of the large breasts in patients under 50 years old and 100% of the breasts in patients older than 50 years. There were few complications, and none required early reoperation. This series proves that vertical mammaplasty can be used in all cases of breast reduction, producing consistently good, stable results with limited scars. The adjunctive use of liposuction in fatty breasts can be considered safe and efficient.

6. Hall-Findlay EJ. A simplified vertical reduction mammaplasty: shortening the learning curve. *Plast Reconstr Surg*. 1999;104:748–763.

7. Hall-Findlay EJ. Pedicles in vertical breast reduction and mastopexy. *Clin Plast Surg*. 2002;29(3):379–391.

15. von Heimburg D, Exner K, Kruft S, et al. The tuberous breast deformity: classification and treatment. *Br J Plast Surg*. 1996;49:339–345.

16. Spear SL, Kassan M, Little JW. Guidelines in concentric mastopexy. *Plast Reconstr Surg.* 1990;85(6):961–966.

In an effort to limit complications associated with periareolar mastopexy techniques, Spear et al. designed a series of rules to follow. Rule 1: $D_{outside}$ ($\leq D_{original} + (D_{original} - D_{inside})$). The amount of nonpigmented skin excised should be less than the amount of pigmented skin excised. This should prevent a postoperative areola larger than the original. Rule 2: $D_{outside} < 2\times D_{inside}$: The design of the outside diameter should be no more than two times the inside diameter in order to minimize the discrepancy in circle sizes, thereby reducing tension on the closure. This should prevent an overly ambitious plan to remove skin, and, as a result, limit the risk of poor scars and overly-flattened breasts. Rule 3: $D_{final} = \frac{1}{2}(D_{outside} + D_{inside})$. This final rule helps predict the final areolar size, which is particularly useful in asymmetry cases, as well as those in whom no round block suture is employed.

18. Benelli L. A new periareolar mammaplasty: the "round block" technique. *Aesthetic Plast Surg.* 1990;14:93–100.

The round block acts as a keystone element to support the reshaped breast. The keystone relies on a crisscross mastopexy and by a circular nonresorbable suture of woven nylon included in the periareolar circular dermal scar. The crisscross mastopexy is achieved via dermis-to-dermis, gland-to-gland, and gland-to-musculoperiosteal unions, all of which are fixed definitively with nonresorbable suture. This technique can be used in many different breast cases, such as that for correction of ptosis, hypertrophy, or hypomastia, among others. In cases of hypomastia, the use of the round block technique permits easy access for insertion of the prosthesis as it simultaneously corrects ptosis. In cases of tumor excision, the round block produces a discrete scar and a more regular breast contour. In all types of mammaplasty, the main goal is to limit the scar

20. Góes JC. Periareolar mammaplasty: double skin technique with application of polyglactine or mixed mesh. *Plast Reconstr Surg.* 1996;97(5):959–968.

23. Lassus C. Breast reduction: evolution of a technique. A single vertical scar. *Aesthetic Plast Surg.* 1987;11:107.

Patients had become more critical about the result of a breast reduction operation over the past 20 years. Natural and lasting shape, as well as minimal residual scarring, is now expected by most of the patients undergoing that surgery. In 1969, the author described a vertical technique that achieved reduction and good shape but the end of the vertical scar could be seen below the brassiere line. In 1977, the author modified the technique by adding a small horizontal scar that eliminated the visible part of the vertical scar. In this article, the author demonstrates that the same technique he described in 1969 and modified in 1977 can produce a single residual vertical scar if properly used.

30. Marchac D, Olarte G. Reduction mammaplasty and correction of ptosis with a short inframammary scar. *Plast Reconstr Surg.* 1982;69:45.

37. Wise RJ, Gannon JP, Hill JR. Further experience with reduction mammaplasty. *Plast Reconstr Surg.* 1963;32:12.

In 1955, the senior author (Wise) presented a new technique for reduction mammaplasty using special patterning devices, and this publication demonstrates the further experiences of the authors. The author's technique allows rapid design of skin flaps and predictable size, contour, symmetry, and nipple position, all of which are difficult to achieve using a free-hand design. A four quadrant form is placed after designing and shaping the skin flaps, and the excess breast tissue is removed via wedge-shaped excisions. Care is taken not to remove too much from the central breast axis and the nipple, as well as not to undermine the skin flaps, to maintain perfusion of all these areas. The results allow for correction of varying degrees of ptosis and breast hypertrophy, as evidenced by case examples.

39. Steinberg JP, Braun BI, Hellinger WC, et al. Timing of antimicrobial prophylaxis and the risk of surgical site infections: results from the Trial to Reduce Antimicrobial Prophylaxis Errors. *Ann Surg.* 2009;250(1):10–16.

8.1

Reduction mammaplasty

Jack Fisher and Kent K. Higdon

SYNOPSIS

- Macromastia, or mammary hypertrophy, is a disease process that can result in physical and psychological symptoms.
- Macromastia symptoms rarely improve without surgical intervention, which typically results in significant improvement in the patient's quality of life.
- Reduction mammaplasty techniques have evolved over millennia, with particularly great strides made in the last 100 years.
- Currently, there exist several well-designed techniques based on sound surgical principles to address macromastia via reduction mammaplasty.

Introduction

Patients with mammary hypertrophy can present with a variety of symptoms. Typical complaints include neck and back pain, shoulder grooving from bra-straps indenting the skin, headaches, difficulty finding well-fitted clothes and limited ability to exercise. Psychosocial issues surrounding excessively large breasts also exist, creating a focal point for embarrassment for women, especially teenagers and elderly women. Often, women with mammary hypertrophy experience intertriginous skin maceration and other rashes, as well as infections – all the result of heavy, pendulous breasts.[1] Netscher et al. evince that macromastia patients' symptoms are better defined with regard to the constellation of their symptoms rather than the volume of excess breast tissue

that need be removed. Further, their work shows that disease-specific group of physical and psychosocial complaints are more directly related to large breast size than to being overweight.[2] Kerrigan et al. showed that the symptoms associated with macromastia represent a significant health burden, and that nonsurgical interventions such as weight loss and special bras do not allay these symptoms.[3] The main purpose of breast reduction is to address these symptoms and, in doing so, improve the quality of life of the women who suffer from mammary hypertrophy. Blomqvist et al.[4] investigated the health status and quality of life of patients who underwent reduction mammoplasty. They conducted a prospective questionnaire study in 49 women who were 20 years or older, using preoperative and postoperative assessments at 6 and 12 months. The questionnaire included four parts: part I assessed pain in the neck, shoulders, back, breast, bra strap indention, and head, whereas part II assessed effects of breast size and weight on body posture, sleep, choice of clothing, sexual relations, and working capacity; part III assessed preoperative expectations for the operation in comparison with postoperative result using a scale of 1–6; part IV consisted of an international health-related quality-of-life questionnaire, the SF-36, which was standardized for the Swedish women queried in the study. The authors found that reduction mammaplasty provided significant reduction of pain in all locations ($p < 0.001$), with an average weight of resected tissue being 1052 g.

Furthermore, the improvements continued up to 12 months postoperatively. The patients' main subjective problems related to the size and weight of the breast were body posture and choice of clothing, and the authors demonstrated significant improvements of all subjective problems ($p < 0.001$) except sleep. The patients' expectations were met to a high extent, and, in some areas such as intimate situations, femininity, and social contacts, the results exceeded the preoperative expectations. Preoperatively, the mammaplasty patients scored significantly lower ($p < 0.05$ to $p < 0.001$, depending on area) in SF-36, which indicated patients had lower quality of life compared with women in the same age group. Postoperatively, patients reported a significantly improved quality of life. These results were similar at 6 and 12 months, indicating long-term improvement. After 1 year, there was no statistically significant difference between the post-reduction patients and the age-matched unoperated women, which suggested those women were normalized in health-related quality of life.[4]

Though the symptomatic improvement of patients suffering from mammary hypertrophy is the primary goal of reduction mammaplasty, there is another goal that is nearly as equally important – creating a more aesthetic breast. In fact, Spear describes the reduction mammaplasty as "the clearest example of the interface between reconstructive plastic surgery and aesthetic plastic surgery."[1]

This chapter seeks to demonstrate the most popular techniques for reduction mammaplasty, with descriptions of each technique's inherent indications, patient selection process, surgical technique, postoperative care, outcomes, complications, and secondary procedures. Each technique may have principles that are somewhat similar or divergent from the others presented. The critical commonalities that exist between and must be employed in all techniques for reduction mammaplasty, however, are sound surgical principles, knowledge of breast anatomy and preservation of perfusion. It is not the intent of this section to promote or advocate one method over another. Rather, the goal is to present each of these techniques so that the plastic surgeon may evaluate and select the one most appropriate for themselves and their patients. Patient and procedural selection are critical components of a successful surgical outcome as well as accomplishing consistent and optimal results. Each surgeon, through their own experience, learns methods of enhancing results which may work with one technique but not another. The key point for choosing the reduction mammoplasty technique is finding what works for you, the surgeon, and what gives your patients the best results.

As breast reduction procedures have evolved, certain goals have been consistent. Among these are an aesthetic, natural breast shape and maintaining that shape long term. Another important goal has been reducing scar length. Of these goals, however, aesthetic breast shape remains of paramount importance; an operation that creates a breast with an unacceptable shape, despite using short scars, is not a success. Unlike many surgical procedures, breast reduction has a long, established history. Thus, it is relevant to review some of the history to understand how we have arrived at today's procedures.

History

One of the earliest descriptions of breast reduction is from the writings of Paulus Aegenita, who described a detailed account of what is thought to be the first surgical correction of gynecomastia in the 7th century AD.[5] Adams' translation from Greek of Aegenita's treatment of gynecomastia is illustrative:

Wherefore, as this deformity has the reproach of effeminacy, it is proper to operate upon it. Having, therefore, made a lunated incision below breast, and dissected away the skin, we unite the parts by sutures. If the breast incline downward, owing perhaps to its magnitude, we make in it two lunated incisions, meeting together at the extremities, so that smaller may be comprehended by the larger, dissecting away the intermediate skin, removing the fat, we use sutures in like manner.[6]

One of the first cases of reduction mammoplasty in a female patient was submitted by Dieffenbach in 1848,[7] who reduced the lower two-thirds of the breast via an inframammary fold incision. Later in the 19th century, Pousson described a superior wedge resection technique that addressed both ptosis and excessive mammary parenchyma in cases of macromastia.[8] From the end of the 19th century to the beginning of the 20th century, there were many approaches to reducing

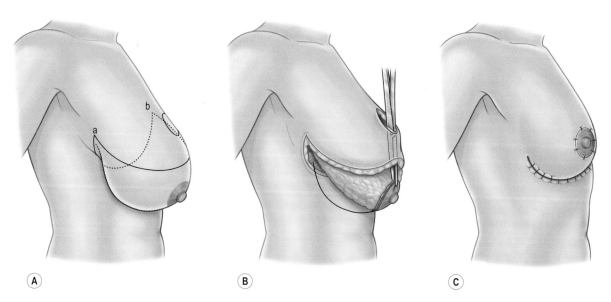

Fig. 8.1.1 Passot technique of nipple transposition. **(A)** Preoperative markings. The solid lines mark the incisions on the anterior breast skin and proposed nipple transposition site; the hatched lines mark incisions along the inframammary fold; points a and b mark the lateral and medial extents of these incisions for the anterior breast as well as for the inframammary fold. **(B)** The breast after parenchymal resection and deepithelialization of the inferior pedicle carrying the nipple-areola complex. The nipple-areola complex is being delivered into the position for final inset, which was marked preoperatively and has since been excised as a circular core of tissue. **(C)** After final closure and inset of the nipple-areolar complex, the result is a reduced breast with periareolar and inframammary fold sutures and no vertical scar. (Redrawn after Lickstein LH, Shestak KC. The conceptual evolution of modern reduction mammaplasty. Operat Tech Plast Reconstr Surg 1999; 6:88–96.)

breast tissue, which, more often than not, actually attempted to correct breast ptosis. Various techniques for skin and parenchymal resections were used, but none employed transposition of the nipple-areola until Morestin in 1909.[9] Resections of up to 1400 g were being reported in this time frame, mostly using an inframammary approach, such as that described by Morestin and Guinard.[10]

The 1920s saw the advent of more reliable operations in the work of Thorek, Aubert, and Passot.[11–13] Thorek published his breast amputation technique in 1922, which consisted of a lower pole amputation and free nipple graft. His technique is still used with some modifications even today for extremely large breasts.[11] The next year, Aubert put forth his technique for reduction mammoplasty, which emphasized the import of minimizing dissection of the skin overlying the breast parenchyma to minimize vascular complications.[12] In 1925, Passot described transposition of the nipple-areolar complex into a buttonhole incision more cephalically on the breast mound, which results in no vertical scar on the reduced breast *(Fig. 8.1.1)*.[13] The late 1920s and early 1930s continued to offer technical advances in reduction mammoplasty. Schwarzmann posited that the perfusion and viability of the nipple-areolar complex could be improved if a ring of dermal tissue was left around it, thereby allowing more successful transposition of the

nipple-areola. This innovative idea is the forerunner of the various reduction mammoplasty techniques used today that base the nipple-areola on a dermoglandular pedicle *(Fig. 8.1.2)*.[14] Another vanguard event in the history of breast reduction came with Biesenberger, who was the first to develop a reproducible parenchymal pedicle-based technique with a "cut as you go" skin resection pattern *(Fig. 8.1.3)*.[15] The procedure results in an inverted-T scar and relies heavily on wide subcutaneous undermining with folding of the breast pedicle. Though it was lauded for its reproducibility, Biesenberger's technique resulted in high rates of skin and nipple necrosis. Yet it remained one of the most popular techniques well into the mid-20th century.

Advances in reduction mammoplasty continued in the 1940s and 1950s with the concept of preoperative planning being brought to the forefront by Aufricht, Bames, and Penn.[16–18] In 1949, Aufricht stressed preoperative geometric planning for parenchymal resections, rather than working free-hand intraoperatively. His technique centered on a superior parenchymal resection, supplying the nipple-areola on an inferior pedicle but preserving lateral and medial pillars and their inherent perforators. Further, he emphasized the importance of redraping the skin after parenchymal resections in reduction mammoplasty.[16] Bames reported his experience with a similar technique, noting the significance of

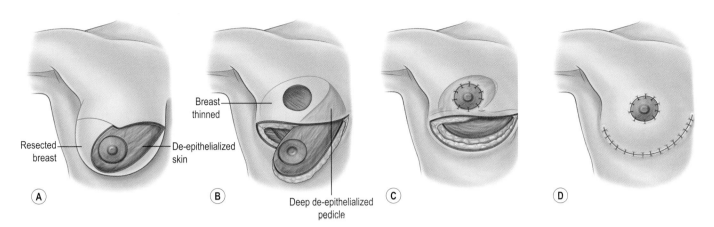

Fig. 8.1.2 (A–D) Schwarzmann reduction with superomedial dermoglandular pedicle. (Redrawn after Lickstein LH, Shestak KC. The conceptual evolution of modern reduction mammoplasty. Operat Tech Plast Reconstr Surg 1999; 6:88–96.)

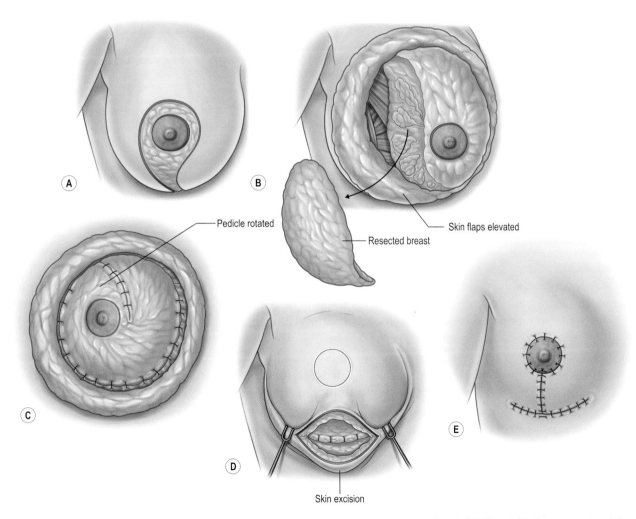

Fig. 8.1.3 (A–E) Biesenberger reduction – degloving the breast with inverted T closure. (Redrawn after Lickstein LH, Shestak KC. The conceptual evolution of modern reduction mammoplasty. Operat Tech Plast Reconstr Surg 1999; 6:88–96.)

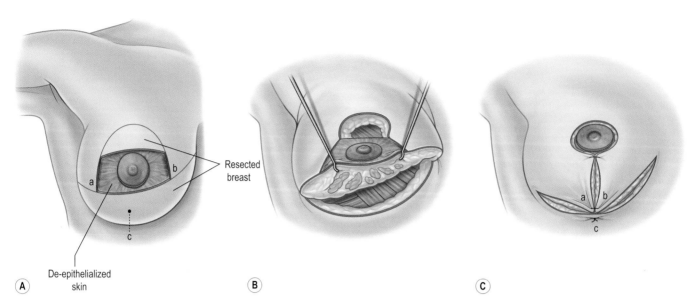

Fig. 8.1.4 Strombeck horizontal bipedicle technique. **(A)** The creation of a horizontal bipedicle allows for resection of parenchyma above and below the pedicle. The image depicts the deepithelialized horizontal bipedicle shown in pink on either side of the nipple-areolar complex. The solid semilunar line above the horizontal bipedicle and the parenchyma below the horizontal bipedicle will be resected. Point a, the confluence of the horizontal and vertical incisions of the lateral breast; point b, the medial breast analog; point c, the point along the inframammary fold incision at the breast meridian. **(B)** The breast after superior and inferior parenchymal resection, creating a horizontal bipedicle to carry the nipple areolar complex, before inset and closure. **(C)** Inset of the nipple-areolar complex into the area of superior parenchymal resection. The skin of the remaining breast after resection is brought together to cone the breast and allow for final closure. This is accomplished by suturing in an inverted-T type closure the tip of the lateral breast skin flap (point a) to that of the medial breast skin flap (point b) and finally to point c on the inframammary fold. Inframammary fold, periareolar, and vertical incision final sutures complete the closure. (Redrawn after Lickstein LH, Shestak KC. The conceptual evolution of modern reduction mammoplasty. Operat Tech Plast Reconstr Surg 1999; 6:88–96.)

preoperative markings in planning parenchymal resections.[17] Aesthetic concepts of nipple areolar complex position were introduced by Penn in 1955, noting that sternal notch-to-nipple distances should be 21 cm and the nipple-to-nipple distance should be the same – to form an equilateral triangle.[18] In 1956, Wise employed these concepts of preoperative marking, geometric parenchymal resections, and nipple-areolar complex placement, when he introduced his keyhole pattern of skin resection. Ultimately resulting in an anchor or inverted-T shape, the Wise pattern of breast reduction became the most reliable and reproducible breast reduction technique and remains one of the most popular techniques to this day.[19]

The 1960s and 1970s saw vast and different approaches toward the end of improving the pedicle in breast reductions. Strombeck demonstrated a horizontal bipedicled flap to maintain the nipple-areolar complex in 1960, thereby capitalizing on the work of Aufricht and Bames (medial and lateral perforators for perfusion, as well as innervation) and Schwarzmann (dermoglandular pedicle) *(Fig. 8.1.4)*.[20] The superolateral dermoglandular pedicle was described by Skoog in 1963, whereas Pitanguy and Weiner described superiorly-based dermoglandular pedicle some 10 years later in 1973 *(Fig. 8.1.5)*.[21–23] Orlando and Guthrie devised the technique of the superomedial dermoglandular pedicle shortly thereafter in 1975, with an eye on maintaining upper pole volume.[24] In 1977, Courtiss and Goldwyn, and Georgiade, among others, made advances in inferior pedicle techniques *(Fig. 8.1.6)*.[25–28] Five years prior, McKissock modified Strombeck's horizontal bipedicle technique into a vertical bipedicle technique. This required thinning of the superior and inferior portions of the bipedicled flap to allow folding, and resultingly does not have as much perfusion as other techniques *(Fig. 8.1.7)*.[29]

The result of the previous decades' developments in breast reduction surgery – Wise pattern skin resection with multiple pedicle options – was labeled in the 1980s as the "gold standard" because the results obtained were reliable, reproducible, and useful for breasts of nearly all shapes and sizes. Modifications and additions were still being made to the cadre of pedicle options for the Wise pattern skin resection technique of breast reduction in the 1980s, such as Hester's central mound technique *(Fig. 8.1.8)*.[30] But the years of experience and

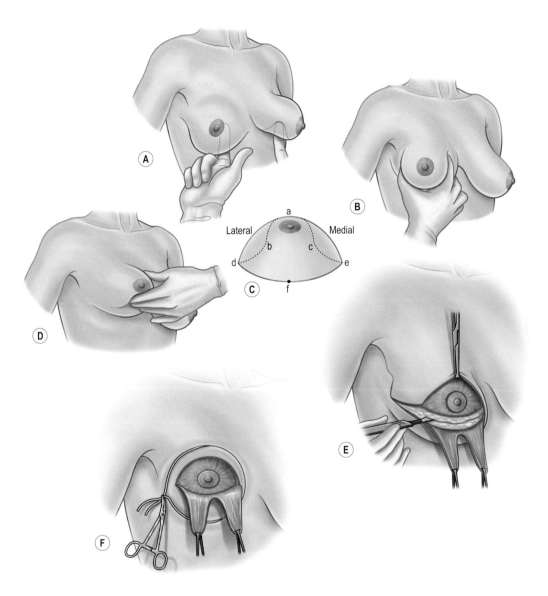

Fig. 8.1.5 McKissock vertical bipedicled dermoglandular flap with Wise-pattern skin excision. (Redrawn after Lickstein LH, Shestak KC. The conceptual evolution of modern reduction mammoplasty. Operat Tech Plast Reconstr Surg 1999; 6:88–96.)

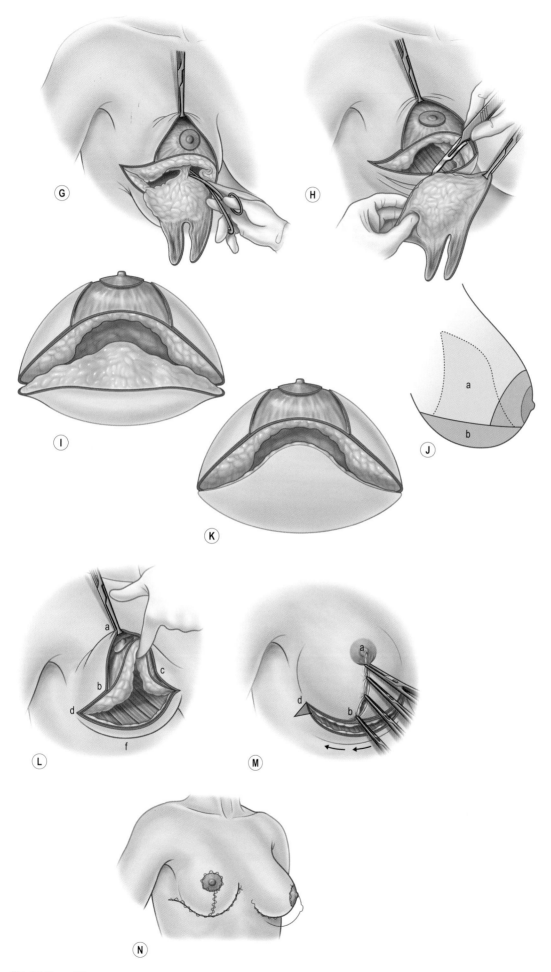

Fig. 8.1.5, cont'd

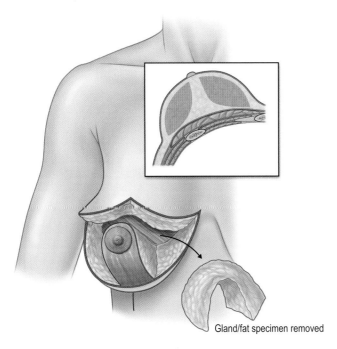

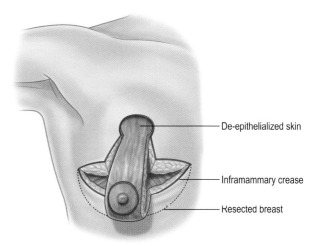

Fig. 8.1.7 Inferior pedicle technique with Wise pattern excision. (Redrawn after Lickstein LH, Shestak KC. The conceptual evolution of modern reduction mammoplasty. *Operat Tech Plast Reconstr Surg* 1999;6:88–96.)

Gland/fat specimen removed

Fig. 8.1.6 Inferior pedicle technique with Wise-pattern skin excision.

follow-up after these reduction procedures demonstrated that the reduced breasts tended to bottom out and lose upper pole fullness *(Fig. 8.1.9)*. This problem actually had been anticipated in previous decades. Orlando and Guthrie, originators of the superomedial pedicle, had devised their approach in an effort to augment the upper pole and thereby reduce bottoming out *(Fig. 8.1.10)*. Another surgeon had devised a technique along the lines of the same ideology – reducing the lower pole to prevent descent. But when Claude Lassus developed his technique in 1970, he did so using a vertical scar with no transverse skin component. Initially, Lassus noticed that the caudal extent of his vertical tended to migrate below the new inframammary fold of the reduced breast.[31] He later added a small horizontal scar along the inframammary fold, but subsequently noticed that the small "T" at the caudal extent of the vertical limb ultimately contracted cephalically onto the lower pole of the breast. Lassus then made a second revision of his technique to leave only a vertical scar that would remain above the inframammary fold.[32,33]

Many other plastic surgeons worldwide began to develop techniques for reduction mammoplasty using short scar and superiorly-based pedicles through the 1980s and 1990s, such as Lejour, Marchac, Peixoto, Góes, and Benelli, among others.[34–39] Techniques to avert the vertical scar, such as the technique of Passot, have been "rediscovered" by various authors in the 1990s and 2000s, including Lalonde, Matloub, and Pribaz.[40–42] Hammond's SPAIR technique for breast reduction employs a short scar skin technique but does use an inferior pedicle, whereas nearly all other short scar techniques implement a superior or superomedial pedicle. Hall-Findlay's variation of the Lejour technique modifies the placement of the nipple-areolar complex pedicle from the superior position to the medially-placed position and uses no skin undermining or adjunctive liposuction.[43] These techniques have helped reduce the tendency of "bottoming out" as well as create breasts with projection and minimal to no transverse scars at the inframammary folds.[9]

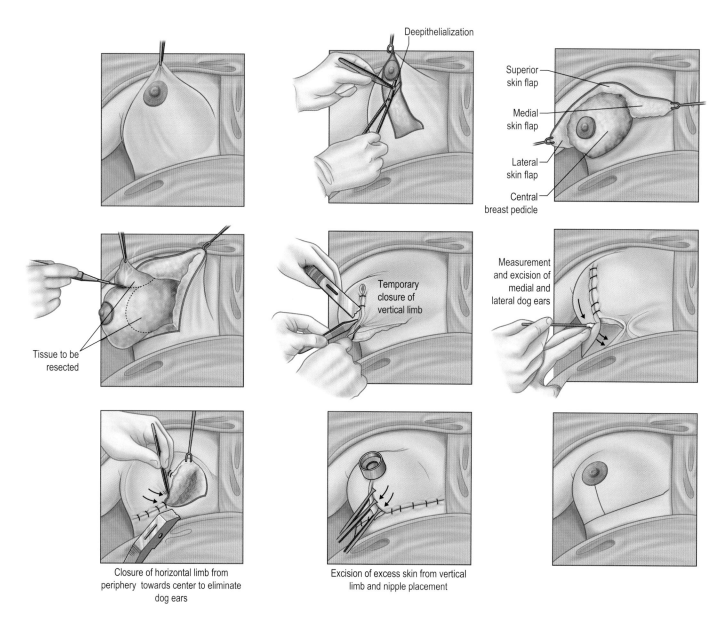

Fig. 8.1.8 Central mound technique popularized by Hester. (Redrawn from Hester TR Jr, Bostwick J III, Miller L. Breast reduction utilizing the maximally vascularized central pedicle. Plast Reconstr Surg 1985; 76:890–900.)

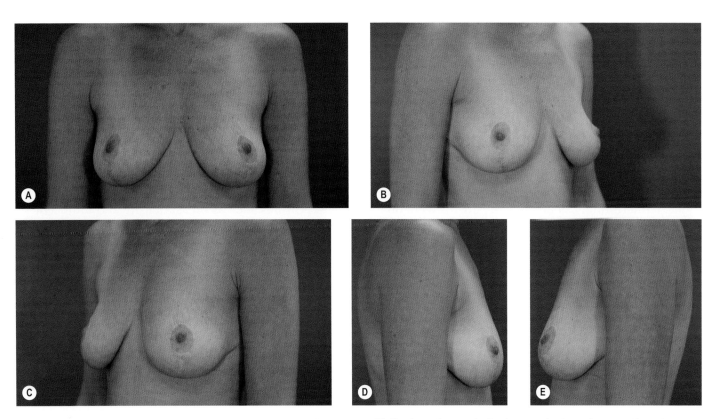

Fig. 8.1.9 (A–E) Postoperative view of a young woman after inferior pedicle with Inverted-T skin closure breast reduction demonstrating bottoming out and loss of upper pole fullness.

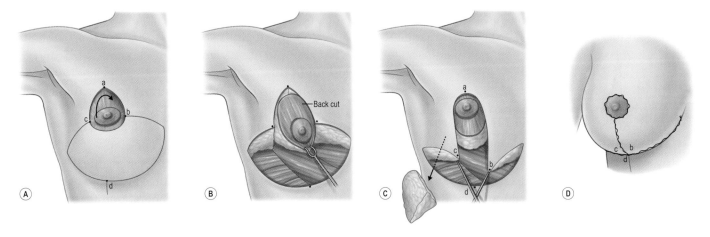

Fig. 8.1.10 (A–D) Superomedial pedicle with Wise-pattern skin closure.

Basic science

Mammary hypertrophy

The pathophysiology of mammary hypertrophy is thought to be the result of an abnormal response of the breast to circulating estrogens, causing breast prolifera-tion which is predominantly fibrous tissue, fat, and, to a lesser degree, glandular tissue. Most women with mammary hypertrophy have normal circulating levels of estrogen as well as normal numbers of estrogen receptors in the breast tissue.[44,45] Details with regard to the embryologic development and anatomy of the breast are detailed elsewhere in this book.

Eliasen *et al.* demonstrated a predominance of atypical ductal hyperplasia in nine patients with macromastia, who ranged in age from 18 to 26 years (average 21 years). Though unable to find any significant gross abnormalities within the resected breast tissue except for two fibroadenomas, the authors were able to demonstrate that each case had a continuum of microscopic ductal changes, which ranged from partial to complete involvement by micropapillary and lactiform epithelial hyperplasia. These changes were sometimes markedly atypical. Interestingly, none of these patients went on to infiltrating ductal carcinoma, with a follow-up that averaged 39 months.[46] In cases of obesity, however, there is an association with increased oncologic risk.[9,47]

Cases of juvenile virginal hypertrophy of the breast can be seen as early as late childhood and often is present in the age range of 11–14 years of age.[9,45] Durston is credited with reporting the first case of juvenile virginal breast hypertrophy in 1670. The young woman in this case actually died at age 24, and, upon post-mortem examination, she was found to have a right breast that weighed 64 pounds and had no evidence of disease.[48,49] Gigantomastia is a condition in patients with mammary hypertrophy that is defined by their need to have over 1800 g of tissue resected. The treatment for these patients is surgical reduction. Recurrence in these patients also poses a significant risk, and the standard treatment in such cases is secondary reduction mammoplasty.[9,45]

Diagnosis/patient presentation

Patient evaluation

Careful consideration of the factors that compel patients to seek reduction mammaplasty are key in the plastic surgeon's assessment of patients with mammary hypertrophy. As noted previously, patient complaints can range from the psychologic, with embarrassment or even depression, or somatic, with neck or back pains, rashes, etc. A thorough history of symptoms associated with mammary hyperplasia should be undertaken. A personal and family history of breast disease and surgery should be taken, and the results of any testing, such as mammography, breast ultrasound or MRI, and BRCA testing should be obtained prior to surgical intervention. Current data shows mammography to be

the only screening tool proven in randomized controlled trials to decrease mortality rates from breast cancer. The American Cancer Society's guidelines for early detection of breast cancer recommend annual mammograms starting at age 40 and continuing for as long as a woman is in good health. A clinical breast examination (CBE) is recommended annually for women 40 and over, and every 3 years for women in their 20s and 30s.[50] Mammography has been criticized as having a low sensitivity, potentially not detecting up to 35% of malignant cases. Features such as breast density and multicentricity or multifocal lesions are thought to be the cause.[51] Though able to provide adjunctive information to mammograms, as well as enabling guidance in biopsy techniques, ultrasound has been proven inferior to mammography as a screening tool. This stems from a high false-positive rate, operator variability and no standardized technique, as well as inability to demonstrate micorcalcifications.[52] The American Cancer Society recommends some women be screened with MRI in addition to mammograms, especially in cases of strong family history or genetic tendency such as breast cancer gene (*BRCA*) mutation positivity, as it is more sensitive than mammography, ultrasound, and clinical breast examination alone.[50,53] Cancer detection in women with silicone augmentations can be challenging, as silicone-induced mastopathy can be mistaken for malignant changes, and vice versa. In these cases, MRI may be useful to differentiate the changes associated with silicone implants from those resulting from malignancy.[54]

In addition to screening, a thorough physical examination should be performed as well, noting any relevant points of the patient's general condition as well as an examination of the breast. At least in the USA, only some breast reduction procedures are considered medically necessary. Such salient general points relate to the patient's height, weight, and habitus, and these measures are often mandatory for insurers to calculate the amount of breast tissue they require for the reduction procedure to be covered. This amount of tissue can, however, vary from state to state and from insurer to insurer. Some insurers use an absolute mass for resection based on the patient's height. Others use calculations using the patient's height and weight, such as the Schnur Sliding Scale, to approve or reject patient's insurance claims for breast reduction. The Schnur Sliding Scale was developed using the findings reported by

Schnur *et al.* in 1991 after analyzing the surveys of plastic surgeons looking. In their study, 92 of 220 plastic surgeons that responded to their survey included information (height, weight, and amount of breast tissue removed) from 600 women regarding the last 15–20 reduction mammaplasties by each surgeon. A second survey followed to estimate percentages of women who sought reduction mammaplasties for purely cosmetic reasons, for mixed reasons, and for purely medical reasons, and 132 of the same 220 surgeons responded. The second survey showed that all women whose removed breast weight was <5th percentile sought the procedure for purely cosmetic reasons, and all women whose breast weight was >22nd percentile sought the procedure for medical reasons. Women whose parenchymal resections fell between the 5th and the 22nd percentiles had mixed reasons for requesting the procedure.[55] It is common for many US health insurers, as a result, to only approve patients whose resected weights fall above the 22nd percentile based on the Schnur Sliding Scale or some modification thereof. Most plastic surgeons agree that the basis of this formulaic approach is flawed as a result of the inaccuracies inherent in merely using height and weight to calculate resection masses. In fact, other formulas have been derived to allow a more precise estimation of weights. Appel *et al.* performed a retrospective analysis of 348 patients undergoing bilateral reduction mammaplasty (696 breasts) between October 2001 and March 2009. The association between resection weight and sternal notch to nipple distance (SNN), inframammary fold to nipple distance (IMFN), and body mass index (BMI) was assessed. Using regression analysis, Appel *et al.* demonstrated a strong correlation between resection weight and SNN distance ($r = 0.672, p < 0.001$); IMFN distance ($r = 0.467; p < 0.001$), and BMI ($r = 0.510, p < 0.001$). The strongest correlation, however, was observed after incorporating all three parameters ($r = 0.740, p < 0.001$), and this enabled the calculation of a formula to predict resection weight: predicted weight = 40.0(SNN) + 24.7(IMFN) + 17.7(BMI) − 1443. They concluded that resection weight correlates strongly with SNN, IMFN, and BMI in patients undergoing reduction mammoplasty, and, when considered together, resection weight can be predicted with a great degree of accuracy.[56]

A focal breast examination is mandatory as well, evaluating for any masses of the breast, axilla, and supra- and infraclavicular fossae. The nipple-areolar complex should be assessed for changes or discharge, as well as its preoperative sensitivity. Some women have decreased sensitivity due to prior surgery, but often there is decreased sensitivity due to the excess weight of the breast causing traction injury to the cutaneous innervation of the nipple-areolar complex. The skin of the breast should be scrutinized to assess for stigmata of previous operations or physiologic changes, such as scars or striae, which should be pointed out to the patient preoperatively. The scars are important for surgical planning or pedicles and skin resections, and striae can often become even more visible post reduction mammoplasty. Finally, shape and symmetry of the breasts preoperatively must also be assessed and pointed out to the patient, especially in cases of very large breasts, because some degree of asymmetry will virtually always remain postoperatively. This is typically not a source of major concern to most patients, as they are happy to have the burden of the excess breast weight removed, especially when the preoperative asymmetry has been demonstrated to them before surgery. Breast measurements, such as the sternal notch to nipple distance, the nipple to inframammary fold distance, and the nipple to nipple distance, must be documented preoperatively. This allows the surgeon to appreciate subtleties of symmetry and size that may have otherwise gone unnoticed. The ideal numbers for the breast are derived from the Penn numbers described earlier in this chapter. Typically, the ideal sternal notch to nipple distance usually is between 19 and 22 cm, though it can be more than twice as much or larger in cases of severe macromastia. Increasing sternal notch to nipple distances portend a decreased likelihood for success using a superiorly-based pedicle. Along the same lines, longer inframammary fold to nipple distances ultimately may preclude the use of an inferior pedicle technique. Vertical short-scar techniques can be performed comfortably if the sternal notch to nipple distance is <38 cm. If the inframammary fold to nipple distance is >22 cm, there may be difficulty with inferior pedicle or central mound techniques. In cases where the sternal notch to nipple distance exceeds 40 cm, plastic surgeons should seriously consider lower pole breast amputation via a Wise pattern skin resection with either free nipple grafting or immediate nipple reconstruction with subsequent tattoo of the areola.[9,45]

Access the complete references list online at **http://www.expertconsult.com**

2. Netscher DT, Meade RA, Goodman CM, et al. Physical and psychosocial symptoms among 88 volunteer subjects compared to patients seeking plastic surgery procedures to the breast. *Plast Reconstr Surg.* 2000;105:2366–2373.

Netscher investigated the relationship between macromastia and physical and psychosocial symptoms. A total of 21 augmentation mammaplasty patients and 31 breast reduction patients were graded on their somatic and psychosocial symptoms and compared with a control group of 88 female university students. The study's purpose was to discover which complaints were most common among women presenting for reduction mammaplasty and to determine whether body mass index and chest measurements affected their symptoms. The authors concluded that patients who present with symptomatic macromastia seeking reduction mammaplasty have a disease-specific group of physical and psychosocial complaints that are more directly related to large breast size than to being overweight.

4. Blomqvist L, Eriksson A, Brandberg Y. Reduction mammaplasty provides long-term improvement in health status and quality of life. *Plast Reconstr Surg.* 2000;106(5):991–997.

Blomqvist et al. investigated the health status and quality of life of patients who underwent reduction mammoplasty. They conducted a prospective four part questionnaire study in 49 women who were ≥20 years, using preoperative and postoperative assessments at 6 and 12 months. The authors found that reduction mammaplasty provided significant reduction of pain in all locations (p < 0.001), with an average weight of resected tissue being 1052 g, and the improvements continued up to 12 months postoperatively. Postoperatively, patients reported a significantly improved quality of life. After 1 year, there was no statistically significant difference between the post-reduction patients and the age-matched unoperated women, which suggested those women were normalized in health-related quality of life.

6. Adams F. *The seven books of Paulus Aegineta.* [Translated from the Greek.] With a commentary embracing a complete view of the knowledge possessed by the Greeks, Romans, and Arabians on all subjects connected with medicine and surgery. Vol 2. London: Kessinger; 2009;(1844–1847):334–335.

7. Dieffenbach JF. *Die operative chirurgerie.* Vol 2. Leipzig: Brockhaus; 1848:370.

13. Passot R. La correction esthetique du prolapsus mammaire par le procede de la transposition du mamelon. *Presse Med.* 1925;33:317.

18. Penn J. Breast reduction. *Br J Plast Surg.* 1955;7:357.

19. Wise RJ. A preliminary report on a method of planning the mammaplasty. *Plast Reconstr Surg.* 1956;17:367.

22. Pitanguy I. Surgical correction of breast hypertrophy. *Br J Plast Surg.* 1967;20:78.

24. Orlando JC, Guthrie Jr RH. The superomedial pedicle for nipple transposition. *Br J Plast Surg.* 1975;28:42.

30. Hester Jr TR, Bostwick III J, Miller L. Breast reduction utilizing the maximally vascularized central pedicle. *Plast Reconstr Surg.* 1985;76:890.

33. Lassus C. Breast reduction: evolution of a technique – a single vertical scar. *Aesthetic Plast Surg.* 1987;11(2):107–112.

34. Lejour M, Abboud M. Vertical mammaplasty without inframammary scar and with breast liposuction. *Perspect Plast Surg.* 1990;4:67.

39. Benelli L. A new periareolar mammaplasty: round block technique. *Aesthetic Plast Surg.* 1990;14:93.

43. Hall-Findlay EJ. A simplified vertical reduction mammaplasty: shortening the learning curve. *Plast Reconstr Surg.* 1999;104 (3):748–763.

46. Eliasen CA, Cranor ML, Rosen PP. Atypical duct hyperplasia of the breast in young females. *Am J Surg Pathol.* 1992;16(3):246–251.

Eliasen et al. demonstrated a predominance of atypical ductal hyperplasia in nine patients with macromastia, who ranged in age from 18 to 26 years (average 21 years). Though unable to find any significant gross abnormalities within the resected breast tissue except for two fibroadenomas, the authors were able to demonstrate that each case had a continuum of microscopic ductal changes, which ranged from partial to complete involvement by micropapillary and lactiform epithelial hyperplasia.

55. Schnur PL, Hoehn JG, Ilstrup DM, et al. Reduction mammaplasty: cosmetic or reconstructive procedure? *Ann Plast Surg.* 1991;27(3):232–237.

In the study by Schnur et al., 92 of 220 plastic surgeons that responded to their survey included information (height, weight, and amount of breast tissue removed) from 600 women regarding the last 15–20 reduction mammaplasties by each surgeon. A second survey followed to estimate percentages of women who sought reduction mammaplasties for purely cosmetic reasons, for mixed reasons, and for purely medical reasons, and 132 of the same 220 surgeons responded.

56. Appel 3rd JZ, Wendel JJ, Zellner EG, et al. Association between preoperative measurements and resection weight in patients undergoing reduction mammaplasty. *Ann Plast Surg.* 2010;64(5):512–515.

Appel et al. performed a retrospective analysis of 348 patients undergoing bilateral reduction mammaplasty (696 breasts) between October 2001 and March 2009. The association between resection weight and sternal notch to nipple distance (SNN), inframammary fold to nipple distance (IMFN), and body mass index (BMI) was assessed. The authors concluded that resection weight correlates strongly with SNN, IMFN, and BMI in patients undergoing reduction mammoplasty, and, when considered together, resection weight can be predicted with a great degree of accuracy.

8.2

Inferior pedicle breast reduction

Jack Fisher

SYNOPSIS

- The inferior pedicle procedure remains one of the most common techniques employed for breast reduction surgery.
- Key to a successful outcome with the inferior pedicle procedure is proper shaping of the pedicle.
- One of the benefits of the inverted T procedure is reducing the amount of skin between the bottom of the areola and the inframammary fold.
- Patients that may benefit from this operation are those with wide, boxy breasts.
- Key to the procedure is not carrying the transverse scar close to the midline or laterally beyond the anterior axillary fold.
- Although modifications are performed intraoperatively, the majority of the procedure is based on the preoperative patient's markings.
- Key steps include leaving the bulk of tissue underneath the nipple-areolar complex, limiting the amount of breast tissue in the lower portion of the pedicle, keeping a thick superior flap.

Evolution of the technique

Breast reduction remains one of the most common procedures related to breast surgery, second only to augmentation mammoplasty. Numerous procedures have been developed specifically for breast reduction surgery, and the inferior pedicle technique has been performed for over three decades.[1-4] Many procedures have been developed to reduce scar length and enhance breast shape. With the development of several short scar breast reduction techniques, some surgeons either no longer employ or limit the patients in whom they perform inferior pedicle procedures.

The inferior pedicle procedure is associated with an inverted T incision and still remains one of the most common techniques employed for breast reduction surgery.[5-8] The length of the horizontal incision can frequently be kept short, and, in the past, this was considered one of the primary negative aspects of this procedure. Key to a successful outcome with the inferior pedicle procedure is proper shaping of the pedicle to minimize recurrent ptosis and bottoming out. With proper patient selection and proper design, the length of that horizontal incision frequently can be kept short. This technique is particularly suited for very large breasts when there is a large discrepancy between skin envelope volume and breast tissue.

This section discusses those factors associated with a successful outcome, including proper patient selection and proper design of both the pedicle and the skin envelope. Specific areas that will be addressed in the evolution of this technique relate to the application of the inverted T inferior pedicle to very large and pendulous breasts. It will be demonstrated that scars, particularly in the horizontal plane along the inframammary fold, frequently can be kept short, avoiding any visible medial or lateral scarring.

One important aspect is modifying the shape of the pedicle itself, so that the bulk of the tissue is centrally located under the nipple-areolar complex with minimal tissue along the lower border of the inferior pedicle. Hester was one of the first to suggest this concept.[9] By keeping the bulk of the tissue centrally and minimizing the tissue along the inferior aspect, secondary problems of bottoming out can be reduced.[10,11]

Also important in the design of this technique has been the realization that the superior flap needs to be kept relatively thick in order to maintain as much superior fullness as possible. If a significant amount of the remaining breast tissue is left attached to the superior flap, then it is less likely to migrate inferiorly over time. This is another maneuver to reduce the effects of gravity in an attempt to minimize the major problem of bottoming out. Also, by leaving the superior flap thick, this helps reduce the common problem of superior flattening after the surgery which is an issue with many patterns in reduction mammoplasty.

Although many variations are popular today, the inferior pedicle with an inverted T has now been utilized for over 30 years and remains a mainstay procedure for many surgeons. Certainly minimizing scar length is a major goal; however, creating a breast with proper contour and shape is the most important component of the surgery, and in selected patients with very large, long breasts, the inverted T with a modified inferior pedicle can give excellent results.

Patient selection

As will be demonstrated, in patients who have very long or large, pendulous breasts, one of the benefits of the inverted T procedure is reducing the amount of skin between the bottom of the areola and the inframammary fold. Some patients can have an exaggerated distance between the inframammary fold and the areola and yet the areola is not in a markedly ptotic location. When trying to reduce this amount of lower pole skin, a transverse incision can enhance the shape and contour of the breast.

Another group of patients that may benefit from this operation are those with a wide, boxy breast where the upper pole and lower pole of the breast are of similar width. In these patients, taking out transverse skin again can often enhance the result. The key to the procedure is not carrying the transverse scar close to the midline or laterally beyond the anterior axillary fold.

This maneuver minimizes not only a very visible scar but a potential hypertrophic scar. Patients with transverse incisions that develop thickened or hypertrophic scars usually have the majority of their problems at the most medial and lateral extent, while the central portion under the breast frequently has the best appearance. This fact is probably due to the pressure of the overlying breast tissue compressing and flattening the scar.

Details of planning and marking

Details of planning

As with any surgical procedure, the two most important components are proper patient selection and proper planning of the procedure. With this technique, although modifications are performed intraoperatively, the majority of the procedure is based on the preoperative patient's markings. With the patient in the upright position, the initial marking consists of creating a line along the midclavicular plane starting from the clavicle down to a projection point through the inframammary fold where the new nipple-areolar complex will be located. Since in many patients, the nipple-areolar complex does not sit in the midclavicular plane, it is important to create this line, ignoring the actual nipple location if it is too lateral or too medial. After creating the midclavicular lines on both sides, another mark is made in the midline to make sure that these lines are symmetrically placed an equidistance from the midline *(Fig. 8.2.1A)*.

Creating an equilateral triangle

Beginning at the lower extension of the midclavicular line at the point where the nipple projection was created based upon the inframammary fold, an equilateral triangle is created. In smaller patients, it may be in the 7 cm range, while in relatively large patients, frequently it can be anywhere from 8–9 cm in length *(Fig. 8.2.1B)*. In patients with a very wide, boxy breast the base of the triangle should be made slightly longer than either side to help narrow and cone the breast and reduce the boxy appearance. Once these equilateral triangles have been created the next step will be creating the transverse

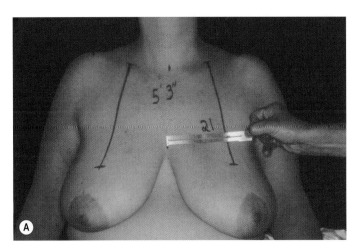

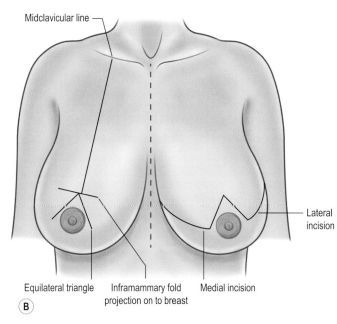

Fig. 8.2.1 (A,B) Patient preoperative marking. With the patient in an upright position, the midclavicular line is drawn. The nipple location is determined by a projection through the breast from the inframammary fold. This is marked at the bottom of the midclavicular line. Symmetry is confirmed by using a ruler to compare the distance of each midclavicular line from the midline.

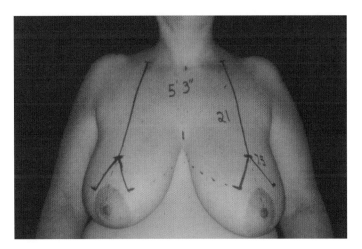

Fig. 8.2.2 Equilateral triangles are drawn extending from the proposed nipple location. These typically vary anywhere from 7 to 8 cm per side. In a wide breast, the base of the triangle may need to be slightly wider than the sides in order to narrow the breast.

incision lines extending from the lower limbs of the triangle *(Fig. 8.2.2)*.

Marking of the transverse incisions at the base of the triangle

Originally, many surgeons using this technique made a very exaggerated or serpentine "S" shape for the medial and lateral transverse incisions. This tended to give a somewhat abnormal shape to the breast. The current technique consists of a very gentle, sloping curve starting at either side of the base of the triangles and extending to the medial inframammary fold and the lateral inframammary fold. One area that may be easily modified intraoperatively to enhance the shape of the breast, is the medial marking. Once the breast is tailor-tacked, it is easy to adjust the medial breast shape if excess skin is present. But an extreme S-shaped curve should be avoided because of the abnormal shape that results.

Marking of the inframammary fold

With the patient in the upright position, the inframammary fold is marked. It is important to mark the fold without putting significant traction on the breast superiorly. It is very easy to distort the fold if too much elevation of the breast is performed. The breast is gently held in one hand, while the fold is marked with the other. After completing the marking of the fold, a projection is made extending the midclavicular line down to and crossing over the inframammary fold for location of the apical closure.

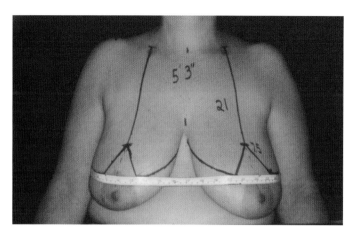

Fig. 8.2.3 With the patient in the upright position, a tape measure is placed marking the bottom of the equilateral triangles. This assists in identifying any breast asymmetry which may not be immediately apparent. In this case, there is significantly more breast tissue below the markings on the left breast with also a lower location of the nipple-areolar complex.

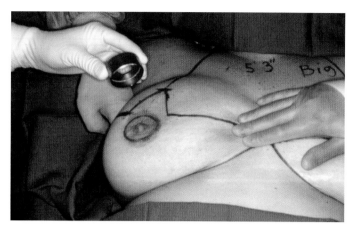

Fig. 8.2.4 With the patient asleep and with the markings in location, a nipple marker is placed to outline the incision for the nipple-areolar complex. This varies anywhere from 38–42 mm in diameter.

Assessing symmetry of markings

Next, with the patient in the upright position, all these marks are compared. Using a tape measure as a pendulum based from the clavicle, the markings of the nipple-areolar complex, the bottom of the triangles, and the medial and lateral extents of the transverse incisions are all compared for symmetry. Frequently, with asymmetric breasts, it can be difficult to evaluate your markings.

Visualizing or examining the asymmetric patient

One trick is to take a tape measure and have the patient hold it under their arms against their chest wall and place it transversely along the base of each triangle. As demonstrated in *Figure 8.2.3*, it is obvious that the patient's left breast is not only larger but the nipple-areolar complex is lower. Having a transverse tape measure helps one visualize any asymmetry *(Fig. 8.2.3)*.

This completes the basic markings and in this technique the areolar will be brought out secondarily based upon the shape of the breast, therefore, no marking of the areola is made at this time.

Detailed description of technical procedure

With the patient in the operating room, there are several important aspects in patient positioning. The arms are

on arm boards but should not be at an extreme right angle, since this can distort the breast shape at the time of closure. The arms are well-secured with slight elevation. The patient is prepped and draped in a manner where all the markings are readily visible. A dilute solution of saline/epinephrine is injected, avoiding injection into the site of the inferior pedicle. The first step consists of marking the nipple-areolar complex *(Fig. 8.2.4)*. With this technique, no traction is applied to the nipple-areolar complex as the cookie cutter is applied to the skin. One problem with applying to much tension at the time of marking is that it could lead to a very tight closure with potential healing problems. Also, having the areola being tight and smooth can result in an artificial appearance. After the marking is made, with the areolar tissue at rest, symmetry is compared and proper location of the cookie cutter incision is evaluated.

Next, the areola is incised, followed by an incision marking out the limits of the inferior pedicle. The inferior pedicle is de-epithelialized by the appropriate method. This author makes superficial cuts with the knife and completes the de-epithelialization with scissors *(Fig. 8.2.5A)*. All skin lines are then incised with the knife, again confirming symmetry. Initially the medial segments of skin and breast tissue are resected, making sure to leave some breast tissue present on the pectoralis fascia *(Fig. 8.2.5B)*. One way to avoid any artificial flattening of the medial breast is to leave some tissue attached medially on the pectoralis.

The other important aspect is to not apply excessive traction, pulling laterally on the pedicle as it is being

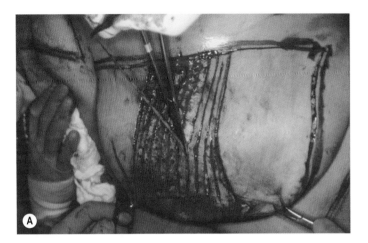

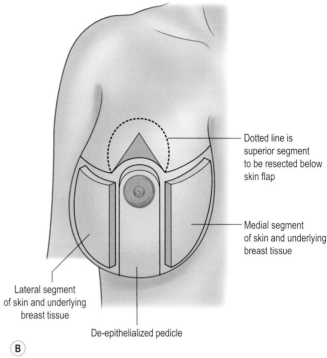

Dotted line is
superior segment
to be resected below
skin flap

Medial segment
of skin and underlying
breast tissue

Lateral segment
of skin and underlying
breast tissue

De-epithelialized pedicle

(A)

(B)

Fig. 8.2.5 (A) The inferior pedicle has been de-epithelialized. This can be done either with sharp dissection with a knife or, as demonstrated here, excising strips with the scissors. **(B)** Outline of the three segments to be resected the medial, lateral and superior.

dissected, since this can cause extensive undermining of the medial portion of the inferior pedicle. The medial triangle is held gently as it is resected. Also, the superior edge of the medial segment undergoes slight undermining in order to start thinning out the residual medial skin flap. In a similar manner, the lateral segments are resected. The majority of tissue reduction of the breast volume comes from the lateral segment of the breast. In most patients, at least two-thirds of the bulk of the breast tissue is located laterally, especially in excessively large cases. Care is taken not to apply too much traction laterally while holding the lateral segment to avoid excessive undermining of the inferior pedicle. Also, along the lateral segment's superior incision, undermining is begun to create the appropriate thickness of the superior flap.

In many patients who are overweight or with very large breasts, the breast extends laterally extensively under their arm. Although liposuction can enhance flattening of this area, it is also easy while resecting the lateral segment to remove some of the lateral tissue beyond the breast underneath the patient's arm.

This will reduce some of the bulkiness postoperatively and enhance the final result. Once the lateral segments are resected, they are compared for symmetry, evaluating the amount of tissue that has been removed from each side. The remaining volumes of the inferior pedicles are now compared *(Fig. 8.2.6)*. Although it is useful to compare the tissue being removed from each side, the amount left behind is far more important *(Fig. 8.2.7)*.

The third phase consists of elevating the superior flap *(Fig. 8.2.8)*. Although originally in the description of this procedure, many people made the superior flap relatively thin to allow it to advance, the problem with creating a thin superior flap is that it will create hollowness in the upper pole of the breast. In this technique, the superior flap is kept relatively thick. Just above the nipple-areolar complex the dissection continues angled slightly superiorly but mostly down toward the pectoralis. The flap can always be thinned secondarily, but maintaining a significant amount of breast tissue under the superior flap allows for two benefits: (1) it minimizes the flatness superiorly and (2) by keeping the

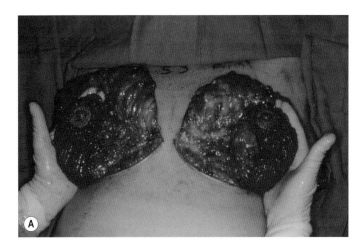

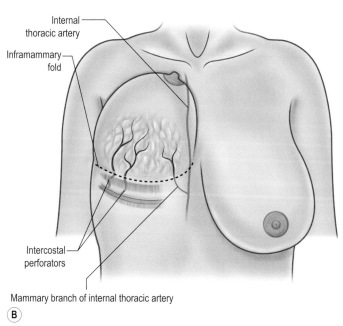

Fig. 8.2.6 (A) The medial and lateral triangles have already been excised consisting of the skin and underlying breast tissue. The hand is being used to palpate and compare the size of the remaining pedicle. **(B)** Blood supply of the inferior pedicle.

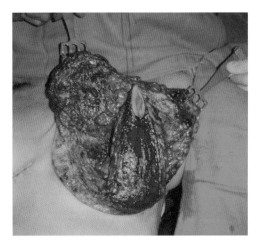

Fig. 8.2.7 It is also important to assess the thickness of the flaps in order to ensure symmetry. The flaps in both medial and lateral segments of the new breast are being evaluated for thickness.

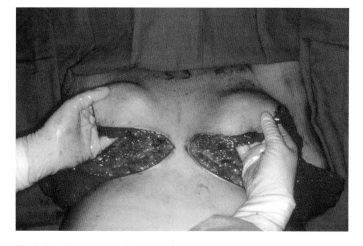

Fig. 8.2.8 Maintaining a relatively thick superior flap.

bulk of the breast tissue attached to the superior flap, it puts less mechanical load on the lower portion of the breast, hopefully reducing secondary bottoming out. Once the superior flap is dissected down close to the pectoralis, the dissection continues superiorly. In most patients, it is unnecessary to completely elevate the superior flap toward the clavicle. This will (1) compromise the blood supply to the superior flap if it is over-dissected, and (2) it will allow that superior flap to drop

over time. Leaving the bulk of the superior flap attached to the pectoralis fascia is another way of enhancing the superior fullness.

Now that all three areas have been resected, consisting of medial, lateral, and superior segments, the next step is getting excellent hemostasis throughout and comparing the residual tissue. Since the majority of patients are asymmetric, just looking at the amount of tissue resected is often inadequate. The best way to

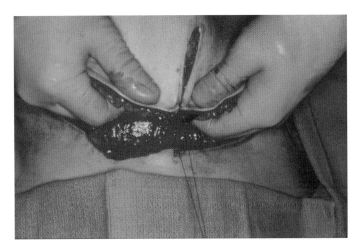

Fig. 8.2.9 In order to reduce shearing forces separating the underlying fat from the skin in the apex, as the apical suture is being tied the medial and lateral flaps with their underlying fat are advanced into the defect. This tends to reduce any shearing of the fat from the underlying skin.

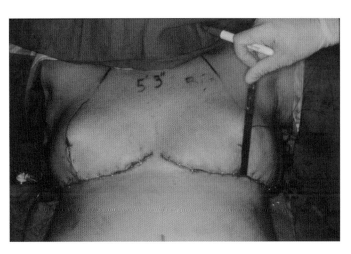

Fig. 8.2.10 Locating the new nipple-areolar complex location. Typically, this is anywhere from 3.5 to 4.0 cm from the inframammary fold. The lower the nipple location, the fewer long-term problems.

ensure postoperative symmetry is by feeling the width of the pedicle, the amount of central tissue, and the thickness of the superior flap – medially, superiorly, and laterally.

The final phase now consists of thinning out carefully the lower portion of the inferior pedicle. This technique is probably as much of a central mound as it is an inferior pedicle. Maintaining the bulk of breast tissue immediately under the nipple-areolar complex can help minimize bottoming out. If the bulk of the breast tissue is left immediately adjacent to the lower pole of the inferior pedicle, then bottoming out and distortion of the lower pole of the breast is more likely to occur.

Once it is ensured that the residual tissues are now symmetrical, closure over a drain is now performed. Initially, an apical suture is used to bring the medial and lateral flaps down to the appropriate point in the mid-clavicular line. One of the problems with the inverted T technique is the possible shearing of the subcutaneous breast tissue off the medial and lateral flaps as the apical stitch is tied. This problem can lead to be skin necrosis at the apical closure. By holding ones hands, as seen in *Figure 8.2.9*, and holding the breast tissue to the overlying skin flaps, this shearing force can be minimized *(Fig. 8.2.9)*. Excessive tension at the apical closure needs to be avoided. Just like in a facelift where the pre-auricular skin should be closed under minimal tension, so should the apical closure.

The vertical and horizontal incisions are temporarily tailor-tacked with a stapler. The patient is placed in the upright position and symmetry and shape is confirmed. Once this has been confirmed, a few 3-0 and mostly 4-0 Vicryls are placed in the appropriate deep layer. Although one hears frequently of 3-0 sutures spitting in incisions, it probably is more related to the depth at which it is placed. The 3-0 Vicryl needs to be relatively deep in the tissues. Only a few 3-0 Vicryls are inserted and by going to primarily 4-0 Vicryls, any potential spitting is minimized.

Once the sutures are in, followed by a 4-0 Monocryl subcuticular, the patient is placed in the upright position and, using the original either 38–42 mm cookie cutter, the nipple-areolar complex location is identified. In most patients, this is 4 cm at the most above the inframammary fold *(Fig. 8.2.10)*. Originally, many authors described at least 5 cm from the bottom of the areola to the inframammary fold. This is too great a distance when the patient is seen 3–6 months postoperatively. By keeping the distance between the inframammary fold and the nipple-areolar complex short, the result will be enhanced long term *(Fig. 8.2.11)*. Another method to evaluate nipple areolar location is to use a pendulum suture based on the sternal notch to help evaluate symmetrical positioning *(Fig. 8.2.12)*. This author has not found methods that identify nipple location based on measurements from the clavicle or mid-arm useful in determining the new NAC location.

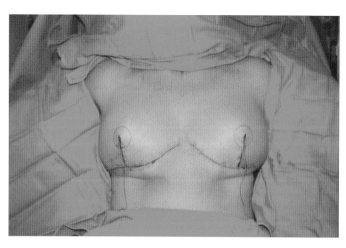

Fig. 8.2.11 With the patient in an upright position, symmetry of the breast mounds is compared prior to excising skin for nipple-areolar complex location.

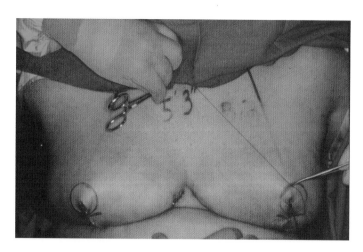

Fig. 8.2.12 A suture at the sternal notch is used as a pendulum to compare symmetry of the nipple markings before the skin is incised.

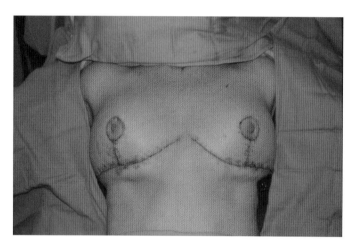

Fig. 8.2.13 Good symmetry based upon these principles with the nipple-areolar complexes brought out approximately 4 cm above the inframammary fold.

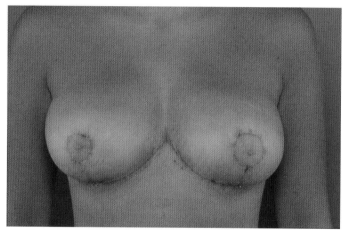

Fig. 8.2.14 Result within first week of surgery showing low NAC location and tight lower pole.

Upon completion of the procedure, the nipple should be slightly low and slightly lateral *(Fig. 8.2.13)*. It is always obvious when the nipples are either too high or too medial. A slightly low and lateral nipple-areolar complex looks more natural in the majority of patients. The drains are sutured in placed, the patient is placed in a light surgical bra, and this completes the surgical technique.

In the early postoperative phase, it is important for the lower pole of the breast to be somewhat flat with the bottom of the nipple areolar complex no more than 4 cm above the inframammary fold *(Fig. 8.2.14)*.

With proper planning and execution of a reduction mammoplasty as described, the patient should have a long-term result maintaining a natural shape *(Fig. 8.2.15)*.

Case examples

Identifying patients suited for an inverted T inferior pedicle procedure is an important first step in the proper patient/procedure selection process. This author's preference for this procedure on patients with long, pendulous, and large breasts is based on the opinion that the patients benefit from excision of skin in the transverse plane. Removal of skin transversely in patients where the distance from the nipple-areolar complex to the

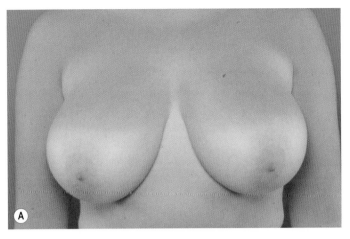
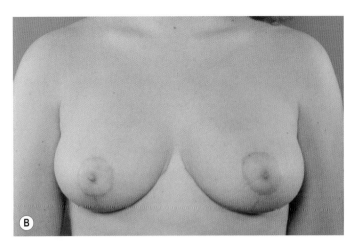

Fig. 8.2.15 (A,B) Before and after photographs of a patient demonstrating follow-up at 2 years. The patient maintains good contour as well as appropriate nipple areolar location.

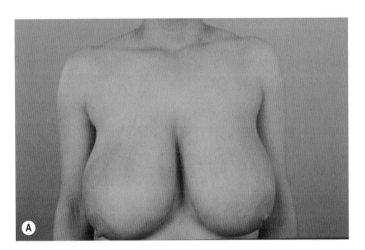
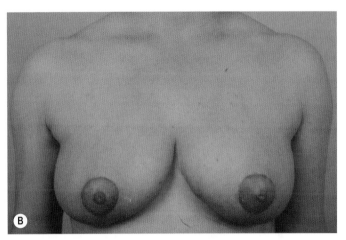

Fig. 8.2.16 (A) A patient with large, pendulous breasts, in which approximately 1300 g of tissue was removed from each side. **(B)** The postoperative result in the same patient at 3 months, demonstrating the relatively low nipple-areolar complex location at this period of time to minimize any effects of bottoming out.

inframammary fold is excessive can enhance the breast shaping process. *Figure 8.2.16* demonstrates a patient with very large and pendulous breasts. The nipples sit low and lateral. In this case, to properly position the nipple-areolar complex it is necessary to move them not only superiorly but medially. This case is a good example in which preoperative markings are critical since the surgeon needs to identify the midclavicular line preoperatively and ignore the actual nipple-areolar complex location. One benefit of the inferior pedicle technique is the wide arc of rotation of the pedicle allowing for nipple repositioning. In this case the nipples were moved medially by a significant distance putting them in the proper midclavicular line.

At 3 weeks postoperatively, the patient's nipple-areolar complexes are relatively low *(Fig. 8.2.16B)*. The nipple-areolar complexes have been moved medially to correct their orientation relatively to the midclavicular line. Over time, there will be some bottoming out but this will be minimized by three components of the original procedure. First, the majority of the breast tissue is located beneath the nipple-areolar complex limiting the amount at the base of the pedicle. Second, the superior flap is left relatively thick keeping the breast tissue adherent to the flap thus limiting inferior descent. Finally, third, the nipple-areolar complex at the time of the procedure is placed low on the breast mount anywhere from 3.5 to 4 cm

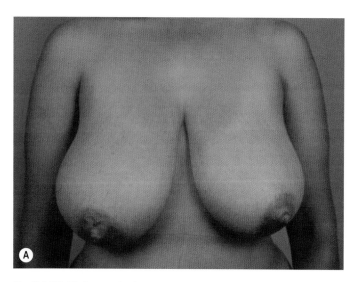 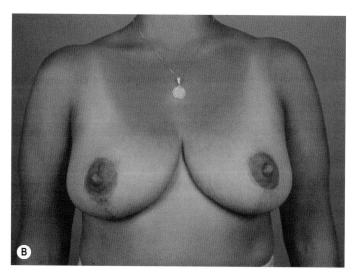

Fig. 8.2.17 (A) Preoperative frontal view of a patient with large pendulous breast with proper position of the nipple-areolar complex. **(B)** The same patient at 2 years postoperatively. The patient has maintained a good contour with minimal bottoming out. Also, the scars around the areola are excellent and the NAC, which were slightly too lateral, are now in the proper mid clavicular line.

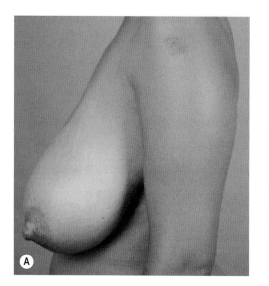 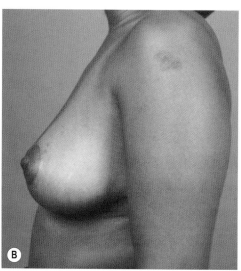

Fig. 8.2.18 (A) On preoperative lateral view the NAC is almost at the level of the elbow. **(B)** At 2 years postoperatively, the patient maintains an excellent contour with minimal lower pole fullness and good NAC position. The breast also has adequate projection.

from the lower edge of the areolar to the inframammary fold.

Another patient with very large and pendulous breasts underwent an inverted T inferior pedicle procedure as described. This patient has darkly pigmented skin and scar appearance is always important but especially in patients with dark skin of any race. Here, because of the degree of ptosis, an inverted T procedure

was selected. The inframammary transverse scar was kept as short as possible, but in this case needed to extend under the patient's arm. Fortunately the patient formed excellent scars and at two years had an excellent result *(Fig. 8.2.17)*. One of the reported detractions of the inferior pedicle technique is that it reportedly creates a boxy flat breast. *Figure 8.2.18* shows a side view of the patient before and after surgery with a 2-year follow up.

It can be seen that she has maintained good projection with an aesthetically pleasing teardrop contour on lateral view. She also has minimal bottoming out. Keeping the superior flap thick, the lower portion of the pedicle thin, and positioning the nipple-areolar complex low intraoperatively are all components of maintaining a long-term satisfactory result.

Complications and how to handle them

Probably the most common complication associated with the inferior pedicle technique is necrosis at the apical closure.[12] As stated previously, this can be minimized by reducing the shearing forces placed on the breast tissue and fat immediately underneath the medial and lateral triangles adjacent to the apex. Also, one should limit or not create too thin a flap in this area. If there is some necrosis at the apex, this is usually treated with Silvadene or wet-to-dry dressings, and in the majority of patients heals without any problems.

One of the benefits of this technique is that in very large patients, if at the end of the procedure it appears that the nipple-areolar complex may have some vascular compromise, it is still possible to do free nipple areolar grafts. The reason this is possible is the skin is still intact in the area to receive the nipple areolar complex. This situation can be handled by closure of all the incisions and then marking of the nipple-areolar complex. The nipples can now be removed as free grafts, and applied to the de-epithelialized area.

The actual number of patients that need free nipple grafts, in my opinion, is relatively small, because it is not the distance from the clavicle to the nipple that is the key determinant; it is the distance from the inframammary fold to the nipple-areolar complex. In many patients with very large, pendulous breasts the actual distance from the inframammary fold to the nipple-areolar complex is fairly short and, therefore, the pedicle itself is not that long.

Other complications that can be seen with any breast surgery such as infection or hematoma need to be treated in the traditional manner. Since the breasts were injected with epinephrine/saline solution prior to the incisions, one needs to make sure at closure that the patient's blood pressure is adequate and assess any potential bleeding sites since as the epinephrine wears off, there could be secondary bleeding.

Postoperative care is relatively simple. The drains come out the next day and the patient has few sutures that need to be trimmed postoperatively since the closure has been primarily accomplished with a running Monocryl suture.

Summary

Although there are many new procedures for breast reduction, I believe there is still an excellent role for the inverted T inferior pedicle when it is properly designed and patients are properly selected, especially in very large, pendulous breasts. The key consists of several steps, including leaving the bulk of tissue underneath the nipple-areolar complex, limiting the amount of breast tissue in the lower portion of the pedicle, keeping a thick superior flap, and minimizing the length of the transverse horizontal scar. With these modifications, this can be an excellent procedure in appropriately selected patients.

 Access the complete references list online at **http://www.expertconsult.com**

3. Courtiss EH, Goldwyn RM. Reduction mammoplasty by the inferior pedicle technique. An alternative to free nipple and areola grafting for severe macromastia or extreme ptosis. *Plast Reconstr Surg.* 1977;59:500–507.

Early description of the inferior pedicle breast reduction technique. The paper describes patients with severe macromastia that previously would have been considered candidates for free nipple grafts but with the inferior pedicle method are able to keep the nipple areolar complex attached to a pedicle with a rich blood supply. They also report improved

sensation of the nipple areolar complex compared to free nipple areolar grafting.

4. Georgiade NG, Serafin D, Morris R, et al. Reduction mammoplasty utilizing an inferior pedicle nipple areolar flap. *Ann Plast Surg.* 1979;3:211–218.

The authors report on the benefits of the inferior pedicle technique. The advantages include predictable breast shape, excellent visualization of the resection areas. Also retention of normal nipple ductal tissue and improved nipple areolar complex sensation with adequate blood supply. They report excellent results in both minimal and extensive tissue resections with this technique.

5. Bernard R, Morello DC. Inferior pedicle breast reduction. In: Mimis C, ed. *Mastery and art of plastic reconstructive and aesthetic surgery.* Boston: Little, Brown and Co; 1994:2114–2125.

7. Maxwell GP, White DJ. Inferior pedicle technique of breast reduction. In: Jurkiewicz MJ, Culbertson JH, eds. Operative techniques in plastic and reconstructive surgery. Vol 3. Philadelphia: Saunders; 1996:170–185.

    The authors present their specific technique using the inferior pedicle method for breast reduction. They discuss its popularity in the United States. They discuss its application over a wide range of breast reduction sizes as well as maintenance of the neuro vascular supply to the nipple areolar complex. The paper includes specific details of the surgical techniques using both text and photographs. Complications are presented, with the most common being healing problems at the T-junction site.

8. Ahmed OA, Kolhe PS. Comparison of nipple and areolar sensation after breast reduction by free nipple graft and inferior pedicle techniques. *Br J Plast Surg.* 2000;53:126–129.

This paper compares two groups of patients with massive breasts undergoing reduction mammoplasty. One group had a reduction with free nipple grafts while the other had reduction with an inferior pedicle technique. The purpose was to compare nipple areolar complex sensation postoperatively with at least 12 months recovery. The evaluation showed both groups had similar areolar sensation but the inferior pedicle group had superior nipple sensation.

12. Mandrekas AD, Zambacos GJ, Anastasopoulos A, et al. Reduction mammaplasty with the inferior pedicle technique: early and late complications in 371 patients. *Br J Plast Surg.* 1996;49:442–446.

The authors reviewed their results in 371 inferior pedicle reduction mammoplasties. Most cases were of large volume reduction averaging 870 g of tissue removed per side. There was an 11.4% complication rate. The most common was wound dehiscence at the T-junction with an incidence of 4.6%. All wounds healed by secondary intention. The next most common was a hypertrophic scar at 3.3%. Fat necrosis and nipple areolar necrosis occurred at equal frequency of 0.8%. Overall 88.6% of patients had no complications with the inferior pedicle breast reduction technique.

8.3

Superior or medial pedicle

Frank Lista and Jamil Ahmad

SYNOPSIS

- Vertical scar reduction mammaplasty using a superior or medial pedicle has the advantage of improved long-term projection of the breasts, along with less scarring than inverted-T scar/inferior pedicle breast reduction techniques.
- A unique aspect of our technique is the use of a superior or medial dermoglandular pedicle for transposition of the nipple-areola complex, depending on its position with respect to the mosque dome skin marking pattern.
- Our method of pedicle selection and design has likely prevented complete nipple loss, and we have not had any necrosis of the nipple-areola complex either.

Evolution of the technique

Vertical scar reduction mammaplasty using a superior or medial pedicle has the advantage of improved long-term projection of the breasts, along with less scarring than inverted-T scar/inferior pedicle breast reduction techniques. We believe that it is the inferior wedge resection of the redundant breast tissue that contributed to breast ptosis, and subsequent suturing of the medial and lateral pillars that result in coning of the breast and are responsible for the long-term shape.[1] In particular, the parenchymal pillar sutures through the superficial fascial system are critical for providing support for the remaining breast tissue, and likely help to prevent pseudoptosis.[2,3] In addition, vertical scar techniques do not violate the structural integrity of the inframammary crease, thus preventing downward migration of the inframammary crease and subsequent pseudoptosis, a problem commonly seen with breast reduction techniques that involve a horizontal scar.[3]

Reduction mammaplasty finishing with a vertical scar was first described by Arie in 1957.[4] However, this technique did not gain popularity because the vertical scar often extended below the inframammary crease leaving an unsightly scar. Years later, Lassus[5–7] and Lejour[8–10] renewed interest in vertical scar reduction mammaplasty and are responsible for much of the pioneering work. In 1969, Lassus[5–7] developed a technique using a superior dermoglandular pedicle for transposition of the nipple-areola complex; a central *en bloc* excision of skin, fat, and gland; and a vertical scar to finish. The shape of the breast was produced by reapproximating the medial and lateral pillars with only suturing of the skin. In 1994, Lejour[8–10] described a modification of Lassus' technique in which pre-excision liposuction was used to eliminate fat contributing to breast volume; the skin surrounding the excised area was undermined to facilitate gathering of the vertical scar; the superior dermoglandular pedicle was sutured to the pectoralis fascia; and sutures were used in the breast parenchyma to reapproximate the pillars producing a more durable breast shape. Gathering of the skin of the vertical wound was used to keep the scar above the inframammary crease. In 1999, Hall-Findlay[11–14] described a modification of Lejour's technique using a mosque dome skin marking pattern; a full thickness medial dermoglandular pedicle to transpose the nipple-areola complex; no skin undermining; no suturing of the pedicle to the pectoralis fascia; and liposuction only rarely to reduce breast volume. Hall-Findlay's technique has since become the most commonly performed limited incision breast reduction technique as reflected in the 2002 American Society for Aesthetic Plastic Surgery[15] and 2006 American Society of Plastic Surgeons surveys[16] of board-certified plastic surgeons. These findings were echoed by a survey of members of the Canadian Society of Plastic Surgeons in 2008.[17]

In 2006, we described our technique for vertical scar reduction mammaplasty that uses a mosque dome skin marking pattern; transposition of the nipple-areola complex on a superior or medial dermoglandular pedicle, depending on its position with respect to the skin markings; an *en bloc* excision of skin, fat, and gland; postexcision liposuction; and wound closure in two planes, including parenchymal pillar sutures and gathering of the skin of the vertical wound using four-point box stitches *(Table 8.3.1)*.[1] Since 1989, we have performed this technique on over 2000 patients requiring breast reduction resulting in consistently good breast shape, while leaving less scarring than in more commonly performed breast reduction techniques. Initially, we performed breast reduction techniques utilizing a variety of pedicles in combination with an inverted-T scar. However, as our practice demographic evolved, we saw younger women presenting for breast reduction, who were not only interested in experiencing relief of their symptoms secondary to mammary hypertrophy but who were also concerned with the amount of scarring that resulted from the procedure and the long-term appearance of their breasts. This necessitated a critical re-evaluation of our approach to breast reduction and an evolution to our technique for vertical scar reduction mammaplasty to address these issues. These concerns have also been studied by other authors[18-20] who have reported that women undergoing breast reduction prefer less scarring and are more dissatisfied with the horizontal component of the inverted-T scar than the vertical component following breast reduction.[20] In 2008, we reported our results at long-term follow-up, showing that pseudoptosis does not occur, attesting to the maintenance of breast shape and projection following this procedure.[2] In this study, three measurements were recorded at each visit: the shortest distance between the inferior edge of the clavicle and the planned postoperative position of the superior border of the nipple-areola complex, the shortest

Table 8.3.1 Comparison of different techniques for vertical scar reduction mammaplasty

	Lassus	Lejour	Hall-Findlay	Lista
Skin markings	Elliptical pattern	Mosque dome pattern, rounded inferiorly	Mosque dome pattern, rounded inferiorly	Mosque dome pattern, pointed inferiorly
Pedicle selection	Superior (or lateral)	Superior	Medial	Superior or medial
Pedicle thickness	5 mm	2–3 cm	Full-thickness	2.5 cm
Design of excision	Central with superior and inferior extensions	Central with superior, inferomedial and inferolateral extensions	Central with superior, lateral and inferior extensions	Central with superior, lateral and inferior extensions
Liposuction	Limited	Extensive pre-excision	Limited	Extensive post-excision, if required
Skin undermining	No	Yes	No	No
Pedicle sutured to chest wall	No	Yes	No	No
Breast shaping	Only skin of medial and lateral pillars sutured together	Skin and parenchyma of medial and lateral pillars sutured together	Skin and parenchyma of medial and lateral pillars sutured together	Skin and parenchyma of medial and lateral pillars sutured together

(Adapted with permission from Lista F, Ahmad J. Vertical scar reduction mammaplasty: 15-year experience including a review of 250 consecutive cases. *Plast Reconstr Surg*. 2006;117(7):2152–2169.)

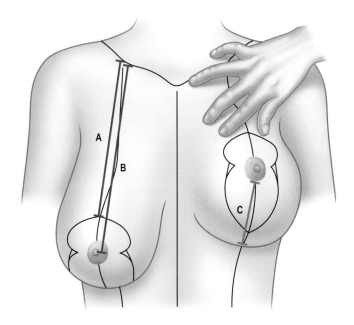

Fig. 8.3.1 Studying the fate of nipple-areola complex position and inferior pole length following vertical scar reduction mammaplasty. (A) The shortest distance between the inferior edge of the clavicle and planned postoperative position of the superior border of the nipple-areola complex. (B) The shortest distance between the inferior edge of the clavicle and the nipple. (C) The distance between the inframammary crease and the inferior border of the nipple-areola complex. (Redrawn from Ahmad J, Lista F. Vertical scar reduction mammaplasty: The fate of nipple-areola complex position and inferior pole length. *Plast Reconstr Surg.* 2008;121(4):1084–1091.)

distance between the inferior edge of the clavicle and the nipple, and the distance between the inframammary crease and the inferior border of the nipple-areola complex *(Fig. 8.3.1)*. Compared with preoperative skin markings, the nipple-areola complex was located significantly higher at both early and long-term follow-up.[2] We attribute the superior movement of the nipple-areola complex to excision of central and inferior pole breast tissue that unweights the remaining breast tissue including the nipple-areola complex allowing for elastic recoil of the superior pole skin. In addition, suturing of the medial and lateral pillars produces coning of the breast and pushes the nipple superiorly. This coning effect also causes the lax skin of the superior aspect of the breast to be distributed in a circumhorizontal direction as opposed to distribution in an inferior direction, as would be the case for breast reductions performed using the inverted-T scar pattern.[2] To accommodate for this, we adjusted the skin marking technique so that the superior border of the nipple-areola complex is marked at the level of the inframammary crease. At 4 years, the

distance from the inframammary crease to the inferior border of the nipple-areola complex was significantly shorter, confirming that pseudoptosis does not occur after vertical scar reduction mammaplasty.[2]

A unique aspect of our technique is the use of a superior or medial dermoglandular pedicle for transposition of the nipple-areola complex, depending on its position with respect to the mosque dome skin marking pattern. Our method of pedicle selection and design has likely prevented complete nipple loss, and we have not had any necrosis of the nipple-areola complex either. A closer study of the blood supply to the nipple-areola complex provides a better understanding of why the selection of a superior or medial pedicle provides a reliable blood supply for transposition of the nipple-areola complex. Many varying observations of the blood supply to the breast have been given since Manchot's[21] 1889 description. More recently, van Deventer[22] performed anatomical studies on 15 female cadavers in an attempt to further clarify the blood supply to the nipple-areola complex and found a large variation in the pattern of its blood supply. An important observation was that in all breasts, the nipple-areola complex received a blood supply medially or superiorly from one or more perforating arteries from the superior four perforating branches of the internal thoracic artery. The third perforator most frequently contributed blood supply to the nipple-areola complex in 47.5% of breasts, while the second perforator contributed in 25%, the first perforator in 15% and the fourth perforator in 12.5%. There were abundant anastomoses around the nipple-areola complex. From this study, van Deventer et al.[23] concluded that the nipple-areola complex generally has a dual blood supply with the internal thoracic-anterior intercostal artery system providing blood supply from medio-inferiorly and the lateral thoracic artery and other minor contributors providing blood supply from latero-superiorly, with the most reliable source of blood supply arising from the internal thoracic artery. Information from this study would lead us to believe that a superior pedicle may have either an axial or random blood supply while a medial pedicle is more likely to have an axial blood supply. Our method of pedicle selection limits the length of the superior pedicle allowing it to provide a reliable blood supply to the nipple-areola complex whether it happens to be axial or random. The use of a superior pedicle is limited to nipple-areola complexes lying within the roof of the mosque dome, allowing this pedicle to receive superior, medial and lateral blood supplies. This reliable superior pedicle was the most commonly utilized pedicle in our series.[1] In cases of mammary hypertrophy with greater degrees of ptosis, we use a medial pedicle, which is more likely to have an axial blood supply to reliably perfuse the nipple-areola complex when it must be transposed greater distances. Another anatomical study by Michelle le Roux et al.[24] examined the neurovascular anatomy on 11 female cadaveric breasts. They reported that the arterial supply to the superomedial pedicle originated from a single dominant vessel while the venous drainage was through an extensive branching network. Along with intercostal nerve branches that innervated the pedicle, the blood supply coursed through the pedicle in a superficial plane. They concluded that deepithelialization or thinning of the superficial aspect of the superomedial pedicle could lead to vascular compromise or denervation of the nipple-areola complex. Instead, they recommended resection should be done from the deep surface or the base of the pedicle if needed. This study supports the safety of the partial thickness superior or medial pedicle design which we use in our technique. The use of a full thickness pedicle can be cumbersome, not only preventing adequate volume reduction but also causing difficulty transposing the nipple-areola complex to its new location. In addition, a full thickness pedicle can become kinked or tethered leading to vascular compromise of the nipple-areola complex; the partial thickness pedicle design transposes the nipple-areola complex easily to its new location.

Patient selection

Symptoms

Kerrigan et al.[25] reported an evidence-based definition of medical necessity for breast reduction in an effort to establish clear, practical, objective, and fair criteria that could be applied by physicians to help differentiate women seeking breast reduction primarily for symptom relief versus aesthetic improvement. They identified seven symptoms specific to breast hypertrophy: upper back pain, rashes, bra strap grooves, neck pain, shoulder pain, numbness, and arm pain. Results of this study established that women reporting at least two of seven physical symptoms all or most of the time improved to a significantly greater extent than women reporting less than two symptoms all or most of the time. Their data suggested that women reporting at least one of seven physical symptoms may also report greater improvement than those with no symptoms all or most of the time. We have found this definition of medical necessity useful in evaluating patients that will benefit most from breast reduction by reduction of their symptoms associated with mammary hypertrophy.

Patient characteristics

We have performed vertical scar reduction mammaplasty exclusively on over 2000 patients presenting for breast reduction. In 2006, we published our experience with 250 consecutive patients treated between November of 2000 and December of 2003.[1] In this clinical series, the average age of the patients was 38.5 years (range, 15–76 years) and the average body mass index was 28.8 kg/m^2 (range, 17.3–46.3 kg/m^2). The average weight of tissue excised per breast was 526 g (range, 10–2020 g). Liposuction was performed in 78.4% of cases and the average volume liposuctioned per breast was 140 ml (range, 50–500 ml). The average total reduction per breast (including liposuction when performed) was 636 g (range, 60–2020 g).

In addition, we analyzed complications based on body mass index, amount of reduction, pedicle selection, and use of liposuction.[1] Although there was no statistically significant difference in the rate of complications between groups for amount of reduction, pedicle selection, and use of liposuction, there was a statistically significant difference between groups for body mass index with complications occurring less frequently in patients of normal weight (body mass index, 18.5–25.0 kg/m^2). These findings have also be corroborated by other authors.[26,27] Since this study was published, we have limited performing this procedure to patients with a body mass index <35 kg/m^2. Patients presenting for breast reduction with a body mass index >35 kg/m^2 are advised to lose weight prior to undergoing this procedure to decrease their risk for complications including superficial wound dehiscence and fat necrosis.

Along with other authors,[7,11] we recommend learning this technique by initially operating on patients with mild to moderate hypertrophy and good skin quality. As more experience is gained, one can progress to performing this technique on patients with greater degrees of mammary hypertrophy and poorer skin quality. Although it is possible to perform this technique on patients with extremely large breasts, it is important for these patients to realize that their postoperative breast size will likely remain larger when compared to other techniques because of the amount of skin preserved with a vertical scar breast reduction. In patients with severe mammary hypertrophy desiring a very small postoperative breast size, this technique is not suitable.

Details of planning and marking

General perioperative care

We routinely perform vertical scar reduction mammaplasty as a day surgery procedure. The average operating time is <70 min.[1] Multiple authors have shown that there is no increased risk of complications following breast reduction as a day surgery procedure.[27–30] In addition, Buenaventura et al.[30] estimated between US$1500 and US$2500 were saved when breast reduction surgery was performed as a day surgery procedure as opposed to requiring inpatient admission, while Nelson et al.[17] reported an estimated cost savings of C$873.

The American Society of Plastic Surgeons Patient Safety Committee evidence-based patient safety advisory provides an overview of perioperative steps that should be completed to ensure appropriate patient selection for the ambulatory surgery setting.[31] In addition, guidelines for perioperative cardiovascular evaluation,[32,33] prevention of pulmonary complications,[34,35] and venous thromboembolism prophylaxis[36,37] are also available.

Skin marking

The patient is marked preoperatively. In the sitting position, the midline of the chest and the inframammary creases are marked *(Fig. 8.3.2)*. The central axis of the breast is drawn by extending a straight line from the midpoint of the clavicle through the nipple to intersect with the inframammary crease. One hand is inserted behind the breast to the level of the inframammary crease, and this point is projected anteriorly onto the breast and marked (A). This point will be the new location of the superior border of the areola. Since the

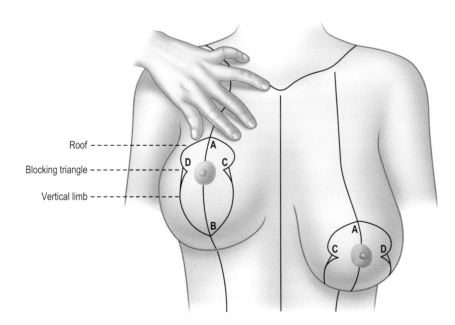

Roof

Blocking triangle

Vertical limb

Fig. 8.3.2 Mosque dome skin marking pattern. Point A is at the level of the anterior projection of the inframammary crease on the breast. Point A will be the new location of the superior border of the areola. Point B is the inferior limit of the skin excision. Point B is 2–4 cm above the inframammary crease along the central axis of the breast. Blocking triangles are extended from points C and D. (Redrawn from Lista F, Ahmad J. Vertical scar reduction mammaplasty: 15-year experience including a review of 250 consecutive cases. *Plast Reconstr Surg.* 2006;117(7):2152–2169.)

nipple-areola complex is located significantly higher compared with preoperative skin markings, at both early and long-term follow-up after this procedure, *(Fig. 8.3.3)* the planned postoperative position of the nipple-areola complex in this technique is approximately 2 cm lower than it would be using an inverted-T scar/inferior pedicle breast reduction technique.[2] The inferior limit of the skin excision is marked B, 2–4 cm above the inframammary crease, depending on the size of the reduction. This distance is shorter in smaller reductions and longer in larger reductions. The inframammary crease moves up after vertical scar breast reduction techniques and this phenomenon accounts for the vertical scar extending onto the chest wall in earlier vertical scar techniques. Limiting the inferior end of the vertical scar to a point above the inframammary crease prevents this problem. A mosque dome pattern is used. The roof of the mosque dome pattern is drawn by extending curved lines from point A to points C and D to form the border of the new nipple-areola complex. The roof is drawn so that when points C and D are brought together, the roof will form a circle. The vertical limbs of the mosque dome pattern are constructed by extending curved lines from point B to points C and D to form the margins of the skin to be excised. The inferior extent of the skin resection is marked in the shape of a "V" instead of a "U" as described in other techniques.[1,11] We feel that this allows for easier skin closure and believe that this helps to prevent the formation of a dog ear at the inferior extent of the vertical scar. Blocking triangles are drawn from point C and point D, toward the central axis of the breast, to prevent the formation of the teardrop deformity of the areola.

The areas where liposuction will be performed at the axillary area and along the lateral chest wall are marked. The new nipple-areola complex and pedicle selection and marking are done after induction of anesthesia.

Detailed description of the technical procedure

Anesthesia and positioning

We perform breast reduction surgery under general anesthesia. The patient is in the supine position with both shoulders abducted to 90° to allow for liposuction of the tail of the breast and lateral chest wall, when necessary. With this technique, we do not sit the patient up during surgery as the breasts have a distorted appearance with flattening of the inferior pole and exaggerated superior pole fullness which can be misleading. Instead, we assess the patient for symmetry of shape and volume in the supine position. In addition, we do not perform any tacking sutures from the breast parenchyma to the pectoralis fascia for breast shaping as is done in other techniques; tacking sutures necessitate sitting the patient up to assess breast shape as these sutures can cause unwanted tethering of the breast.

Selection of the pedicle

After the patient has been anesthetized and placed in the supine position, a tourniquet is applied to the breast to keep the skin taut. The nipple-areola complex is outlined using a metal washer, 4.5 cm in diameter, centered over the nipple. At this point in the operation, we select the type of pedicle to be used to transpose the nipple-areola complex *(Fig. 8.3.4)*. If any part of the new areola lies superior to a line joining the blocking triangles, a superior dermoglandular pedicle is used; if all of the areola lies inferior to this line, a medial dermoglandular pedicle is used *(Fig. 8.3.5)*. This rule limits pedicle length and helps to avoid vascular compromise of the nipple-areola complex. The superior pedicle is drawn from the blocking triangles inferiorly, leaving a 2.5 cm border around the nipple-areola complex. The medial pedicle can be drawn with a base that is partially in the roof and in the vertical limb or completely in the vertical limb of the mosque dome, depending on the location of the nipple-areola complex. A 2.5 cm border is left around the nipple-areola complex. The base of the medial pedicle should be wide enough to maintain a pedicle width-to-length ratio of no less than 1:2 to preserve its blood supply but should be narrow enough to allow easy rotation and insetting of the nipple-areola complex into the roof of the mosque dome.

Infiltration

A small incision is made superior to point B through the skin that will later be excised. Infiltration is performed just deep to the skin and then within the breast parenchyma. Each breast is infiltrated with 500 ml of a

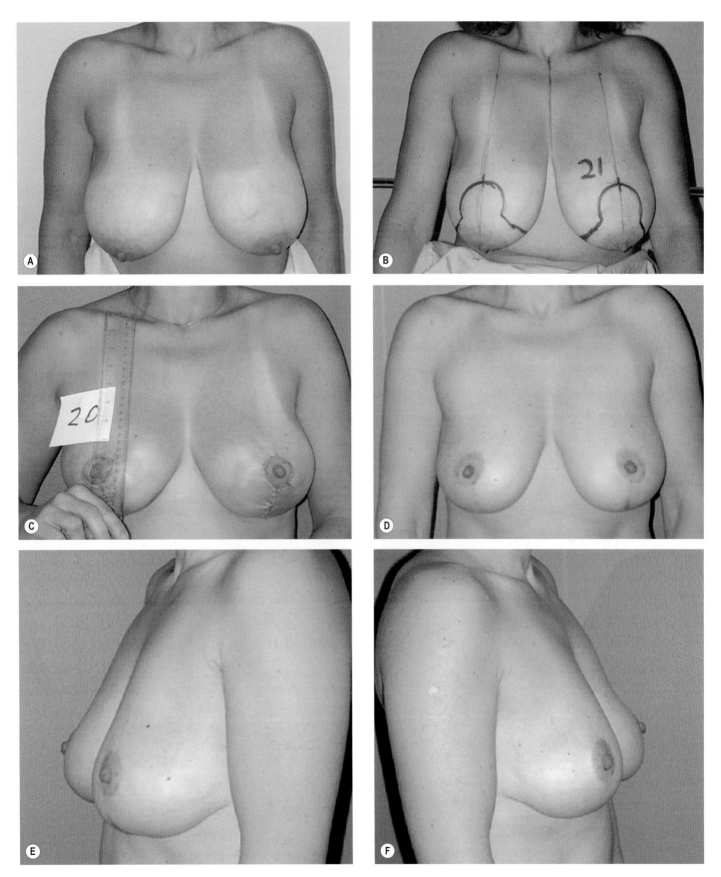

Fig. 8.3.3 (A,B) A 38-year-old woman underwent vertical scar reduction mammaplasty using bilateral superior pedicles. A total of 375 g was excised from the right breast and 325 g from the left. **(C)** Preoperatively, the distance from the inferior edge of the clavicle to the level of the planned postoperative position of the superior border of the nipple-areola complex was 21 cm. **(D)** At 5 days postoperatively, the distance from the inferior edge of the clavicle to the superior border of the nipple-areola complex is 20 cm, resulting in a difference of 1 cm. **(E,F)** At 4 years follow-up, the distance from the inframammary crease to the inferior border of the nipple-areola complex was unchanged. (Reproduced with permission from Ahmad J, Lista F. Vertical scar reduction mammaplasty: The fate of nipple-areola complex position and inferior pole length. *Plast Reconstr Surg.* 2008;121(4):1084–1091.)

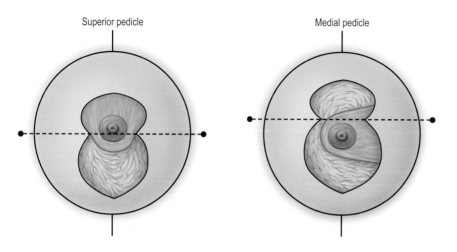

Superior pedicle   Medial pedicle

Fig. 8.3.4 Approach for pedicle selection. A superior pedicle is used if any part of the new areola lies superior to a line joining the blocking triangles (left), and a medial pedicle if all of the areola lies inferior to this line (right). (Redrawn from Lista F, Ahmad J. Vertical scar reduction mammaplasty: 15-year experience including a review of 250 consecutive cases. *Plast Reconstr Surg.* 2006;117(7): 2152–2169.)

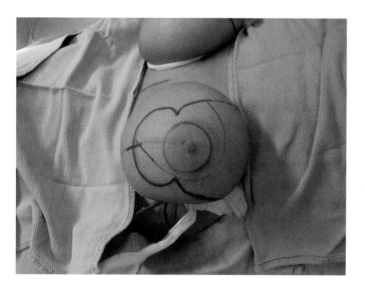

Fig. 8.3.5 Mosque dome skin marking pattern with medial pedicle.

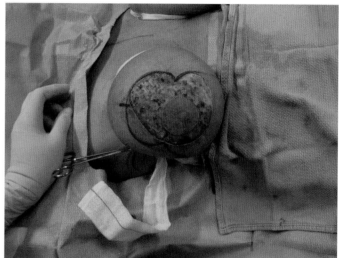

Fig. 8.3.6 Medial pedicle de-epithelialized.

solution composed of 1000 ml of Ringer's lactate solution, 40 ml of 2% lidocaine and 1 ml of 1:1000 epinephrine.

Deepithelialization

To facilitate de-epithelialization of the pedicle, a tourniquet is applied to the base of the breast to increase tension of the skin overlying the breast. Before de-epithelialization, the nipple-areola complex and the pedicle are marked, as explained previously. To prevent damage to the blood vessels travelling superficial through the pedicle, it is important to leave the deep dermis intact when deepithelializing as opposed to removing the skin full thickness *(Fig. 8.3.6)*.

Surgical excision

Surgical excision en bloc of skin, fat, and gland is performed as outlined by the skin markings. Modification of these skin markings intraoperatively is not necessary, removing a great deal of "intuitiveness" from this operation. The excision is extended down to the chest wall, leaving a layer of breast tissue over the pectoralis fascia to prevent bleeding and postoperative pain. If more volume reduction is needed, the excision may be extended in superior *(Fig. 8.3.7A)* and lateral *(Fig. 8.3.7B)* directions deep to the skin to encompass more breast tissue. This leaves more breast fullness medially leading to a more pleasing breast shape *(Fig. 8.3.7D)*. When excising tissue deep to the pedicle, it is important to

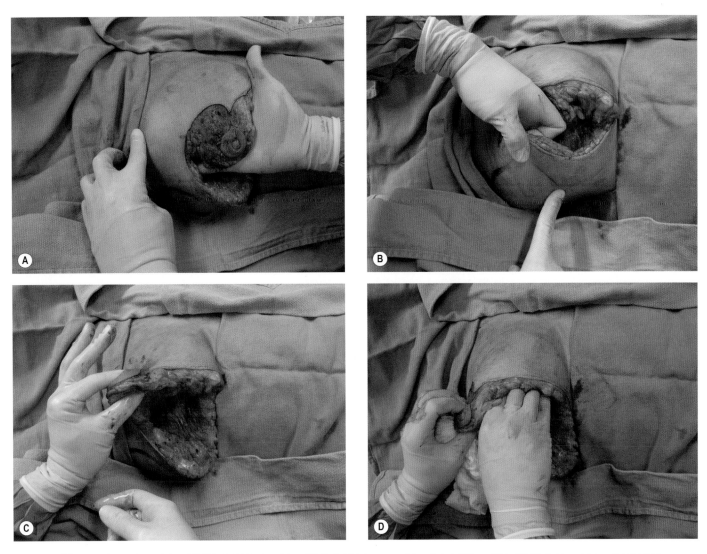

Fig. 8.3.7 **(A)** Extent of superior excision. **(B)** Extent of lateral excision. **(C)** Partial thickness medial pedicle is 2.5 cm thick. **(D)** Medial breast tissue is left intact preserving medial fullness.

leave the pedicle at least 2.5 cm thick to preserve its blood and nerve supply *(Fig. 8.3.7C)*. When excising breast tissue laterally and superiorly, the flaps should be maintained 2.5 cm thick throughout their length *(Fig. 8.3.8)*. The tissue between the end of the vertical wound and the inframammary crease is thinned to prevent a dog-ear from forming *(Fig. 8.3.9)*. We have not found it necessary to perform any excisional modification of the skin in this region to control dog-ear formation or redundant skin folds. When using a superior pedicle, a superficial incision can be extended 2 cm superiorly from each blocking triangle to facilitate the insetting of the nipple-areola complex.

Liposuction

Liposuction is performed after excision because it is very difficult to accurately assess the composition of the breast preoperatively by clinical examination. When necessary, post-excision liposuction is performed using a 4-mm, three-hole blunt cannula for volume reduction of the axillary area of the breast and contouring of the lateral chest wall. In excessively fatty breasts, liposuction can be performed on the superior half of the breast for volume reduction. Access to these areas is through the medial and lateral pillars created by the surgical excision.

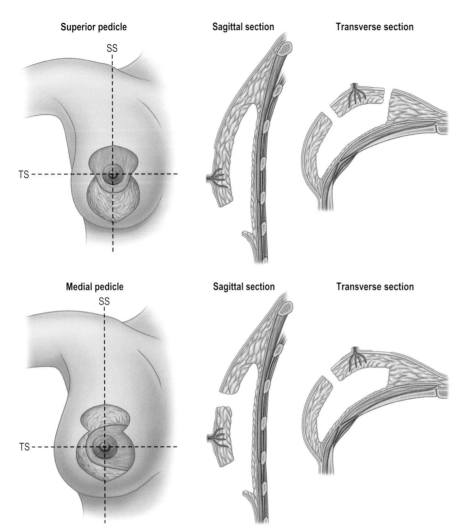

Superior pedicle   **Sagittal section**   **Transverse section**

Medial pedicle   **Sagittal section**   **Transverse section**

Fig. 8.3.8 Extent of breast tissue excision using a superior pedicle (above) and medial pedicle (below) shown in sagittal (SS) and transverse sections (TS).

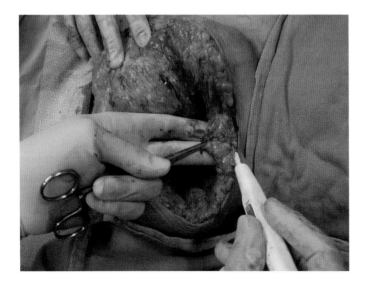

Fig. 8.3.9 Excision of breast tissue between the end of the vertical wound and the inframammary crease to prevent a dog-ear from forming.

Breast shaping

Wound closure is performed in two planes, including parenchymal pillar sutures and gathering of the skin of the vertical wound using box stitches. Inverted 1-0 Vicryl sutures (Ethicon Inc, Somerville, NJ) placed through the superficial fascial system are used to reapproximate the medial and lateral pillars of the breast parenchyma *(Fig. 8.3.10)*. These parenchymal pillar sutures may contribute to improved long-term projection of the breasts following this procedure preventing pseudoptosis or "bottoming out" of the breast.[2] Usually, two parenchymal pillar sutures are used, but the inferior most suture should be placed no closer than 4 cm from the inferior end of the incision. Placing the pillar sutures too close to the inferior end of the vertical wound may lead to the formation a dog-ear. Temporary skin staples are used to close the vertical wound while suturing the skin.

Wound closure

All suturing of the skin is performed using a 4-0 Monocryl suture (Ethicon Inc, Somerville, NJ). A four-point box stitch is used to gather the skin of the vertical wound *(Fig. 8.3.11)*. Use of this box stitch allows selective gathering of the vertical wound leading to more control of the vertical scar. The skin is gathered

beginning at the inframammary crease. Gathering of the skin assists in eliminating dog-ears close to the inferior end of the vertical scar. Skin within 1 cm of the areola is not gathered to prevent distortion of the areola. After gathering of the skin, there may be gaping of the horizontal pleats caused by the box stitches along the vertical wound *(Fig. 8.3.12)*. These are corrected using a deep

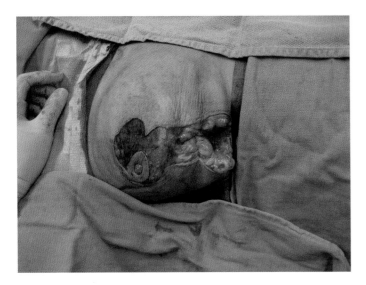

Fig. 8.3.10 Parenchymal pillar sutures.

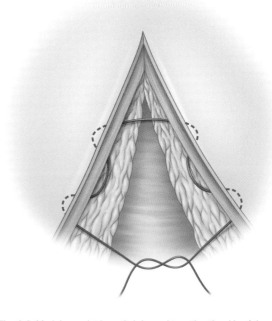

Fig. 8.3.11 A four-point box stitch is used to gather the skin of the vertical wound.

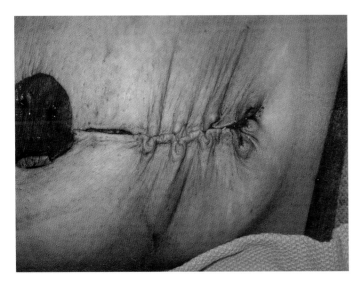

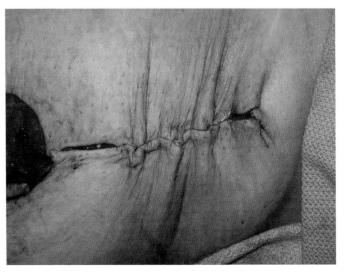

Fig. 8.3.12 (A) The vertical wound has been gathered using four-point box stitches resulting in gaping of the gathered wound edges. **(B)** Correcting gaping of the horizontal pleats using inverted deep dermal sutures.

dermal, inverted suture. Correction of horizontal pleats is essential because they do not settle with time and lead to small horizontal scars within the larger vertical scar.

Using box stitches, the skin can be gathered several centimeters so that the vertical scar ≤8 cm. However, the vertical scar can measure >8 cm after larger breast reductions. With inverted-T scar reductions, it is necessary to keep the length of the vertical scar to <5.5 cm.[12] Limiting this length will accommodate for the pseudoptosis that occurs following inferior pedicle/inverted-T scar breast reduction techniques. However, in vertical scar reduction mammaplasty, a much longer vertical scar is acceptable. Lassus[6] measured the distance between the inferior border of the areola and the inframammary crease in young women with beautiful breasts and found measurements ranging from 4.5 to 10 cm. Lassus[6] concluded that the distance was relative to the size of the breast. Lassus[5] reported vertical scar lengths up to 9 cm in large reductions. Hall-Findlay[11] showed results where this distance was up to 12 cm. Along with other authors,[10] we have observed that the length of the vertical scar does not increase over time after vertical scar reduction mammaplasty.[2] Cutaneous wrinkling of the vertical scar associated with gathering of the skin will disappear by 6 months postoperatively.[38]

Skin staples are used along the vertical wound for final closure *(Fig. 8.3.13)*. Deep dermal, inverted sutures are used to inset the nipple-areola complex. Intradermal, continuous sutures are used for closer approximation of skin edges of the periareolar wound.

We do not routinely use drains. Along with other authors,[39,40] we do not feel that drain placement is necessary following breast reduction. Wrye et al.[40] reported that performing reduction mammaplasty without the use of closed suction drainage does not increase complications and is preferred by patients.

Dressings and wound care

Each breast is injected with 10 ml of 0.5% 1:200000 bupivacaine for postoperative pain relief. The wounds are dressed with paraffin gauze, followed by dry gauze, and finally by abdominal pads. These are held in place by the patient's bra.

General postoperative instructions and follow-up

Patients should wear a bra at all times for 3 weeks following surgery. On postoperative day 1, they are instructed to shower and wash their wounds with soap and water and dress them with dry gauze. Patients are seen on postoperative day 5 for removal of skin staples and Steri-Strips (3M, St Paul, MN) are applied. We typically see patients again at 1 month and 3 months postoperatively. Patients may return to their normal level of activity 3 weeks postoperatively and can begin physically demanding activity one month following surgery.

Examples of superior and medial pedicle breast reductions

Vertical scar reduction mammaplasty has been applied to breast reductions of all sizes and has consistently produced good breast shape with less scarring that inverted-T scar breast reduction techniques.

Superior pedicle breast reduction

Figure 8.3.14 shows a 19-year-old woman who underwent vertical scar reduction mammaplasty using bilateral superior pedicles. 420 g was excised from the right

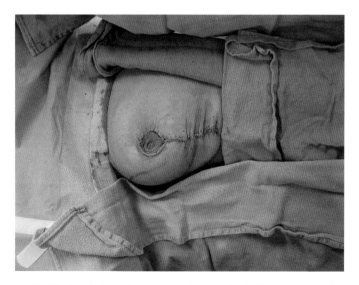

Fig. 8.3.13 The nipple-areola complex has been inset and skin staples are used along the vertical wound for final closure.

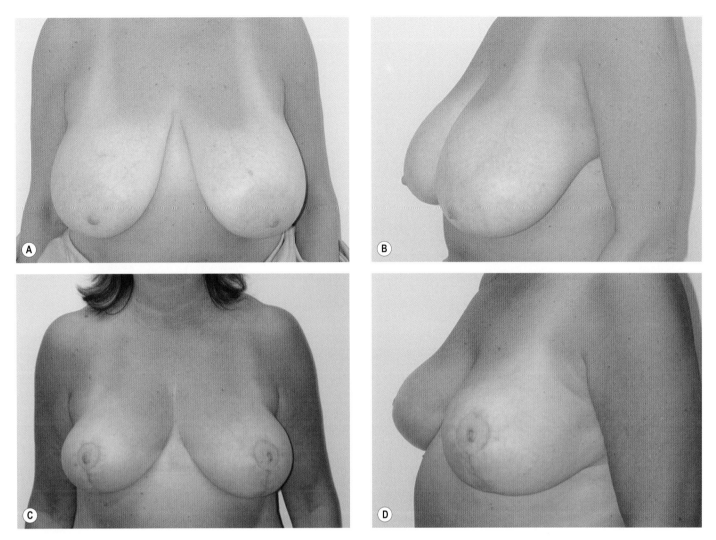

Fig. 8.3.14 (A–D) A 19-year-old woman who underwent vertical scar reduction mammaplasty using bilateral superior pedicles. A total of 420 g was excised from the right breast and 400 g from the left; 50 ml was liposuctioned from the right breast and 100 ml from the left. Results 3 months postoperatively are shown.

breast and 400 g from the left. 50 ml was liposuctioned from the right breast and 100 ml from the left. Results 3 months postoperatively are shown.

Medial pedicle breast reduction

Figure 8.3.15 shows 54-year-old woman who underwent vertical scar reduction mammaplasty using bilateral medial pedicles; 460 g was excised from each breast; 200 ml was liposuctioned from the right breast and 250 ml from the left. Results 6 months postoperatively are shown.

Complications and how to handle them

In our 2006 review of 250 consecutive cases, the complication rate was 5.6% of breasts *(Table 8.3.2)*.[1] Complications were analyzed by body mass index, amount of reduction, pedicle selection, and use of liposuction. A modified χ^2-test was used to analyze complications based on body mass index, amount of reduction, pedicle selection, and use of liposuction. With a value of $p < 0.05$, there was no statistically significant difference between groups for amount of reduction ($p = 0.107$), pedicle selection ($p = 0.662$), and use of liposuction

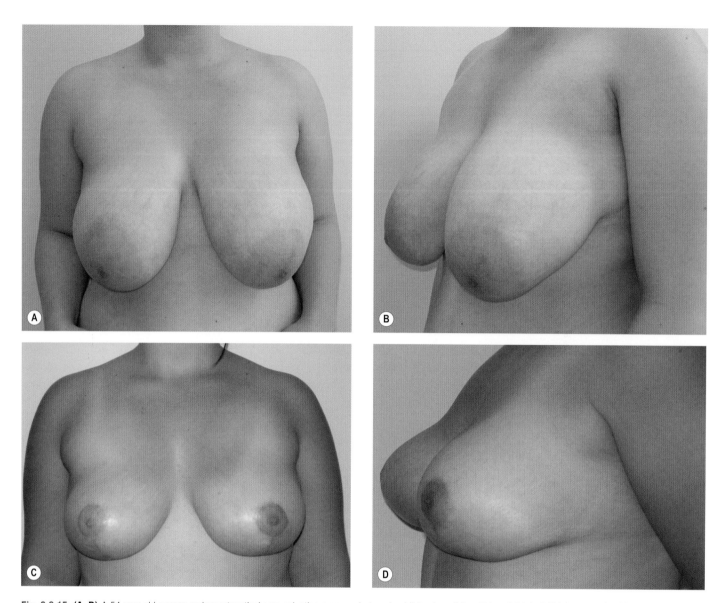

Fig. 8.3.15 (A–D) A 54-year-old woman underwent vertical scar reduction mammaplasty using bilateral medial pedicles. A total of 460 g was excised from each breast; 200 ml was liposuctioned from the right breast and 250 ml from the left. Results 6 months postoperatively are shown.

($p=0.831$). However, there was a marginally statistically significant difference between groups for body mass index ($p=0.048$), with complications occurring less frequently in patients of normal weight (BMI 18.5–25.0).[1]

Healing of the vertical scar

The early appearance of the vertical scar can be a common concern for patients following this procedure. The best way to mitigate these concerns is to discuss this preoperatively with patients. They should understand that, initially, there will be horizontal pleats along the vertical scar and that these typically flatten out by 3 months. Postoperatively, the patient should be reminded that these horizontal pleats are normal for several weeks to months and they should be reassured that the horizontal pleats will resolve. Another important issue is that the staples should be removed between 5 and 7 days after surgery, but no later as the staples may leave additional scars (*Fig. 8.3.16*).

Table 8.3.2 Frequency of complications after vertical scar reduction mammaplasty in 250 patients

	Number of breasts	(%)
Superficial wound dehiscence	11	2.2
Hematoma	6	1.2
Fat necrosis	4	0.8
Seroma	2	0.4
Repeat reduction	2	0.4
Glandular infection	1	0.2
Inverted nipple	1	0.2
Scar revision	1	0.2
Areola necrosis	0	0.0
Nipple loss	0	0.0
Blood transfusion	0	0.0

(Adapted with permission from Lista F, Ahmad J. Vertical scar reduction mammaplasty: 15-year experience including a review of 250 consecutive cases. *Plast Reconstr Surg.* 2006;117(7):2152–2169.)

Wound dehiscence

Superficial wound dehiscence was the most frequent complication in our review of 250 consecutive cases; it occurred in 2.2% of breasts. The area where this occurs is typically at the middle portion of the vertical wound as this is the area under greatest tension. Although other authors[8,11] have described using a continuous intradermal suture to gather the skin of the vertical wound, it may be a source of wound healing problems because of constriction of the blood supply to the skin edges. Using the four-point box stitch gathers the skin of the vertical wound effectively while causing less ischemia to the skin edges. In addition, staples provide further approximation of the skin edges without causing additional ischemia.

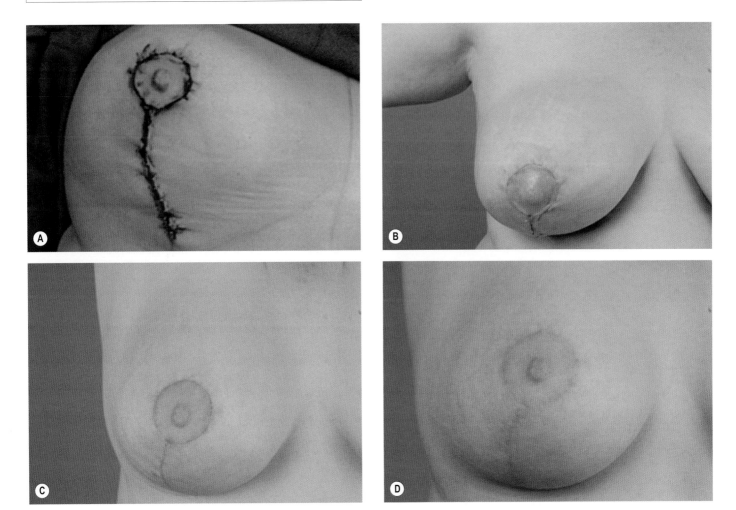

Fig. 8.3.16 Vertical scar with staples (A). Postoperative appearance of vertical scar at 6 days (B), 6 weeks (C) and 6 months (D).

Under-resection

Vertical scar/superior or medial pedicle breast reduction techniques have been criticized because it can be difficult to assess the adequacy of the reduction because the endpoint of the operation is unfamiliar to those who normally perform inferior pedicle/inverted-T scar breast reduction techniques.[41] At the end of the operation, there is exaggerated superior pole fullness, inferior pole flatness, and indrawing of the nipple with which one must become familiar. Although vertical scar breast reductions have a characteristically unusual appearance on the operating room table at the end of the procedure, they invariably give a much more aesthetically pleasing result postoperatively.

While learning this technique, there is a tendency for under-resection because inadequate tissue is resected laterally and superiorly. However, with the simple design of the excision in this technique, increased reduction can be safely achieved by excising breast tissue laterally to the anterior axillary line and superiorly deep to the pedicle, if necessary. Provided that the thickness of the pedicle and skin flaps is 2.5 cm, it is possible to resect more tissue without compromising the blood supply of the pedicle or skin of the vertical wound.

In our 2006 review of 250 consecutive patients, we had to perform secondary breast reduction in one patient.[1] A total of 1412 g of tissue was excised bilaterally during the first breast reduction. Liposuction was not used. Subsequently, the patient felt that her breasts were still too large, so a second breast reduction was performed 10 months later; 1085 g of tissue was excised and 500 cc was liposuctioned bilaterally to achieve the desired result.

Summary

In our over 20-years' experience of more than 2000 patients, we have found that vertical scar reduction mammaplasty using a superior or medial pedicle to transpose the nipple-areola complex, allowing for the critical inferior wedge resection and subsequent suturing of the medial and lateral pillars, results in a narrower, more projecting breast, superomedial breast fullness, minimal scar burden, and long-lasting breast shape, which are the *sine quibus non* of aesthetic breast surgery.

Access the complete reference list online at **http://www.expertconsult.com**

1. Lista F, Ahmad J. Vertical scar reduction mammaplasty: 15-year experience including a review of 250 consecutive cases. *Plast Reconstr Surg.* 2006;117(7):2152–2169.

   We describe our technique for vertical scar reduction mammaplasty using a superior or medial pedicle. We performed a review of 250 consecutive patients including an analysis of complications. Technical considerations are discussed in detail and a review of previously described techniques of vertical scar reduction mammaplasty is included.

2. Ahmad J, Lista F. Vertical scar reduction mammaplasty: The fate of nipple-areola complex position and inferior pole length. *Plast Reconstr Surg.* 2008;121(4): 1084–1091.

   We report on the early and long-term fate of the nipple-areola complex position and inferior pole length. Compared with preoperative skin markings, the nipple-areola complex was located significantly higher at both early and long-term follow-up. Based on these findings, we adjusted their skin marking technique so that the superior border of the nipple-areola complex is marked at the level of the inframammary crease. We also observed that at 4 years, the distance from the inframammary crease to the inferior border of the nipple-areola complex was significantly shorter, and pseudoptosis did not occur after vertical scar reduction mammaplasty.

6. Lassus C. A 30-year experience with vertical mammaplasty. *Plast Reconstr Surg.* 1996;97(2):373–380.

8. Lejour M. Vertical mammaplasty and liposuction of the breast. *Plast Reconstr Surg.* 1994;94(1):100–114.

11. Hall-Findlay EJ. A simplified vertical reduction mammaplasty: Shortening the learning curve. *Plast Reconstr Surg.* 1999;104(3):748–763.

13. Hall-Findlay EJ. Pedicles in vertical breast reduction and mastopexy. *Clin Plast Surg.* 2002;29(3):379–391.

   A succinct review of various breast reduction techniques and the pedicles that are used to transpose the nipple-areola complex. Dr Hall-Findlay describes her technique for vertical scar reduction mammaplasty in detail.

23. van Deventer PV, Page BJ, Graewe FR. The safety of pedicles in breast reduction and mastopexy procedures. *Aesthetic Plast Surg.* 2008;32(2):307–312.

A thorough review of the blood supply to the nipple-areola complex and the implications on pedicle choice and design during breast reduction surgery.

24. Michelle le Roux C, Kiil BJ, Pan WR, et al. Preserving the neurovascular supply in the Hall-Findlay superomedial pedicle breast reduction: An anatomical study. *J Plast Reconstr Aesthet Surg*. 2010;63(4):655–662.

25. Kerrigan CL, Collins ED, Kim HM, et al. Reduction mammaplasty: Defining medical necessity. *Med Decis Making*. 2002;22(3):208–217.

An evidence-based definition of medical necessity for breast reduction is described in an effort to establish clear, practical, objective, and fair criteria that could be applied by physicians to help differentiate women seeking breast reduction primarily for symptom relief versus aesthetic improvement.

27. Stevens WG, Gear AJ, Stoker DA, et al. Outpatient reduction mammaplasty: An eleven-year experience. *Aesthet Surg J*. 2008;28(2):171–179.

8.4

Short scar periareolar inferior pedicle reduction (SPAIR) mammaplasty

Dennis C. Hammond

SYNOPSIS

- Evolution of SPAIR mammaplasty
- Patient selection: creating the best result
- Surgical planning and marking for SPAIR mammaplasty
- Surgical technique
- Results: for small, moderate and large breast reduction
- Complications specific to SPAIR mammaplasty

Evolution of technique

The short scar periareolar inferior pedicle reduction (SPAIR) mammaplasty was developed in an attempt to eliminate the major complications related to the use of the inverted T pattern inferior pedicle technique for breast reduction. As experience was gained using the inverted T or "Wise pattern" approach, it soon became clear that the extensive scar burden was a significant drawback for many patients and in particular for younger women undergoing this procedure. In addition, every patient who undergoes this procedure experiences a progressive change in the shape of the breast over time with expansion of the lower pole breast contour and a gradual shift of the breast volume progressively into the lower pole. When this change occurs to excess, the aesthetic result is variably compromised leading to the well recognized phenomenon of

"bottoming out". In these patients, the upper pole of the breast appears hollowed out and the inframammary fold scar actually becomes positioned up onto the breast as the breast itself migrates down the chest wall incorporating upper abdominal skin into the formation of the skin envelope of the lower pole of the breast. One frequent admonition for young surgeons is to plan for this occurrence and at the time of placement of the nipple and areola complex (NAC), it is very common to artificially place the NAC in a low position in preparation for the "bottoming out" phenomenon to occur. It is likely that division of Scarpa's fascia at the level of the fold during dissection of the breast along with disruption of the internal fascial scaffold of the breast predisposes to "bottoming out". Therefore, despite the fact that the inverted T inferior pedicle technique for breast reduction has been the standard method used around the globe for many years, the scar burden and the shape change over time are disadvantages that certainly justify the search for alternative techniques of breast reduction.

In evaluating other techniques designed to reduce the scar burden associated with breast reduction, two contrasting methods stand out. First, based on the work of Benelli,[1] attempts to limit the scar to just the periareolar area have been described. Here the inherent "dog-ear" that is created by the use of a large periareolar incision and a smaller areolar incision places great stress on the subsequent skin closure. Therefore, while the scar can be limited to just the periareolar incision when this technique is used, severe drawbacks include compromise of the size, shape, and position of the areola, stippling and irregularity in the periareolar scar, and shape distortion with flattening of the breast itself. As a result, this technique can be reliably utilized only in small reductions of 200 g at most and where the skin envelope is only minimally redundant. In contrast to strictly periareolar techniques stands the classical vertical mammaplasty of Lassus and Lejour.[2-10] Here, the defect created for the NAC is designed to more or less match the dimensions of the incision made around the areola. As a result, the inherent "dog-ear" that is created with the application of the vertical segment is entirely limited to the area between the inferior portion of the areola and the inframammary fold. For a breast of any size, the stress placed on this portion of the breast both in scar quality and healing can be significant. As well, because the parenchymal removal is performed in the inferior pole of the breast, not only is the internal scaffold of the breast disrupted but the entire inframammary fold is released. As a result, and as with the inverted T approach, the breast will "bottom out" or change shape over time. In fact, it is commonly recommended that the shape of the breast appears significantly distorted at the end of the procedure such that the upper pole is over-filled and the lower pole appear flattened in preparation for this shape change to take place. Therefore, rather than eliminating bottoming out as has been claimed by some, the final result actually depends on bottoming out to create the final breast shape. Another significant drawback related to limiting the skin removal to the vertical segment involves the final shape of the breast. For larger breast reductions, plicating the lower pole of the breast in a vertical fashion from the areola down to the fold simply results in a vertical scar that is too long. The distance from the areola to the fold becomes excessive and the breast appears "bottomed out" with a nipple position that is too high. As well, due to irregular tissue approximation at the level of the inframammary fold (IMF), wound breakdown, unsightly scars, and shape distortion can also occur. Often times, these complications become manifest only when the patient raises her arms over shoulder level. In an attempt to manage this aspect of the pattern, various strategies for creating scar contracture at the level of the fold have been described including the use of purse-string sutures

and aggressive liposuction however these issues continue to be responsible for many revisions in patients undergoing vertical mammaplasty. For these reasons, the vertical mammaplasty is best applied to smaller breast reductions of ≤400 g. Using the technique in larger patients may risk unfavorable results with an unacceptably high revision rate.

Despite the disadvantages associated with these various procedures, there are very effective strategic design elements of each that can be combined to provide a versatile and widely applicable technique of breast reduction. From the inverted T experience comes the reliability noted with the use of the inferior pedicle to maintain the vascularity of the NAC even in extreme circumstances. Also, by keeping this centrally located mound of tissue directly under the NAC, the shape of the breast can be better controlled and very importantly, the dissection can be modified to allow the structure of the IMF to remain intact. From the periareolar experience comes the realization that the size of the periareolar incision can exceed that of the areolar incision up to point and still provide a controlled and aesthetic periareolar shape and scar. From the vertical experience comes the observation that the addition of a vertical segment to the skin pattern is a powerful and effective shaping maneuver that can offset the disadvantages associated with purely periareolar techniques. Therefore by using an inferior pedicle technique for management of the vascularity to the NAC with a combined and slightly modified vertical and periareolar or circumvertical skin pattern, the dog-ear inherent in the skin envelope management strategy is distributed over the entire incision as opposed to just around the areola (i.e., Benelli) or just to the vertical segment (i.e., vertical mammaplasty). The result is a very effective, reliable, and widely applicable technique for breast reduction. This is the basis for the SPAIR procedure.[11-14]

Patient selection

After utilizing the SPAIR mammaplasty for the past 14 years, it is clear that the pattern can be applied to a breast of basically any shape, size, or volume. However, as with all short scar techniques, the quality of the aesthetic result will be inversely proportional to the preoperative size of the breast and the redundancy of the skin enveloped. In other words, the technique provides outstanding results for less severe cases of mastopexy or breast reduction up to approximately 800 g per side. Between 800 and 1200 g per side, the technical challenges of the procedure are better handled by those experienced with the procedure, and for reductions over 1200 g, some compromise in shape or scar is likely to result as compared to smaller reductions. In spite of that, the compromises are less troublesome than with other techniques and even in cases of gigantomastia, aesthetic and effective results can be obtained.

Surgical planning and marking

Video
1

The patient is marked in the upright position. Basic landmarks, including the location of the inframammary fold, the breast meridian, and the midsternal line are drawn in. By communicating the level of the inframammary fold across the midline, the location of the fold can be directly seen without the need to manipulate the breast and potentially skew the apparent location of the fold. An 8 cm pedicle is diagrammed on the lower pole of the breast centered on the breast meridian. Measuring up from the inframammary fold on either side of the pedicle a distance of 8–10 cm is measured and then marked. For smaller reductions, the 8 cm measurement is used with the 10 cm measurement being used for larger reductions. Communicating these points identifies the lower portion of the periareolar pattern. The top of the periareolar pattern is drawn 4 cm above the inframammary fold line. This means that the nipple will be located 2 cm above the fold. This is the desired location given that the location of the fold will not change as a result of the dissection. To artificially position the NAC in any other location in an attempt to accommodate for suspected changes in the shape of the breast is unnecessary and will risk NAC malposition. To determine then the medial and lateral extent of the periareolar pattern, the breast is transposed first up and out and then up and in and the breast meridian is ghosted onto the newly transposed breast at the level of the nipple. The four cardinal points of the pattern are then joined with a smooth line and the inferior pedicle is drawn in skirting the top of the periareolar pattern by a distance of 2 cm. This completes the marking process *(Fig. 8.4.1)*.

Technique

With the patient supine, the proposed areas of de-epithelialization are infiltrated with a diluted solution of lidocaine with epinephrine. With the breast under tourniquet tension, an areolar diameter of 40–44 mm is marked and the areolar and periareolar incisions are made. The intervening skin is de-epithelialized and the dermis around the periareolar incision 5 mm inside the incision edge is divided so as to create a small dermal shelf. This shelf will serve as the soft tissue architectural support for the subsequent interlocking PTFE suture. The tourniquet is released and the breast flaps are then sculpted such that the initial flap edge is quite thin with the flap then getting progressively thicker until the chest wall is reached. Initially the dissection proceeds directly under the dermis, however at the level of the chest wall, the flap is 4–6 cm thick. This describes the medial and superior flap dissection. Laterally the flap is dissected down to the lateral border mark made preoperatively at the level of the breast fascia and, as a result, the lateral flap is noticeably thinner than the superior or medial flaps. This is required as there is a tendency for the breast to be excessively full laterally if too much tissue is left at this phase of the dissection. As the lateral flap development then moves superolaterally, the dissection gradually merges with the thicker flap superiorly to create a smooth transition.

Once the flaps have been created, the inferior pedicle is skeletonized. This is done by peeling the redundant breast tissue away from the inferior pedicle moving from medial to superior to lateral. Care is taken to avoid undermining the pedicle so that the breast septum with its associated vascular mesentery located in the midportion of the pedicle is left intact. Care must also be taken to ensure that the removal of tissue extends completely from the inferomedial corner of the dissection space all the way around the pedicle to the inferolateral corner of the breast. In this fashion, enough breast parenchyma will be sufficiently removed to ensure that the base diameter of the breast is narrowed enough to create an aesthetic contour. Trimming can be done as needed to create smooth contours in the flaps and the pedicle to ensure a smooth even result once the skin envelope is reduced.

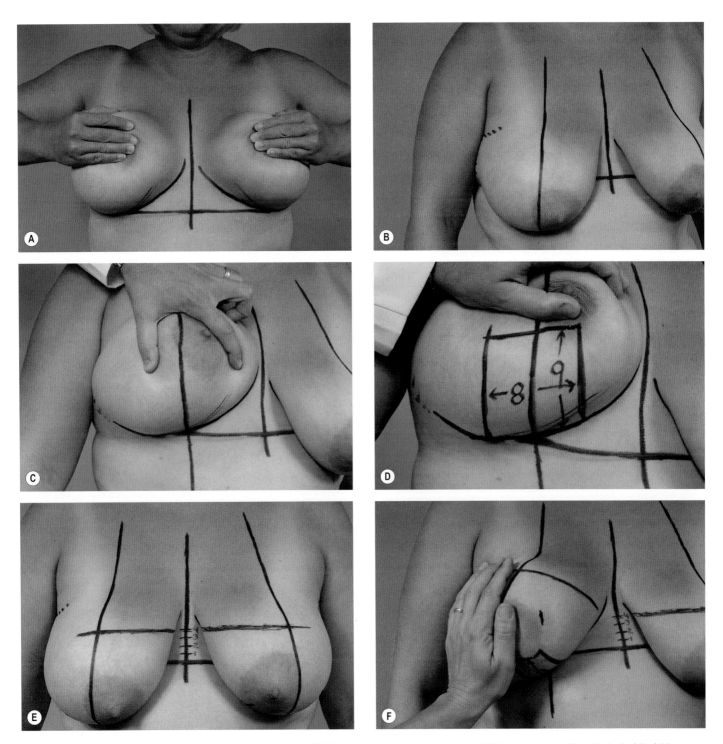

Fig. 8.4.1 **(A)** The mid-sternal line and inframammary fold are marked. **(B)** By communicating the inframammary fold line across the midline, the level of the fold can seen from the front without the need to manipulate the breast. **(C)** A breast meridian is then diagrammed extending down onto the abdominal wall. **(D)** An 8 cm inferior pedicle is centered in the breast meridian and a pedicle length of 8–10 cm is marked. In this patient, a 9 cm length was chosen. This mark identifies the inferior aspect of the periareolar pattern. **(E)** Line paralleling the inframammary fold line 4 cm above the fold is chosen and marked. Where this line intersects the breast meridian marks the superior aspect of the periareolar pattern. **(F,G)** By transposing the breast first up and out, and then up and in and ghosting the meridian onto the breast, the medial and lateral extent of the periareolar pattern can be identified.

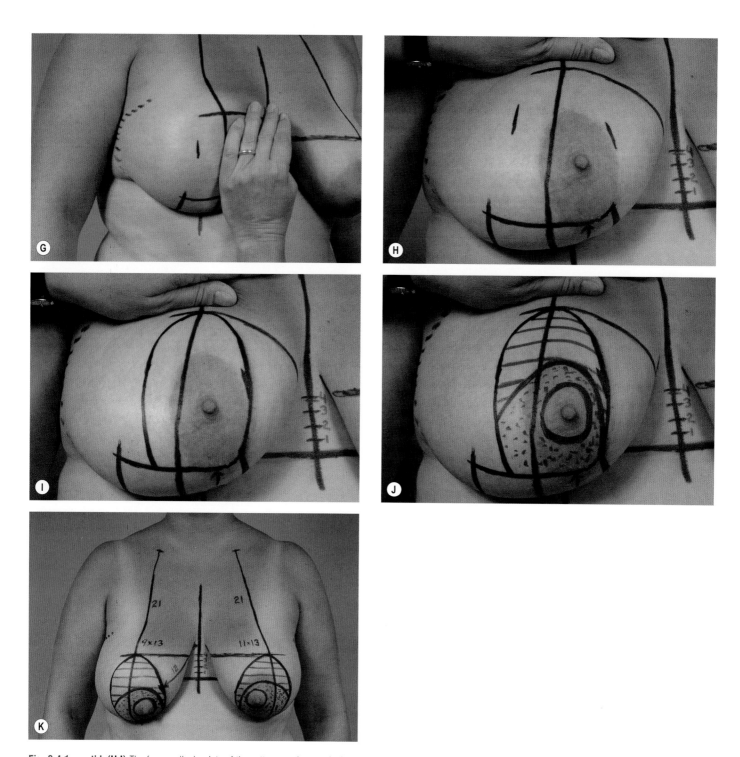

Fig. 8.4.1, cont'd (H,I) The four cardinal points of the pattern are then marked to create an elongated oval. **(J)** The inferior pedicle is drawn in skirting the top of the areola by a distance of 2 cm. **(K)** Final appearance after the marking is completed.

After the breast has been reduced, the skin envelope must be retailored to match the reduced breast volume. This is accomplished by first placing the key staple. By grasping the distal tip of the inferior pedicle and pulling upwards, two small folds will form at either side of the pedicle along the periareolar skin incision. By grasping these two points and stapling them together, the start of the vertical plication pattern can be accurately positioned. By then grasping the deepithelialized dermis on either side of this staple with hemostats and pulling with firm upward traction, the lower pole skin envelope will be seen to variably fold on itself in a line that extends from the key staple downward in a slightly laterally curving arc. By stapling this line together a pleasing lower pole contour will be created. The NAC is then temporarily stapled into the periareolar defect and the patient is placed in the upright position on the operating table where the shape of the resulting breast can be assessed. Further tightening, loosening or infero-lateral extension of the staple line can be performed as needed to create the most aesthetic shape possible. The extent of the skin plication required to create a pleasing shape depends on many factors including how redundant the skin envelope is to begin with, the elasticity of the skin, where the NAC is positioned, and where the breast sits on the chest wall. Basically for each patient, the slightly angled vertical plication is tightened until a pleasing shape is obtained. Care must be taken not to allow the plication line to extend past the IMF down onto the upper abdomen. Rather, the plication line is curved out inferolaterally along the fold to take up any remaining redundancy. For smaller reductions, this plication line will have only a slight lateral cant at the IMF. For larger reductions there will be a more extensive lateral plication extending out along the fold. This represents the only difference in technique for breasts of different volumes. All other aspects of the marking and the dissection are the same except for the fact the in larger reductions, the plication line extends further laterally along the IMF.

Once a pleasing shape has been created, the plication line is marked with a surgical marker and the patient is placed back supine on the operating table. Orientation lines are added and the staples are removed. The skin that sits on the pedicle as defined by the plication pattern is deepithelialized and the excess skin on either side of the pedicle is removed. Typically along the medial side

this amounts to a small wedge of tissue. Laterally however the resection line extends down the entire lateral border of the pedicle. This accomplishes two goals. First, additional volume is removed which can be helpful in assuring that a sufficient reduction in breast volume is performed to ensure relief of symptoms. Second, by fully releasing the lateral flap, advancement medially over to the medial incision on top of the inferior pedicle is more easily performed without creating any tissue bunching or distortion. The vertical incision is then closed using absorbable monofilament sutures. Drains are placed in the larger reductions of approximately ≥800 g and it is at this point that the drain is positioned to run from medial to lateral across the top of the dissection space exiting the breast just lateral to the distal end of the vertical plication.

The final task is to now manage the periareolar closure.[15] Again with the patient upright, the shape of the periareolar opening is assessed. It is very common for this opening to exhibit an oval shape with the long axis running from superomedial to inferolateral, which could predispose to the creation of a less than circular areolar shape postoperatively. For this reason, the periareolar opening is trimmed to create a circular opening to better match the circular areolar incision. Care is taken to be sure a small dermal cuff is left behind as was done initially to ensure a proper platform for placement of the PTFE suture. At this point the interlocking PTFE suture is placed. Eight cardinal points are diagrammed onto the areolar and periareolar incision edges. Using the 3-0 PTFE Teflon suture attached to a straight Keith needle, the pattern is begun at the most medial extent of the opening. This point is chosen for the position of the knot as it will form a substantial mass of suture. In the unusual case of infection related to the permanent PTFE suture, it is far easier to remove the suture if the knot can be reliably located. For this reason, it is always placed medially. The needle is passed from deep to superficial through the dermal shelf. At the corresponding location on the areola, a small bite of areolar dermis is then taken with the needle and the suture is then passed back over to the dermal shelf right next to where the initial pass entered the dermis. The needle is then run through the dermal shelf directly along the incision until the next cardinal point is reached. Here again, the need is passed medially to take a small bite of areolar dermis and then it is passed back over again to the periareolar dermal shelf. This process is repeated around the entire circumference of the periareolar incision joining the eight cardinal points in an interlocking fashion. At the junction of the vertical incision with the periareolar incision, the needle is passed down into the vertical incision as it is woven past this point. Then, when the suture is pulled tight it will have a lifting effect on this critical point where the vertical incision meets the periareolar incision and help prevent this point from being pulled inferiorly thus creating a small teardrop deformity in the shape of the areola. When the starting point in the pattern has been reached, the needle is passed from superficial to deep to ensure that the

subsequent knot will be buried under the medial edge of the dermal shelf. Once the suture has been successfully woven into position it is pulled tight until the incision edges are approximated and the desired size and shape of the areola has been created. It is here that the utility of the Teflon suture becomes evident. No other suture material will pass through this extensive woven pattern with as much ease or control. The handling characteristics of Teflon and its permanent nature make it the ideal material for use in managing large periareolar defects. About 8–10 throws are required to keep the knot from slipping. The suture ends are cut short and the knot is slipped under the dermal shelf to

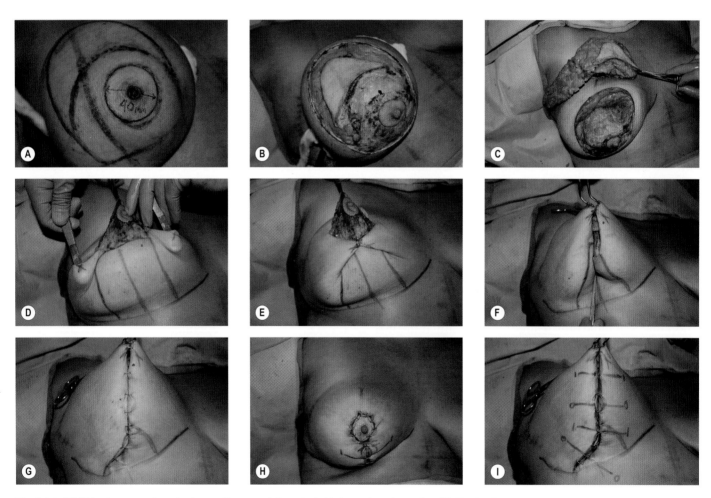

Fig. 8.4.2 (A) With a breast tourniquet in place, a 40 mm areola is marked with the areola under tension. **(B)** The dermis around the periareolar incision is divided leaving a small dermal shelf. The superior aspect of the pedicle is also incised. **(C)** Appearance of the breast after skeletonization of the pedicle. The breast has been reduced by removing a "C" shaped segment of tissue from around the sides and top of the pedicle. The flaps have been left sufficiently full to help assist on the shaping of the breast. **(D)** By applying traction on the tip of the pedicle, two folds will form in the skin pattern on either side of the pedicle. **(E)** These two points are joined together with the placement of the "key" staple. **(F–H)** By applying upward traction on the pattern, the redundant skin envelope of the breast can be plicated to create a rounded lower pole. Note that the inferior end of the plication begins to cant laterally along the inframammary fold. **(I)** Once a pleasing shape has been created, the margins of the plication line are marked and orientation lines are added to assist in closure once the incisions have been made.

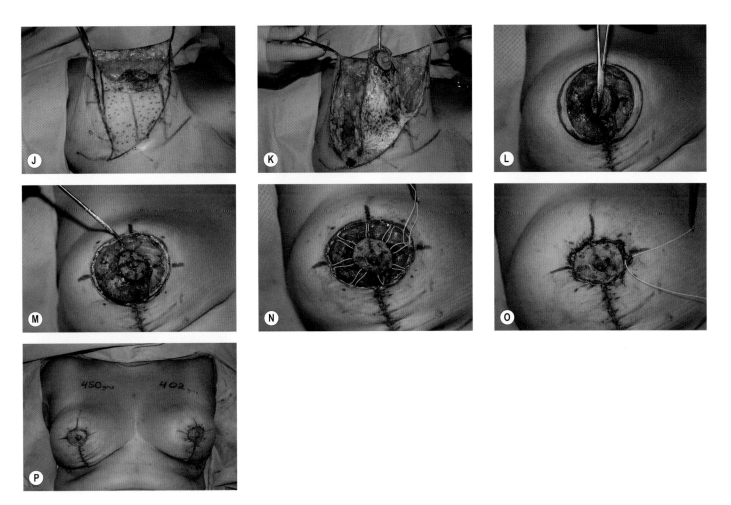

Fig. 8.4.2, cont'd (J) With the staples now removed, the extent of the vertical pattern can be seen. The stippled area represents the inferior pedicle. **(K)** Appearance after deepithelialization of the inferior pedicle and removal of redundant tissue medial and lateral to the pedicle. **(L)** With the patient upright, the now reduced periareolar opening is redrawn to approximate a perfect circle. **(M)** Eight cardinal points are marked on the periareolar as well as the areolar incision to guide placement of the interlocking purse-string Teflon suture. **(N)** A polytetrafluoroethylene (PTFE) or Teflon suture attached to a straight Keith needle is placed in such a manner as to join the eight cardinal points of the two incisions. **(O)** As a result of the smooth surface and easy handling characteristics of the suture, it can be easily pulled down to create the desired areolar diameter. **(P)** Final result after the removal of 450 g of tissue from the right and 402 from the left.

prevent any possibility of subsequent erosion with exposure. If at this point, the shape of the areola is not circular with the patient upright, additional skin is carefully deepithelialized as need to create circular opening. The areola is then inset into the periareolar opening using only a 3-0 monofilament barbed (Quill) suture. The barbed suture adds an additional layer of support to the closure to help prevent postoperative spreading of the areola. The incision lines are dressed with tissue glue and OpSite dressings and a support garment is applied *(Fig. 8.4.2)*.

Postoperative care is very straightforward. The support garment is worn to comfort. The OpSite dressings are removed at 1 week and scar management with a vitamin E-based ointment covered with paper tape is instituted for a total of 6 weeks. The drains are removed at the first postoperative visit, which occurs at about 7 days. The patient is then seen back at 6 weeks and 1 year, where she is then discharged from care and seen back only if there are any complications or questions.

Results

Small breast reduction (≤400 g): As with any short scar technique, the results obtained with small breast reductions are outstanding. It is not difficult at all to apply

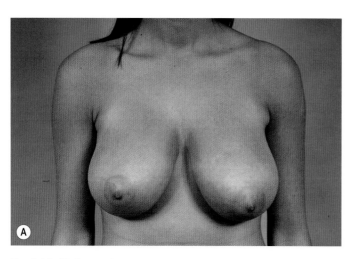 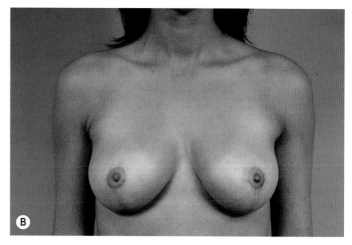

Fig. 8.4.3 (A) Preoperative appearance of a 26-year-old woman in preparation for breast reduction using the SPAIR technique. **(B)** Postoperative appearance at 7 months after the removal of 425 g of tissue from the left breast and 300 g from the right.

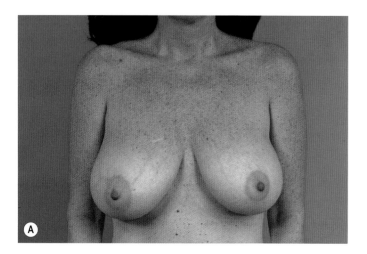 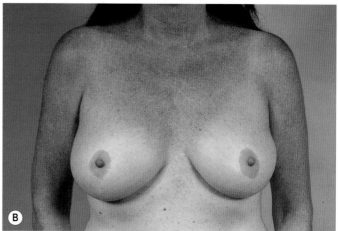

Fig. 8.4.4 (A) Preoperative appearance of a 52-year-old woman in preparation for breast reduction using the SPAIR technique. **(B)** Postoperative appearance at 6 years after the removal of 327 g of tissue from the left breast and 415 g from the right.

the circumvertical pattern and little stress is placed on the periareolar closure. The only difficulty lies in the fact that the periareolar opening can be somewhat limiting during the dissection making accurate flap creation and pedicle skeletonization somewhat tedious. However, the results are worth the effort as the aesthetics of the reduced breast are remarkable and the result is maintained for years *(Figs 8.4.3, 8.4.4)*.

Modest breast reduction (400–800 g): As the preoperative size of the breast increases, it becomes easier to technically perform the procedure. Patients who present in this category are the best patients to begin applying the procedure to for the novice SPAIR surgeon. The periareolar pattern is big enough to easily dissect the

flaps, yet the skin envelope is still easily managed using the circumvertical pattern. As with smaller reductions, the results are outstanding and maintain an aesthetic appearance over time *(Fig. 8.4.5)*.

Large breast reduction (>800 g): In these cases, it is helpful to have experience using the circumvertical pattern as intraoperative adjustments of the pattern become more important. Flap dissection and pedicle skeletonization are very straightforward due to the size of the periareolar pattern. However, ultimately making sure the dimensions of the skin envelope match the remaining volume of the breast requires the greatest skill and artistry on the part of the surgeon as opposed to smaller breast reductions. Despite the technical

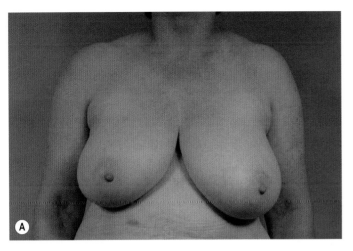 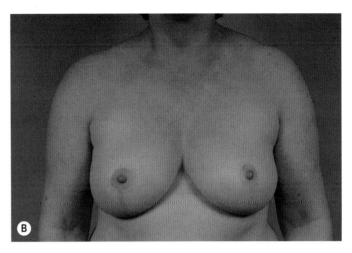

Fig. 8.4.5 (A) Preoperative appearance of a 58-year-old woman in preparation for breast reduction using the SPAIR technique. **(B)** Postoperative appearance at 13 months after the removal of 645 g of tissue from the left breast and 436 g from the right.

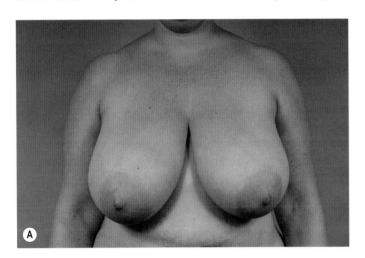 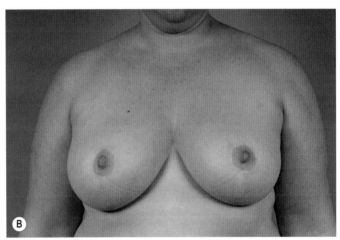

Fig. 8.4.6 (A) Preoperative appearance of a 50-year-old woman in preparation for breast reduction using the SPAIR technique. **(B)** Postoperative appearance at 1 year after the removal of 961 g of tissue from the left breast and 1004 g from the right.

requirements of the procedure, outstanding results are obtained with few complications. It is this facet of the procedure that ultimately is very appealing. This group of patients is the very group that is prone to complications using other techniques, however with the SPAIR complications are few and when they do occur are easily managed *(Fig. 8.4.6)*.

Complications

The complications noted with the SPAIR mammaplasty generally mirror those noted with other techniques however several issues specific to this technique merit specific comment.

Fat necrosis

Despite preservation of the underside of the inferior pedicle and the attachments to the septum, there can be a relative ischemia to the most distal end near the areola. Postoperatively the presence of ischemic and/or necrotic fat can be identified as firmness that can be easily identified via palpation along the superior border of the periareolar scar. The best option is to wait for this process to stabilize over a period of 6–12 months to allow the necrotic fat to completely demarcate. Early attempts to remove this fat will result in the removal of additional viable parenchyma due to the inflammation still present in the wound making it difficult to discern living from necrotic tissue. Once the swelling has completely resolved and the fat has fully demarcated, removal is usually very straightforward and only rarely will affect the eventual shape of the breast. No matter how extensive, excisional biopsy of this necrotic fat is recommended to allow subsequent breast cancer surveillance to be performed without difficulty or confusion.

Shape distortion

Despite every effort to maximize symmetry as well as the quality of the overall aesthetic result, instances of asymmetry or shape distortion will occur. These can range from differences in volume, to asymmetries in NAC position, to distortion in either the shape of the areola or the shape of the breast itself. No matter what the specific problem is, almost any problem related to asymmetry or shape can be managed by re-applying the circumvertical pattern with or without excision of additional volume. Simply as a result of the effect that the combined periareolar and vertical skin management strategy has on the shape of the breast, a great deal of control over the results is provided that can be reliably predicted simply by tailor-tacking the skin together. In this fashion, areolar position and shape as well as breast width and lower pole contour can all be reconfigured as needed to address specific concerns. It is actually this aspect of the circumvertical pattern that affords such satisfaction as the quality of the result will be determined in part by the artistic abilities of the operating surgeon.

One particular shape problem that has been encountered rarely relates to the development of a seroma postoperatively. In selected cases this seroma, which surrounds the deep superior aspect of the pedicle, may not be obvious early and the appearance of the breast can be quite normal to about the 6-week mark. However, as the seroma gradually reabsorbs and the cavity contracts, the surrounding parenchyma is pulled inward with the end result being a flattened and blunted breast apex with distorted fullness around the upper pole. If this does not resolve over a period of 6–12 months, surgical intervention is required. By entering the breast through the periareolar incision, the old seroma cavity is resected allowing the breast to re-expand into a pleasing shape.

Areolar spreading

In selected cases, there can be either spreading or distortion of the shape of the areola, particularly in those cases where the diameter of the periareolar defect prior to placing the interlocking PTFE suture was >10 cm. This complication is actually very simply addressed by re-applying the interlocking technique. Even under local anesthesia if desired, the new areolar diameter is diagrammed with the aid of an areolar template and a second incision is made outside the existing periareolar scar. The intervening skin is de-epithelialized and the old PTFE suture removed. Placing the new PTFE suture in an interlocking fashion allows the shape and size of the areolar to be reconfigured to the desired dimensions. A side benefit of this approach is that any persistent stippling that may have been present along the scar is removed as well leaving behind a better appearing scar.

PTFE infection/exposure

Despite efforts to bury the PTFE suture and knot under the skin flaps, some patients will present with an erythematous hue around the areola usually with small pinpoint openings along the scar that drain a clear fluid. This is the hallmark of an infected PTFE suture. Although it is tempting to treat this condition with antibiotics alone, the best approach is to simply remove the PTFE suture remembering that that knot is located at the medial aspect of the areola. This can easily be done using local anesthesia as needed. Oral antibiotics for routine skin flora are administered as well. At this point there is then a risk that the areolar diameter could spread with the support of the PTFE suture now gone. If after 6 months there is spreading of the areola, a repeat periareolar procedure using the interlocking PTFE suture technique can be applied to create the desired areolar diameter and shape.

Recurrence of hypertrophy

Occasionally, patients will present with re-hypertrophy of the breast over time and request re-reduction. Also, some patients may present with dissatisfaction with the original procedure feeling that they were not reduced enough. In either instance it is possible to simply reapply the SPAIR procedure taking car to preserve the integrity of the inferior pedicle as much as possible. However, a simpler and less invasive approach is to utilize standard liposuction technique to reduce the volume of the breast and then tighten the skin envelope by re-applying the circumvertical pattern as needed to create the desired shape. In this fashion, the breast can re-reduced to good effect with little chance devascularizing the NAC.

Summary

While the overriding goal of breast reduction is to reduce the volume of the breast to relieve the stress placed on the upper torso, it is inescapable that there is a significant aesthetic component to the procedure. Any technique used to treat the hypertrophied breast must allow volume reduction and yet preserve the blood supply to the NAC and yield an aesthetic shape that maintains itself over time. The SPAIR mammaplasty accomplishes these goals with a minimum of complications. By combining an inferior pedicle approach with a circumvertical skin pattern, the volume of the breast is effectively reduced leaving behind roughly half the scar burden associated with standard inferior pedicle techniques. The quality of the aesthetic result is outstanding and these results are maintained over the long term. Incorporating the concepts associated with the SPAIR mammaplasty will enhance the breast reduction experience, not only for the patient, but for the surgeon as well.

 Access the complete reference list online at **http://www.expertconsult.com**

2. Lassus C. A 30-year experience with vertical mammaplasty. *Plast Reconstr Surg*. 1996;97(2):373–380.

   Claude Lassus can be called the "father" of the vertical mammaplasty. His work provided the modern stimulus for all others to re-examine the issue of not only reduced scars, but better shape as well. This paper distills his 30-year experience. True students of breast reduction must be familiar with this paper.

3. Lassus C. Update on vertical mammaplasty. *Plast Reconstr Surg*. 1999;104(7):2289–2298.

   As variants of the vertical mammaplasty concept began to be described, Dr Lassus provided a summary of his technique and contrasted it with these other modifications. This paper summarizes the differences and provides further understanding of how the vertical incision shapes the breast.

4. Lejour M. Vertical mammaplasty. *Plast Reconstr Surg*. 1993;92(5):985–986.

   While Dr Lassus can be credited with describing the basics of the vertical mammaplasty, Dr Lejour is largely responsible for popularizing it. Although she introduced some modifications in technique, the basic operative strategy is the same and it was her work that served to be the tipping point in introducing the concepts to the rest of the world.

11. Hammond DC. Short scar periareolar inferior pedicle reduction (SPAIR) mammaplasty. *Plast Reconstr Surg*. 1999;103(3):890–901.

    While the Lassus type of vertical mammaplasty was really revolutionary in design, certain complications unique to the technique became well recognized. In an attempt to eliminate these complications, the SPAIR technique was developed. By combining a more aggressive circumvertical approach with an inferior pedicle technique, a versatile procedure was developed that largely eliminates the potential for wound breakdown at the inferior end of the vertical incision. This paper was the first description of this technique.

15. Hammond DC, Khuthaila DK, Kim J. The interlocking Gore-Tex suture for control of areolar diameter and shape. *Plast Reconstr Surg*. 2007;119(3):804–809.

    This paper describes an extremely effective and versatile technique for control of the periareolar defect in all types of aesthetic and reconstructive breast surgery. It provides for an effective method of minimizing postoperative spreading and shape distortion in periareolar surgery. Every serious student of surgery of the breast will find the concepts described in this paper useful.

8.5

The L short-scar mammaplasty

Armando Chiari Jr.

SYNOPSIS

- The technique principle: "what is most important is what remains, not what is removed."
- The resulting L scars are used for small, medium and large reductions. The mini-L scars are used for mastopexies with the associated use of prosthesis.
- The technique uses a superomedial transposition pedicle and resects middle and inferior portions of the breast while preserving the third, fourth and fifth lateral intercostal nerves.
- In short-scar mammaplasties, the resection of a large amount of skin at the top of the mammary cone leads to areola enlargement, bad periareolar scars and early ptosis relapse.
- By marking the skin that will remain, the L short-scar mammaplasty makes possible larger resections at the middle and inferior parts of breasts, making large removals of periareolar skin unnecessary.
- With reduced scars, this technique creates good shape with excellent long-term results.

Evolution of the technique and patient selection

The L short-scar mammaplasty is a reduced scar technique, which seeks to maximize the utilization of the principle that what is most important is what remains, not what is removed.[1]

The author's previous publications showed the variants of the L short-scar mammaplasty with very small resulting scars – vertical and mini-L scars – with simplified markings.[2,3] He tried to use these variants in most of the cases, but late evaluation showed ptosis relapse and areola enlargement in the cases of larger and more ptosed breasts. At that time, the 'L short-scar' or Chiari reduction was best suited for women with mild (resections up to 300 g) and moderate (300–600 g) hypertrophies. This fact instigated a reversion to indicating marking with a resulting scar in the shape of an L for most of his cases. With some improvements from years of practice, this has helped enable surgeons to perform large hypertrophies operations (resections of 600–900 g) or very large (≥900–1200 g), if the breast skin elasticity is sufficient (see *Fig. 8.5.6*).

The author has indicated the variants of the technique, with vertical or mini-L resulting scars to patients,[2,3] the results being ptosis relapse and areola enlargement for the cases of more hypertrophy and ptosis, especially the ones whose mammary content was fatter and the skin was less elastic. In these cases, there was apparent good accommodation of the skin in the operation room, but time and gravity caused a curvature of the inferior poles and areola enlargement. Routine indication of suture in periareolar pouch[4] with colorless 4-0 Mononylon® minimized, but did not solve the problem. The author reverted to indicating the technique with resulting "L" scars to patients (see *Figs 8.5.6–8.5.10*), with a more simplified marking (see *Fig. 8.5.1A*) than described in the original publication.[1] Today, the markings of the variants with mini-L and vertical scars[2,3] are indicated, especially for mastopexies with the associated use of prosthesis.

One of the most important indications of this technique is asymmetry (see *Fig. 8.5.9*). For symmetry it is better to mark and resect directly to preserve similar portions of the breast, than to mark and resect different breast portions and only as a consequence, reach similar portions that will result in symmetry.

Since 1988, the author has performed 1287 operations using the L short-scar technique,[1–3,5,6] which uses a superomedial transposition pedicle, an extensive undermining from the thoracic wall, and resects middle and inferior portions of the breast while preserving the third, fourth and fifth lateral intercostal nerves. The steps of the technique are described below.

Planning and marking

This technique's marking is more concerned with the skin that will remain than the skin that will be removed. Markings are based on the midsternal line, the inframammary fold and its projection on the anterior surface of the breast (point A), rather than on a predetermined pattern.[1] Therefore, we delimit the amount of skin strictly necessary (see *Fig. 8.5.1*) for reshaping the medial (line *BC*) and the lateral (line *B′C′*) portions of the breasts. After resection, the breast is reshaped by suturing together lines *BC* and *B′C′*, originating the upright stem of the L scar (see *Fig. 8.5.1*).

With the patient standing, the mid-mammary and midsternal lines are marked. Point A is marked on the projection of the submammary sulcus, on the mid-mammary line, and point A′ is marked 2 cm above it. Afterwards, the patient is set in dorsal decubitus and *all the following marks are made on a stretched skin.*[1–3,5]

Point C is marked 8 cm from the midsternal line and 2 cm (for larger breasts) from the submammary sulcus (see *Fig. 8.5.1*). Point B is marked 10 cm from the midsternal line and 8 cm from point A. *The larger and more ptosed the breast is, the longer line BC will be* (see *Fig. 8.5.1A,B*). In bigger patients or in those whose chests are wider, the distance from points C and B to the midsternal line should increase from 8 cm and 10 cm to 9 cm and 11 cm or to 10 cm and 12 cm, respectively.

Point B′ (see *Fig. 8.5.1A*) is marked between the nipple and point A, *the larger and more ptosed the breast is, the closer point B′ should be from point A* (see *Fig. 8.5.1A,B*). The lateral distance from the areola is determined by trial and error: the formation of a new mammary cone with good projection and without tension is sought by uniting points B and B′ with bidigital maneuvers.[1–3,5] Point C′ is marked 7 cm from point B′, forming line B′C′, with breast skin stretched medially and upwards (see *Fig. 8.5.2*). Point D is marked 3.0 cm (for larger breasts, see *Figs 8.5.1B and 8.5.6*), from the submammary sulcus, at the end of the skin fold that is formed by the union of lines BC and B′C′, by the use of bidigital maneuvers.[1–3,5] For patients whose breasts are smaller (see *Figs 8.5.8–8.5.10*), the distances from points C and D to the submammary sulcus are 1.0 cm and 1.5 cm, respectively.

Technical procedure

The operation starts with patients in a supine position. The skin around the areola is de-epithelialized *(Figs 8.5.1, 8.5.2)*, after marking the new areola within 4.3 cm. The skin is incised along line CD and the adipose capsule is dissected 1.0 cm caudally. This dissection is extended slantwise up, until above the inferior border of the pectoralis muscle, preserving the mammary tissue adhered to the muscle fascia – enough to avoid retractions on line CD.

Then the breast is extensively detached from the pectoralis muscle up to the breast superior border. That detachment is prolonged medially and laterally, up to two resistant fascial structures. Laterally, this fascial structure is surgically isolated by using a blunt detacher. The chest anterolateral wall skin is detached about 6 cm horizontally, from the end of the incisions that originated the "L" scar lateral branch. That detachment should go beyond the anterior axillary line. From that point, the skin detachment is vertically turned aside, towards the correspondent axilla, about 7 cm. That isolated structure is called the breast lateral neurovascular pedicle[1,7] and contains the anterior divisions of the lateral cutaneous branches of the third, fourth and fifth intercostal nerves,[1,7–9] important for nipple-areola sensitivity. In all techniques, incisions, resections and detachments at the level of the anterior axillary line

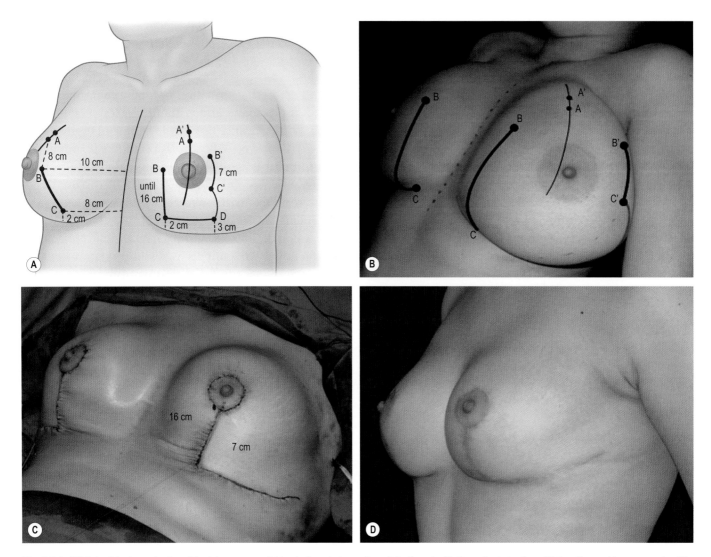

Fig. 8.5.1 (A) Point A is the projection of the inframammary fold onto the anterior surface of the breast, with the patient standing. All the other markings are made with the patient in a supine position, with the skin on stretch. The main medial markings, line BC, refer to the midsternal line, to the inframammary sulcus and to the point A. *The larger and more ptosed the breast is, the longer line BC will be.* **(B)** Markings in the operating room, in the patient of *Figure 8.5.6* (resections of 1258 g and 1252 g). *The larger and more ptosed the breast is, the longer line BC will be (16 cm in this patient). The larger and more ptosed the breast is, the closer point B' should be from point A,* with its lateral distance from the areola determined by trial and error: the formation of a adequate mammary cone is sought by uniting points B and B' with bidigital maneuvers.[1–3,5] **(C)** Same patient as in *Figure 8.5.6*, result in the operating room (resections of 1258 g and 1252 g). The lateral line B'C', which was 7 cm long, was sutured to line BC, which was 16 cm long, originating the upright stem of the L scar, with some compensation folds. **(D)** Same patients as in *Figures 8.5.1B,C and 8.5.6*, result 3 months after operation. The compensation folds that result from the vertical skin compensation disappear around the third postoperative month.

and beyond it involve a higher risk of lesions to this pedicle.

Next, patients are set in a semi-sitting position and the breasts are pulled upwards, from point A. Mammary resection starts through an incision made along line C'D, which continues vertically towards the chest. From lines BC and B'C', the incisions in mammary tissue converge at 60° towards the chest *(Fig. 8.5.3)*.[1–3,5] An incision or a resection of the necessary mammary tissue is made

in the superior pole,[1–3,5] between the areola and point B' *(Fig. 8.5.3)*. Thus, two mammary tissue pillars are formed; a medial one, which corresponds to line BC projection, and a lateral one, which corresponds to line B'C' projection. The bases of the pillars formed are resected, making them 7 cm high, on average *(Fig. 8.5.4)*. When performing this maneuver, great care should be taken in order to preserve the breast lateral neurovascular pedicle.[1,7,8]

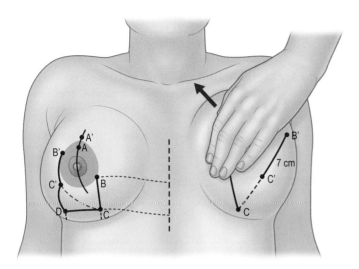

Fig. 8.5.2 Point B′ is marked between the nipple and point A. *The larger and more ptosed the breast is, the closer point B′ should be from point A.* Point C′ is marked 7 cm from point B′, forming line B′C′C, with breast skin stretched medially and upwards.

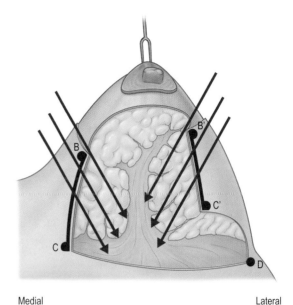

Medial   Lateral

Fig. 8.5.3 From lines BC and B′C′, the incisions in mammary tissue converge at 60° towards the chest.[1–3,5] An incision or a resection of the necessary mammary tissue is made in the superior pole,[1–3,5] between the areola and point B′.

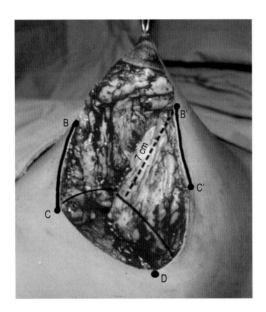

Fig. 8.5.4 Left breast with the main slanting incisions in mammary tissue performed. The bases of the pillars formed are resected at the horizontal blue lines, making them 7 cm high.

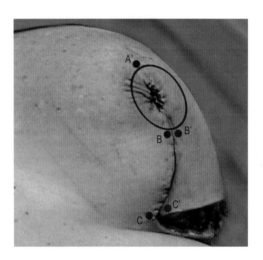

Fig. 8.5.5 The lateral line B′C′ was sutured to the medial line BC originating the upright stem of the L scar. A temporary skin compensation pouch is made using more medial skin,[1–3,5] in order to achieve a well-projected mammary cone top. The new areola position is marked within 3.6 cm and de-epithelialized with A′ as the vertex.[1–3,5]

After careful hemostasis, the medial and lateral pillar bases are sutured together, as well as lines BC and B′C′, forming the L scar vertical stem *(Fig. 8.5.5)*. When it comes to large breasts, the lateral line B′C′, which is 7 cm long, is sutured to the much longer line BC (see *Fig. 8.5.1A–C)*; the compensation folds that result from this skin compensation disappear around the third postoperative month *(Fig. 8.5.1D)*.

A temporary skin compensation pouch is made using more medial skin,[1–3,5] in order to achieve a well-projected mammary cone top, without tension *(Fig. 8.5.5)*. The new areola position is marked within 3.6 cm and de-epithelialized with A′ as the vertex.[1–3,5] The removal of periareolar skin is small, being much bigger in the middle and inferior parts of the breast. A continuous circular intradermal suture[4,5] is done with colorless 4-0

Monocryl® fixed within 4.3 cm, to prevent areolar enlargements and to rotate the skin that remains at the top of the mammary cone from medial to lateral. The areola is placed in the limits of the four cardinal points.

At the lateral skin fold superior margin, a skin triangle is resected to place the L scar horizontal stem more superiorly.[1,5]

Examples of large, medium, and small reductions

Markings of the skin that will remain make possible the indication of this reduced scar technique for small, medium and large hypertrophies, and for breast asymmetries (*Figs 8.5.6–8.5.10*).

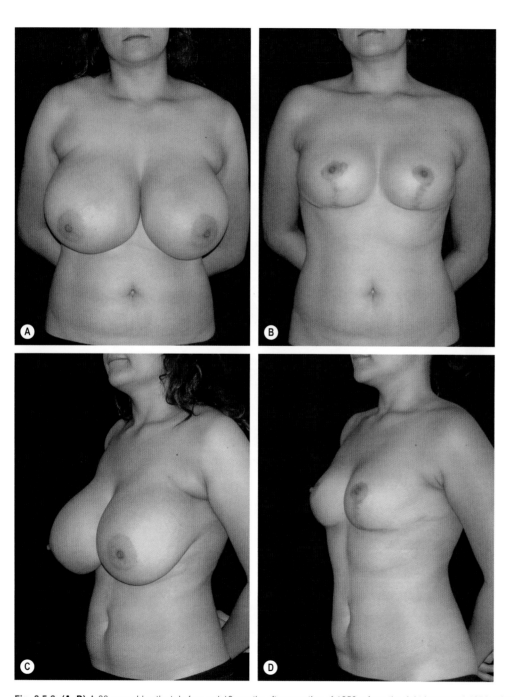

Fig. 8.5.6 (A–D) A 23-year-old patient, before and 12 months after resection of 1258 g from the right breast and 1252 g from the left breast, with resulting "L" scars.

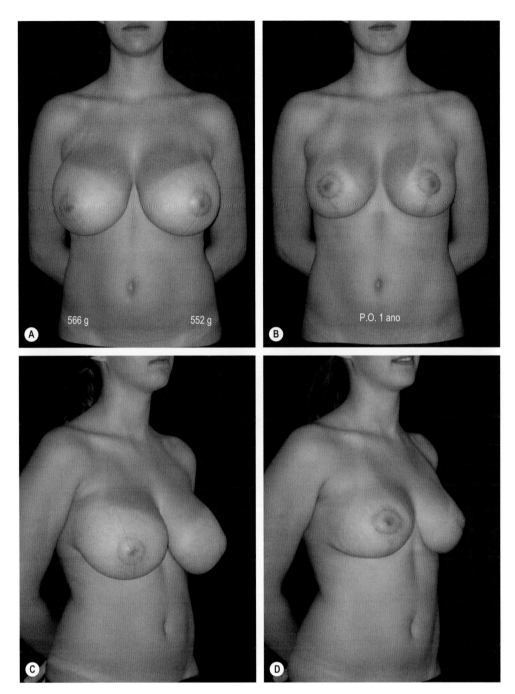

Fig. 8.5.7 (A–D) An 18-year-old patient, before and 12 months after resection of 566 g from the right breast and 552 g from the left breast, with resulting "L" scars.

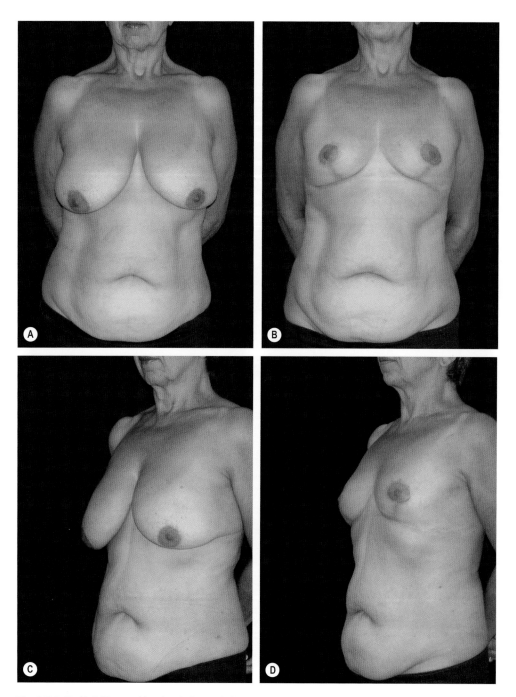

Fig. 8.5.8 (A–D) A 56-year-old patient, before and 12 months after resection of 450 g from the left breast and 405 g from the right breast, with resulting "L" scars.

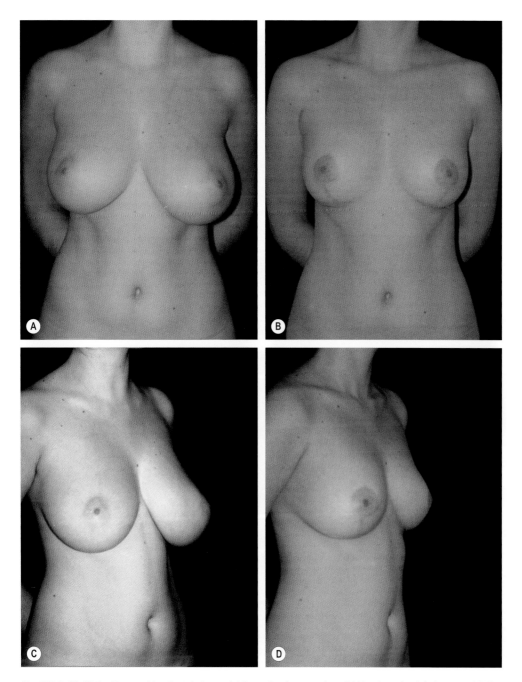

Fig. 8.5.9 (A–D) An 18-year-old patient, before and 24 months after resection of 240 g from the right breast and 350 g from the left breast, with resulting "L" scars.

Complications

Areola enlargement, bad periareolar scars and early ptosis relapse are avoided by resection of a small amount of skin at the top of the mammary cone. Sensitivity of the NAC has been consistently preserved by maneuvers adopted to protect the lateral cutaneous nerves.[7] No hematomas develop, as good hemostasis is essential. Small slough of areolas rarely may occur, especially in very large hypertrophies with great ptosis, and are treated conservatively with daily dressings with effective lubrication, and carboxytherapy.

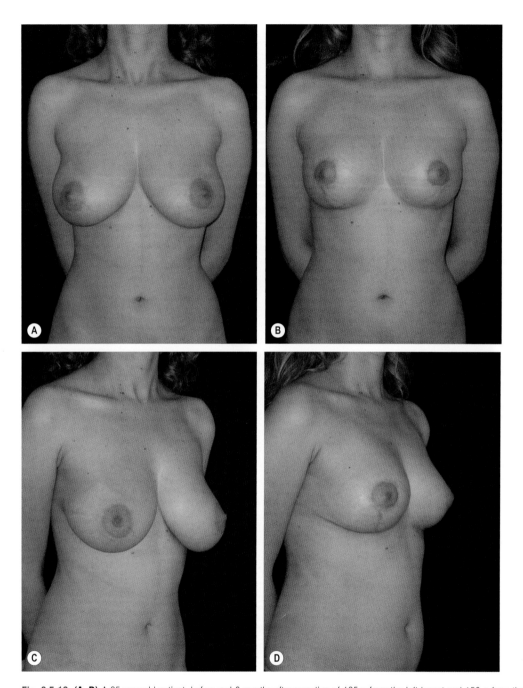

Fig. 8.5.10 (A–D) A 25-year-old patient, before and 6 months after resection of 195 g from the left breast and 150 g from the right breast, with resulting "L" scars.

Summary

In short-scar mammaplasties, the resection of a large amount of skin at the top of the mammary cone leads to areola enlargement, bad periareolar scars and early ptosis relapse, specially for larger breasts.

By marking the skin that will remain, the L short-scar mammaplasty makes possible larger resections at the middle and inferior parts of breasts, making large removals of periareolar skin unnecessary. With reduced scars, this technique creates good shape with excellent long-term results *(Figs 8.5.6–8.5.10)*, preserving breast sensitivity in patients, including large-breasted ones *(Fig. 8.5.6)*.

This technique uses a superomedial transposition pedicle, extensive undermining from the thoracic wall and resects middle and inferior portions of the breast.

References

1. Chiari Jr A. The L short-scar mammaplasty: a new approach. *Plast Reconstr Surg.* 1992;90:233–246.
   Original work, establishing the principles of the technique, its anatomic basis and indications.

2. Chiari Jr A. The L short-scar mammaplasty: 12 years later. *Plast Reconstr Surg.* 2001;108:489–495.
   Presents a variant of this technique with even smaller scars – with vertical and mini-L scars.

3. Chiari Jr A. The L short-scar mammaplasty. *Clin Plast Surg.* 2002;29:401–409.

4. Benelli L. A new periareolar mammaplasty: the "round block" technique. *Aesthet Plast Surg.* 1990;14:93–100.

5. Chiari Jr A, Grotting J. The L short-scar mammaplasty. In: Spear SL, ed. *Surgery of the breast: principles and art.* 3rd ed. Philadelphia: Lippincott Williams & Wilkins; 2011:1128–1143.

6. McCulley SJ, Rousseau TE. A modified Chiari L short-scar mammoplasty – the technique and results. *Br J Plast Surg.* 1999;52:112–117.
   A good example of how any surgeon can adapt the technique, obtaining good results.

7. Chiari Jr A, Nunes TA, Grotting JC, et al. Breast sensitivity before and after the L short-scar mammaplasty. *Aesthet Plast Surg.* 2011; June 3rd [Epub ahead of print].

8. Würinger E, Mader N, Posch E, et al. Nerve and vessel supplying ligamentous suspension of the mammary gland. *Plast Reconstr Surg.* 1998;101:1486–1493.
   Work based on anatomical dissection, which confirmed the innervation described in the original publication of this technique.

9. Sarhadi NS, Shaw Dunn J, Lee FD, et al. An anatomical study of the nerve supply of the breast, including the nipple and areola. *Br J Plast Surg.* 1996;49:156–164.
   Anatomical study that describes the innervation of the breast, including historical perspective on the classical study by Cooper.

8.6

Periareolar technique with mesh support

Joao Carlos Sampaio Góes

SYNOPSIS

- The chapter describes a technique based on reshaping the breast parenchyma and treating the glandular mound separately from the skin.
- The skin is redraped over the new breast architecture, though the periareolar approach, and the new breast is assembled through glandular flap rotation and fixation to the anterior pectoral fascia.
- The cutaneous lining is duplicated using a circular dermal flap with the central pedicle in the areolar region.
- The addition of the mixed mesh to the original technique, applied as a sandwich between the two layers of cutaneous lining, was performed to obtain a longer-lasting aesthetic result based on a resistant supporting system.
- This would maintain the ideal position of the gland after surgery and permit adequate fixation of the tissues into place.

Evolution of the technique

The areolar surgical approach has always been of great interest to the authors, as it enables surgical access to the whole breast; the glandular mound can be treated separately from the skin coverage, and the surgery results in minimal scars, avoiding the unpleasant 'surgical' appearance. In 1976, the authors described the areolar mammary quadrant resection, with plastic repair using two internally rotated glandular flaps detached from the skin.[1]

This technique, which is currently used in oncological quadrantectomies, was the basis for the development of Góes' periareolar technique, first published in 1989.[2–9] Periareolar mammoplasty was initially intended to reposition the glandular mound and provide a new positioning in relation to the thorax and a new aesthetic format.[10–16] The skin cover, initially detached from the gland, only covers the repositioned gland, leaving one scar in the periareolar region. Excessive periareolar skin is de-epithelialized and used as an internal flap, working as an internal bra to support the new breast.

In early postoperative follow-up, it was observed that this tissue structure was insufficient to maintain ideal conic format of the remodeled breast for a prolonged period, and therefore a permanent internal support system is required to provide stability and avoid distension of tissues in a centrifugal direction, thus avoiding expansion of the breast base and the diameter of the areola. In order to create stability, Góes started using a support mesh sandwiched between the two skin layers, the external layer and the de-epithelialized internal layer.

This system provides a long-lasting aesthetic result based on a more resistant support system. It helps maintain the ideal position of the gland after surgery and enables adequate fixation of the tissues into place, counterbalancing the forces of gravity.

Different kinds of materials have been used for the support system. A polyglactin 910 mesh was initially used in 55 cases. Because it is an absorbable material, there was a partial loss of the aesthetic result after 2 years of follow-up.[4,5]

To obtain a long-lasting result, a mixed-mesh of polyglactin 910 and polyester was used in 172 cases, providing excellent results which were maintained in the late follow-up for several years. Other partially absorbable materials were also used and with delicate permanent components, which we consider important to maintain the ideal format of the breast, such as Vypro made of polypropylene and polyglactin and presently, we are using ULTRAPRO made of polypropylene and monocryl.[6,7]

It is important to emphasize that the nonabsorbable material used is the same as that of suture threads usually used in surgeries in general. There were no complications resulting from their use after hundreds of surgeries.

Patient selection

Patient selection is a fundamental principle because the technique is not ideal for all patients. Resection limits, breast dimensions, tissue quality, and the presence of thoracic wall deformities are important factors that must be taken into consideration. Tissue quality is important because eventual scars produced by the mesh and skin retraction are responsible for the end result. Therefore, patients with thicker and more elastic skin have better retraction, less postoperative periareolar wrinkles, and longer-lasting maintenance of the newly shaped breast.

Breasts with greater proportions of glandular tissue (i.e., younger patients) are ideal for this operation because the newly shaped gland is more consistent and more firmly supported. Obese patients with fatty breasts have a worse result because there might be greater tissue displacement in relation to the thoracic wall, resulting in variable loss of anterior projection.

In terms of resection limits, satisfactory results can be obtained when resections of up to one-third of the breast volume are used. In addition, when ample periareolar skin resections are required, there is a higher rate of postoperative periareolar wrinkles. Finally, glandular reassembly may be technically difficult in patients with exaggerated breast ptosis and a narrow breast base.

Technique

The technique consists of separately treating the skin coverage of the breast gland, involving the construction of an internal support system (internal-bra) using the following anatomical elements:

1. Anterior pectoral fascia
2. Intramammary connective ligaments
3. Periareolar dermal flap as the internal skin layer
4. Use of mixed mesh sandwiched between the two skin layers
5. Skin coverage forming the external layer.

Marking

Preoperative planning and marking must be carefully performed so that the correct amount of skin is present to cover the reassembled gland without tension (*Fig. 8.6.1*). Insufficient skin at any point tends to pull the

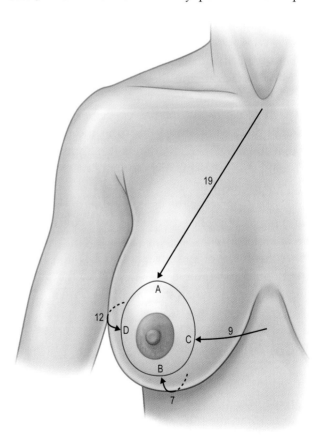

Fig. 8.6.1 Preoperative marking of the patient.

areola, leading to loss of anterior projection and compromising the final result.

An important observation is that the position of the NAC in relation to the breast and thorax is not taken into consideration during marking. Because the markings are based on fixed points on the thorax (sternal notch, midline, inframammary fold (IMF), and lateral breast border) and not on the breast's anatomic structure, gland asymmetries lead to asymmetric markings. Also, the resulting teardrop is larger in larger breasts, reflecting the increased amount of tissue to be resected.

Marking is carried out by defining the four cardinal points that will automatically bring the nipple-areola complex (NAC) to its new position.

Point A (superior cardinal point) defines the upper border of the future NAC and is located 2 cm above the projection of IMF on the breast surface. Its precise location depends on individual thoracic shape and lies anywhere between 16 and 18 cm from the sternal notch.

Point B corresponds to the inferior border of the future NAC and is normally placed 7 cm from the IMF. In patients with <7 cm of skin available in the lower hemisphere (e.g., in tuberous breasts), more skin may be harvested by advancing the dissection inferiorly to the IMF.

Point C represents the medial border of the future NAC and should be at least 9 cm from the midline to ensure that the new NAC maintains its slightly lateralized normal positions. This distance may reach 10.5 cm in patients with large breasts.

Point D corresponds to the lateral border of the future NAC and should be placed at least 12–13 cm from the breast's lateral border.

Due to the force of gravity, the final shape of the marking should resemble a teardrop with the patient standing and a circle when the patent lies down.

Surgical technique

The procedure begins by defining the diameter of the future areola, which is normally 4.5–5 cm and should be 0.5 cm larger than the purse-string suture placed at the end of the operation. This produces a slightly projected and convex areola in relation to the new breast. If these

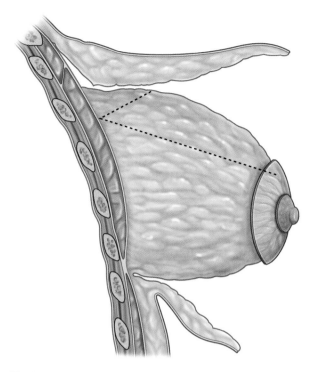

Fig. 8.6.2 Subcutaneous dissection to the pectoralis major fascia.

dimensions are made equal, there is a slight tension on the suture during the early postoperative period with a tendency to flatten the NAC.

The region between the areola and the teardrop markings is de-epithelialized. Dissection of the upper skin flap is beveled, so that the thickness of adipose tissue attached to the skin increases progressively. This maneuver enhances the upper pole fullness since the thickened flap overlaps the newly assembled gland at the end of the operation. The first 4–5 cm are dissected, leaving a 0.5 cm layer of subcutaneous adipose tissue attached to the dermis, which preserves the subdermal vascular plexus responsible for flap viability. From then on, flap thickness increases until the anterior pectoral fascia appears. Dissection continues superiorly for approximately 4 cm or until the ideal position of the future upper breast pole is reached *(Fig. 8.6.2)*.

The medial flap is kept uniformly thin throughout its elevation, and dissection is interrupted 2 cm before reaching the muscle fascia to preserve the perforating vessels that supply the flap and the central gland. The inferior flap is also kept thin until dissection reaches the IMF, which should be preserved. Dissection should only continue caudally when harvesting larger amounts of skin for the lower hemisphere is required.

The lateral flap is dissected until the lateral border of the breast is reached; dissection then progresses upward until the lateral border of the pectoralis major appears and there is communication with the dissection of the upper pole. The dermal flap is dissected and disconnected from the gland leaving some adipose tissue attached to the dermis. Dissection should be interrupted 1–1.5 cm before the border of the NAC to preserve its blood supply.

The volume of resected tissue is larger in the upper hemisphere, which results in a slightly triangular breast after reassembly. This way, the lateral and medial sides are slightly convex at the end of the operation, and the natural accommodation of tissues in the postoperative period will only slightly increase this convexity (without inducing an excessively rounded breast shape), maintaining an elegant and projected breast shape (*Fig. 8.6.3*).

Reduction is performed initially in the upper pole by resecting a large U-shaped wedge of tissue from the central region, which shortens the radius of the upper

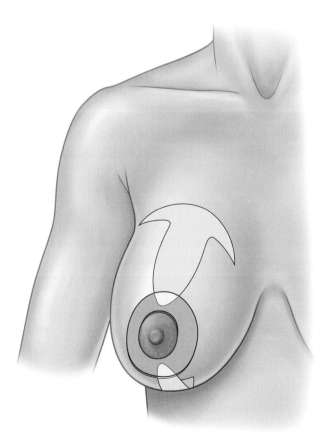

Fig. 8.6.3 Radial resection in both hemispheres.

hemisphere. In the lower hemisphere, one may resect another central wedge of tissue without detaching the base of the breast, where the perforating vessels are located. The volume to be resected is assessed by manually tacking excess tissue in, thus defining the precise limits of the mastopexy (*Fig. 8.6.4*).

Assembly is carried out in both breast hemispheres. In the upper hemisphere, rotation is performed superiorly by suturing the central extremities of the glandular flaps to the anterior pectoral fascia, suspending the breast to a higher position (*Fig. 8.6.5*). Therefore, the upper pole of the breast is filled and lifted to the ideal future superior breast pole. Complementary sutures may be used to fixate the rest of the superior pole to the thoracic wall.

In the lower hemisphere, excess tissue is either resected or tucked under the NAC to enhance anterior projection. Mastopexy is performed by suturing the resultant flaps to the anterior pectoral fascia; the flaps should be slightly rotated medially to decrease the base diameter of the breast. The constructed breast cone should have a height of 8–9 cm, which is slightly longer than the 7 cm of skin available to cover the inferior breast pole. This maneuver places slight pressure on the NAC giving it a convex shape. Complementary sutures are placed to fixate the gland's inferior border to the IMF. Final modeling of the breast can be performed by resecting the adipose tissue attached to the gland's parenchyma and/or under the skin flaps.

The circular dermal flap is sutured onto the top of the breast cone and to the breast's connective ligaments, providing the internal cutaneous lining. Adequate projection of the NAC can be obtained by applying slight tension to these circumferential sutures.

Mesh application

The synthetic mesh is applied over the dermal flap as a brassiere and is then sutured to the anterior pectoral fascia using interrupted 4-0 nylon sutures or titanium clips (*Fig. 8.6.5*). Fixation begins centrally at the IMF and ascends along both lateral and medial breast borders to provide an ideal conical shape and induce a slight elevation of the breast.

In the upper pole, a 2 cm excess of mesh can be left over the muscle fascia so fibrous tissue proliferates in this area, providing further support (*Fig. 8.6.6*). The two

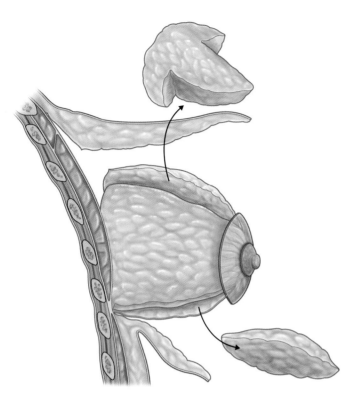

Fig. 8.6.4 Radial resection in both hemispheres.

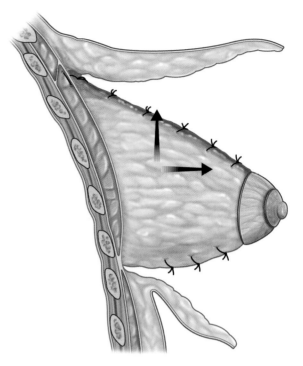

Fig. 8.6.5 Gland assembly. Lift the superior pole after detachment from the thoracic wall. Perform inferior mastopexy to project the mammary cone.

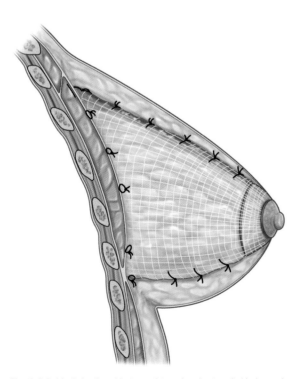

Fig. 8.6.6 Mesh is placed between internal and external skin layers in a sandwich.

extremities of mesh join in the central part of the upper hemisphere and are sutured together so the breast is entirely covered with mesh *(Fig. 8.6.7)*. Suction drains are placed either through the axilla or through the lateral border of the IMF.

The quality of the periareolar scar depends fundamentally on the amount of tension on the suture. Therefore, the external skin coverage should be abundant to prevent widening of the areola and breast flattening with loss of projection. There is a trend towards areolar projection, which gradually decreases over time, leading to tissue accommodation and reabsorption of edema. Therefore, projection should be slightly exaggerated during surgery to ensure an adequate and natural projection.

Skin closure is carried out using two layers of sutures *(Fig. 8.6.8)*. The external cutaneous lining, which determines the diameter of the new areola, is closed using a seamless Mersilene 3-0 purse-string suture. A straight 7 cm needle is used to keep the suture line in an intradermal position. As already mentioned, this suture should be tied around a 4.5 cm tube so the resulting

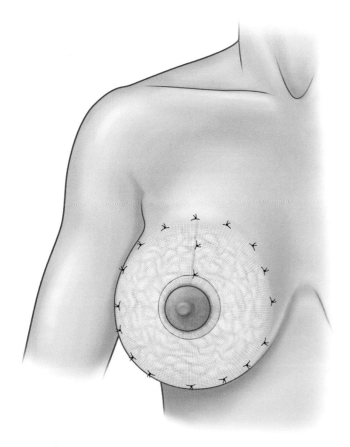

Fig. 8.6.7 Mixed mesh support.

shape of the NAC (whose diameter is 5 cm) is slightly convex. Finally, the areola is sutured to the external cutaneous lining using a seamless Monocryl 4-0 intradermal suture.

This suture should be distributed at a ratio of 4 mm of external tissue to 1 mm of NAC dermis to minimize the formation of periareolar wrinkles. Dermabond is used to seal the suture.

Tegaderm dressing is placed over the entire breast and is left in place for 5 days, constructing a triangular support system. The dressing also compresses the skin flaps against the underlying tissue, improving healing and adherence. The drains are left in place for at least 5 days and should only be replaced when the discharge is serous and <20 mL/day.

Antibiotics, non-steroidal anti-inflammatory drugs, and analgesics are given for 10 days. Patients with residual edema can be treated with variable doses of cortisone. Clinical results are shown in the following cases *(Figs 8.6.9–8.6.12)*.

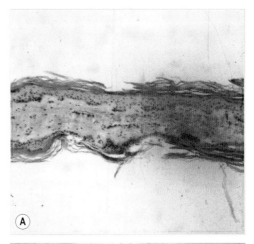

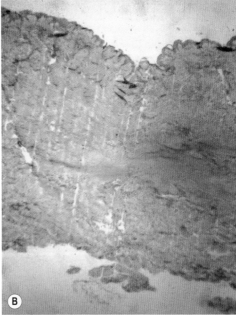

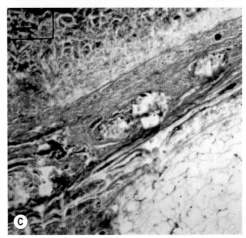

Fig. 8.6.8 **(A)** Normal skin pathology. **(B)** Doubled skin. **(C)** Mesh integration with laminar scarring.

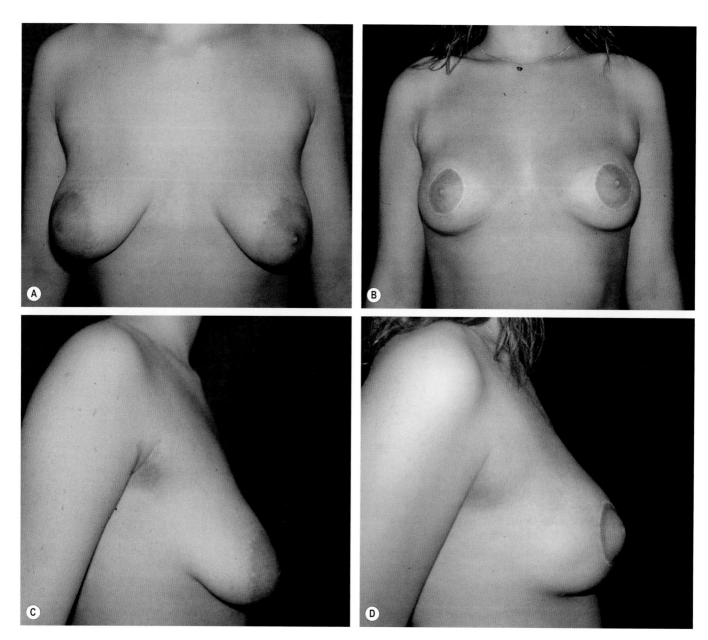

Fig. 8.6.9 Patient, aged 30. **(A,C)** Preoperative view. **(B,D)** View 2 years postoperatively.

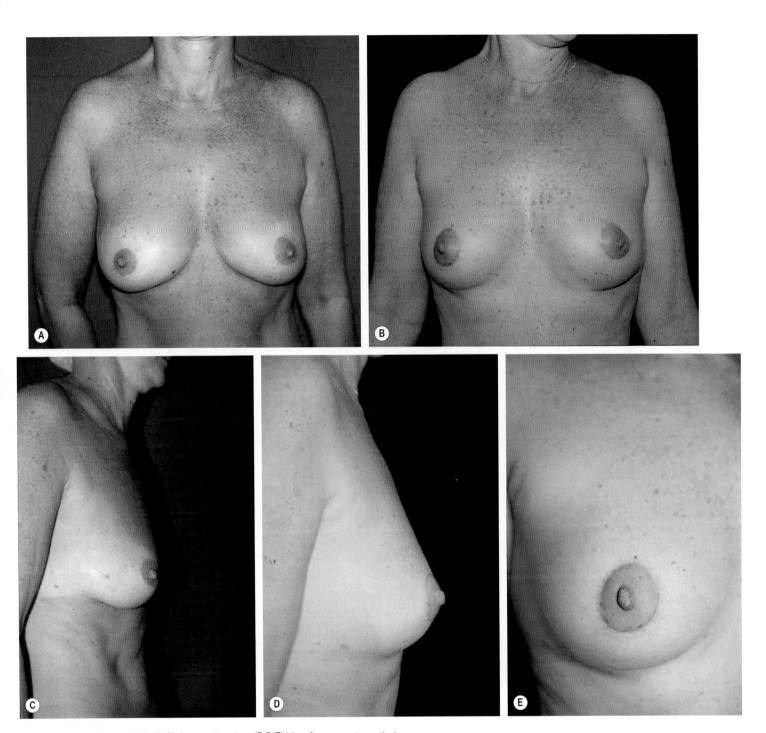

Fig. 8.6.10 Patient, aged 40. **(A,C)** Preoperative view. **(B,D,E)** View 2 years postoperatively.

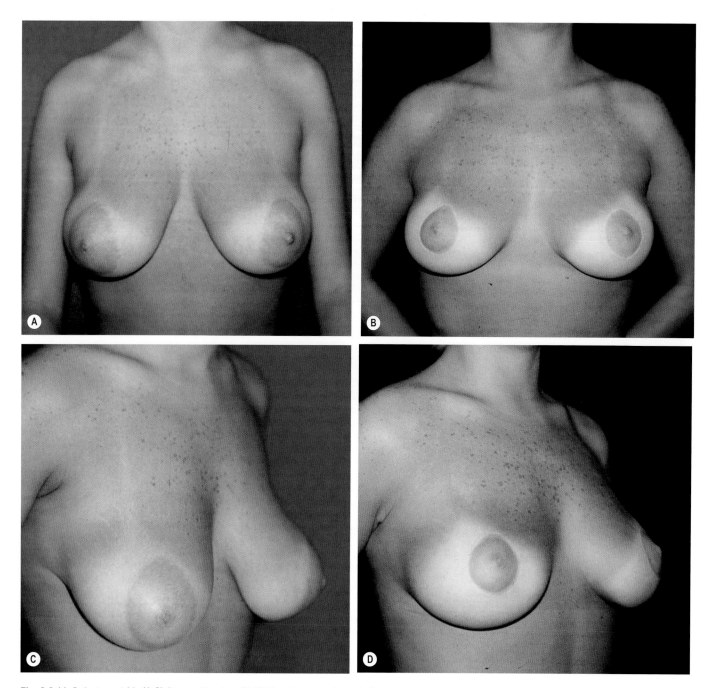

Fig. 8.6.11 Patient, aged 30. **(A,C)** Preoperative view. **(B,D)** View 4 years postoperatively.

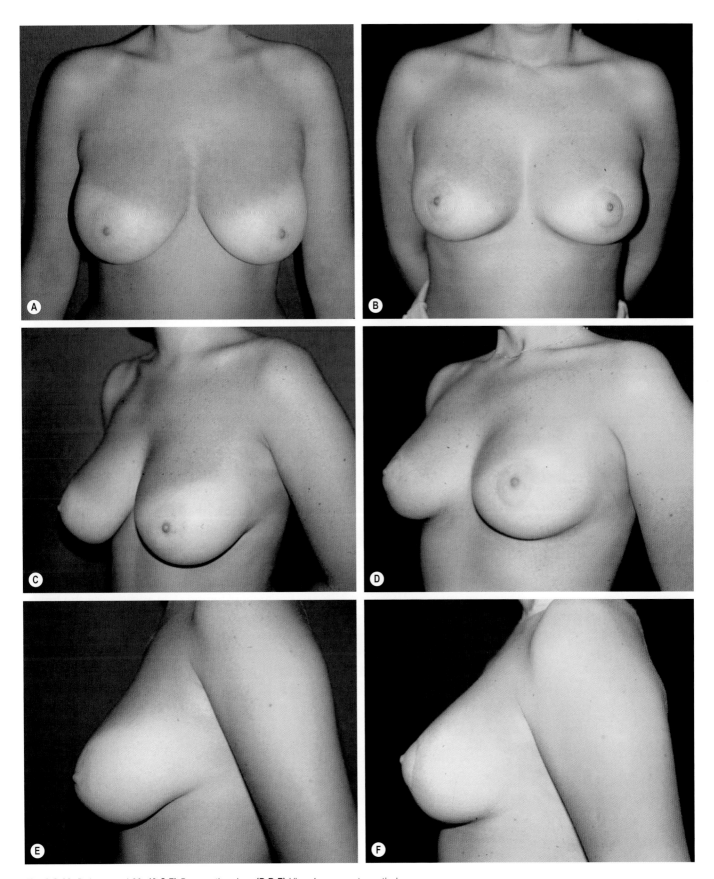

Fig. 8.6.12 Patient, aged 30. **(A,C,E)** Preoperative view. **(B,D,F)** View 4 years postoperatively.

Table 8.6.1 Complications of periareolar technique with mixed mesh in clinical series of 385 patients

	n	(%)
Infection	2	0.5
Retraction	2	0.5
Mesh extrusion	0	0
Vascular hyperemia (smokers)	4	1.0
Skin necrosis	0	0
Seroma	5	1.3
Hematoma	2	0.5
Fat necrosis	8	2.0
Areolar paresthesia	11	2.8

(Reproduced with permission from: Góes JCS. Periareolar mammaplasty: double-skin technique with application of mesh support. In: Spear SL *et al.*, eds. Surgery of the breast: principles and art, Vol. 2, 2nd edn. Lippincott Williams & Wilkins; 2006:991–1007.)

Complications

The rate of complications has been very low, due to careful patient selection and rigorous postoperative care *(Table 8.6.1)*. Caffeine, anticoagulant substances, and especially smoking are discontinued at least 10 days before surgery to optimize blood flow to the healing tissues.

The most frequent complications were seromas and/or hematomas. These tend to occur in younger patients due to excessive movement in the early postoperative period causing rupture of pectoralis major muscle tissue in the areas of mesh fixation. There was no need for reoperation in these cases and the final aesthetic result was not impaired. There was one case of infection which was easily controlled with antibiotics and local wound care.

Residual edema may take place in older patients, probably due to the absorbable component of the mesh.

These patients respond very favorably to three to four doses of cortisone, and compressive Micropore dressings for 20–30 days may be required, especially in the lower pole. Two patients had allergic reactions to the Mersilene purse-string suture, and satisfactory healing was only observed after its replacement. There were no cases of skin necrosis, retraction, or mesh extrusion. One patient who had been previously submitted to liposuction of the breast and two patients who had been submitted to benign tumor resection had signs of low blood perfusion on the NAC. Therefore, patients with a history of procedures which may have disrupted vascularization (central pedicle) of the NAC are not candidates for this technique.

Sensitivity is totally resumed in 96% of patients after approximately 30 days. This high rate is attributed to meticulous preservation of the fourth intercostal nerve, which innervates the NAC.

Summary

Our experience with periareolar breast surgery leads us to conclude that redraping skin alone does not avoid late ptosis. This has led to the development of our technique based on reshaping the breast parenchyma and treating the glandular mound separately from the skin, which is then redraped over the new breast architecture, though the periareolar approach, and the new breast is assembled through glandular flap rotation and fixation to the anterior pectoral fascia. The cutaneous lining is duplicated using a circular dermal flap with the central pedicle in the areolar region. The addition of the mixed mesh to the original technique, applied as a sandwich between the two layers of cutaneous lining, was performed to obtain a longer-lasting aesthetic result based on a resistant supporting system. This would maintain the ideal position of the gland after surgery and permit adequate fixation of the tissues into place.

 Access the complete references list online at **http://www.expertconsult.com**

4. Góes JCS. Periareolar mammaplasty: double skin technique with application of polyglactin 910 mesh. *Rev Soc Bras Cir Plast*. 1992;7:1–3.
    This article shows the first mesh application to support a periareolar mammaplasty. An absorbable mesh was used with good results, increasing the late support for a longer *follow-up time. Also a pathology study of the mesh integration was made.*

5. Góes JCS, Bostwick III J, Benelli L, et al. Minimizing scars in breast surgery (Expert Exchange). *Perspect Plast Surg*. 1993;7(2):59–85.

This paper brings an interesting discussion about different techniques using minimal scars, applied by experts.

6. Góes JCS. Periareolar mammaplasty: double-skin technique with application of mesh support. *Clin Plast Surg.* 2002;29(3):349–364.

The increasing demand for reduced scars has led to the development of numerous minimal incision procedures, which constitute the most recent and exciting advances in breast surgery. Numerous different periareolar techniques are described in an attempt to eliminate scars on the breast surface by restricting them to the interface between the areola and the skin. These conclusions show a clear evolution of the technique as well as an improvement in the obtained aesthetic results. The author has developed new techniques for periareolar mammaplasty based on repositioning the breast parenchyma and maintaining this new architecture with a stronger and more durable supporting system. The development of new materials, technical refinements in the technique, and increased experience will undoubtedly lead to even better results in the future.

8. Góes JCS. The application of mesh support in periareolar breast surgery: clinical and mammographic evaluation. *Aesthet Plast Surg.* 2004;28:268–274.

Some surgeons have been reluctant to apply any kind of prosthetic material to the breast, fearing inflammation, an unfavorable aesthetic outcome, palpable or visible deformities, and/or interference with mammographic evaluation of breast cancer. This study analyzed the aesthetic, clinical, and mammographic implications of using mesh as a supportive device in periareolar breast surgery.

15. Góes JCS. Periareolar mammaplasty: double skin technique. *Rev Soc Bras Cir Plast.* 1989;4:55–63.

The author's first publication describing his concept of treating the gland independent to the skin. In this article, the author did not use a mesh support system, but was able to obtain a nice breast shape in the early follow-up for 3 years.

8.7

Sculpted pillar vertical reduction mammaplasty

Kent K. Higdon and James C. Grotting

SYNOPSIS

- The sculpted pillar technique gives the most consistently good results, with a minimum number of complications.
- It is easy to learn and most who try it adapt it into their breast practices.
- It has the advantage of narrowing the base of the breast, leaving fullness in the superior pole, which is virtually never resected, and reducing the height of the column of breast tissue left behind.

Evolution of technique

The sculpted pillar technique evolved from a constellation of maneuvers all aimed at creating a stable breast cone built from two pyramids of carefully shaped breast tissue. It has been said about other techniques that what is important is the tissue that is left behind rather than what is resected, and that axiom certainly applies to the sculpted pillar technique as well. In general, the superior pedicle popularized by Lassus with a vertical approach is the same as the sculpted pillar. Only when the nipple areolar complex cannot be physically manipulated to its new position on a gliding plane do we convert to the superomedial pedicle of Hall-Findlay. The "A point" is selected from the anterior reflection of the inframammary fold, the humeral midpoint, and the visual most projecting point of the new simulated breast

shape. The position selected is the top of the areola rather than the actual new nipple position.

The shaping sutures used in the sculpted pillar have been described previously by Marchac, but the lateral shaping sutures were introduced by Alex de Souza, a Brazilian plastic surgeon, in an unpublished communication. The shaping of the pillars themselves is done using concepts described by Armando Chiari, but the gland is not rotated as in the Chiari technique, fully outlined later in this chapter. We have gradually improved the sculpted pillar method since 1999 and have used it on hundreds of patients up to the present time.

Patient selection

Ideal patients for the sculpted pillar technique are those with moderate breast hypertrophy or smaller. Individual breast weights of approximately ≤1000 g lend themselves well to this method. Young patients with more fibrous parenchyma and normal skin without striae are ideal, although if the breast is too large, the superior pedicle may have difficulty folding on itself and will require more thinning. Therefore, in this group of patients, a superomedial pedicle may be a better choice. Even with larger breasted patients, we prefer to approach the reduction using this technique. Because the gland and the skin are handled separately, the larger patients will most often benefit by an inverted T skin resection, so the scar will be longer. The smaller reduction or moderate ones in patients with normal skin can always be handled with a vertical scar only in addition to the periareolar closure.

Patients who have true gigantomastia, the elderly, or active smokers must be approached cautiously. Some are better treated with either an inferior pedicle or free nipple graft technique. Smokers should be encouraged to quit at least four weeks prior to the procedure to reduce the risk of wound healing problems.

Planning and markings

The markings are performed with the patient in the standing position (*Fig. 8.7.1*). The future nipple position is determined right at the reflection of the inframammary fold on the anterior surface of the breast (the A-point or Pitanguy point). This is checked against the visual midpoint of the acromion to humerus distance, as well as other visual landmarks. Typically, this point is about 2 cm lower than the point chosen for inverted T techniques. It is preferable to use the standard superior pedicle for the nipple-areolar complex, but if the density of the gland or distance of elevation appears restrictive, the superomedial pedicle recommended by Hall-Findlay is used.[1,2] The medial and lateral pillar lines are drawn by manually distracting the breast tissue medially and laterally. The volume to be left behind is approximated, and the resulting shape is visualized (*Fig. 8.7.2*). These lines should anticipate the parenchyma to be removed and should be adjusted in or out on the basis of the planned volume of resection. These lines mark the anterior-most projections of what will be, after resection of the intervening parenchyma, the vertical pillars of this technique. Inferiorly, the bottom of the V should be at least 2–3 cm above the native inframammary fold (*Fig. 8.7.3*). It is also preferable to mark on the skin surface the glandular tissue that will be resected at the caudal extent of the planned medial and lateral pillars, much the same way as one would mark this in a Wise pattern reduction. This will indicate the level of base resection for the medial and lateral vertical pillars, which, when approximated later in the procedure, will stabilize the construct of the new breast on the chest wall via these adjoined medial and lateral solid pyramids.

Technique

Local anesthetic with epinephrine is infiltrated in the intended lines of incision, in the dermis of the skin to be de-epithelialized, as well as beneath the gland. The superiorly-based dermoglandular pedicle is completely de-epithelialized after incising the newly-marked areolar diameter, which typically is measured with a

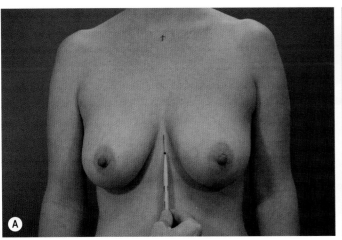
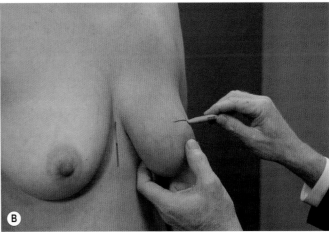

Fig. 8.7.1 Preferred modification of vertical technique preoperative markings. Point A is the location of the new nipple. Points C and D will become the bottom of the new areola. The dashed line represents the new areola boundary and is usually 12–14 cm in length.

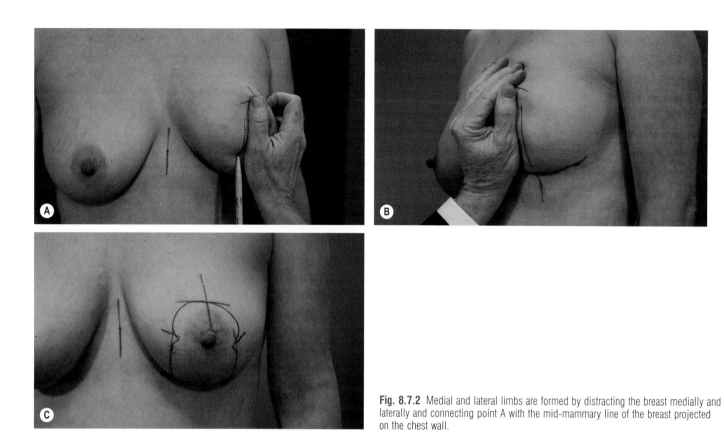

Fig. 8.7.2 Medial and lateral limbs are formed by distracting the breast medially and laterally and connecting point A with the mid-mammary line of the breast projected on the chest wall.

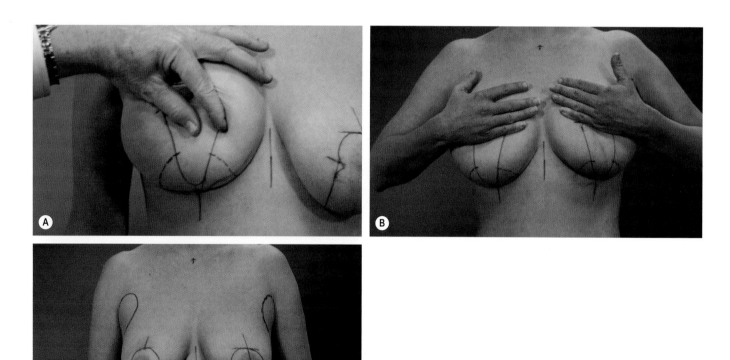

Fig. 8.7.3 Note the bottom of the incision line coming to a V approximately 2–3 cm above the inframammary fold (point B). The hatched lines show the location of the glandular resection or the superiorly based inferior flap if it is retained for upper pole fill.

38–45 mm nipple marker. The lower pole of the breast is then incised along the marks, and electrocautery is used to obtain hemostasis with any subcutaneous vessels that may require electrocoagulation. The parenchyma is then sharply dissected in the mastectomy plane, typically using facelift scissors, from the skin of the lower pole along the anterior aspects of the bases of the proposed vertical pillars. This represents the parenchyma that is marked out in the inferomedial and inferolateral aspects of the inverted-T reduction, with the difference being that the skin is not excised. The gland is initially elevated off the muscular fascia of the pectoralis using electrocautery and then bluntly undermined via manual dissection in the subglandular plane up to the superior pole to establish a space. A laparotomy pad is then placed into this newly-created subglandular space upon completion of its dissection. Often, there is a large perforator, which is usually the fifth intercostal perforator, which may require electrocoagulation or suture ligature.

The breast is then distracted medially, and the lateral pillar is then created by incising the breast parenchyma down to the laparotomy pad. This incision can be beveled medially or laterally to incorporate more or less tissue into the lateral pillar, as is indicated by the volume of reduction required. Similarly, the breast is then distracted laterally, and the medial pillar is then created by incising through the parenchyma to the laparotomy pad. Again, this incision can be beveled medially or laterally to incorporate more or less tissue into the medial pillar, as is indicated. The superiorly-based flap created as a result of this dissection is ovoid or tongue-shaped, and remains attached to the inferior extent of the superior pedicle including the de-epithelialized nipple-areolar complex. This parenchymal flap is then resected caudal to the nipple-areolar complex, which again is usually based on a superior dermoglandular pedicle. It should be noted that a superomedial dermoglandular pedicle can be implemented with this technique in cases where significant (>8 cm) nipple-areolar complex elevation is required. This simply requires not incising the medial vertical pillar and resecting tissue superolaterally, laterally, and inferiorly. Care must be taken to leave intact the superomedial tissues that are part of the superomedial pedicle, especially while undermining in the subglandular plane. In either the superiorly-based or superomedially-based pedicle

technique, the flap should be carefully thinned to not less than 2 cm thick. The superomedial technique, with its superior parenchymal resections, requires a thicker pedicle to preserve internal mammary arterial perforators. When using the superiorly-based pedicle technique, a keel-shaped wedge of tissue can be resected from beneath the flap if necessary.

Closure

After hemostasis is ensured, a 2-0 Vicryl suture is placed from the undersurface of the gland cephalic to the level of the nipple-areola complex to the pectoral fascia as high up in the upper pole as possible. This superior shaping suture imparts roundness and fullness to the upper pole. In the superomedial pedicle technique, this suture is placed beneath the glandular tissue of the superior flap and sutured to the pectoralis fascia, and the pedicle is then rotated into place.

The superior aspect of the transposed areola is then temporarily stapled in place to the new 12-o'clock position of the breast skin. An Adair clamp is then placed into the dermis just beneath this and the dissected breast is held by the assistant to facilitate coning of the remaining pillars. The bases of the lateral and medial pillars are then resected 5–7 cm from the top of the vertical limb down to the base of the pillar in order to decrease projection. Appropriate projection of the gland left behind prevents recurrence of ptosis.

The key suture is placed to reapproximate the pillars at the top of the vertical limbs at the 6-o'clock position of the areola. Laterally, at the base of the lateral sculpted pillar, another shaping suture is used to bring the lateral parenchyma at the anterior axillary fold toward the midline of the breast. This creates an aesthetic curve to the lateral portion of the breast. The medial and lateral pillars are then reapproximated with 2-0 Vicryl sutures in the parenchyma and 3-0 polydioxanone as a layered and running skin closure. The nipple-areola complex is exteriorized in its corrected position with the patient sitting up in the operating room (*Fig. 8.7.4*). The areola can be reassessed prior to exteriorization at this point, and any adjustments to achieve aesthetic circular shape can be achieved by remarking with the appropriately-sized nipple-areolar marker templates in the upright position. After completing any additional indicated de-epithelialization, the nipple-areolar complex is then

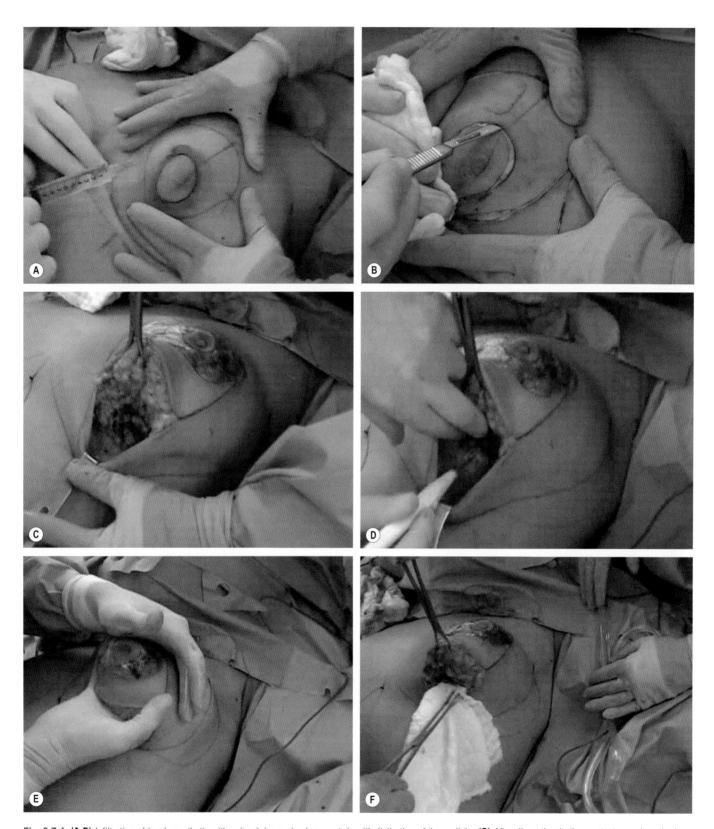

Fig. 8.7.4 **(A,B)** Infiltration of local anesthetic with epinephrine and subsequent deepithelialization of the pedicle. **(C)** After dissection in the mastectomy plane the lower pole skin from the anterior bases of the pillars. **(D–F)** Subglandular dissection, both with electrocautery and then blunt manual dissection, and laprotomy pad placement into the subglandular pocket.

inset with eight half-buried horizontal mattress sutures of 4-0 nylon at the four cardinal points and four points between those points. The skin closure of the nipple-areolar complex is then completed with a running, subcuticular 4-0 polydioxanone. At the completion of the operation, the "on table" shape is usually one of a slightly-flattened lower pole and a rounded upper pole, with the nipple pointing slightly inferiorly, creating the so-called "upside-down breast" *(Fig. 8.7.5)*. It is recommended that a drain be left overnight, especially in cases of large parenchymal resections as well as when adjunctive liposuction is used to thin the lateral chest, axillary, and tail of the breast areas. The use of Tegaderm to support the final shape is an important aspect of postoperative care *(Fig. 8.7.6)*. It should be left on for up to 2 weeks, at which point a bra should be used day and night for 6–8 weeks. Half-buried periareolar sutures are removed at approximately one week postoperatively.

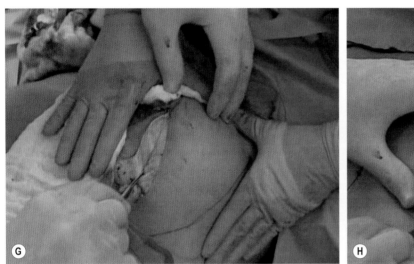
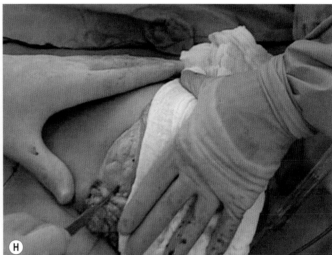

Fig. 8.7.4, cont'd (G,H) Sharp dissection of lateral and medial vertical pillars.

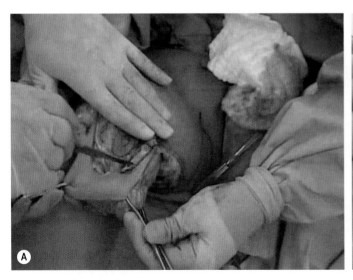
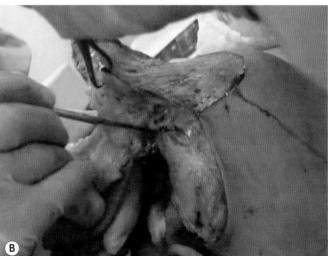

Fig. 8.7.5 (A,B) Sharp dissection of a 2 cm thick pedicle for the nipple areolar complex.

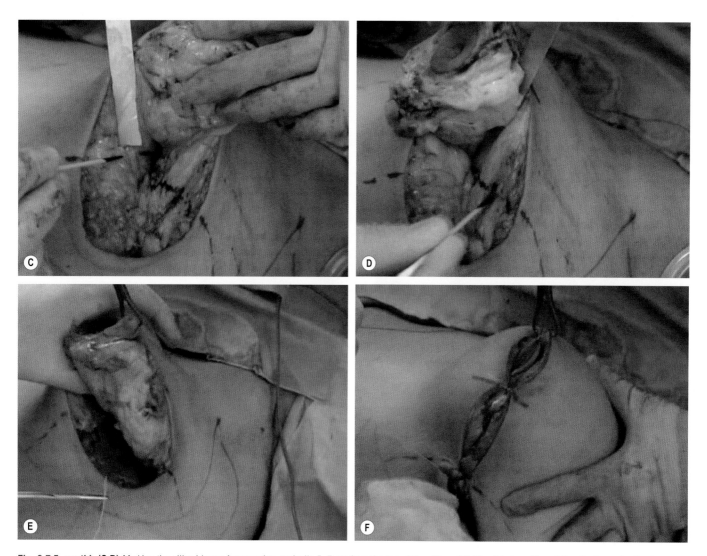

Fig. 8.7.5, cont'd (C,D) Marking the pillars' bases for resection, typically 5–7 cm from the top of the pillars. **(E)** Simulated position of the nipple areola after base resection. **(F)** Closure of the cephalic and caudal extents of the pillars after placing a superior shaping suture.

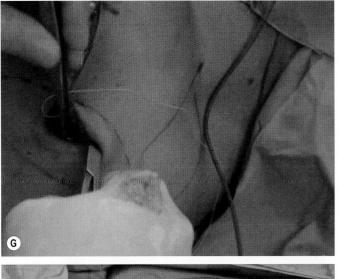

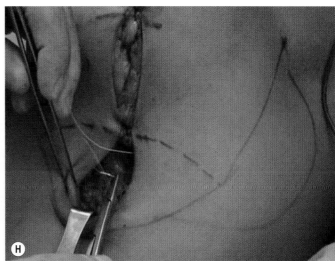

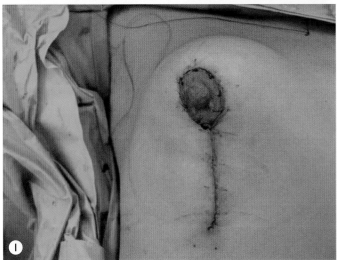

Fig. 8.7.5, cont'd (G,H) Placement of a lateral shaping suture. **(I)** Authors' preferred technique after closure and inset of nipple areolar complex. Rounded superior pole, flat lower pole, and slightly downward pointing nipple.

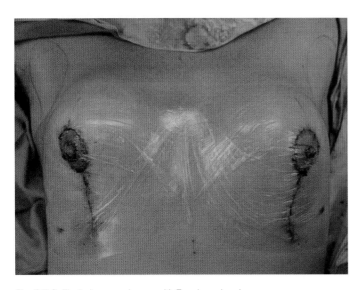

Fig. 8.7.6 Final closure and cover with Tegaderm dressing.

Walking is encouraged in the first week after surgery, and light exercise, such as stationary biking and use of elliptical trainers without the adjunctive use of upper extremity modalities, can be initiated at three weeks postoperatively. Full exercise is begun at 8 weeks postoperatively.

Patient examples: small, medium, and large reductions

Case 1: small breast reduction

A 31-year-old female with reasonably symmetric size D breasts underwent vertical sculpted pillar reduction mammaplasty. Parenchymal resections of 273 g on the right and 225 g on the left were performed *(Fig. 8.7.7)*.

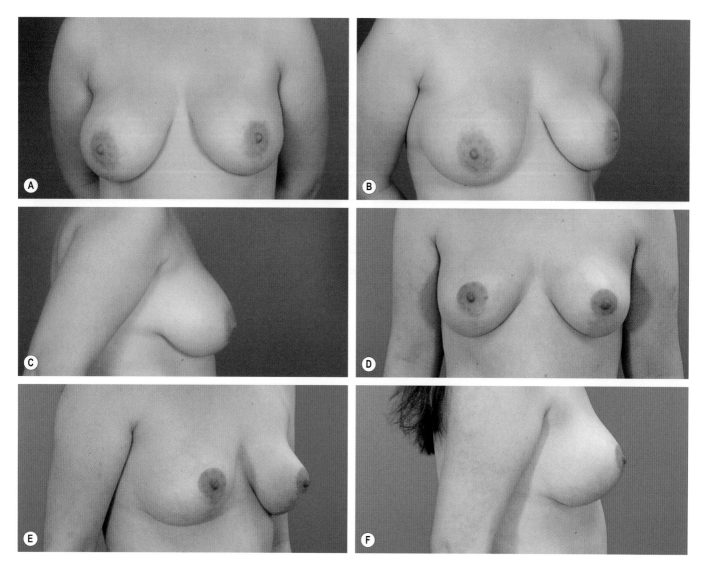

Fig. 8.7.7 (A–E) Small breast reduction. **(A–C)** Preoperative: A 31-year-old female with reasonably symmetric size D breasts who underwent vertical sculpted pillar reduction mammaplasty. **(D,E)** Postoperative: parenchymal resections of 273 g on the right and 225 g on the left were performed.

Case 2: moderate breast reduction

A 57-year-old female with breast asymmetry and size 36DDD breasts underwent vertical sculpted pillar reduction mammaplasty. Parenchymal resections of 552 g on the right and 789 g on the left were performed *(Fig. 8.7.8)*.

Case 3: large breast reduction

A 61-year-old female with slight breast asymmetry and size 44G breasts underwent vertical sculpted pillar reduction mammaplasty. Parenchymal resections of 1332 g on the right and 1237 g on the left were performed *(Fig. 8.7.9)*.

Complications

Hematoma formation can occur as an early or late complication. Vessels in spasm as a result of the tissue resection or from the effect of epinephrine may relax and lead to early hematoma formation. On the other hand, late hematomas can form with severe coughing or retching fits that strain tissues and sutures near vessels, from drain removal, or for other reasons. The incidence is

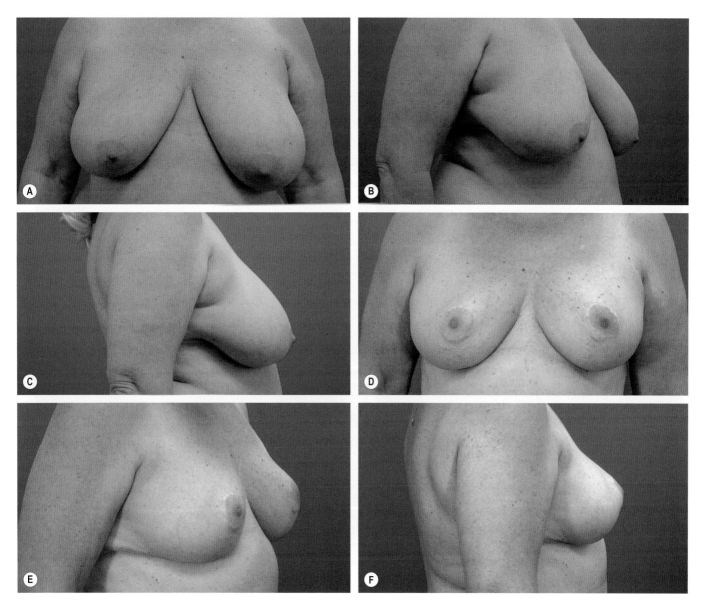

Fig. 8.7.8 (A–E) Moderate breast reduction. **(A–C)** Preoperative: A 57-year-old female with breast asymmetry and size 36DDD breasts who underwent vertical sculpted pillar reduction mammaplasty. **(D,E)** Postoperative: parenchymal resections of 552 g on the right and 789 g on the left were performed.

quite low and reported as being <1%. Hematomas are typically best treated with operative exploration, evacuation, and ligation if active bleeding is present.

Infection can manifest as a spectrum of clinical entities, from subclinical infections, such as suture abscesses or "spitting" sutures, to frank abscess. Suture spitting is typically treated by removing the offending suture and allowing the area to heal with topical antibiotic ointment. Cellulitis is usually managed with oral

antibiotics, and cases of abscess formation are treated with incision, drainage, and appropriate antibiotic therapy. In routine cases of reduction mammaplasty, one dose of a perioperative antibiotic is recommended for prophylaxis and is the practice of these authors.

Seroma formation is a not infrequent complication in reduction mammaplasty. Although some authors advocate conservative management of seromas with observation and allowing the tissues to resorb the fluid,

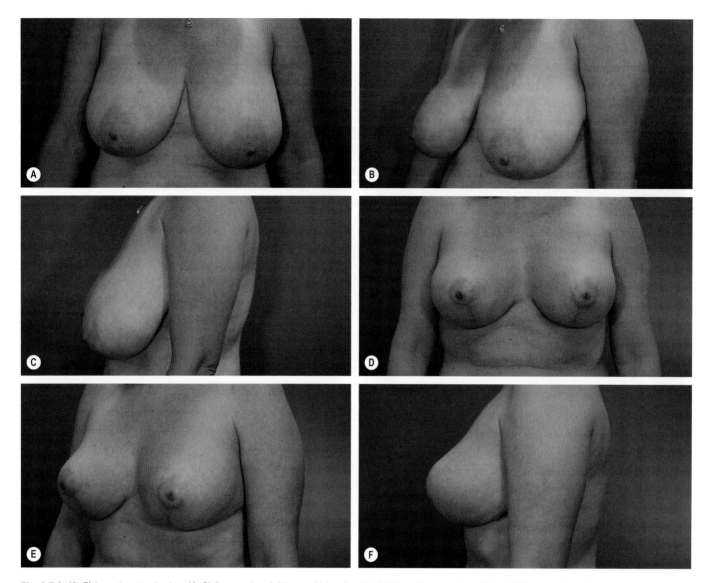

Fig. 8.7.9 (A–E) Large breast reduction. **(A–C)** Preoperative: A 61-year-old female with slight breast asymmetry and size 44G breasts who underwent vertical sculpted pillar reduction mammaplasty. **(D,E)** Postoperative: parenchymal resections of 1332 g on the right and 1237 g on the left were performed.

these authors typically aspirate under sterile conditions any seromas that are clinically apparent.

Dehiscence and wound healing complications may result from excessive tension on the approximated tissues, suture failure, infection, fat necrosis, or inadequate perfusion of the tissues. The etiology of the dehiscence must be ascertained, but typically this is treated conservatively. Any tissue necrosis is debrided sharply to healthy bleeding tissue, and local wound care is performed until the wound is healed.

Revisions are then usually performed as a secondary procedure.

Fat necrosis can occur when there is inadequate perfusion of the tissues around the pedicle or other areas, but most commonly it is due to large suture bites of the pillars when they are being reapproximated with tension. Treatment consists of drainage or excision of the areas of fat necrosis *(Fig. 8.7.10)*.

Nipple loss is an infrequent complication, usually the result of inadequate arterial inflow or venous outflow to the nipple areolar complex. Usually, this is recognized intraoperatively or immediately postoperatively. Intraoperative assessment of a potentially ischemic nipple involves release of any sutures which may be constricting inflow and assessment of bleeding of the tissues. Intraoperative use of fluorescein and a Woods lamp is an adjunctive modality for perfusion assessment, but it carries potential risk for anaphylaxis, can stain the patient's urine, and can be less useful in darker-skinned populations. Indocyanine green injection and assessment with the SPY device, made by Novadaq Technologies, Mississauga, Ontario, Canada, is an alternative means of assessing perfusion but has potential for cost and resulting availability issues. Venous congestion is often self-limited, but other times flaps cannot be salvaged with even the most aggressive maneuvers. These are typically the result of poor pedicle design. A useful adjunct, however, is the medicinal leech, Hirudo medicinalis, which is indigenous to Southeast Asia and Europe. A less common risk factor for nipple necrosis is the sickle-cell trait. The 31-year-old female in *Figure 8.7.11* underwent bilateral reduction mammaplasty with parenchymal resections measuring 1039 g on the left and 1161 g on the right. She presented with necrosis of both nipple-areolar complexes 3 weeks postoperatively and required debridement and nipple reconstruction.

Summary

Of all the techniques that we have used, we find the sculpted pillar to give the most consistently good results, with a minimum number of complications. It is easy to learn and most who try it adapt it into their breast practices. It has the advantage of narrowing the base of the breast, leaving fullness in the superior pole, which is virtually never resected, and reducing the height of the column of breast tissue left behind. Although the shape evolves over several weeks, we have not found this to be of any concern to the patients during recovery. We have found it to be reliable and with the short final scar, patients tend to refer their friends and acquaintances for the same procedure. The accompanying video demonstrates the nuances of the vertical sculpted pillar breast reduction technique.

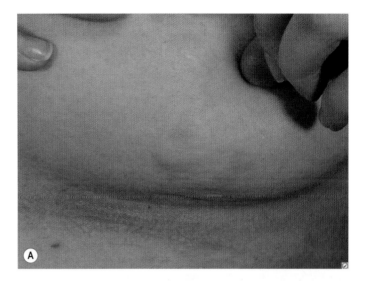

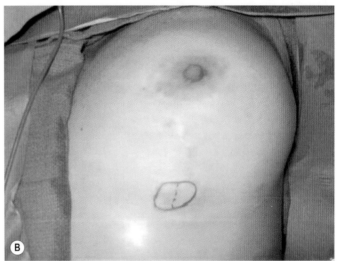

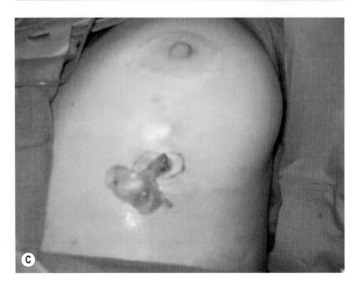

Fig. 8.7.10 Oily cyst presenting 4 years postoperatively as a persistent subdermal mass located in the line of incision.

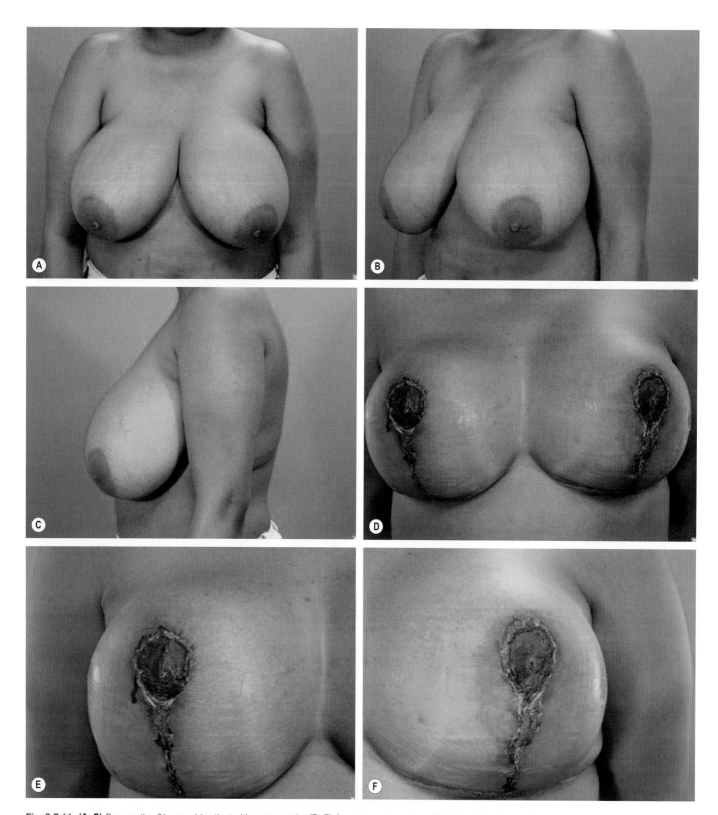

Fig. 8.7.11 (A–C) Preoperative 31-year-old patient with macromastia. **(D–F)** 3 weeks postoperative with bilateral nipple necrosis;

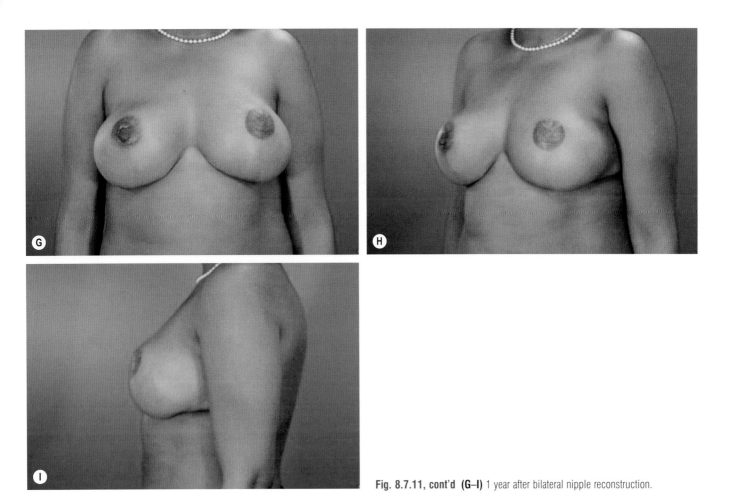

Fig. 8.7.11, cont'd (G–I) 1 year after bilateral nipple reconstruction.

References

1. Hall-Findlay EJ. A simplified vertical reduction mammaplasty: shortening the learning curve. *Plast Reconstr Surg.* 1999;104:748–763.

    This article describes modifications to the standard Lejour vertical reduction mammaplasty that simplify the technique and make it more reliable and easier to perform. These modifications include using a medial (or lateral) dermoglandular pedicle, not undermining the skin, using liposuction only rarely to reduce breast volume, and not using pectoralis fascia sutures; the modified technique has been used in a series of 400 vertical breast reductions. In this series, scarring was reduced and the technique was easily learned and applied. It is useful for both small and large breast reductions, with a series average of 525 g removed per breast (range, 100–1425 g). By using these modifications, scarring in reduction mammaplasty was effectively reduced while the nipple and areola were safely transposed on a medial or lateral dermoglandular pedicle.

2. Hall-Findlay EJ. Pedicles in vertical breast reduction and mastopexy. *Clin Plast Surg.* 2002;29:379–391.

    The pattern of skin resection should be considered separately from the pedicle design. There are numerous combinations available, and different situations will determine which combination is preferable. The author performed a standard inferior pedicle Wise pattern technique for the first 11 years of her practice and has now used variations of the vertical technique for the past 8 years. She has personally found that the medial pedicle gives the best breast reduction results in her hands. On the other hand, a lateral pedicle is used for mastopexies so that the inferior and lateral tissue can be rotated up under the areola. When faced with a re-reduction of a previous inferior pedicle, the vertical technique can still be used, and an adaptation of the inferior pedicle can be very acceptable. The superior pedicle is reserved mainly for very small reductions or mastopexies, but the author still finds the medial pedicle allows better lateral resection even in small reductions, and the lateral pedicle with recruitment of tissue allows for some auto-augmentation in mastopexies.

9

Revision surgery following breast reduction and mastopexy

Kenneth C. Shestak

SYNOPSIS

- The plastic surgeon should know the pedicle created in the first operation and reuse it.
- "Tailor-tacking" (or skin staple tacking) is a powerful tool for simulating breast shape changes which are best evaluated with the patient sitting at 90° on the operating room table.
- Wide de-epithelialization of the peri-areola tissues with preservation of the subdermal plexus and the use of the interlocking Gore-Tex® suture technique is helpful where additional movement of the nipple is necessary in revision cases.
- Be extremely cautious in performing a mastopexy following a previous subglandular breast augmentation.
- Do not perform these procedures in patients who smoke.

Revision surgery following a breast reduction has been relatively uncommon in the author's practice experience over the past 25 years – probably in the range of 2–3%. The main reasons patients seek or have revision surgery at various time points in the wound healing continuum are listed under the headings of sub-acute and long-term complications of breast reduction, listed in *Table 9.1*.

This chapter focuses on the conditions listed under the long-term complications section. It also comments on two acute complications, namely hematoma and nipple areola ischemia, since these complications should be addressed acutely and require revision of the original surgical procedure.

Introduction

Breast reduction is a popular procedure worldwide. It most often results in relief of the presenting symptoms in the patients seeking it. The postoperative appearance of the breasts is generally improved since they are uplifted and re-shaped from the standpoint of improved projection and the manner in which they relate to the torso of a given patient. Therefore in a real sense, the operation is both a functional and cosmetic procedure. The vast majority of patients who experience relief from their macromastia symptoms will readily accept the "trade-off" of "scars for shape".

Patient history

The history, biologic processes related to wound healing, postoperative management and potential complications should be carefully reviewed with every patient undergoing a surgical procedure. These elements of patient care are of critical importance in being considered for elective reoperative or revision surgery, including revision of breast reduction, and revision of mastopexy. There is significant overlap of these elements for these two procedures, which must be sought out by the plastic surgeon, analyzed, and discussed with the patient prior to any revisional surgery procedure. Because of this

Table 9.1 Complications of breast reduction
Acute complications
Hematoma
Seroma
Imperfect healing with wound separation and open wounds
Infection – cellulitis or abscess
Nipple areola ischemia
Sub-acute complications
Asymmetry
Hypertrophic scars
Fat necrosis
Long-term complications
Contour deformities – dog ears
Sub-optimal scars – hypertrophic
Loss of shape – bottoming out loss of upper pole projection
Nipple malposition
Partial nipple loss
Complete nipple loss
Asymmetry(ies) – volume, NAC complex
Under resection
Over resection
Pain

overlap, these elements are presented here prior to describing the specific conditions noted below.

The revision of augmentation-mastopexy entails the additional element of a breast implant, which has its own particular set of potential complications and inherent risks (capsular contracture, implant failure, and unplanned additional surgery considerations), which must also be discussed with the patient prior to a revision procedure.

The history is an extremely important element of the patient evaluation in all cases of revision breast reduction, mastopexy and augmentation mastopexy. It is a critical determinant of *whether to reoperate* (a patient may have a problem which can be improved by surgery or unrealistic expectations for improvement) or *when to reoperate*. The latter is determined by a satisfactory degree of wound healing or the return of softness and suppleness to the tissues of the breast. This wound healing or maturation is influenced by the time elapsed since the previous surgery(ies) and whether the previous procedure resulted in a surgical complication, the nature of the complication and the patient's recovery. In general, reoperation is best delayed at least 6 months following the previous procedure.

Reoperative surgical procedures in all areas of plastic surgery require an in-depth understanding of the problem from the standpoint of anatomy, aesthetic appearance, concerns of the patient, and as mentioned above, the time which has elapsed relative to the previous procedure(s). Regardless of whether the surgeon is operating to treat a problem in one of his or her own patients or is planning to treat a patient operated on elsewhere, carefully obtaining an accurate history and performing a thorough physical examination is essential.

Particular attention is paid to the patient's chief complaint. It is critical to understand what she is most bothered by and therefore focus on her chief complaint as much as possible. Is the patient dissatisfied with: the scar appearance; contour problems; asymmetry(ies); nipple areola position or appearance; masses of lumps in the breast; under-reduction with persistence of symptoms; over-reduction; loss of shape, or pain? Is it a combination of these symptoms? A key element of successful revision procedures is to understand what the patient is most bothered by and then to communicate with the patient about what can and cannot be made better.

It is essential that the surgeon planning a reoperative procedure following breast reduction have as precise an understanding as possible about the blood supply to the nipple areola complex, as a revision surgery procedure may entail moving the NAC on a pedicle or altering breast shape adjacent to it.[1] This is also true for revision of mastopexy and augmentation-mastopexy procedures. This information is most accurately obtained from a review of the previous operative record(s). The greatest margin of safety for ensuring nipple areola complex viability is obtained by using the previously developed pedicle. In patients you are evaluating after surgery performed elsewhere, these records can be obtained by asking the patient to request them in writing from the previous surgeon. In most US states, the law requires that permission must be given by the patient before you can speak with the previous surgeon.

It is important to comment on breast pain following previous surgery. Mastodynia or pain in the breast is multifactorial in etiology and moreover, the exact cause is often not possible to identify, especially when scars have been added to the various etiologies. *Moreover the author's experience has shown that it is most often not possible to completely cure such pain with a scalpel. Therefore* no guarantees should be made about pain relief in virtually any circumstance. Instead, inform each patient that their pain may be unchanged, may be made better, or may even be made worse by a revision surgery procedure.

Preoperative patient evaluation

Diagnosis/patient presentation

Physical examination includes a careful visual inspection and aesthetic analysis along with thorough palpation of the breast tissues. Careful notes are made regarding the symmetry of volume, breast parenchyma, the position of the breast on the chest wall, and any contour abnormalities. Also of importance is the position of the nipple areola complex (NAC) related to the maximal projecting point of the breast mounds and the relationship of the NAC to the inframammary (IM) folds along with their shape, size, symmetry, and nipple projection that are all noted and compared from the perspective of symmetry. Overall skin quality and position of the scars is noted.

A tactile examination of the breast is performed to evaluate the quality of the skin, breast parenchyma and scars. In addition, any masses, areas of thickening, tenderness, and scar adhesions are noted. Although there are occasional exceptions, in general, reoperative breast surgery procedures should not be undertaken until there is a return of mobility of the breast tissue over the underlying chest wall structures and it should not be done until the skin of the breast has reacquired its mobility over the underlying breast tissue and the scars have begun to soften.

Finally, surface measurements of key aesthetic features of the breast from fixed anatomic points on the chest wall are made with the patient standing. This includes the supra-sternal notch to nipple distance, the distance from nipple to IM fold and to the mid-sternum and lateral breast fold, along with the inferior areola to IM fold dimension. The base width of the breast is also measured. All of these surface measurements are recorded on a standardized diagram or worksheet used for breast procedures. Photographs are then taken, cropped the same way on all patients using a digital camera, including AP, lateral, and oblique views. When

necessary, include supine views or photographs taken from above the patient (what the patient would see when she is looking down at her breasts). Refer to both the diagrams and photographs when planning all surgical procedures.

Mammographic examination of the breasts is ordered as necessary. These are especially helpful when there is a mass in the breast. Breast ultrasound (sonography) is often a helpful adjunct to mammography in many patients. Reviewing these studies directly with the radiologist can be very helpful in more complex cases. For any problems involving a mass in the breast or an abnormal mammogram, additional consultations with a radiologist or oncologic breast should be sought as needed.

Basic science

The basic science/wound healing elements relate to the condition of the breast tissue, which includes skin and parenchymal tissue elasticity, degree of scar tissue present and maturation of scar. The surgeon must pay particular attention to the mobility of the skin over the underlying tissue and the softness and distensibility of scar or lack thereof.

Postoperative management

The postoperative management includes appropriate perioperative pain medication, antibiotic therapy, along with drain placement and care. The patient and their family should be instructed in how to manage the suction drains, and a system of communication between the surgeon's office and the patient regarding 24 h drain output should be set in place.

All patients are asked to refrain from vigorous physical exertion (high impact activity and anything that causes their breast to bounce) for at least a month following surgery. This includes running, especially running on a treadmill. In an attempt to support the breast during the acute and sub-acute phase of internal wound healing patients should wear a "snug fitting" sports bra for support of their breasts on a 24 h a day basis for 4–6 weeks following surgery.

Patients' questions received by telephone should be answered promptly when they have concerns about potential healing issues. This makes the patient feel better and builds on the trust that began in the preoperative period.

Outcomes/prognosis/complications

The potential risks and complications of the revision surgery should be thoroughly reviewed with the patient preoperatively. The author has adopted a standardized approach reviewing the wound healing issues and cosmetic issues related to each procedure under these specific headings. These explanations are reflected in the typed office consent document, which the patient reviews and signs at the time of these explanations, confirming her receipt of this information. Highlights of the patient–doctor routine discussions are outlined below.

Wound healing is not completely predictable following surgery, especially in revision procedures. Unanticipated wound separation, open wounds, prolonged time to healing of these wounds and sub-optimal scarring occurs. Patients need to be aware of this – especially patients who have sustained a similar complication in the past. **It has been established that wound healing in all fields of surgery is negatively impacted by cigarette smoking. For this reason, the author will not perform elective plastic surgery procedures involving skin elevation, flap advancement and skin tightening at the line of closure (often exactly what is entailed in revision breast reduction, revision mastopexy, and revision augmentation mastopexy) in patients who smoke.** Loss of sensation in the skin or NAC is possible in all cases of breast surgery especially when the NAC is being moved. As noted previously, relief of pain by surgical intervention almost never completely occurs and this is explained to the patient and their family or other support team preoperatively. It is important to repeat this several times during a consultation and document that the patient has been told about this.

A discussion of complications is also important. It is best to convert this to a time for informing and teaching the patient, explaining what may be done to minimize the likelihood of unwanted events. The patient's questions must be addressed and answered to the best of the surgeon's knowledge. The patient should be issued with a copy of the informed consent document to take home to read, and she should discuss it with their family and support team. They should be informed that they can call the surgeon with any questions that they may have regarding anything in the consent or anything discussed during the consultation.

The surgeon should outline and disclose to the patient in writing, his or her policy for unplanned additional surgery from the standpoint of professional fees, facility fees, and fees for ancillary services (e.g., anesthesia). This should be outlined for unplanned surgical intervention in the acute postoperative period (e.g., drainage of a hematoma following a procedure) or for long-term sequelae (recurrent breast ptosis). Making sure that patients understand this uncommon but potential reality is important.

Finally, an overall aesthetic improvement, while expected and realized in most cases, can never be guaranteed. This arena of revision for significant problems following breast reduction, mastopexy, and augmentation mastopexy is one where it is best for the plastic surgeon to "under promise but over deliver."

Surgical re-intervention for acute problems

Hematoma

Reoperation in this setting is relatively rare. It mainly entails drainage of hematomas when they occur. The hematoma rate is $\leq$1–2%. It is marked by swelling, ecchymosis, and pain. It can occur at any location in the breast. For localized, nonexpanding and liquefied hematoma problems, a percutaneous aspiration may suffice *(Fig. 9.1)*. It is essential to aspirate or drain hematomas since they may threaten the viability of the overlying skin[3] and/or result in long-term palpable abnormalities and asymmetries in the breast(s). Any existing coagulopathies that may not have been identified preoperatively (e.g., von Willebrand's disease[4]) must be sought and corrected.

For situations where the process is more diffuse or the hematoma may be expanding, re-exploration is often indicated. Re-opening the incisions provides excellent access to the entire operative field. Most commonly, a defined bleeding point is not found with the exception of large branches from the internal mammary or

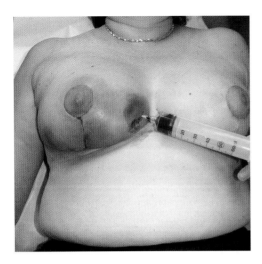

Fig. 9.1 Aspiration of liquefied hematoma in lateral aspect of breast on postoperative day 10.

external mammary (lateral thoracic) arteries. The wound is copiously irrigated and a drain is inserted.

Skin flap necrosis

Minimizing wound problems related to skin flap necrosis requires careful planning in terms of skin flap design, surgical precision in terms of flap elevation and sufficient pedicle resection such that the flaps can be redraped without excess tension in the line of closure. By the very nature of the Wise pattern (inverted T) incision, and other patterns used for breast reduction, the skin flaps are sutured with some degree of tightness at the line of closure. However, at present, most breast surgeons do not believe that the skin closure contributes significantly to breast shape. Rather, the pedicle configuration and the manner in which the reduced pedicle "fits" the skin envelope is the key component contributing to long-term breast shape. Therefore, if there is excessive tension at the line of closure at completion of a breast reduction, then additional tissue should be resected from the pedicle to lessen the tightness at the incision line. Such tightness often leads to scar spreading or to frank skin loss with unfavorable scars and at times, loss of breast shape.

Skin flap ischemia is rarely noted at surgery but rather it appears in the immediate postoperative period. In my experience, it is much more common in patients who smoke as is delayed healing of open wounds, wider scars, and fat necrosis. The author believes that

this must be mentioned to all patients preoperatively, and a strong plea made to smoking patients to completely stop for 4 weeks prior to surgery.[3] The incidence of complications following breast reduction has been linked to elevated BMI (>30), hypertension, previous breast incisions, and the amount of tissue resected.[3]

Some degree of imperfect healing and wound separation along the course of the incisions in a breast reduction is not uncommon. Generally, this will lead to wound separation that will necessitate the institution of dressing application or wound ointments to help with healing. The most common location is at the "T" junction in the Wise pattern breast reduction. It is usually seen on the distal aspect of the lateral flap. This random pattern flap has a much longer length to width ratio and the distal edge is further away from branches of the lateral thoracic nutrient vascular system.

Postoperative care

Such wounds will heal by the processes of epithelialization and contraction and it is decidedly rare to reoperate to facilitate wound healing. It is important to remove all foreign bodies (suture material) from such open incisions, for the patient to perform daily wound care by water pulsed mechanical irrigation of the wounds in the shower on a twice a day basis, and for surgeons to perform judicious debridements during periodic follow-up visits to the office. Keeping such wounds slightly moist with the application of saline moistened gauze sponges or antibiotic impregnated ointments applied topically will usually hasten the wound healing. The scars resulting from such secondary wound healing tend to be larger, usually hypo-pigmented, thinner in texture and more depressed relative to the skin surface than the remainder of the scars. The vast majority of patients do not request surgical revision of such wound scars even when they are extensive.

Wound excision and re-closure

Unattractive scarring is probably the most common adverse consequence of breast reduction. The problem is most commonly related to scar hypertrophy or to a wide depressed scar after skin loss noted during the acute and sub-acute phases of wound healing. Both can be improved by a well-timed and properly executed wound excision and re-closure.

Scars all go through a life cycle. In general, they appear more favorable as time passes. Therefore it is preferable not to perform any type of scar revision surgery for at least 1 year following surgery. In the case of significant scar hypertrophy, especially laterally after a Wise pattern incision, the intra-scar injection of Kenalog 10 mg/mL mixed with 1% Xylocaine is helpful. The author performs a single injection and then allows 3 months to elapse before performing an additional injection if requested. It must be borne in mind that color changes in the scars, especially hypo-pigmentation are not uncommon with this approach. In addition, injections should be into the scar itself and not into the subcutaneous tissue. Injecting the subcutaneous tissue will cause tissue atrophy and can produce a "sunken appearance" of the scars.

If after a year the patient has significantly spread scars, and other conditions are favorable, then a scar excision and re-closure is an option. It should be carefully explained to the patient that a definite improvement in the scar condition cannot be guaranteed. The keys to perform this type of approach would be to excise through the skin at a right angle. Excise tissue deep to the scar and limit the actual undermining of the skin tissue. A layered closure of the wound with a coated polyglycolic acid suture (4-0 PDS) with buried knots is the author's suture of choice and has not routinely used the permanent suture in this situation, although some surgeons feel that it may confer an advantage in terms of long-term maintenance of a narrower scar. The author recommends that patients apply paper tape to their wounds. Although this has not been studied in a scientifically, it appears that it has some benefit. This is continued for 3 months. Subsequent to this, scar massage is performed twice a day, along with the topical application of vitamin E cream.

Contour abnormalities at the end of incisions

Contour abnormalities at the end of incision probably represent the most common reoperative procedure performed in patients seeking additional surgery following breast reduction. These excisions can be performed in an office setting as an outpatient. These "dog-ears" can be addressed in the operating room at the end of the procedure if they appear at the end of the wound closure. If they are not addressed at this stage, then they can be addressed in the office as a brief outpatient surgical operation.

Nipple areola ischemia

Ischemia of the NAC is a dreaded but fortunately rare potential complication of every pedicled breast reduction procedure (probably in the range of 1%). It is most often related to arterial insufficiency, and it usually occurs in the setting of a large breast reduction (>1000 g resection), where a long pedicle is created to carry the circulation to the NAC, often with associated co-morbidities such as obesity and diabetes mellitus.[2] Folding such a pedicle during closure additionally stresses the circulation. Therefore, in cases where NAC is suspected, the incision should be opened and the pedicle examined. If it is too bulky, it should be reduced in volume and the circulation re-evaluated. If this improves the situation, then re-closure of the wounds is attempted. If re-closure again causes a decrease in circulation, the pedicle might be trimmed further, the skin flaps might be made thinner, or some of the incisions may be left open.

If this still does not adequately address the problem, then consideration is given to removing the nipple from its position on the pedicle, resecting the distal pedicle, and applying the nipple as a full thickness skin graft more proximally on the pedicle itself *(Fig. 9.2C,D)*. It is important for the surgeon to realize that the circulation to the pedicle beneath the NAC is compromised and therefore in all likelihood, this tissue will need to be resected. Alternatively, the "free nipple graft" can be placed on the skin of the breasts after the skin flaps have been re-approximated *(Fig. 9.2A,B)*.

These possible contingencies should be reviewed with every patient preoperatively during the discussion of the potential risks and complications of breast reduction. Approaches to removing the nipple areola complex and replacing it as a full thickness graft are detailed below.

Depending on the incisions made at the outset of the procedure, the strategies for applying the NAC as a full

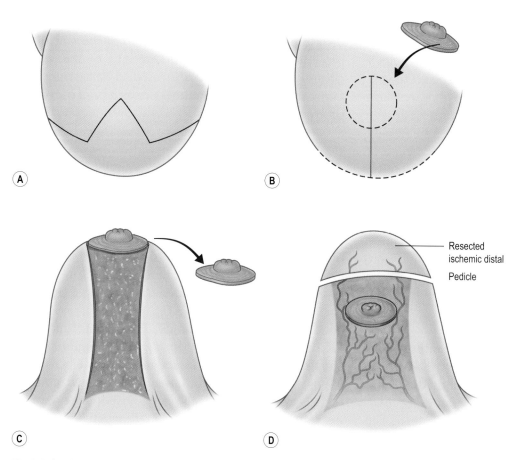

Fig. 9.2 (A–D) Removing the nipple and areola complex (NAC) from its present position and replacing it on more proximally on the breast pedicle as a full thickness skin graft. The nipple graft can also be placed on a de-epithelialized area of the breast skin flaps **(A,B)**.

thickness graft may be different. If the circular incision for insetting the NAC has been made, then either the pedicle will need to be advanced such that the nipple full thickness NAC graft can be re-inserted through the cut-out or the cut-out must be closed in a purse-string fashion *(Fig. 9.3)*. The skin is then de-epithelialized at the level of the superficial dermis and the NAC is applied and fixed with a tie over bolster dressing.

If the circular cut-out for the areola has not been established then no purse-string is needed and the skin at the site of the desired new areola position is simply de-epithelialized and the graft is applied as illustrated above *(Fig. 9.2A,B)*.

Areola deformities

Deformities of the nipple areola complex are not uncommon. These vary from asymmetries to a "teardrop"

deformity related to separation of the wound edges in the superior aspect of the vertical incision or the use of a three point suture at the junction of the 6 o'clock position of the areola and the vertical incision.

Patients will not infrequently be bothered by an elongated appearance of the lower aspect of the areola. This relates to areola healing to an area of separation between the medial and lateral skin flaps.

The correction is straightforward. The procedure requires excision of the previous vertical skin scar at its junction with the areola which has been pulled inferiorly along with elevation of the areola at the level of the dermis from the 4 o'clock to the 8 o'clock position with approximately 1 cm of undermining. The medial and lateral skin flaps on either side of this incision are elevated for a short distance with advancement and re-closure of this central incision. A small portion of the most superior aspect of these flaps is de-epithelialized re-cutting the skin in the configuration of a circle. This

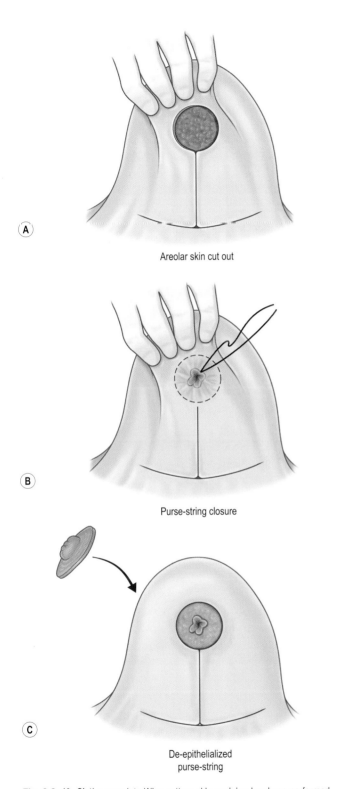

(A) Areolar skin cut out

(B) Purse-string closure

(C) De-epithelialized purse-string

Fig. 9.3 (A–C) If a complete Wise pattern skin excision has been performed including the circular "cut-out" for the nipple and the NAC requires replacement on the skin then the circular cut out can be closed with a purse-string suture and de-epithelialized in order to optimally position the NAC.

allows the elevated areola to be "set down" on a de-epithelialized skin platform and to re-establish a circular configuration. Closure is then proceeds in a tension free manner and healing normally proceeds in a fashion that will result in a circular contour of the areola.

Asymmetries of the areola are also not uncommon. Most commonly, one areola is larger than the other. Patients are frequently bothered by the larger areola shape.

The goal is to reduce the size of larger areola *(Fig. 9.4A)*. An incision, in a circular manner, is inscribed on the areola *(Fig. 9.4B)*. This "downsizing" results from the resection of the excess areola tissue in a "washer-shaped" configuration at the periphery of the wound (stippled area of *Fig. 9.4B*). The edges of the skin wound must be managed and "brought together" in order to achieve good healing.

The introduction of the "interlocking Gore-Tex® technique" by Hammond[2] has been a major advance in controlling the diameter of the new areola and peri-areola skin in peri-areola surgery. The technique utilizes a CV-2 Gore-Tex® suture on a Keith needle and taking care to keep the Gore-Tex® in the deep portions of the dermis. Approximately two bites in the peripheral skin are taken for every single bite in the areola itself. By suturing both sides of the wound, the size of the skin opening can be reduced and stabilized. Repair of the more superficial skin wound is performed with absorbable 4-0 Polysorb sutures. A stable long-term correction can usually be achieved. Such a case is illustrated in *Figure 9.4*. This patient had undergone a breast reduction elsewhere and presented with a marked asymmetry of the NAC with the left side being larger than the right. A previous attempt at correction was inadequate. She then underwent a reduction of the size of the NAC and a repositioning of the NAC using the interlocking Gore-Tex® technique *(Figs. 9.4C–E)*. This is a powerful technique for controlling the areola size and for simultaneously repositioning it on the breast surface *(Fig. 9.4F)*.[2] This technique is illustrated in the video that accompanies this chapter.

Areola hypopigmentation

It is not uncommon for some of the areola to develop hypopigmentation following a breast reduction. This is

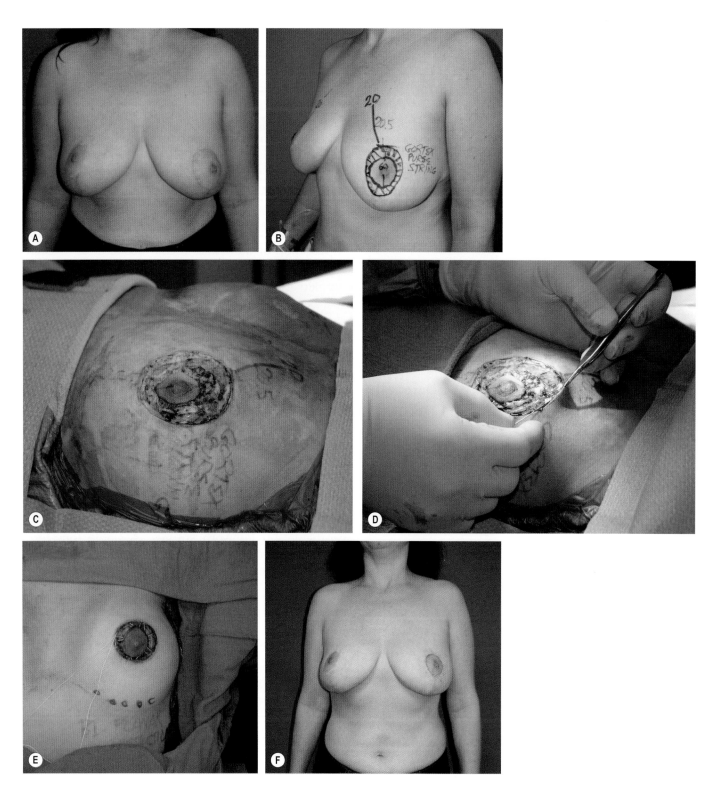

Fig. 9.4 (A) Significant postoperative asymmetry in the size of the NAC following a breast reduction done 1 year previously. The LEFT side is much larger than the right. **(B)** Preoperative plan for reducing the diameter of the NAC and repositioning it on the breast by moving it superiorly. The stippled area of areola and adjacent skin will be discarded. **(C)** The sequence of steps includes de-epithelialization of the skin peripheral to the new areola dimension **(D)** incising through the dermis peripherally to allow placement of the Gore-Tex® suture in the deepest aspect of the dermis keeping it as far away from the skin surface as possible and **(E)** the Gore-Tex® suture which engages the peripheral skin and the areola itself. Two bites are taken peripherally to every bite placed in the areola. **(F)** Postoperative appearance showing much improved symmetry between the nipple areola complexes.

especially true in patients undergoing breast augmentation with a resection and nipple transplantation technique. Such "blotchy" hypopigmentation can be bothersome to the patient.

An intra-dermal tattoo can be especially helpful in these cases. It is important to match up the color as closely as possible and not to use a pigment that is too dark. In addition, patients must be told that more than one tattoo procedure may be necessary, as these tattoos have a tendency to fade with time.

Fat necrosis

Fat necrosis can occur in any surgical procedure on the breast and is not uncommonly seen in breast reduction. Large areas of fat necrosis result from a significant focal devascularization of the adipose tissue in the breast. This can result in a firm to hard area which is uncomfortable. At times, a visual abnormality can be seen.

The process presents as one of induration, initially. There is a definite thickening of the tissue. When the condition persists past 6–12 months, surgical intervention is often needed to improve it.

In my experience, the preferred treatment is either total or more often, subtotal excision of the area of fat necrosis. This area must be localized with the patient in the sitting position on physical examination. It is important to realize that this is a "space occupying lesion" in the breast. Resecting it will cause a decrease in volume and often a contour abnormality (slight indentation). It is important to mention this to the patient preoperatively. Preoperative breast imaging with a mammogram or ultrasound may also be helpful from the standpoint of understanding the volume of tissue involved. This allows the plastic surgeon to inform the patient about the size of the likely resulting defect.

Surgical planning involves elevation of the skin flaps and dissection of the breast tissue exposing the problematic region. Subtotal excision is a good strategy in many cases with the removal of the most superficial aspects of the necrotic adipose tissue. This has the advantage of improving the visible contour deficit, while minimizing the resulting contour defect.[4] The trade-off of an area of discomfort for less of an area of discomfort is one that many patients will accept.

The author has not performed subsequent adipose free autologous fat grafts into an area of fat necrosis, although this may be an option for patients who have undergone resection. At this point in time, surgical judgment would dictate waiting at least 6 months or perhaps a year before attempting such free adipose cell grafting.

Fat necrosis of significance following a breast reduction is unusual and when it occurs, the areas are small. They tend to occur in the most distal aspects of the pedicle. If they are large, the surgical treatment strategy outlined above will usually result in an improvement.

Asymmetry(ies)

Asymmetries following breast reduction are common. Patients should be routinely told to expect some asymmetry following reduction but that this will not be "lopsidedness". The author tells the patient "if you stare at your breasts in the mirror you will see some element(s) of asymmetry."

Asymmetries can be related to volume, contour asymmetries, asymmetries of the nipple areola position, or the skin envelope and its drape over the breast. All of these asymmetries can be bothersome. Virtually all are amenable to revision. Discrepancies in volume are common. They are usually minor or subtle. Occasionally, they are more obvious.

If the patient has one breast which is much larger than the other, breast correction can be achieved with secondary liposuction. This is a good procedure in a patient whose breasts are significantly replaced with adipose tissue (fat replaced breasts). Careful marking of the area to be reduced is done preoperatively with the patient in the upright position. The author generally uses a wet, "not super wet" technique. Suction of the entire gland is usually necessary as opposed to one specific area. Healing and contraction of the tissues usually result in improvement. Such liposuction can be combined with a tightening of the breast skin to achieve the best possible shape. These decisions can be made peroperatively by a digital manipulation of the skin and breast tissues with the patient in the sitting position. Alternatively, open resection of adipose tissue can be done.

Nipple retraction

Nipple retraction can be seen in breast reduction. The etiology is insufficient volume deep to the nipple to support its projection anteriorly. To avoid this deformity, a concerted effort must be made not to resect breast tissue beneath the nipple areola complex at the time of the initial procedure. If this happens however, it is possible to re-make the incisions and to recruit additional tissue to the pedicle during this procedure. The surrounding skin can then be tightened around the nipple areola complex in such a way as to narrow the "periareola skin cut-out". This will then allow the nipple to be inset onto the skin with the skin serving as a platform. Relatively good corrections of nipple retraction can be achieved in this way.

Nipple malposition

Nipple malposition is quoted as one of the most common long-term complications of breast reduction. This results from the fact that the nipple actually stays in the position that it was initially placed but the tissue surrounding the nipple (the parenchyma) descends. There is excess volume in the lower part of the gland accompanied by a stretch deformity of the skin which is in excess. The treatment involves repositioning the underlying parenchyma. This can be done by elevating the inferior aspect of the breast parenchyma and "in folding" it behind the gland as a method of "auto-augmenting" the parenchyma *(Fig. 9.5)*. The lower skin and breast tissue is elevated off of the chest above the infra-mammary fold and the skin is de-epithelialized prior to "in folding" it behind the breast gland. This maneuver can increase the apparent volume in the upper pole, thereby creating the illusion of less of superiorly malpositioned NAC *(Fig. 9.6)*.

The NAC can also be too low. If the top of the areola on one side is lower than the top of the areola on the other side by ≤1.5 cm, then a crescentic excision *(Fig. 9.5A,B)* of skin can be done and the upper portion of the NAC can be elevated.[4] If this maneuver is used when the discrepancy between the upper portion of the areola is >1.5 cm, then an elongation of the NAC is likely to

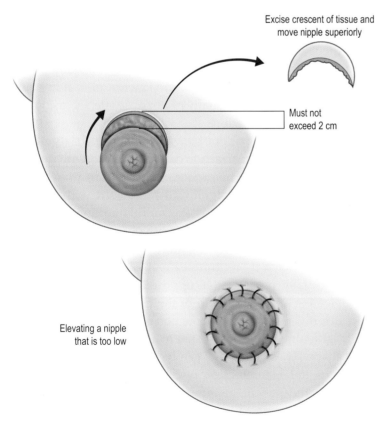

Excise crescent of tissue and move nipple superiorly

Must not exceed 2 cm

Elevating a nipple that is too low

Fig. 9.5 The approach to addressing "bottoming out" with loss of volume in the upper pole of the breast. **(A)** The excess lower pole tissue is identified and de-epithelialized. This tissue is elevated off of the underlying chest wall for a variable distance superiorly. It may be necessary to convert an inferior pedicle to a central pedicle with this maneuver. **(B)** The lower pole tissue is then folded under the elevated breast and fixed to the chest wall. This will provide an apparent increase in volume to the breast and an improved shape.

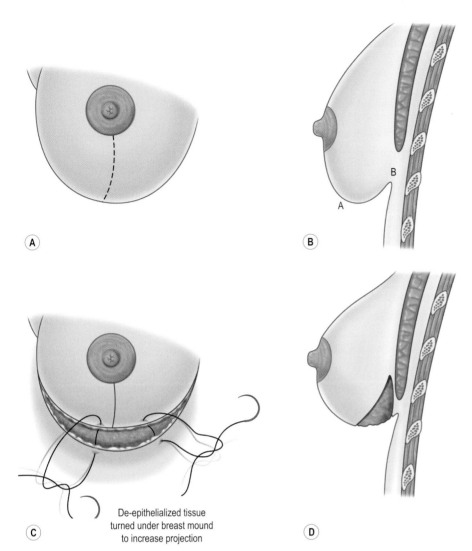

Fig. 9.6 Elevation of NAC which is slightly low (<1.5 cm) is achieved by crescentic skin excision above the junction of NAC with breast skin between the 10-o'clock, 9-o'clock and 3-o'clock position.

De-epithelialized tissue turned under breast mound to increase projection

occur giving the NAC an ovoid shape. A similar strategy can be used to lower the inferior aspect of the NAC that is felt to be too high, or it can be used to restore a smooth convex downward curve to the NAC at the 6:00 position in situations where it is too flat. When >2 cm of nipple elevation is desired, then the strategy illustrated in *Figure 9.4* can be utilized. It may be combined with advancement of the skin flaps skin on either side of the vertical incisions.

Nipple loss

Nipple loss is a devastating complication following breast reduction. It occurs with a frequency of approximately 1%. This should be mentioned in the discussion with all patients who are being seen in consultation for a breast reduction.

Nipple ischemia can sometimes be recognized at the time of surgery but not always. This is especially true in patients of color (African-American and some Hispanic or Asian patients). If it is recognized, the maneuvers to address it are outlined above.

There are patients who sustain nipple loss following a breast reduction, however. For these individuals, a nipple reconstruction with additional intra-areola tattoo may be a good option to bring the appearance of the breast closer to normal.

There are many techniques available but my preference is the modified star flap or "C to V" flap.[4] This technique can be used to augment the nipple which has lost much of its projection, or it can be used to restore the nipple in cases of complete nipple loss. The author prefers this to the procedure of nipple sharing in this setting *(Fig. 9.7)*.

Re-do breast reduction

Patients who have undergone a breast reduction can present much later in life with "recurrent" breast hypertrophy. This is usually related to weight gain, with a corresponding increase in the adipose tissue content of the breast that increases the size. A recurrence of previous symptoms can occur and their breast once again can represent an encumbrance to all or most of their activities of daily living.

Although a decidedly uncommon occurrence (probably one patient per decade), patients requesting re-do breast reduction will present for evaluation. The surgeon should know and understand their specific goals. A careful history includes the patient's recollection of her recovery from the previous operation, keying in on problems with healing and other issues such as sensory changes or any problems with anesthesia. Any intervening breast problems such as mammographic abnormalities, any additional breast surgical procedures such as biopsies or previous revisions of the initial operation must be sought out prior to surgery. The surgeon should have a precise understanding of what pedicle was used in the first operation to carry the nipple areola complex. Although there are reports to the contrary, most surgeons believe that it is most advisable to develop the same pedicle that was used in the first procedure.[1]

Many of these patients can be managed by aggressive liposuction of the breast tissue and a skin tightening in the form of tailor-tacking. Relatively minimal elevation of the nipple areola complex should be undertaken, and this should be carried out on a broad de-epithelialized dermal pedicle.

In cases where a more significant reduction is requested, then re-developing the same pedicle[1] *(Fig. 9.8C)* with resection of tissue peripheral to it coupled with tightening of the skin envelope using "tailor-tacking" *(Fig. 9.8D)* is the preferred approach. This planning and operative sequence is illustrated in *Figure 9.8*. The patient is marked preoperatively in the standing position to site the nipple position *(Fig. 9.8A)*. It is essential that the patient is placed in the sitting position at

90° on the operating table before committing to final nipple position and to the skin excision, which is suggested by the tailor-tacking maneuver. These basic technical approaches can lead to successful outcomes in major revisions of a previous breast reduction.

Revision of mastopexy

Mastopexy is a procedure that reshapes the breast by elevating and re-contouring the breast parenchyma along with repositioning the nipple areola complex (NAC) in a more cosmetically desirable location. The challenge that all plastic surgeons performing this procedure face, is elevating the breast tissue and keeping it in a more superior location with parenchymal sutures, pillar support or, more commonly, skin support. Recent advances in technique have focused on parenchymal re-shaping and fixation more than skin support. The duration of the benefit derived from the initial procedure depends on a number of factors, including: the degree of existing ptosis; the elasticity of the skin and breast parenchyma; the patient's heredity; weight stability and limitations of weight fluctuation and her overall health. Patients with advanced ptosis at an early age without an obvious etiologic factor (e.g., large and frequent fluctuations in weight) are more prone to relapse after a mastopexy procedure. Finally, every patient must understand the "trade-off" of scars for shape and the fact that, although the scars are permanent after breast uplift, an undeniable sequelae of every mastopexy is recurrent ptosis.

The most common reasons for reoperation following mastopexy are dissatisfaction with breast shape due to recurrent ptosis, inadequate breast fullness, suboptimal scarring and nipple areola complex asymmetry or malposition. My personal experience in revision surgery following mastopexy, includes patients who have undergone mastopexy alone and patients who have had a previous augmentation mastopexy. In the latter group of patients, the problem may be with implant in the form of capsular contracture or implant malposition. Alternatively, it may be related to the soft tissue envelope, which has a tendency to "settle away" from the implant in the lower pole breast or has problems with the NAC aesthetics or the scars on the breast. Not infrequently, there a combination of factors which

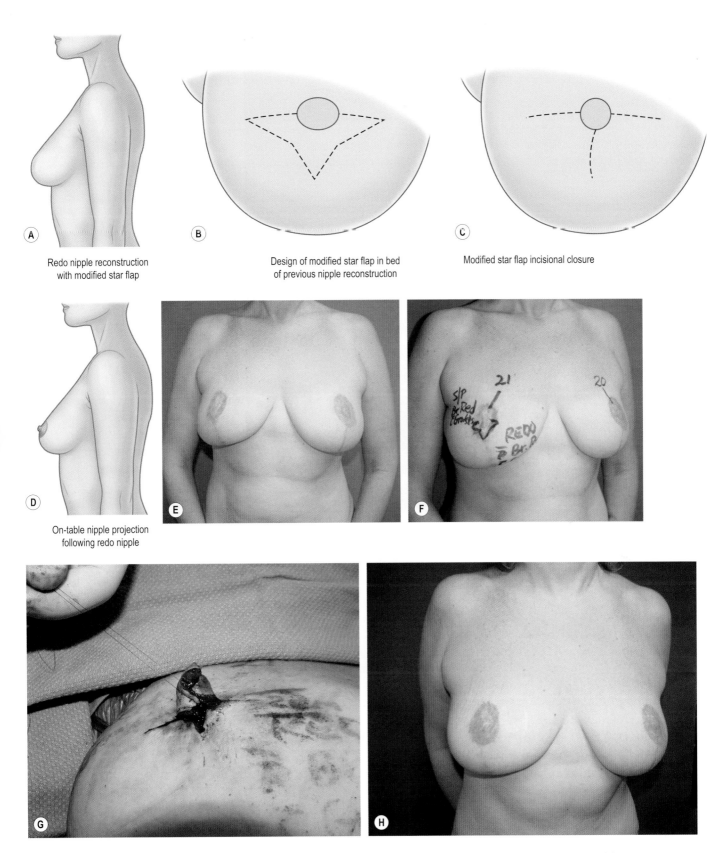

Redo nipple reconstruction
with modified star flap

Design of modified star flap in bed
of previous nipple reconstruction

Modified star flap incisional closure

On-table nipple projection
following redo nipple

Fig. 9.7 (A–D) Technique of modified star flap or "C-to-V flap" elevation. **(E)** Clinical case showing nipple loss after previous breast reduction. **(F)** Plan for a modified star or C-to-V flap reconstruction. **(G)** The flap elevated. **(H)** A 1 year postoperative photograph showing increased nipple projection.

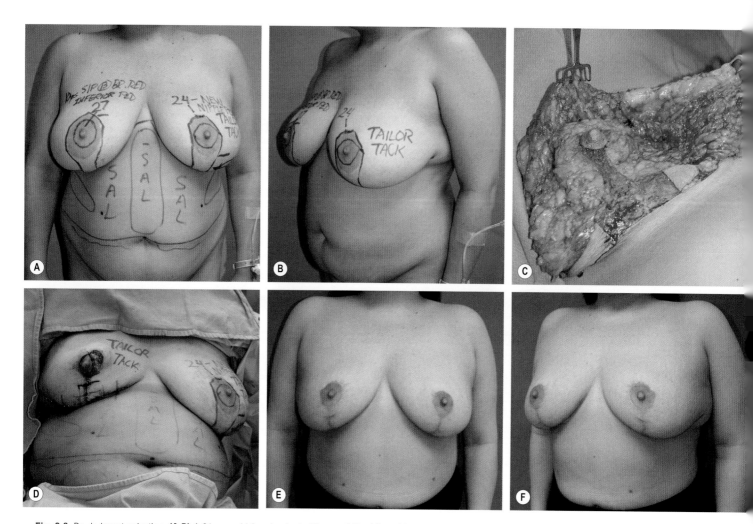

Fig. 9.8 Re-do breast reduction. **(A,B)** A 31-year-old female who is 10 years S/P a bilateral breast reduction using an inferior pedicle and a Wise pattern skin excision. She has gained 80 pounds and her breast size is a "DD cup". She desires reduction to a "C" cup and requests concomitant liposuction of the abdominal wall. **(C)** The previous inferior pedicle is recreated with preservation of the dermis. **(D)** "Tailor-tacking" of the skin helps to confirm nipple position and the appropriate resection of the skin flaps. **(E,F)** The patient is pictured 8 months postoperatively, showing a good shape to the breasts which have been reduced to a "C cup" in size.

must be sorted out and analyzed preoperatively by the surgeon after a careful discussion with the patient about what is bothering her the most. As mentioned above, it is essential to have the patient articulate her "chief complaint" related to her breast appearance. This allows the surgeon to make a determination about the degree of correction that can be achieved with a surgical intervention and to communicate this to the patient.

As with patients who are undergoing revision procedures after breast reduction, it is important for the surgeon to be aware of exactly what pedicle was used in the original operation to support the vascularity of the NAC. This is most accurately determined by reading the previous operative report. Very frequently, the same incisions will be used and when moving the NAC it may be helpful to widely de-epithelialize the skin around the areola and to use broad cutaneous and breast pedicles whenever possible.[5] In cases of previous subglandular or pre-pectoral breast augmentation done with a mastopexy, the surgeon must be aware of the fact that the vascularity of the NAC has already been reduced, again underlining precautions regarding developing narrow pedicles of skin and breast paren-chyma.[5] *Finally, extreme caution must be exercised when considering or offering the procedure to patients who smoke. This author personally will not do revision mastopexy or breast reduction in these patients.*

The following two cases illustrate surgical revisions of a previous mastopexy and augmentation mastopexy and illustrate the surgical approach to both situations. The first patient was a 36-year-old nulliparous physical fitness enthusiast who stood 5'6" and weighed 135 pounds, with a BMI of 27. She used a 36C bra cup but her breasts demonstrated profound grade III mammary ptosis *(Fig. 9.9A,B)*. There was markedly decreased elasticity of the skin and breast tissue, as evidenced by striae on the breasts bilaterally. She desired breast rejuvenation without the use of an implant. The operative plan was for a superior dermoglandular vertical mastopexy with a vertical skin excision. That provided the optimal chance for fixation of the breast parenchyma to the superior chest region *(Fig. 9.9C)*. There was a good shape change noted in the operating room following the completion of the right side *(Fig. 9.9D)* The vertical skin excision depicted in the preoperative plan *(Fig. 9.9C)* was perhaps over aggressive. The procedure improved the breast shape as seen at a 2-week postoperative visit *(Fig. 9.9E)* but epidermolysis of the peripheral areola region and of the medial aspect of the lateral flap of the right breast was evident 2 weeks following surgery. This culminated in spreading of the NAC, widened cosmetically unacceptable scars *(Fig. 9.9F,G)* and compromise in shape with loss of upper pole fullness *(Fig. 9.9H)* as illustrated in the 18-month postoperative views.

The plan was to re-do the mastopexy by re-elevation of the superior pedicle, fixation to the pectoralis fascia with two rows of 2-0 Polyglycolic acid "pexy" sutures with a conservative (limited to 2 cm) skin excision and the re-do of pillar approximation inferiorly. The markings *(Fig. 9.9I)* and intraoperative AP view after correction of the left side *(Fig. 9.9J)* illustrated improved shape largely due to the "pexy" sutures in the upper pectoralis major muscle area along with improved nipple areola aesthetics. The patient had an uneventful recovery and maintains a very good correction 6 years following surgery *(Fig. 9.9K,L)*.

This case is instructive for a variety of reasons. The preoperative presentation illustrates a patient who is at great risk for relapse following a ptosis correction of any type. The initial procedure did not emphasize pedicle fixation by the use of sufficient "pexy" sutures to fix the parenchyma to the pectoralis major muscle (PMM) fascia in the upper chest but instead relied too heavily on skin suturing with tension. Using sutures to fix the undersurface of the dermoglandular superior pedicle to the pectoralis fascia is an important maneuver and the author virtually always uses a minimum of two rows of sutures (usually 3–4 in each row) to achieve this fixation to PMM fascia. Also important is to realize that this is a parenchymal re-shaping procedure and that pillar apposition in the lower breast supports the "fixed" pedicle in the upper pole of the re-shaped breast and it also should eliminate tension on the skin closure. When using a superior dermoglandular pedicle the central breast pedicle is "telescoped" superiorly after "scoring" the breast parenchyma with the electrocautery device on coagulation mode incising its deep surface through the posterior breast fascia into the deep breast parenchyma. The pedicle is fixed in its new superior position by the "pexy" sutures. This produces immediate on-table upper pole breast fullness. However, it is bringing the pillars together in the midline with 3 or 4 pillar sutures of 2-0 Polyglycolic acid that "locks" the pillars together below the pedicle and forms that most important part of the pedicle stabilization.

Every vertical mastopexy procedure is far more dependent on parenchymal re-shaping rather than a tight skin closure to maintain the correction. The latter maneuver routinely leads to wide unattractive scars or open wounds and should be avoided. In the author's opinion, the vertical technique is the most powerful breast re-shaping tool available to plastic surgeons. Other methods of pedicle stabilization have employed de-epithelialized extensions of the skin from the pedicle which can be tacked to the chest wall, for example when an inferior pedicle is mobilized and placed in a more superior position on the chest wall. Support from the skin envelope closure is of secondary importance in all of these cases.

Revision of augmentation-mastopexy is more complex because of the effect of the implant on breast appearance and the tissues themselves. The surgeon must carefully analyze the breast from the standpoint of implant position relative to the breast parenchyma and the location of the NAC. The amount of upper pole breast fullness

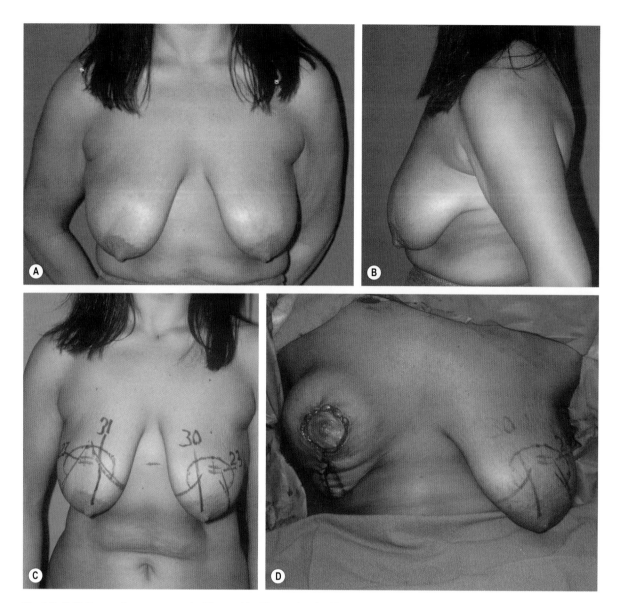

Fig. 9.9 **(A,B)** Preoperative appearance of a 36-year-old nulliparous female with grade III ptosis and generalized laxity of her skin. **(C)** Markings for a superior dermoglandular pedicle vertical mastopexy. **(D)** Intraoperative AP view showing marked shape change of the right breast after this side is completed. **(E)** The 2-week postoperative AP view shows improved appearance but peripheral epidermolysis of the right NAC and marginal ischemia of the lateral flap of the right breast. **(F–H)** At 18 months following surgery there is some loss of ptosis correction and unacceptable appearance of the breast scars. **(I)** Preoperative marking for revision of mastopexy using the same superior pedicle **(J)** The intraoperative view showing correction of the left breast. We have used two rows of 2-0 Polyglycolic acid sutures to "pexy" the deep portion of the breast gland to the upper pectoralis major muscle and underlying fascia. **(K,L)** The patient is seen 6 years following surgery with maintenance of a good correction.

is critical to assess. The patient is examined in the upright and supine positions and the mobility of implant under the influence of gravity is noted in both positions. The implant is then digitally manipulated in the sitting position to ascertain its mobility or lack of mobility in the peri-prosthetic capsular space (PPCS). If the PPCS is too low or too lateral the upper pole fullness of the breast is most often sub-optimal and the space should be altered by either suture capsulorraphy or mirror image capsulectomies of the anterior and posterior capsule tissue and suture repair. The implant is then replaced into the capsule which has been modified by repositioning it superiorly and medially. If on the other hand, capsular contracture is suspected and is

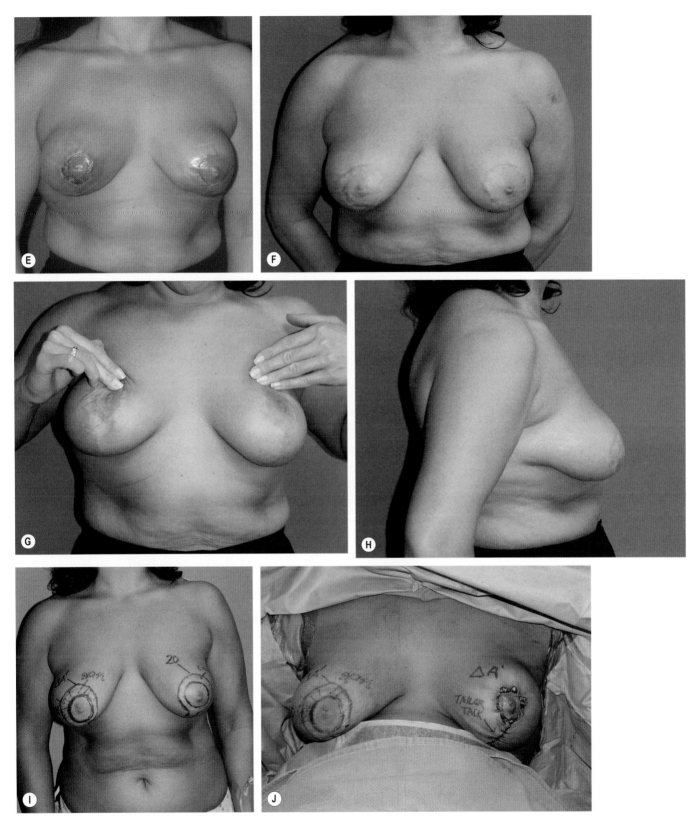

Fig. 9.9, cont'd

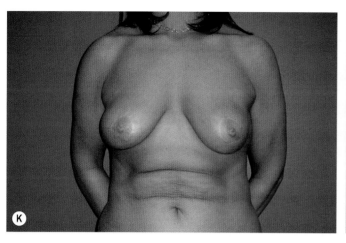
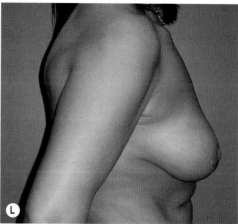

Fig. 9.9, cont'd

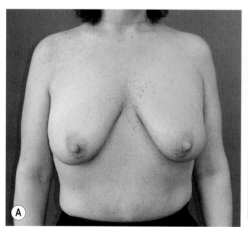
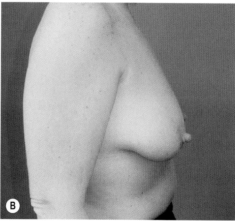

Fig. 9.10 (A,B) Preoperative appearance of 36-year-old nulliparous patient with bilateral breast ptosis. She desires an uplift and increased breast volume.

producing an unwanted appearance, the preferred approach is usually to perform a total capsulectomy prior to replacing an implant. With the implant providing sufficient volume and upper pole fullness, the soft tissue envelope is then altered using a "tailor-tacking" maneuver. This is obviously a critical technique for giving the surgeon a true "plasticity" in maximizing aesthetics.

In the situation of a sub-optimal breast shape following a previous augmentation-mastopexy, the problem may relate to: skin scar deformity; stretching of the lower pole secondary to the effects of gravitational settling of the implant in either an inferior or lateral direction (frequently in both directions); the potential effect of capsular contracture on the production of deformity and asymmetry; gravitational settling of the lower pole tissues away from the implant, especially in cases of capsular contracture. Again the surgeon must be wary of a possible decrease in the blood supply of the breast and to the NAC from the previous surgical procedure. This is more important in cases where a previous subglandular or pre-pectoral approach has been used for breast augmentation.[5] As noted previously, in such a case, it is wise to maintain as much dermal tissue peripheral to the NAC as possible.

The patient in *Figure 9.10* is also a 36-year-old nulliparous woman, with grade II mammary ptosis *(Fig. 9.10)* and a generalized looseness of her skin and decreased elasticity of her breast parenchyma. The plan was for an augmentation-mastopexy with the placement of a saline implant in a dual plane position with a vertical mammaplasty approach. The plan *(Fig. 9.11)* was to place the nipple at least 3 cm above the inframammary fold (IMF). A 300 cc smooth surface moderate profile saline implant was placed first through a short vertical incision and a "tailor-tacking" of the skin *(Fig. 9.12)* was done to simulate the optimal breast shape. At a 3-month postoperative visit, the patient demonstrated good breast aesthetics *(Fig. 9.13)* but at a 2-year follow-up, she developed a stretch deformity of the lower pole and a slight inferior implant mal-position and loss of upper pole fullness *(Fig. 9.14)*, which compromised the upper pole fullness and overall breast aesthetics. She requested revision. This was accomplished by using a suture capsulorraphy to raise the level of the lower breast capsule fold by 1 cm. A slightly larger silicone gel implant was placed 350 cc, the patient underwent peri-areola skin tightening *(Fig. 9.15)* along with resection of skin from the lower pole to address the stretch deformity. She is shown 3 years following this procedure with improved breast appearance in *Figure 9.16*.

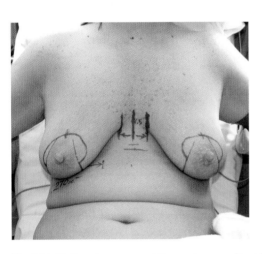

Fig. 9.11 Markings for an augmentation mastopexy performed with a vertical mastopexy approach.

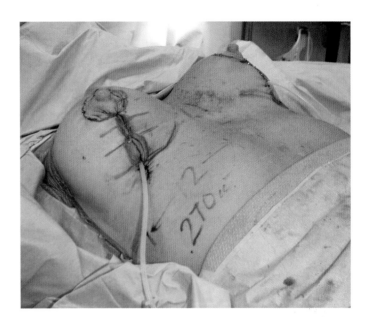

Fig. 9.12 On-table view of a 330 moderate profile saline implant in place and tailor-tacking completed to guide skin excision and nipple position.

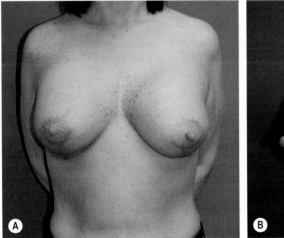
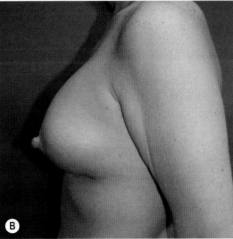

Fig. 9.13 (A,B) The 3-month postoperative appearance shows volume augmentation and good nipple position and an overall good early outcome of the procedure.

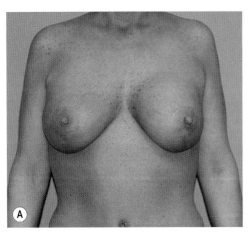
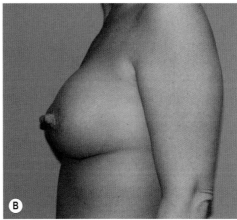

Fig. 9.14 (A,B) At 23 months postoperatively, the patient shows a stretch deformity of the lower pole of the breast, slight inferior implant malposition and some loss of upper pole fullness of the breasts.

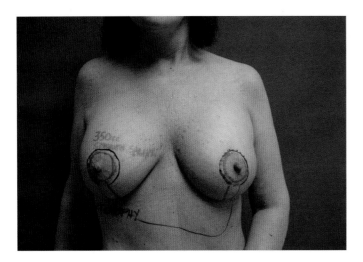

Fig. 9.15 The plan for a inferior capsulorraphy, resection of lower pole breast tissue and exchange of the current implant to a 350 cc moderate profile silicone gel device.

Revision mastopexy

Postoperative care

The postoperative care of patients undergoing revision mastopexy is very similar to that of patients undergoing breast reduction. If drains are used (this is an uncommon practice in mastopexy), they are removed on a schedule indicated above. A "snug fitting" jogging bra is worn on a 24 h basis for a 4–6 week period. The patients are asked to refrain from vigorous activities following surgery for at least 1 month. They are especially asked to minimize any activities that involve

bouncing such as running on a treadmill or high impact aerobic exercise.

Revision augmentation/mastopexy

Postoperative care

The care of these patients is very similar to the patients undergoing revision mastopexy. If drains were employed, they are removed on the schedule noted above. Support of the breast is important and the patient is asked to wear a "snug fitting" jogging bra for a 4–6 week period after surgery. This is worn both during the daytime and at night on a "24/7" basis for this time period. The patient is asked to refrain from vigorous activities (any high impact activities, especially those in which bouncing is involved).

The obvious difference in these patients is the use of a breast implant. In this case, implant displacement exercises are instituted as soon as the patient is comfortable, and generally this is 24–48 h following surgery. Patients are instructed to methodically move their implants "in and out" and also "up and down"; 10 repetitions of each movement twice a day. It is most conveniently done in the morning upon rising and in the evening prior to sleep. Initially, the activity is performed gently but it becomes more vigorous as the time from surgery becomes more remote. This limits the incidence of capsular contracture.

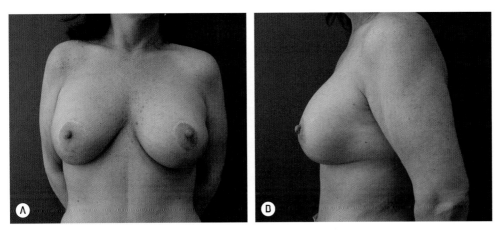

Fig. 9.16 (A,B) The patient's 3 year postoperative AP and lateral views show a markedly improved breast appearance.

Patients should not sleep on their stomachs, since this can promote lateral implant movement and can also lead to lateral implant malposition. Patients are seen at follow-up at 2 weeks, 1 month, 3 months, and 6 months postoperatively. They are then seen at yearly intervals. Implant integrity is monitored by high resolution ultrasonography of the breast, performed every 4 years. If there are any abnormalities noted with this study, an MRI is employed for additional imaging specificity.

Complications

Complications related to revision augmentation/ mastopexy are a combination of those related to the breast augmentation and those related to the mastopexy. Many of these (lower pole stretch deformity, loss of shape) are demonstrated in a case presented below.

As noted previously, complications are routinely explained to patients for augmentation/mastopexy, in terms of three general categories.

Wound healing issues: bleeding, hematoma, seroma, infection, wound separation, implant exposure, sensory loss to the skin or the NAC, pain, hypertrophic scars, painful scars and animation deformity in the situation where the implant was placed in the subpectoral space. Extreme vigilance is exercised at the time of surgery to minimize infection in every case. This includes intravenous perioperative antibiotics as well as a triple antibiotic solution used to irrigate and bathe the dissection space at the time of surgery. This solution is a combination of 1 g Ancef, 100 mg of Gentamicin and 50 000 units of Bacitracin placed in 500 cc of saline as described by Adams.

Any sign of infection (erythema, incisional pain, and fever accompanied by implant discomfort) should be aggressively evaluated and treated. Infections usually respond to treatment with appropriate broad spectrum antibiotics. The patient is commonly started on Keflex 500 mg QID. If bacteriology is available it may be helpful in directing antibiotic treatment. Return to the operating room is indicated by severity of infection or failure to respond to intravenous antibiotic therapy. Some of these implants maybe salvaged if soft tissue coverage is adequate and if there is no evidence of gross purulence (pus) in the peri-prosthetic capsular space. At surgery, it is necessary to aggressively irrigate and curette the peri-prosthetic capsular space. The author finds that a uterine curette is an excellent instrument for removing biofilms while minimally injuring the peri-prosthetic capsule tissues. A suction drain is used. An excellent discussion related to the salvage of such implants has been published by Spear.[1]

Aesthetic complications include: asymmetries of all types, which encompass breast shape, breast volume, position of the NAC, position of the surgical scars. If any of these are significant, a revision procedure may be employed. In addition, implant malposition along with the presence of ripples, ridges and folds from the implant can also occur. These most commonly relate to the quality and thickness of the overlying covering tissue that includes the patient's skin and subcutaneous tissue and breast parenchymal layer. It is important to assess the upper pole of the breast in every patient for the "pinch thickness". If this area of tissue is <2 cm in thickness it is best to place the implant in the subpectoral position. Patients with thin covering tissues in this area are more prone to the development of rippling.

In addition to the tissue factors just mentioned, it is important to realize that the implant itself often produces stretching of the peri-prosthetic capsule tissue and the overlying breast parenchyma and skin. In addition, the "stretch" imposed on the peri-prosthetic capsule by the implant increases the volume of the peri-prosthetic capsular space. The implant volume however, remains unchanged, thus creating a "peri-prosthetic capsular space-implant disproportion". When a responsive gel implant is used, this process definitely contributes to the formation of visible folds.

This problem is difficult to completely correct but it can be addressed by surgery on both the peri-prosthetic capsule and by a procedure to augment the overlying soft tissue coverage. Techniques to tighten the capsule tissue and at times reposition it are well described in various texts.[4] They might include capsulorraphy or capsule excision and repair. Most recently, there has been considerable enthusiasm for the use of acellular dermal matrixes from the standpoint of supplying additional support to the capsule repair. In addition to modifying the peri-prosthetic capsule autologous fat grafting can be used to increase the thickness of the overlying soft tissue envelope. This is most consistently done using the micrografting technique introduced and refined by Coleman.

The inherent risks of implants include: capsular contracture, implant failure and unplanned additional surgery. Capsular contracture rates appear to be trending downward for silicone gel implants but are probably still in the range of 10–15% at 3 years (Baker grade III and Baker grade IV). This decrease in capsular contracture rate most probably relates to changes in the implant shell itself and the widespread use of antibiotic irrigation at the time of placement.

Reoperation of capsular contracture carries a good prospect for improvement. Approximately 80% of patients who treated with procedures which involve removing the entire capsule and replacing the pervious implant with a new implant are improved in terms of softness. These surgical procedures include site change, creation of "neo pockets", and the use of acellular dermal matrix-often done in combinations. There is an increasing body of evidence that strongly suggests that multi modality therapy of site change, implant change and the use of acellular dermal matrix may significantly reduce the subsequent reoccurrence of capsular contracture.

Implant failure is a reality of all previously placed implants. Surveillance for silicone gel breast implant integrity is breast accomplished by radiologic imaging performed every 4 years using high resolution ultrasound. The "gold standard" for implant surveillance and for establishing the diagnosis of implant failure remains MRI. In the author's practice, implants that are suspected of having failed, especially if there is evidence of extra capsular silicone, are removed. This is done with a surgical operation that employs a general anesthetic. Drains are uniformly utilized after the capsulectomy procedure is completed. Following drain removal, implant displacement exercises are instituted as described.

All patients who undergo any of the revision procedures described in this chapter must be made aware of the definite likelihood of unplanned additional surgery. For patients undergoing implant placement, this is at least 25% at a 5-year follow-up.

Conclusion

These revision procedures require an assessment of all of the components that contribute to the deformity. After a careful physical examination, the surgeon is then able to formulate a well derived plan for correction. The patient is informed that perfect symmetry is almost never achieved and that the passage of time will usually diminish the improvement achieved at surgery. These procedures are some of the more difficult procedures that challenge the breast plastic surgeon but they frequently result in significant satisfaction for the patient and the surgeon alike. In performing such revisions, it is better for the surgeon "to under promise and over deliver."

References

1. Spear SL. Secondary reduction mammoplasty: is using a different pedicle safe? *Plast Reconstr Surg.* 2000;106(5): 1009–1010.
   Discussion of an article suggesting the safety of using a different pedicle for re-do breast reduction. Dr Spear disagrees

strongly and states that the same pedicle should be used whenever the nipple areola complex is to be moved. This same opinion has been expressed many times by Dr James C. Grotting at various breast surgery symposia.

2. Hammond DC, Khuthaila DK, Kim J. The interlocking Gore-Tex suture for control of areolar diameter and shape. *Plast Reconstr Surg.* 2007;119(3):804–809.

   Description of a powerful operative technique which greatly expands the capability and reliability of peri-areola skin excision and re-distribution on the breast. It has a significant role in both primary and revision mastopexy and augmentation mastopexy.

3. Henry SL, Crawford JL, Puckett CL. Risk factors and complications in reduction mammaplasty: novel associations and preoperative assessment. *Plast Reconstr Surg.* 2009;124(4):1040–1046.

   This an excellent review correlating preoperative risk factors with occurrence of complications following breast reduction.

4. Shestak KC. *Re-operative plastic surgery of the breast.* Philadelphia: Lippincott Williams & Wilkins; 2006:200–202, 219.

   This is a single author textbook, which focuses exclusively on reoperative plastic surgery of the breast. It outlines in much more detail, many of the techniques referred to in the foregoing chapter.

5. Handel N. Secondary mastopexy in the augmented patient: a recipe for disaster. *Plast Reconstr Surg.* 2006;118(7S):152S–163S.

   This is an outstanding overview of the perils and pitfalls of performing revision mastopexy in patients who have undergone previous breast augmentation. The author presents strategies for minimizing complications in this clinical setting. It is a must read for plastic surgeons planning these procedures.

Further reading

Bartsch RH, Weiss G, Kästenbauer T, et al. Crucial aspects of smoking in wound healing after breast reduction surgery. *J Plast Reconstr Aesthet Surg.* 2007;60(9):1045–1049.

Collins ED, Kerrigan CL, Striplin DT, et al. The effectiveness of surgical and non-surgical interventions in relieving the symptoms of macromastia. *Plast Reconstr Surg.* 2002;109:1556–1566.

Kerrigan CL, Collins ED, Striplin DT, et al. The health burden of beast hypertrophy. *Plast Reconstr Surg.* 2001;108:1591–1599.

Losee JE, Elethea H, Caldwell MD, et al. Secondary breast reduction mammaplasty: is using a different pedicle safe? *Plast Reconstr Surg.* 2000;106(5):1009–1010.

Varma SK, Henderson HP. Is it justified to refuse breast reduction to smokers? *J Plast Reconstr Aesthet Surg.* 2007;60(9):1050–1054.

10

Breast cancer: Diagnosis, therapy, and oncoplastic techniques

Elisabeth Beahm and Julie E. Lang

SYNOPSIS

- Breast cancer afflicts one in eight women; screening mammography has been shown to reduce mortality from breast cancer by early detection of disease. Core needle biopsy is the preferred diagnostic strategy.
- Breast cancer is a heterogeneous disease; several unique molecular subtypes of breast cancer have been identified based on the prognostic markers estrogen receptor, progesterone receptor and the HER2/neu oncoprotein.
- Breast conserving surgery plus radiation provides equivalent overall survival to a total mastectomy, if feasible based on extent of disease.
- Decision making for adjuvant chemotherapy and radiation therapy involves tumor and patient specific features. These must be considered preoperatively by the surgical team in order to achieve optimal results.
- Many stage 0, stage I, or stage II breast cancer patients planning for mastectomy and most patients electing for prophylactic mastectomy are candidates for immediate breast reconstruction.

 Access the Historical Perspective sections online at
http://www.expertconsult.com

Introduction

In the United States, breast cancer is the most common noncutaneous malignancy among women.[1] The lifetime incidence of breast cancer for American women is approximately 1 in 8. Male breast cancer represents 1% of all breast cancers. On occasion, a patient will present to the plastic surgeon with breast complaints as well; thus, knowledge of the current diagnostic and therapeutic strategies is essential. The expertise of a plastic surgeon may be called upon regarding screening or the diagnostic evaluation of a previously augmented patient with breast complaints or abnormal imaging. Many patients opt for immediate or delayed reconstruction after mastectomy for breast cancer. It is crucial for plastic surgeons to understand the implications of adjuvant oncologic therapies on the suitability for immediate breast reconstruction. Plastic surgeons are an important part of the multidisciplinary care of the patient with breast cancer.

Basic science

Several unique molecular subtypes of breast cancer have been described by gene expression microarray classification that have implications on prognosis, such as overall survival and distant metastasis recurrence free survival.[4] These molecular profiles provide information in addition to the traditional histopathologic markers estrogen receptor (ER), progesterone receptor (PR), and the HER2/neu oncoprotein. These include the basal subtype (ER, PR, HER2/neu negative, or the so-called triple negative subtype, typically with high grade and high proliferation rates), the luminal A subtype (ER positive, PR positive, HER2 negative, typically with low expression of proliferation related genes) and the luminal B subtype (ER and PR positive but lower expression than luminal A; variable expression of HER2/neu, and high expression of proliferation related genes). While most triple negative tumors are basal-like by microarray, and most basal-like tumors are triple negative, discordance does exist about 30% of the time, which must be kept in mind when comparing studies with different classification strategies.[5] Basal-like cancers are aggressive and share features with tumors arising from BRCA 1 mutation carriers. Triple negative cancers will not benefit from treatment with available targeted therapies, such as endocrine therapy for ER positive disease[6] or trastuzumab, a monoclonal antibody directed at the HER2/neu oncoprotein receptor, for HER2 positive disease.[7] Therefore, triple negative breast cancer patients generally are recommended cytotoxic chemotherapy, based on evidence-based guidelines.[8]

Gene expression predictors such as the Oncotype DX 21 gene recurrence score (Genomic Health, Redwood City, CA) and the Mammaprint 70 gene profile (Agendia, Irvine, CA) are being used increasingly to risk stratify patients regarding the need for adjuvant chemotherapy based on predicted clinical outcomes by primary tumor characteristics.[9,10] These molecular assays are gaining acceptance by the oncology community as decision making tools. The Oncotype DX 21 gene recurrence score has been incorporated into the NCCN guidelines for breast cancer management.[8] The American Society of Clinical Oncology (ASCO) has published guidelines for use of tumor markers in the management of breast cancer.[11]

In recent years, the breast cancer research community has focused much attention on the stem cell theory, which contends that only a small fraction of breast parenchymal cells possess the inherent ability to self-renew, differentiate or cause tumorigenesis.[12] The stem cell theory is in contrast to the traditional clonal evolution, multi-hit theory.[13] Several investigators have made important contributions in recent years in the study of putative breast cancer stem cells. Al-Hajj et al. reported the ability to identify tumorigenic stem cells based on surface markers (CD44 positive, CD24 negative) and showed that as few as 100 of such cells form tumors in immunocompromised mice, whereas tens of thousands of unselected cells typically fail to form tumors.[14] Dontu

et al. developed a suspension cell culture technique that allows for selection of tumorigenic stem cells from tumor specimens.[15] Shackleton et al. demonstrated the ability of a single breast stem cell to generate a functional mammary gland.[16] Understanding the biology of breast stem cells may provide an opportunity to target this refractory population of slow growing stem cells, which are resistant to standard cytotoxic chemotherapy and radiotherapy.

Patients who carry a deleterious BRCA 1 or BRCA 2 mutation have an elevated risk of breast cancer diagnosis – about a 60–80% lifetime risk.[2] Hundreds of known mutations exist and may be detected via a blood test for genetic sequencing. BRCA 1 and BRCA 2 are important for DNA double strand break repair.[17] These patients also have elevated risk of contralateral breast cancers, ovarian cancer, fallopian tube cancer and other types of malignancy due to their inability to repair damaged DNA. For this reason, clinicians are increasingly referring patients to genetic counselors for consideration for genetic testing. Stage for stage, BRCA mutation carriers have equivalent prognosis to non-BRCA carriers, however, BRCA 1 related tumors tend to be of the aggressive basal-like subtype and tend to afflict younger women.

Diagnosis

The benign and malignant conditions of the breast may be subdivided into two diagnostic categories: (1) conditions that present as symptomatic breast disease with clinical signs and symptoms and (2) asymptomatic disease detected by screening mammography.

Clinical breast examination

Despite numerous advances in breast imaging, the clinical breast examination remains of utmost importance in the assessment of the breast and its associated lymph node basins. Like physical examination of all other regions of the body, the clinical breast examination consists of visual inspection followed by physical examination of four key elements: (1) breast parenchyma; (2) nipple-areola complex; (3) skin envelope, and (4) ipsilateral axillary and supraclavicular lymph node basins. The clinical breast examination is a routine part of annual breast screening by primary care physicians as well as an integral part of the breast surgeon's assessment of a patient.

Diagnostic imaging modalities

Mammography

Mammography is a highly effective screening modality. The typical views include a mediolateral oblique view and a craniocaudal view. With questionable lesions, specific magnified views are obtained to better delineate the area of interest. The American Cancer Society (ACS) guidelines recommend beginning screening mammography at age 40 and continuing annually, as long as they are in good health. Although recently recommendations made by the US Preventive Services Task Force based on a systematic review of the literature prompted much controversy and debate,[18] clinically the ACS guidelines continue to be usual practice.[19]

The BIRADS (Breast Imaging Reporting and Data System) classification *(Table 10.1)* is the most commonly used reporting system for mammography.[20] These

Table 10.1 The BIRADS classification is used to classify screening and diagnostic mammograms, breast ultrasounds and breast MRIs; all breast imaging receives a score based on the BIRADS classification, which helps determine if further evaluation and possible biopsy are indicated

BIRADS[a] category	Interpretation
0	Assessment incomplete; needs additional imaging evaluation
1	Negative; routine screening mammogram indicated in 1 year
2	Benign finding; routine screening mammogram indicated in 1 year
3	Probably benign finding; short interval follow-up study (usually 6 months) indicated
4	Suspicious for malignancy; core biopsy recommended at this time
5	Highly suspicious for malignancy; core biopsy recommended at this time
6	Known biopsy proven breast cancer

[a]Breast Imaging Reporting and Data System, developed by The American College of Radiology.
(Reproduced from Balleyguier C, Ayadi S, Van Nguyen K, et al. BIRADS classification in mammography. *Eur J Radiol.* 2007;61(2):192–194.)

standardized criteria provide a means of radiographically risk-stratifying lesions such that the significance of the mammogram is clear to all clinicians. In this classification, BIRADS 4 (suggestive of malignant disease) or BIRADS 5 (highly suggestive) should always prompt biopsy for tissue diagnosis of a mammographic abnormality *(Fig. 10.1)*. The more frequent use of mammography for screening purposes has resulted in increased recommendations for breast biopsies for clinically occult lesions. As a result of screening mammography, many breast cancers may now be detected at an earlier stage; it is estimated that implementation of regular mammography for women older than 50 years can reduce breast cancer mortality significantly for this population.[21]

Ultrasonography

Breast ultrasonography is widely used as a diagnostic modality that typically plays a role in the work-up of all breast masses; moreover, ultrasound interpretations also utilize the BIRADS classification to describe radiographic findings *(Fig. 10.2)*. Other indications include evaluation of palpable masses in young women with radiographically dense breasts, evaluation of masses in conjunction with diagnostic mammography, and guidance for biopsy or evacuation of cysts.[22] Many breast surgeons use focused breast ultrasonography as an extension of the physical examination. Several ultrasonographic criteria help differentiate malignant from benign lesions, including the presence of spiculations, a taller than wide shape, multiple the presence of calcifications, angular margins, a markedly hypoechoic lesion, posterior shadowing, and a heterogeneous internal structure.[23,24]

Magnetic resonance imaging

In recent years, contrast-enhanced magnetic resonance imaging (MRI) has been used for the evaluation of the breast for cancer. One controversial study found that as many as 10% of newly diagnosed breast cancer patients may have a contralateral primary tumor.[25] A prospective randomized controlled trial found no difference in reoperation rate for newly diagnosed breast cancer patients based on whether or not MRI was ordered as part of the diagnostic work-up.[26] A recent consensus conference proposed guidelines for the use

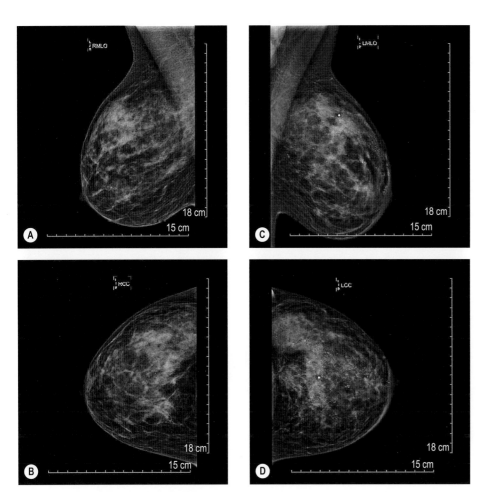

Fig. 10.1 This 45-year-old patient's screening mammogram detected her locally advanced left breast cancer. Her dense breast tissue bilaterally masked the fact that she had an invasive ductal carcinoma occupying most of the left breast. She went on to be treated with neoadjuvant chemotherapy on a clinical trial, followed by a left modified radical mastectomy. She received adjuvant comprehensive radiation therapy to the chest wall, supraclavicular, infraclavicular and axillary fields. She is a candidate for delayed reconstruction about 1 year after completion of her radiation therapy.

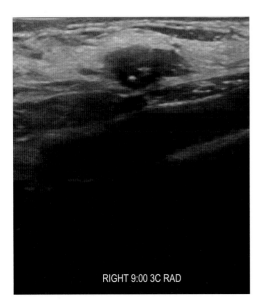

Fig. 10.2 Ultrasound demonstrates a mass in the 9-o'clock position of the right breast. Image guided breast biopsy is indicated for this suspicious finding.

of MRI as a diagnostic and screening tool.[27] MRI is extremely helpful for screening patients at high risk for breast cancer, such as individuals who carry a deleterious BRCA mutation. MRI is also useful in the management of patients with axillary node metastases and unknown primary. The main disadvantages are cost (which precludes widespread use as a screening modality), issues with specificity leading to additional needle biopsies and limited availability compared with mammography or ultrasonography. Several centers have reported increasing mastectomy rates correlating with increasing use of breast MRI.[28] MRI is best reserved as a problem solving tool for specific indications in the diagnostic work-up of breast cancer and may not be necessary for all breast cancer patients. However, the United States Food and Drug Administration recommends monitoring patients with silicone breast implants for occult rupture with breast MRI performed 3 years

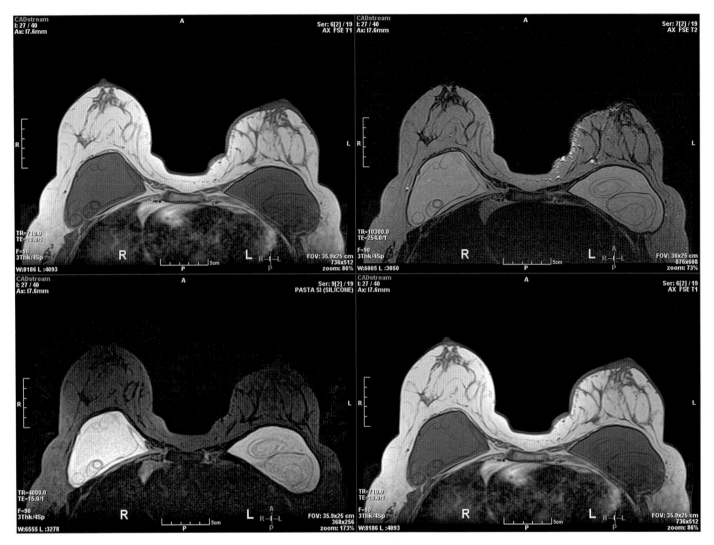

Fig. 10.3 Bilateral linguine signs are noted on breast MRI with gadolinium. This demonstrates rupture of this patient's bilateral silicone breast implants.

postoperatively, then every 2 years thereafter. The "linguine sign" indicates evidence of ruptured silicone breast implants on MRI *(Fig. 10.3)*.

Diagnostic imaging in patients with breast implants

As implants are widely used in both reconstruction and augmentation of the breast, the efficacy of breast cancer screening with mammography is important in this population. A breast implant is radiopaque on mammography and obscures some breast tissue. This, seemingly, may reduce visualization and therefore compromise detection of breast tumors. Efforts to limit the impact of implants on imaging of the breast include submuscular

placement of the device – theoretically allowing better definition and separation from overlying breast tissue – as well as special mammographic techniques. These mammographic approaches include additional surveillance views of the augmented breast tissue and displacement of the implant away from the breast tissue.[29] Mobility of the implant is critical to the efficacy of these techniques. If the implant is not freely mobile, a straight lateral view is obtained in an attempt to more adequately visualize the tissue posterior to the implant. Factors that restrict the mobility of the implant – such as an overly large implant in proportion to the overlying breast tissue, or an implant that has a calcified or contracted and rigid peri-prosthetic capsule – can significantly impair the efficacy of mammography in terms of adequate visualization, particularly the posterior aspect of the breast.

The estimated proportion of breast tissue that is obscured from mammographic examination ranges in the literature from 25% to 80%.[30] However, stage at presentation for augmented patients was no different from that for the patients without implants in two retrospective analyses.[31,32] Holmich *et al.* reported a study of 2955 patients who underwent breast augmentation between 1973–1997;[33] the authors found that women with breast implants on average were diagnosed with breast cancer at the same stage as were control subjects. There was no significant difference in overall survival between the two groups after an average of 6.4 years of follow-up. Several studies have reported that augmented women do not have a higher incidence of breast cancer.[34–36] There has been supposition that patients with breast implants have an enhanced sense of body image and self with a greater percentage of self-reported breast cancers and attention to examination, although these data are somewhat empiric in nature. Recently, Xie *et al.* reported a comparison of a cohort of 24 558 women who underwent bilateral cosmetic breast implants to a cohort of 15 893 women who underwent other types of plastic surgical procedures between 1974–1989.[37] In the largest series to date, the authors reported that women who had undergone prior augmentation mammoplasty were more likely to present with more advanced stage breast carcinoma. This may suggest, in contradistinction to prior study, that breast implants delay detection.[37] Additionally, diagnostic biopsies such as core needle or excisional biopsy may risk rupture of the implant *(Fig. 10.4)*.

Histologic diagnostic modalities

The majority of lesions for which women undergo breast biopsy prove to be benign. In addition, many women must undergo multiple biopsies over the course of their lifetime. No breast biopsy technique has 100% accuracy, however, large gauge image guided core needle biopsy closely approximates results of open surgical excision of breast lesions.[38,39] The most widely used techniques for breast biopsy is percutaneous image guided core needle biopsy.[27] Core biopsy is advantageous in terms

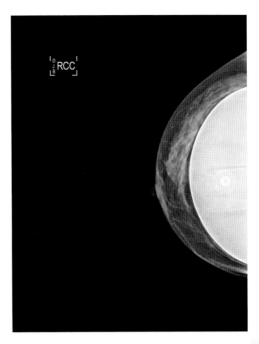

Fig. 10.4 This patient with a history of bilateral breast augmentation required an ultrasound guided core biopsy for suspicious microcalcifications. Pathology showed atypical ductal hyperplasia. Note the titanium marker clip position adjacent to the implant. An excisional breast biopsy was performed which confirmed atypical ductal hyperplasia but no evidence of malignancy. This resection did not enter the capsule of the implant, therefore, the patient was able to safely preserve her implant in this case. Needle biopsy and surgical procedures of the breast do post some risk of implant rupture as part of routine oncologic work-up of image detected or palpable breast abnormalities.

of minimal scar, decreased anatomic deformity permitting improved mammographic surveillance (minimal or no scarring on subsequent mammograms), decreased pain, and significantly decreased cost while diagnostic accuracy is maintained. The diagnosis of cancer is thus generally known preoperatively, facilitating appropriate planning and counseling about treatment options. Furthermore, diagnosis by core biopsy allows for proper surgical planning, including the possibility of a nodal evaluation procedure (if indicated) as well as appropriate planning for resection with adequate margins.

Image-guided core biopsy

Image-guided core biopsy is performed by either stereotactic *(Fig. 10.5)* or ultrasound guidance *(Fig. 10.6)*. Stereotactic biopsy is indicated when planning breast biopsy of lesions only visible mammographically (i.e., calcifications). Ultrasound guidance is increasingly being incorporated into surgical practice in the care of

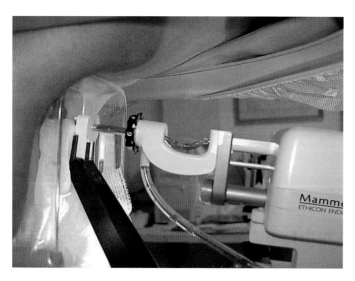

Fig. 10.5 Percutaneous vacuum assisted core needle biopsy allows for excellent accuracy in tissue diagnosis. This approach may be accomplished with stereotactic guidance (as shown here) or with ultrasound guidance. Multiple cores may be obtained via a single small incision with a single needle placement given that the device is equipped with a cutting needle and suction.

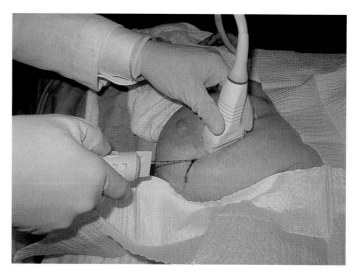

Fig. 10.6 Breast cancer is diagnosed by image guided percutaneous vacuum assisted core needle biopsy. Excisional biopsy should be used only rarely when needle biopsy is not possible technically or is discordant with clinical suspicion.

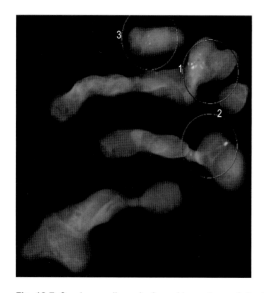

Fig. 10.7 Specimen radiograph of core biopsy demonstrates that the suspicious calcifications were appropriately sampled.

breast disease; it is indicated when planning breast biopsy of lesions well visualized sonographically. Ultrasonography provides excellent guidance for core biopsy, fine-needle aspiration, and drainage of cysts.

Fine-needle aspiration

Fine-needle aspiration (FNA) is performed under guidance by palpation, ultrasonography, or stereotactic

mammography. The examiner places a 20- to 23-gauge needle into the lesion. On aspiration with a syringe, material is sampled with multidirectional passes for cytopathologic examination. The cellular material is placed on slides for review by a cytopathologist. FNA typically does not provide enough tissue architecture for the diagnosis of invasive carcinoma to be made.[40] When atypia is found on FNA, 61% ultimately proves to actually be malignant disease.[41] Therefore, findings of atypia should result in surgical excision. The biggest pitfall to use of FNA is the problem of sampling error; false-negative rates of 2–22% have been reported in the literature.[42,43] FNA provides cytologic diagnoses that must be closely correlated with clinical and imaging findings to improve sensitivity of diagnosis (the so-called triple test of clinical, radiographic, and pathologic findings). In many centers, core needle biopsy has supplanted FNA as the diagnostic breast biopsy of choice due to high accuracy, accurate histopathology with prognostic markers while remaining minimally invasive.

Core needle biopsy

Core needle biopsy involves use of a biopsy device with an 8–14-gauge needle *(Fig. 10.7)*. The needle is positioned by either stereotactic or sonographic guidance *(Fig. 10.8)*.[38] Multiple passes are required to optimize

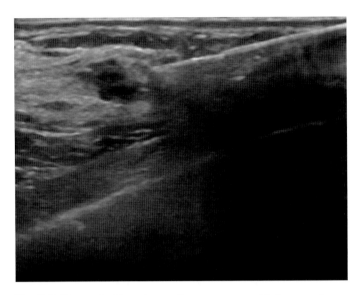

Fig. 10.8 Ultrasound guidance for percutaneous vacuum assisted core needle biopsy of a breast mass.

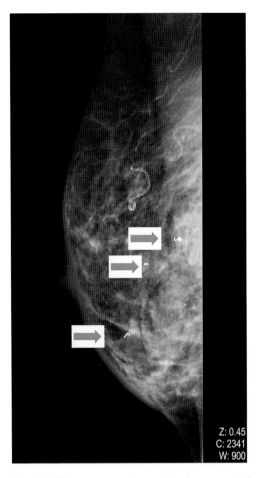

Z: 0.45
C: 2341
W: 900

Fig. 10.9 This mammogram demonstrates three separate sites of tissue marker clip placement after core needle biopsy. Clip placement helps to identify the position of the lesion(s) within the breast. In this case, the patient had multicentric breast cancer. The extent of disease is factored into decision-making for total mastectomy versus segmental mastectomy, as well as treatment decision-making such as neoadjuvant therapy versus a surgery first approach.

sensitivity and to determine histologic grade with accuracy.[44] Often, modern core biopsy devices use vacuum to aspirate tissue into a chamber, where it is sampled. With suction assistance, high-speed oscillating knives pull a cylinder of tissue into a chamber outside the breast. The advantage of these techniques is that multiple passes are accomplished by rotating the needle sequentially rather than by reinsertion; thus, only one needle stick is required. Accuracy of the vacuum-assisted breast biopsy approaches 100%.[38,45] Core biopsy specimen provides enough tissue to analyze estrogen receptor status and the presence of the HER-2/neu oncoprotein, neither of which is normally ascertainable by an FNA specimen. A titanium tissue marker clip is inserted to mark the site of the core needle biopsy; multiple types of clips exist to help demarcate biopsies of different lesions *(Fig. 10.9)*.

Excisional biopsy

With the increasing use of percutaneous image-guided biopsy, indications for excisional biopsy have evolved to include disagreement between the mammographic or clinical impression and histologic findings of percutaneous biopsy; atypical ductal hyperplasia on percutaneous biopsy[46,47]; and radial scar on mammography or percutaneous biopsy.[48] When percutaneous biopsy is nondiagnostic for nonpalpable radiographic lesions,

a needle-localized breast biopsy is recommended. It is important to emphasize that clinical judgment must determine decision-making whether or not to excise radiographically occult breast masses based on clinical grounds. A nonsuspicious fibroadenoma of the breast diagnosed by ultrasound or core biopsy may be observed with serial follow-up; reasons to consider excisional biopsy for a fibroadenomas include patient preference, suspicion of phyllodes tumor, or a growing or painful lesion.

Patient selection

A breast cancer patient's decision making regarding choice of breast surgical procedure is influenced by numerous factors, including ratio of breast size to tumor burden, stage, multicentricity of disease, family history, age, availability of radiation therapy, personal preferences, and biases by her providers. The multi-disciplinary team caring for breast cancer patients includes breast surgical oncologists, medical oncologists, radiation oncologists, radiologists, pathologists, nuclear medicine specialists and plastic surgeons – each with their own meaningful role in the management of breast cancer. Decision making regarding indications for adjuvant chemotherapy and radiation therapy is an important topic but beyond the scope of this chapter; a detailed summary of standard of care evidence based algorithms may be found published in the NCCN guidelines.[8] Patients diagnosed initially with clinically Stage III breast cancers are evaluated with a staging work-up to rule out metastasis prior to initiating systemic therapy or surgical resection *(Fig. 10.10)*. Clinicians and patients may consider neoadjuvant or preoperative systemic therapy (chemotherapy or endocrine therapy) to reduce the tumor burden such that a lumpectomy may be feasible. A neoadjuvant approach also permits determining if a patient responded to the chosen therapy, which provides valuable prognostic information (examples of locally advanced and inflammatory breast cancers are shown in *Figures 10.11–10.14*). In general, there is no survival advantage for a neoadjuvant approach versus surgery first, unless the patient has a pathologic complete response which implies a more favorable prognosis.[49]

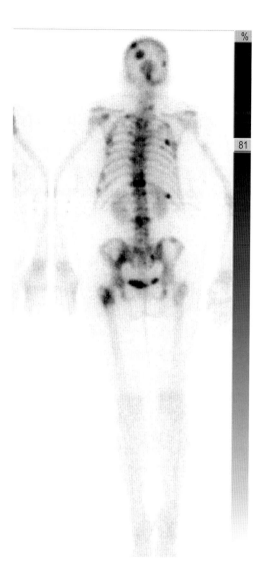

Fig. 10.10 Patients presenting with locally advanced breast cancer require a staging work-up to rule out metastatic disease. This bone scan demonstrates diffuse osseous metastasis in a patient presenting with pathologic fractures of the thoracic and lumbar spine. This patient will require systemic therapy and radiation therapy for her Stage IV disease.

Treatment/surgical technique

Breast conserving surgery

The management of early-stage breast cancer with a partial mastectomy – lumpectomy, quandrantectomy, or segmentectomy – followed by adjuvant radiation therapy is collectively termed "breast conserving therapy" or "breast conserving surgery." This approach is appealing to a number of women. Segmental mastectomy, along with radiation, has been shown to be roughly equivalent to mastectomy in long-term survival in a number of prospective trials. These randomized studies with follow-up periods from 6 to 13 years found no difference in overall or distant disease-free survival between lumpectomy versus mastectomy.[50–52] In the landmark National Surgical Adjuvant Breast/Bowel Project (NSABP) B-06 trial, local recurrence rates for lumpectomy with adjuvant therapy were 14.3%; with lumpectomy without radiation therapy local recurrence rates were 39.2%. Accordingly, these data punctuate the need for adjuvant radiation for successful treatment with partial mastectomy in the majority of patients.[52] The NSABP results may be limited by the definition of margins used in the study. In this report,

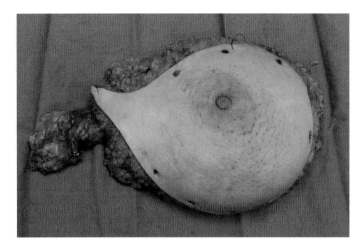

Fig. 10.11 This inflammatory breast cancer patient has obvious residual disease after a lengthy course of neoadjuvant chemotherapy. At the time of her modified radical mastectomy, numerous skin biopsies were taken in an attempt to achieve negative margins. Neither skin sparing nor breast reconstruction would be appropriate for inflammatory breast cancer patients. She will require comprehensive radiation therapy as well.

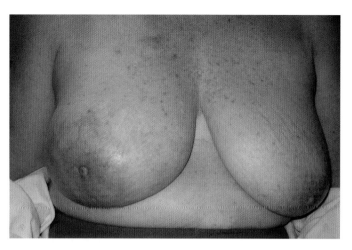

Fig. 10.12 Patients with inflammatory breast cancer (IBC) require an aggressive multimodal approach for these Stage III cancers. Treatment begins with systemic therapy first, followed by modified radical mastectomy and comprehensive radiation therapy if the patient is a candidate. IBC patients are not candidates for immediate breast reconstruction. The 5-year survival for this disease is only 40%, therefore the focus must be on completion of all necessary oncologic treatments.

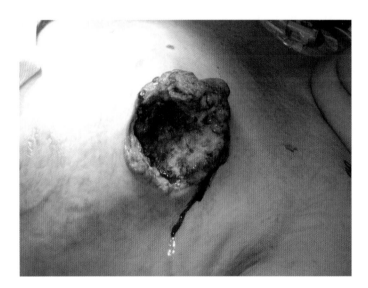

Fig. 10.13 This patient with a locally advanced breast cancer presents with an ulcerating, necrotic tumor wound. Often wound care is required such that patients presenting with these findings may begin systemic therapy prior to definitive surgical intervention.

negative margins were defined as "no tumor on ink," while most surgeons prefer a wider free margin (typically ≥0.2 cm). As several of the studies suggesting a higher recurrence rate with breast conserving approaches did not have well-established negative margin criteria, some of the early reports of higher local-regional recurrence with breast conserving therapies are subject to interpretation.

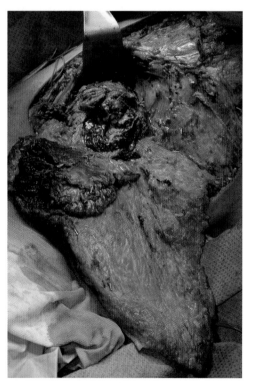

Fig. 10.14 This patient had a poorly-differentiated breast cancer originating in the axillary tail. Her tumor did not respond to neoadjuvant chemotherapy. This locally advanced tumor was adherent to the axillary vein; it involved the breast and axillary nodal basins Levels I–III. A radical mastectomy was performed with negative margins. She received a pedicled latissimus flap to reconstruct the soft tissue defect and permit closure. She went on to receive comprehensive radiation therapy.

Breast cancer recurrence is complex and multifactorial. Factors that contribute to recurrence after breast conserving therapy, such as young age, no systemic therapy, aggressive disease, etc., also predispose the patient to recurrence after mastectomy. Recurrence relates not only to the operative technique, but also to intrinsic tumor characteristics as well as adjuvant and the neoadjuvant therapies utilized. Modern local recurrence rates may be inferred from the Early Breast Cancer Trialists' Collaborative Group overview which found 5-year local recurrence rates of 7% for lumpectomy with radiotherapy compared with 26% for lumpectomy without radiotherapy.[53] This large overview of 78 prospective randomized trials of early breast cancer found that if four breast cancer recurrences could be prevented, one breast cancer related death would be averted.[53]

The oncologic limitation of breast conserving approaches has historically been largely related to concerns that this approach might carry a higher risk of recurrence than a mastectomy for an equivalent disease. The Early Breast Cancer Trial's Collaborative Group demonstrated quite convincingly that avoiding local recurrence translates into a survival advantage and that breast conserving therapy – when properly carried out – is essentially oncologically equivalent to a mastectomy for appropriately selected patients. The increased utilization of segmental mastectomy in lieu of total mastectomy reflects the oncologic parity of the technique in terms of treatment as well as a number of advances in complimentary disciplines, such as imaging and systemic treatment. There has been improved screening with increased early detection, as well as more aggressive use of adjuvant chemotherapy and endocrine therapy lowering the risk of ipsilateral breast disease. Neoadjuvant chemotherapy, with tumor downsizing of those initially considered too large to be treated with a conserving approach, has rendered some of these larger tumors amendable to treatment with partial mastectomy. Additionally, there have been advances in approaches to segmental mastectomy.

Technique

The diagnosis is confirmed by a core biopsy preoperatively, and the patient is re-examined before the operation is commences. The lesion is marked while the patient is awake to facilitate location of the tumor in the operating room. If the lesion is not palpable then wire localization or ultrasound may be used to identify the location of the lesion or biopsy clip. Incision selection is demonstrated in **Figure 10.15**.

After the incision is made, tissue forceps are used to grasp the skin and electrocautery is used to dissect circumferentially around the tumor including a margin of grossly normal tissue. The dissection may continue to the pectoralis fascia for the deep margin, but for small, superficial tumors, this depth of resection may not be necessary. If the tumor is near the skin, an ellipse of skin should be resected to ensure negative margins. The tumor is oriented with marking sutures. The resection specimen is sent for an *ex vivo* radiograph to ascertain whether the calcifications in question were removed. Breast conserving surgery carries with in an inherent risk of close or positive margins microscopically on permanent section histopathology (range 9–32%).[54-57]

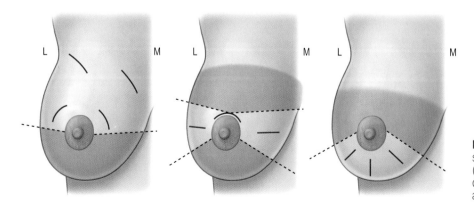

Fig. 10.15 Most of the time, curvilinear incisions are selected for lumpectomy, however, in the keyhole area (6-o'clock) linear incisions work well. For upper outer quadrant tumors a radially oriented incision may provide a better resulting contour after resection.

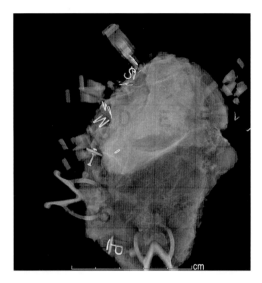

Fig. 10.16 The breast surgeon obtains a specimen radiograph of the lumpectomy specimen to ensure that the target was removed and assess margins radiographically. Note the titanium tissue marker clip from the patient's diagnostic core biopsy. Radio-opaque orientation clips may be used for specimen radiography.

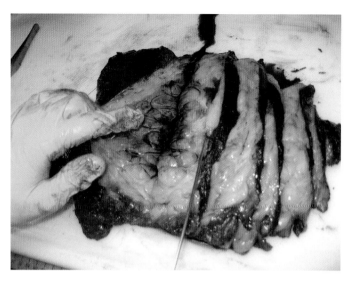

Fig. 10.17 Breast specimens are oriented by the breast surgeon such that the pathologist can assess margin status. Many centers perform intraoperative assessment of resection specimens to avoid a second operation for re-excision for margin control.

Meticulous intraoperative margin assessment must be followed to ensure the best possible outcome in breast conserving procedures. Intraoperative processing of the partial mastectomy is extremely important; needle localization with radiographs *(Fig. 10.16)* and stepwise sectioning *(Fig. 10.17)* have been utilized to decrease the rate of positive margins. This necessitates a team of radiologists and pathologists to ensure that the safest minimal volume of tissue adjacent the tumor is resected – thus enhancing the aesthetic outcome – while optimizing the likelihood that adequate and accurate margins are obtained. While the extensive intraoperative process is time consuming, it can significantly decrease the need for re-excision to achieve negative margins and enhance the aesthetic results.[58] If there is any concern about margins based on surgical, radiographic or pathology input, the lumpectomy cavity is re-excised prior to closure. These re-excision specimens are sent separately from the main specimen for pathologic evaluation. If there are questions regarding margin status, it may be best to delay the plans for reconstruction in conjunction with the conserving surgery to avoid any transposition of local tissues that might confound re-excision.

Oncoplastic surgery

The term Oncoplastic Surgery was introduced in 1993 by Audretsch *et al.*,[59] reflecting techniques of tumor extirpation that might avert aesthetic deformities of the breast resulting from conservation therapy. These techniques draw from a number of principles inherent to plastic surgery procedures on the breast such as breast reduction or mastopexy. Balancing the oncologic and aesthetic imperative has been a growing trend in breast conservation, permitting greater application of the technique. The approaches for oncoplastic surgery range from more favorable scar orientation and/or placement to significant soft tissue rearrangement that may necessitate elective changes to the contralateral normal breast.

Deformities resulting from breast conservation are generally fairly easy to predict *(Figs 10.18, 10.19)*. The location of the tumor, the size of the breast, and the size and orientation of the necessary skin and parenchymal excisions are the most important variables in predicting a postoperative need for reconstruction with a breast conserving approach. With a central segmentectomy, the contour of the breast is preserved but the nipple areolar complex may require reconstruction *(Fig. 10.20)*.

In a smaller volume resection, the orientation of skin incisions can have a significant impact on the aesthetic outcome. From an oncologic perspective, skin incisions should be located directly over the tumor. Periareolar incisions are generally the most favorable as they may be camouflaged by the adjacent areola. Curvilinear

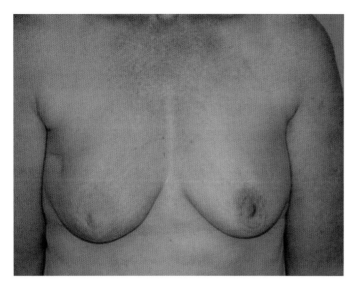

Fig. 10.18 A contour deformity is present in this breast conserving therapy patient, who desired partial breast reconstruction.

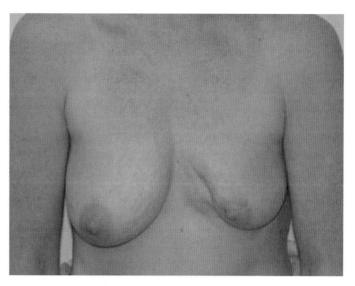

Fig. 10.19 A marked deformity after lumpectomy may be present, rarely. This patient would clearly be a candidate for partial breast reconstruction. A critical aspect is location of the defect. Note that the lateral defect seen in *Fig 10.18* is a similar size but not so deforming. The medial defects are hard to fix, particularly in small breasts, by partial mastectomy. They may require a flap or be better served with a total mastectomy and reconstruction on an aesthetic basis.

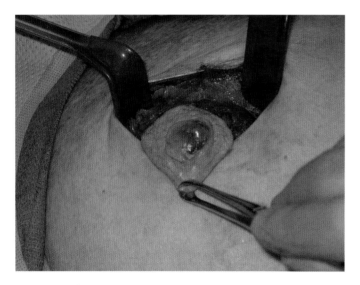

Fig. 10.20 This patient presented with Paget's disease of the nipple. She was found to have ductal carcinoma *in situ* just posterior to the nipple areolar complex. A central segmentectomy achieved negative margins. She required adjuvant radiation therapy.

excision in this region commonly results in the compromising of breast contour and nipple projection and position. Radial incisions such as those used in reduction mammoplasty balance the tissue loss of parenchyma and skin; therefore providing tissue to support the contour of the breast mound and/or nipple-areolar complex and resulting in significantly improved breast aesthetics if there is a significant amount of tissue removed during tumor resection.

Balancing the resection with breast landmarks and shape to preserve breast aesthetics are the fundamentals of oncoplastic surgery.[60] Averting deformity has become an important tenet of modern breast surgery. The timing and approach to reconstruction associated with the breast conserving technique is highly topical and controversial. While the relative merits of specific surgical techniques vary from surgeon to surgeon and across the disciplines of plastic surgeons and oncologic surgeons, there is agreement that breast conservation without consideration of the potential aesthetic sequelae can and will result in deformity and unhappy patients. Surgical cure alone may fall short of anticipated outcomes for many in our patient population. It is estimated that, at minimum, 20–35% of patients treated with a breast conserving approach have unfavorable aesthetic outcomes.

incisions can help to minimize deformity by increasing the surface area limiting the contraction seen in a linear scar over a round structure like the breast. These caveats hold true provided there is not a large accompanying volumetric or skin resection which will most often cause a problematic distortion of breast shape and/or nipple areolar position. Tumors located in the inferior portion of the breast are notoriously prone to deformity. Simple

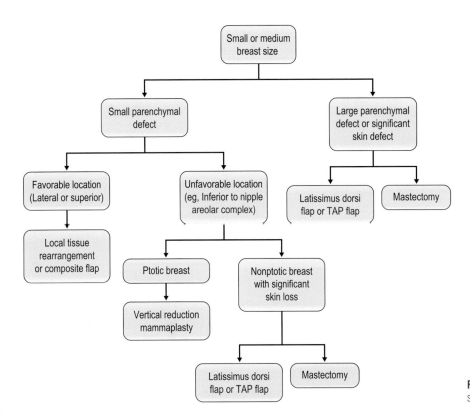

Fig. 10.21 An algorithm for partial breast reconstruction in small or medium-breasted patients is proposed.

While many patients accept these results, a significant portion of these patients are dissatisfied enough to seek corrective surgery. Unfortunately, repairing breast conserving deformities after radiation therapy is far from a straightforward endeavor. The effects of radiotherapy figure heavily into the complexity of an adequate repair. While patients might prefer a simple approach, local tissue rearrangement is generally obviated by the effects of radiotherapy, and use of breast implants often carries prohibitively high rates of fibrous capsule contraction and scarring. Adequate repair of these defects must take into consideration the volume and location of the defect. Correction of established deformities after conservation and radiation necessitate flap reconstruction. These procedures carry attendant donor site scarring and morbidity. Complications are common. This is often not well received by a patient who initially sought a minimally invasive approach. These factors may help to explain why delayed repair of these defects is generally accompanied by poor satisfaction rates of approximately 20–40%. The difficulties of delayed repair underscore the imperative to anticipate and prevent unfavorable results with breast conservation therapy.[61]

The most common causes of an unfavorable result in breast conserving approaches include removal of a large amount of breast parenchyma in a small volume breast, and/or excision in an unfavorable location. A general guideline is that removing 15–20% of breast parenchyma in a small volume A- or B-cup or 30% in a larger breast is going to be accompanied by distortion (*Figs 10.21, 10.22*). Limiting the volume of tissue to be resected appears to greatly improve the result after conserving therapy. Accordingly, patients with larger primary tumors may benefit from neoadjuvant therapy to shrink the tumor and hence the resection. In patients with tumors that are initially too large to allow conserving approaches, neoadjuvant chemotherapy may make breast conservation possible.[62] Careful intraoperative margins analysis can help minimize the volume of the resection. Resection of an aesthetically sensitive area such as a medial superior or medial inferior defect is far less acceptable to a patient than a lateral defect. An excision such as that results in adherence of the underlying pectoralis muscle or fascia will create a severe deformity. Nipple areolar malposition, no matter what the location will prompt patient complaints.

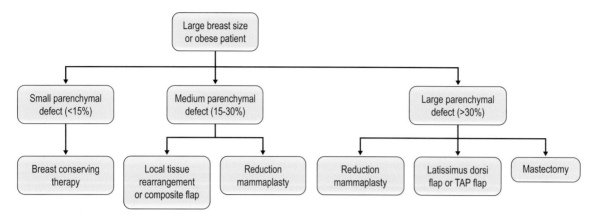

Fig. 10.22 An algorithm for partial breast reconstruction in obese or large breasted patients is proposed.

If breast conservation may be anticipated to result in significant deformity and/or may necessitate a great deal of local tissue rearrangement – including reduction of the contralateral breast – when, on purely aesthetic grounds, should surgeons recommend mastectomy and reconstruction? Several studies compared the outcomes of breast conservation with those of total mastectomy and reconstruction in terms of quality of life, decision making analysis, cost, and aesthetics, yielding conflicting results.[63–70] The appeal of sparing the majority of the breast is attractive to a number of patients and surgeons, if breast conserving therapy is appropriate from an oncologic standpoint. Once oncologic parity is established, then how do we best maximize the surgical outcome of a partial mastectomy versus a total mastectomy?

While there have been a number of studies attempting to establish the superiority of one approach over another in terms of aesthetic outcome, quality of life and patient satisfaction, not surprisingly, consensus has not been achieved, due to the subjective and personal nature of this decision making. As breast conserving approaches preserve the breast mound, skin and nipple areola complex, the conserving approach is believed to have a psychological advantage over a mastectomy. Proponents of mastectomy note that this approach most often avoids the need for, and downsides of, adjuvant radiotherapy. The potential for donor site morbidity with scarring and functional loss inherent to autologous approaches, or the implant related complications such as fibrous capsule contracture, infection, extrusion and device failure associated with

implant-based approaches must all be considered. Proponents of skin-sparing mastectomy with reconstruction suggest that the excellent results that can be achieved with autologous free tissue transfer and the longitudinal reliability of this approach are convincing. Implant-based reconstruction after mastectomy has been endorsed by a number of patients who wish to minimize donor site deformity. Satisfaction studies evaluating outcomes have generally suggested that there is a complex interplay of variables including the patient's age, education, fear of cancer, and pre-morbid psychological status that contribute to the patient's quality of life and satisfaction after breast surgery. Although patients' decisions are often motivated by a number of factors, including breast preservation, cosmetic results, operative morbidity and treatment duration as well as convenience, patients are generally more satisfied if they feel that they have had input in the decision-making process and received the treatment approach they initially desired.[63–67]

Mastectomy: terminology and techniques

The mastectomy procedure has evolved from the Halsted radical mastectomy, a procedure that involved a wide excision of all breast tissue, all overlying skin, and the pectoralis major muscle including a full en bloc dissection of Level I, II, and III nodes. Because of the increased morbidity incurred without any demonstrated benefit in terms of local recurrence or survival, radical mastectomies are rarely performed today.[71] However, rarely there are situations in which a tumor may invade through the chest wall and surgical resection may be appropriate; plastic surgeons may be consulted for reconstruction of these chest wall defects, on rare occasions *(Figs 10.23, 10.24)*. Several types of mastectomy procedures are available to the breast surgeon.

Total mastectomy

The most commonly performed mastectomy is the total mastectomy, which removes all breast tissue including the nipple-areola complex (NAC) and an ellipse of skin adjacent to the nipple-areola complex *(Figs 10.25, 10.26)*.

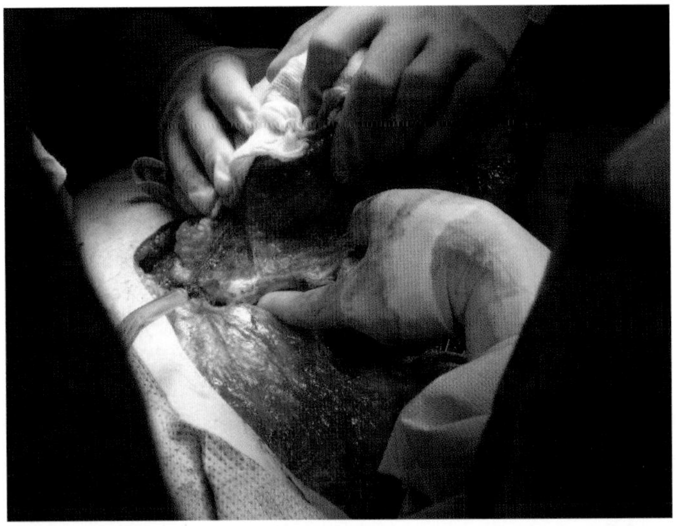

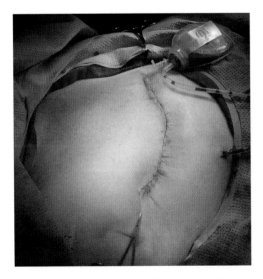

Fig. 10.23 Extended radical mastectomy for tumor invading through chest wall. This patient had a post-radiation sarcoma in the field of her chest wall after being treated for breast cancer 5 years prior. Her sarcoma did not respond to neoadjuvant therapy, therefore an aggressive surgical approach was required. She had a pedicled TRAM reconstruction of this soft tissue defect.

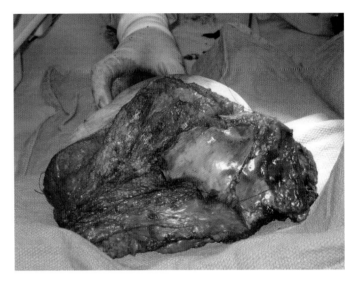

Fig. 10.24 Specimen for extended radical mastectomy. Note that *en bloc* resection of two ribs was required.

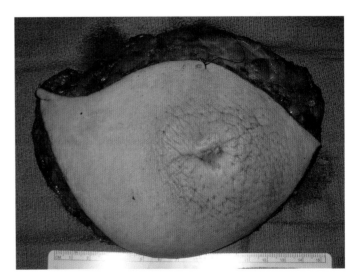

Fig. 10.25 A total mastectomy with no reconstruction for a patient with T3N0 infiltrating ductal carcinoma of the breast. She required adjuvant chemotherapy and radiation therapy. The patient will be able to wear a breast prosthetic if she chooses. She may be offered delayed breast reconstruction 6–12 months after completion of radiation therapy.

Fig. 10.26 A total mastectomy was performed for a bulky breast carcinoma. Primary closure was possible with this T3 lesion in this case, however, surgical oncologists treating locally advanced cancers such as this often consult plastic surgeons for reconstruction of complex post-mastectomy defects.

A total mastectomy is bordered by the clavicle superiorly, sternum medially, anterior axillary line laterally, and inframammary crease inferiorly; the breast is resected en bloc with the pectoralis major fascia posteriorly. A skin-sparing total mastectomy resects all breast tissue through a circumareolar incision including resection of the nipple but preserving the skin envelope, thus facilitating immediate reconstruction. A nipple sparing total mastectomy is a modification of the skin sparing mastectomy that preserves the NAC.

Breast tissue is distributed widely over the anterolateral chest and axilla. Haagensen noted that breast parenchyma protrudes into the underlying pectoral muscles, extends along Cooper ligaments to the skin, may cross the midline, and laterally may reach the apex of the axilla.[72] Temple *et al.* showed that breast tissue extends high into the axilla and is adherent to the pectoralis fascia.[73] It is thus doubtful that any type of mastectomy can completely resect all breast tissue. A total mastectomy removes about 90–95% of the breast tissue.[74]

Skin-sparing mastectomy

Video 1

For women who will require mastectomy as the surgical management of their breast cancer, skin-sparing mastectomy with immediate reconstruction is an excellent choice for complete breast parenchyma resection and acceptable breast mound provided by an implant or flap. This procedure preserves as much of the patient's breast skin as possible – the breast parenchyma, nipple-areola contents are removed through a circumareolar incision (sentinel lymph node dissection may be performed through a separate incision if indicated). By preserving the inframammary fold and native skin envelope, the plastic surgeon can reconstruct a breast that is an excellent match to the contralateral breast in size, color, and shape *(Figs 10.27, 10.28) (Fig. 10.29).*[75] Skin sparing mastectomy has been shown to have equivalent local recurrence rates as conventional mastectomy, given the selection bias of reserving this approach for patients without clinical evidence of locally advanced or inflammatory breast cancer.[76–79] FIG **10.29** APPEARS ONLINE ONLY

The surgical team of general and plastic surgeons mark the skin preoperatively. If the tumor is superficial, the incision is carefully planned to remove any breast skin required to obtain a negative margin (particularly any tumor within 1 cm of breast skin) – this point is imperative. If the tumor is deep within the breast, no additional skin is resected. By use of electrocautery or sharp dissection, the skin flap is elevated circumareolarly with the assistance of skin hooks for skin retraction. The flaps are dissected at a uniform thickness at the junction of the breast parenchyma and subcutaneous adipose tissue and the breast is resected en bloc off the pectoralis major muscle, inclusive of its fascia.

Nipple sparing mastectomy

Nipple sparing mastectomy involves a total mastectomy via a noncentral incision, such as an incision lateral to the areola *(Fig. 10.30)*. Crowe et al. published one of the first modern series with this technique, reporting the technical feasibility of nipple sparing mastectomy.[80] However, concern for somewhat higher than expected local recurrence rates, lack of sensation to the nipple, and issues with nipple necrosis and resultant implant loss were problematic issues.[80] Brachtel *et al.* published an important series noting occult nipple involvement in 36% of those with tumors >2 cm and 30% of women with one to three positive nodes.[81] Factors independently associated with nipple involvement were the size of the primary cancer, the distance between the tumor and the nipple, and amplification of *HER2.*[81] Another concern was that the sensitivity of detecting nipple involvement by histological testing of a single *en face* frozen section of the subareolar tissue was found to be only 80% when malignancy was actually present.[81] For this reason, many surgical oncologists prefer to reserve nipple sparing mastectomies for prophylactic mastectomies and perhaps highly selected early stage patients with tumors remote from the nipple areolar complex.

A subcutaneous mastectomy involves the use of a noncentral incision (such as an inframammary or axillary approach) to perform a mastectomy *(Fig. 10.31)*, thereby preserving the skin, skin envelope, and cutaneous portion of the nipple-areola complex. Subcutaneous mastectomy implies somewhat thicker mastectomy flaps than a modern nipple sparing mastectomy and is not a preferred operation by breast surgical oncologists due to concerns regarding retained breast tissue.

The use of a nipple-sparing mastectomy in terms of aesthetic outcome appears to hold significant promise

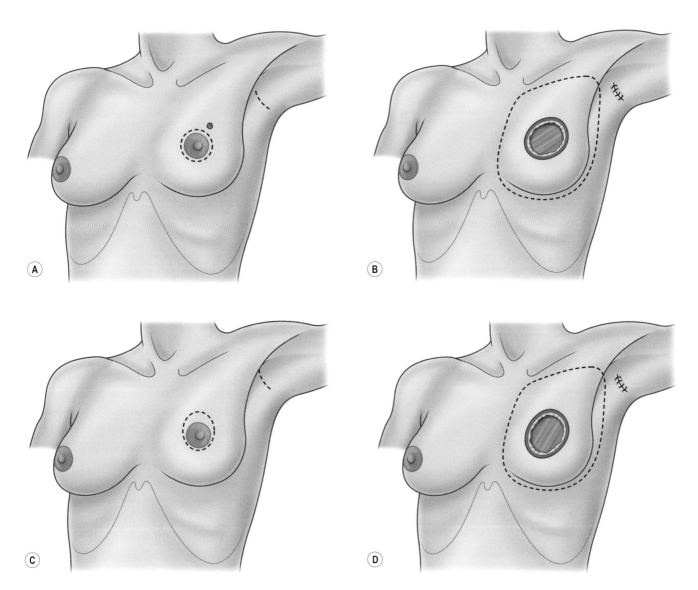

Fig. 10.27 A skin sparing total mastectomy is performed via a periareolar incision, permitting preservation of the skin envelope while the nipple areolar complex is resected along with the breast parenchyma. This approach is typically selected when planning to perform immediate breast reconstruction.

when the outcome is favorable, yet is technically more complex for both the breast surgical oncologist and the reconstructive surgeon. On a technical level, successful preservation of the nipple requires meticulous technique. The presence of the nipple and a remote incision to preserve breast aesthetics, such as an inframammary approach, may somewhat complicate the access to recipient vessels for microsurgery. Several approaches are available, however, generally either a laterally based incision, originating at the areolar verge

or an inframammary approach is most common. The advantage of nipple sparing procedures is most evident in implant-based reconstructions as the point of maximal projection of the breast is best preserved. In general we advocate the use of a two-stage procedure as the nipple may be significantly challenged for a period of time and nipple loss is possible. Patient selection is critical; very large and/or ptotic breasts are not likely to have a good result with this approach. Nipple-sparing mastectomies must undergo prudent oncologic criteria to sample the

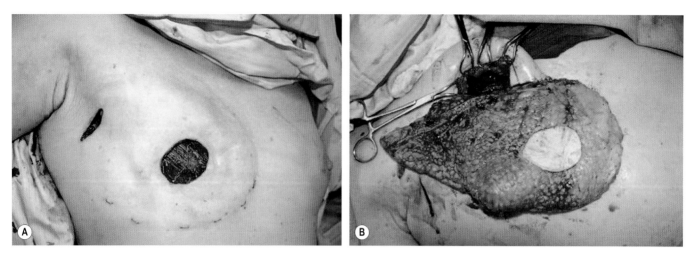

Fig. 10.28 Skin sparing mastectomy via periareolar incision. Skin sparing mastectomy is an excellent choice for a breast cancer patient requiring or opting for mastectomy who is a candidate for immediate reconstruction.

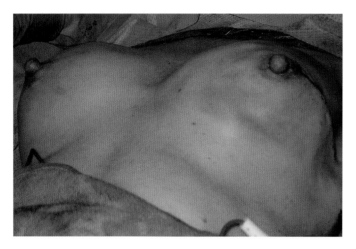

Fig. 10.30 This patient was a carrier of a deleterious BRCA2 mutation. She underwent a prophylactic, risk reducing nipple sparing mastectomy with implant based reconstruction.

nipple and careful informed consent. We advise the patient that the nipple may be lost or removed at the time of the mastectomy due to oncologic reasons, or noted vascular compromise in the peri- or postoperative period due to vascular compromise, or during a secondary procedure if the nipple position or quality appears to be inadequate.

Prophylactic mastectomy

The most common indications for prophylactic mastectomy include women with a known genetic predisposition for breast cancer and those with a unilateral breast cancer desiring contralateral prophylactic mastectomy. The Society of Surgical Oncology established a position statement describing indications for consideration of prophylactic mastectomy.[82] Prophylactic mastectomy itself has no descriptive value regarding the skin envelope and may imply total, skin sparing or nipple sparing mastectomy. In the absence of a deleterious BRCA mutation, the expected incidence of contralateral primary breast cancers is about 0.7% per year of life.[83] Plastic surgeons may be consulted to consider reconstructions in patients requesting contralateral prophylactic mastectomy; therefore, it is important to consider issues of oncologic risk as well as symmetry.

As advances in genetic testing have made it possible to identify patients with a genetic predisposition to breast cancer (most commonly *BRCA1* or *BRCA2*), more patients are now undergoing these tests and seeking recommendations from clinicians concerning the preventive measures available. Breast oncologists, general surgeons, and plastic surgeons will increasingly be asked about the data supporting prophylactic mastectomy. Some 5–10% of breast cancer results from an inheritable genetic mutation. Patients with *BRCA1* or *BRCA2* mutations have a 60–80% lifetime risk for breast cancer and elevated risk of other cancers as well (ovarian, primary peritoneal, colorectal, pancreatic, skin, and prostate cancer in men); these patients may have up to a 30% risk of a contralateral breast malignancy after their first breast cancer.[2] Age at diagnosis of a BRCA mutation should be factored into decision-making.[84]

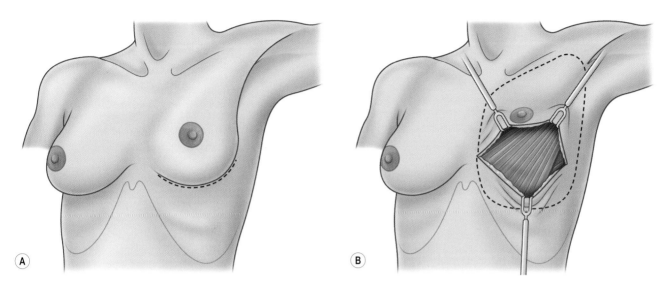

Fig. 10.31 Subcutaneous mastectomies incorporate a noncentral incision, typically in the inframammary crease. This type of mastectomy is not considered oncologically sound given the propensity for thick mastectomy flaps.

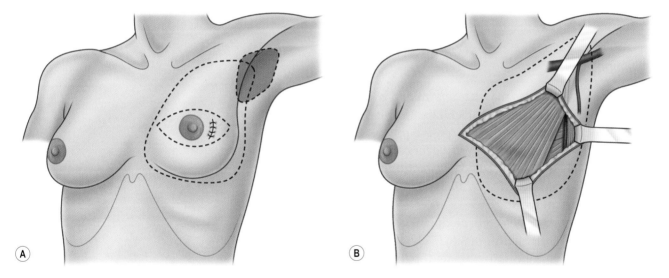

Fig. 10.32 Modified radical mastectomy – total mastectomy with axillary lymph node dissection. The incision may be oriented transversely or obliquely.

Modified radical mastectomy

Modified radical mastectomy removes the breast tissue, the nipple-areola complex, and the Level I–II axillary lymph nodes *en bloc* **(Fig. 10.32)**. The incision is marked as an ellipse to include the nipple-areola complex, any previous biopsy site, and any excess breast skin. Care should be taken to avoid extension of the incision medial to the sternum or lateral to the breast mound because this will produce dog-ears.[85]

Skin edges are elevated with skin hooks while skin flaps are dissected with electrocautery. *En bloc* axillary dissection is performed as part of modified radical mastectomy. The wound is irrigated, and hemostasis is carefully obtained. Closed suction drains are placed and brought out through separate incisions. If no immediate reconstruction is planned, deep dermal sutures are placed to re-approximate the wound followed by a running subcuticular absorbable suture.

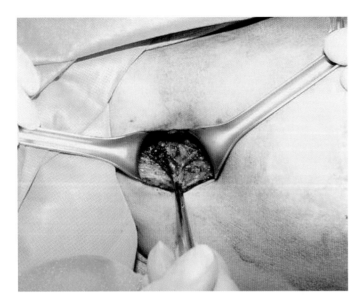

Fig. 10.33 Sentinel lymph node biopsy (SLNB) may be accomplished using Technetium 99 sulfur colloid as radioisotope, with or without a vital blue dye, as shown here. SLNB is 95% as accurate as a complete axillary node dissection but has far less morbidity.

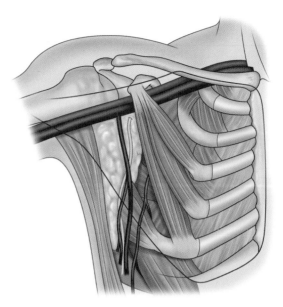

Fig. 10.34 Levels of axillary dissection. An axillary node dissection for breast cancer typically includes removal of the Level I and II lymph nodes. The axilla is defined by the axillary vein superiorly, the latissimus dorsi laterally, the serratus anterior medially and the subscapularis muscle posteriorly. Care is taken to preserve the thoracodorsal and long thoracic nerves along their course.

Nodal evaluation

The status of the axillary nodes may be determined by a sentinel lymph node dissection *(Fig. 10.33)* that is performed at the same operation as the extirpative procedure; or if the nodes were found to be positive for cancer pre- or intraoperatively, an axillary node dissection of Levels I and II may be performed *(Fig. 10.34)*. Level III dissections are rarely required for breast cancer – only if palpable gross disease is detected at operation. A recent clinical trial is potentially practice changing in regards to whether lumpectomy treated patients planned for adjuvant radiation who have 1–2 positive lymph nodes require a completion axillary lymph node dissection or not as no advantage in local recurrence was demonstrated in patients randomized to completion axillary dissection after sentinel node.[86]

Outcomes, prognosis, complications

Breast cancer patients are staged via the American Joint Committee on Cancer (AJCC) staging manual which incorporates the TNM (tumor, nodes, and metastasis) status of each patient. The AJCC Staging Manual is updated periodically (the 7th edition was recently

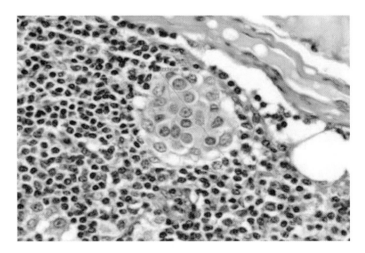

Fig. 10.35 A subcapsular micrometastasis is found on routine H&E analysis of this sentinel node. This would be staged as N1mic, however, clearly a low burden of nodal disease is present. Decision making regarding the need for axillary lymph node dissection would depend on several factors, including number of nodes positive, co-morbidities, use of breast conserving surgery with external beam radiation versus mastectomy, intended adjuvant treatment plan, use of neoadjuvant therapy and patient preferences. The trend in management of minimal nodal burden is towards axillary conserving therapy.

published, in 2010).[87] Notably, the staging for breast cancer currently records minimal amounts of nodal disease on sentinel node biopsy, such as micrometastases (N1mic, 0.2–2 mm) *(Fig. 10.35)* or isolated tumor cell deposits (N0(i+), <0.2 mm) *(Fig. 10.36)*. Recommendations for adjuvant systemic therapy (cytotoxic chemotherapy and or endocrine therapy) and adjuvant radiation therapy *(Fig. 10.37)* are made based on the National Comprehensive Cancer Network (NCCN) guidelines.[8]

Breast reconstruction after mastectomy

Immediate reconstruction

A mastectomy for early stage breast cancer generally obviates the need for radiation therapy and its untoward sequelae. The magnitude of the surgery for a total mastectomy as opposed to a partial mastectomy is generally greater. Critically evaluating the pros and cons of various approaches with the patient and guiding her through this decision-making process, while incorporating primarily oncologic, but also aesthetic and quality of life concerns, is critical to the best possible outcome. Coupling a skin-sparing mastectomy with autologous free-tissue transfer techniques has demonstrated extraordinary outcomes that are reliable and stable over time. Autologous techniques have evolved from pedicled flap based reconstruction *(Figs 10.38, 10.39)* to a perforator type approach *(Fig. 10.40)* in which underlying muscle is spared in an effort to decrease the morbidity of the donor site; perforator flaps represent a major advance in breast reconstruction given their greatly enhanced donor site. ⊚ FIG **10.38** APPEARS ONLINE ONLY

Lower abdominal free flap territories are most commonly used due to the anatomic versatility of the region, the ability to hide the donor site under clothes, and the

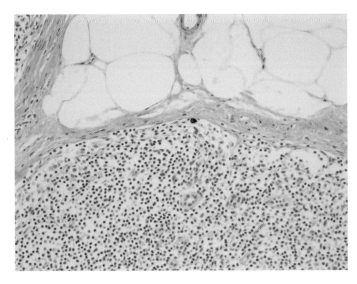

Fig. 10.36 A single isolated tumor cell is found by immunohistochemistry for cytokeratins in this sentinel node. This would be staged as N0(i+). Axillary lymph node dissection would not be recommended following this result.

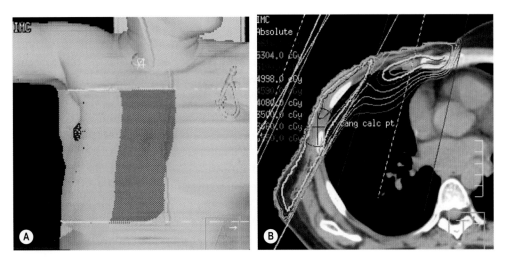

Fig. 10.37 Comprehensive post-mastectomy radiation is required for improved locoregional control in certain locally advanced breast cancers. Patients likely to require post-mastectomy radiation generally are better candidates for delayed breast reconstruction as immediate breast reconstruction risks postoperative complications which would delay appropriate oncologic care. Patients who received post-mastectomy radiation are excellent candidates for flap-based reconstructive strategies.

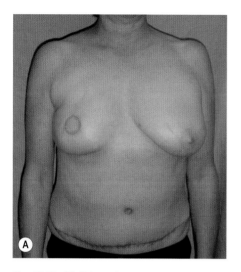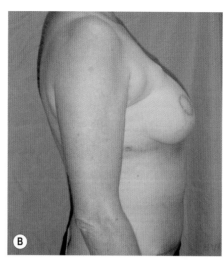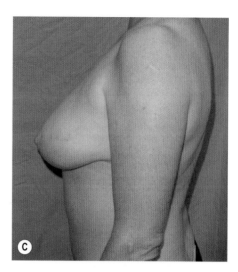

Fig. 10.39 **(A)** Skin sparing mastectomy with pedicled TRAM reconstruction. **(B)** Profile of skin sparing mastectomy with TRAM. **(C)** Profile of unaffected breast.

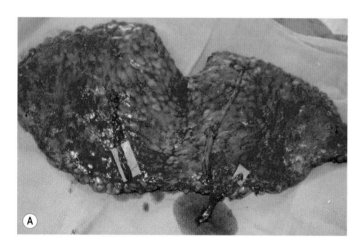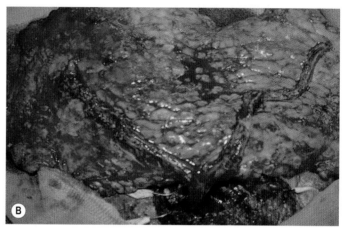

Fig. 10.40 An example of a "supercharged", two pedicled deep inferior epigastric perforator flap is shown. Microvascular anastomosis is required, generally to the internal mammary recipient vessels.

quality and character of the soft tissue and fat that is quite favorable to the requirements of a breast reconstruction. Alternate donor sites such as the gluteal and gracilis territories have undergone a recent resurgence of popularity and increased utility, but are generally utilized when the abdominal territory is unavailable or inadequate. In general, autologous techniques require a sufficient donor site volume as even nonstandard flaps may not yield adequate tissue to meet the reconstructive requirement of the breast in a slender patient. The patient may not wish to undergo the more extensive of surgery or may not be a candidate for it due to medical co-morbidities.

Implant-based reconstruction has been frequently endorsed for patients with minimal donor sites and those wishing to minimize donor deformity. Although the result is generally less natural in appearance and feel than that which can be achieved with an autologous approach – and the potential for temporal instability long term is significant – this approach can provide reasonable results in suitable patients with modest surgical intervention. The use of the latissimus dorsi flap, including modifications such as a perforator flap, can help enhance the appearance of the implant reconstruction. Once the "workhorse" of breast reconstruction, high rates of seroma formation, as well as the significance of the donor site in terms of visible scars and functional loss, has recently limited the application of this approach in breast reconstruction *(Fig 10.41)*.

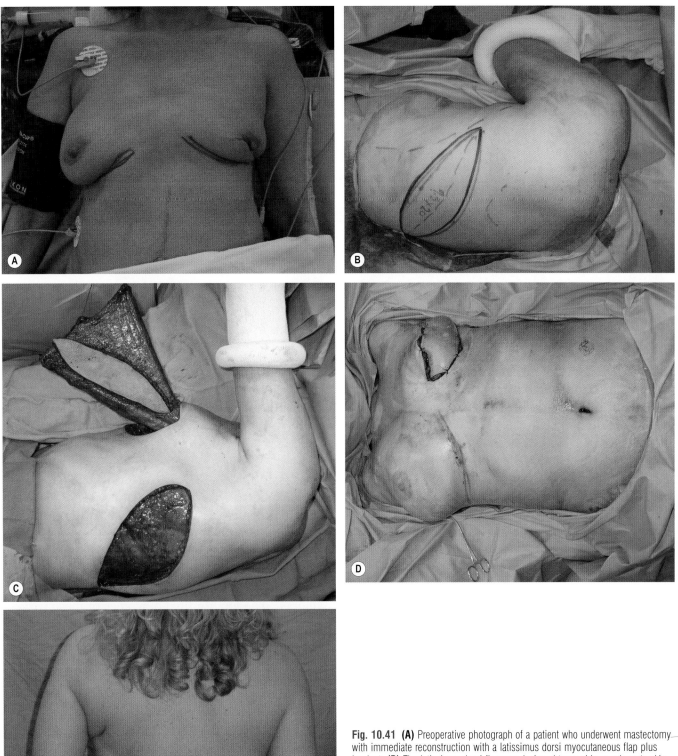

Fig. 10.41 (A) Preoperative photograph of a patient who underwent mastectomy with immediate reconstruction with a latissimus dorsi myocutaneous flap plus implant. **(B)** The latissimus dorsi flap was designed to provide an adequate skin paddle to reconstruct the breast mound. **(C)** A pedicled latissimus dorsi myocutaneous flap was harvested and transposed to reconstruct the breast mound of a patient who desired reconstruction. **(D)** The breast mound was contoured using the latissimus flap, which was inset into the skin sparing mastectomy defect. **(E)** The donor site incision postoperatively from a patient who underwent reconstruction with a latissimus dorsi pedicled flap with an implant for breast reconstruction.

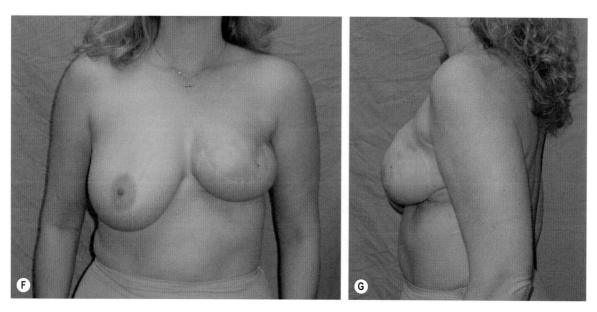

Fig. 10.41, cont'd (F,G) Postoperative photograph of breast reconstruction with a latissimus dorsi flap with an implant.

Many of the aspects critical to outcomes in breast reconstruction are innate to considerations that are out of the hands of the plastic surgeon, including the size of the breast, the skin quality and vascular integrity of the mastectomy skin flaps. The best possible outcomes for reconstruction result after a skin-sparing or nipple-sparing mastectomy, in a moderate sized breast. Very small breasts and very large ones are difficult to duplicate surgically.

The increasing use of adjuvant radiotherapy has greatly affected approaches in breast reconstruction. Applied before, during or after reconstruction of the breast, radiation therapy severely compromises the aesthetic outcome. There is increased scarring, loss of skin coverage and a greatly increased rate of complications with both implant-based and autologous tissue reconstruction in the setting of radiation therapy. Different institutions report various results utilizing implants in the face of radiation therapy, but in general this is felt to be a less reliable approach than autologous tissue. Implant-based reconstructions have a higher implant loss rate and an increased rate of fibrous capsular contracture and infection than nonradiated implants. Radiation of an autologous flap compromises the reconstruction significantly in most cases and necessitates revision – including a second flap in a number of cases. At this juncture the majority of practitioners recommend a delayed reconstruction with autologous tissue if radiation therapy is anticipated.

These issues can confound outcomes in breast reconstruction. If radiation is not needed and a delayed reconstruction is performed, the patient will often lose breast skin – which compromises her aesthetic result, and necessitates an additional operative procedure, and carries a negative psychological impact. There have been a number of protocols endorsed to minimize the effect of radiation on breast reconstruction, such as the use of a delayed-immediate type protocol with the use of a temporary placeholder type approach with a tissue expander implant in an effort to preserve breast skin envelope.[88] The longitudinal outcomes of these various approaches are still under consideration and prospective study. These considerations are particularly acute regarding patients with a T2 breast cancer in which the nodal status is unclear. Options to improve the reliability of preoperative diagnostic strategies – including MRI – and premastectomy sentinel node dissection are evolving. The impetus for these decisions is, of course, the fact that once tissues are irradiated they behave very differently surgically in terms of reconstruction, and the ultimate result is difficult to salvage. While there is controversy as to the effect of radiation on reconstruction, it is felt to be deleterious. This is particularly notable in situations such as a bilateral autologous reconstruction and when the volume of tissue available to create a breast replica is limited. Accordingly, if one or both of these reconstructions is irradiated, there is very little ability to salvage this. More favorable candidates for autologous reconstruction in a patient who may require adjuvant radiation generally require a unilateral reconstruction[89] in which one can overcorrect the breast by a minimum of approximately 20%, as there is an anticipated approximate 20% shrinkage of the flap after radiation therapy. One must not only consider the effect of the radiation on the reconstruction, but of the reconstruction on the radiation.[90]

There are significant differences in the approach to radiotherapy from institution to institution. Some radiotherapists regularly employ radiation over a tissue expander or a fully expanded implant and feel that there is no compromise. Other institutions, such as MD Anderson Cancer Center, at this juncture, feel that radiation of an inflated implant or even an autologous reconstruction may interfere with dosing, particularly of the internal mammary nodes. There are published data to suggest interference in the radiation therapy treatment plan with breast reconstruction,[90] and while

this remains theoretic at present, it prompts careful prospective study.

Delayed reconstruction

Delayed reconstruction is a challenging endeavor *(Fig. 10.42)*. The amount of skin and parenchymal equivalent needed to satisfy the reconstructive requirement is greatly underestimated. The loss of skin inherent to delayed reconstruction compromises the ultimate result of the reconstruction. An expander implant approach can be employed, although the prior scarring will often limit the volume and compromise the shape of an implant based reconstruction, particularly confounding the achievement of an acceptable inframammary fold *(Fig. 10.43)*. Autologous approaches, no matter how accurate the restoration of shape and volume will be plagued with the color and texture mismatch of a large patch of flap skin contrasting with the native chest skin.

The complexity of delayed reconstruction increases greatly in the setting of radiation due to the difficulty of creating a soft and natural appearing mound with the alteration and scarring that is incumbent to radiation

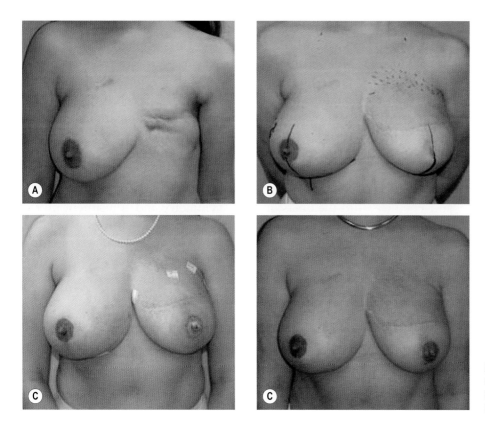

Fig. 10.42 This patient underwent delayed reconstruction with a DIEP flap. Preoperative, postoperative, and post-nipple areolar reconstruction photographs are shown.

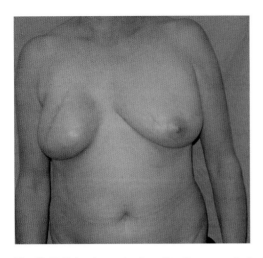

Fig. 10.43 Delayed reconstruction with a tissue expander implant.

injury. We prefer autologous tissue for delayed reconstruction, particularly in the setting of radiation therapy as the introduction of an implant in this setting can result in an exacerbation of the healing response and fibrous capsule contracture to an extraordinarily high degree. Radiation therapy creates the need to place well-vascularized tissue in proximity to this skin as it will behave in a fashion that is quite unfavorable and generally "shrink wrap" around the flap tissue and greatly distort it. Consequently, a very large amount of soft tissue and skin is necessary to replicate a breast, even a moderately sized one.

It is generally advisable to utilize tissue that is equivalent to more than half of the abdomen for one breast. We often employ a bilateral for a unilateral reconstruction as the amount of lower abdominal soft tissue that can be carried on one vascular pedicle is often inadequate.[91] This is done technically by anastomosing the deep system of vessels to an anterograde and retrograde mammary or to an anterograde mammary and a pedicle to each other to afford for a well perfused flap. In a delayed reconstruction the reconstruction will often be compromised aesthetically if the lower abdominal territory is not available. Use of the latissimus dorsi may be utilized in conjunction with an implant, but the amount of skin available is greatly limiting.

Gluteal and gracilis based flaps carry less skin and soft tissue and are best utilized in immediate reconstruction and may pose a significant challenge in a delayed setting. Bilateral reconstructions in which one side has been irradiated are particularly difficult due to the greater demand of soft tissue and skin required in a delayed reconstruction. This scenario greatly increases the operative complexity and morbidity and decreases the aesthetic outcome as use of the abdominal territory may be inadequate. Radiation will alter the response of tissues used in reconstruction and use of implants and flaps, or a combination of flaps from different territories will make symmetry highly problematic. Patients must carefully consider the true benefits of a prophylactic risk-reducing procedure and be adequately informed of their actual risk for a contralateral cancer. The surgical oncologist must help accurately assess the patient's true risk as well as preference in approaches.

Secondary procedures

The end result of breast reconstruction, while a reconstructive endeavor, has a significant aesthetic component. It is incumbent upon the surgeon to seek the best possible aesthetic result and temper this with the demands and expectations of each individual patient. Patient satisfaction is integral to the success of the procedure and a great deal reflects an individual's preferences and considerations. A number of patients are very satisfied with no reconstruction at all, while others wish to have the best possible aesthetic outcome and will endure a number of procedures or more extensive procedures achieve such an outcome. One must thoroughly vet these options with the patient and work with her toward an informed approach for the anticipated treatment.

In general, the best possible outcome for breast reconstruction cannot be achieved in one operative venture. Breast reconstruction is a staged endeavor with creation of the breast mound, symmetry and adjustment procedures as well as nipple areolar reconstruction. Some of these procedures may be obviated if the nipple-sparing approach is undertaken. A contralateral balancing procedure can be undertaken at the time of the initial reconstruction, but may be best if delayed due to of the potential for flap loss, implant loss, need for adjuvant therapy radiation, weight loss and/or gain that can alter factors that are integral to symmetry *(Fig. 10.44)*. It is often best to stage this as a secondary approach once the breast mound by whatever means – implants autologous or a combination therapy – has been undertaken.

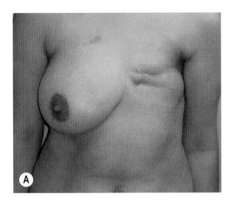

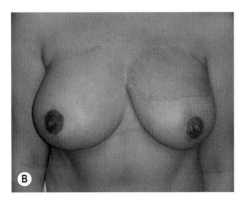

Fig. 10.44 This patient underwent a bilateral DIEP flap for left breast reconstruction. She had a contralateral vertical mastopexy for symmetry.

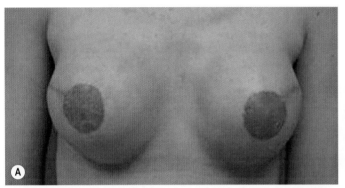

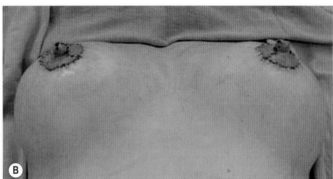

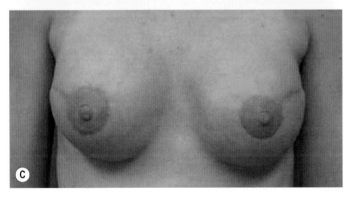

Fig. 10.45 Nipple areolar reconstruction is the last step of the reconstructive process.

Ancillary procedures such as fat grafting have proved to be a great adjunct in improving the contour of both implant and autologous reconstructions.[92,93] Reconstruction of the nipple areolar complex can be undertaken by a number of different approaches that generally involve the creation of the nipple with local skin flaps and the creation of the areola with a tattoo and/or skin graft. We have recently employed the use of a pre-tattoo for a nipple areolar complex to minimize the loss of projection that is often incurred with the placement of a tattoo as well as minimizing the scars. We have found this to be quite efficacious *(Fig. 10.45)*.

The principles governing the approach to revisions and secondary procedures in breast surgery must consider the best possible long term outcome. There are significant aesthetic and functional aspects of the donor sites such as hernia, bulge or contour deformity. These problems can be difficult to repair secondarily and should be adequately addressed in the initial procedure. In autologous reconstruction the approach to the donor site must be meticulous and not relegated to the most junior member of the team. In comparison, the free flap that is performed for the breast must be executed and transferred safely, and excessive manipulation after revascularization can be deleterious to the flap and ultimate result. Factoring in a planned, secondary approach for the revision and shaping of the breast when a free tissue transfer is undertaken is often prudent.

The utilization of an implant-based reconstruction can be done as either a one-stage or two-stage approach. Generally, at our institution, due to the oncologic imperative and the potential for compromise of the mastectomy skin flaps, a two-stage approach is preferred. While the appeal of utilizing an initial implant for reconstruction is undeniable, this must be approached with caution and is most advisable in a favorable setting in which the resecting surgeon and plastic reconstructive surgeon work together a great deal. This approach is likely successful in the setting of prophylactic mastectomy in which the skin flaps will usually be more robust and tolerate the tension incurred with placement of a full sized implant. Improving the aesthetic appearance

and minimizing the time to a full expansion with the use of acellular dermal matrix products has been advocated. Concerns for increased risk of seroma and infection have been raised making this a promising technique, but one currently under study. Currently, reconstructive techniques can provide restoration of the breast at a standard far superior to that previously obtained. Continued refinements in flap harvest and prosthetic quality coupled with progress in attention to patient satisfaction promise to provide our patients with progressively enhanced outcomes in their reconstructive endeavors.

Bonus images for this chapter can be found online at
http://www.expertconsult.com

Fig. 10.29 Skin sparing mastectomy with immediate reconstruction.
Fig. 10.38 Delayed reconstruction may be accomplished by autologous reconstructions, such as a transverse rectus abdominus

 Access the complete references list online at **http://www.expertconsult.com**

4. Sorlie T, Perou CM, Tibshirani R, et al. Gene expression patterns of breast carcinomas distinguish tumor subclasses with clinical implications. *Proc Natl Acad Sci U S A.* 2001;98(19):10869–10874.

   Survival analyses on a subcohort of patients with locally advanced breast cancer uniformly treated in a prospective study showed significantly different outcomes for the patients belonging to the various groups, including a poor prognosis for the basal-like subtype and a significant difference in outcome for the two estrogen receptor-positive groups.

27. Silverstein MJ, Recht A, Lagios MD, et al. Special report: Consensus conference III. Image-detected breast cancer: state-of-the-art diagnosis and treatment. *J Am Coll Surg.* 2009;209(4):504–520.

   An interdisciplinary expert panel reviewed the evidence regarding best practices in the field of breast oncology. This paper reports the panel's conclusions on what is considered state of the art for the diagnosis and therapy of breast cancer as it pertains to breast surgical oncology.

34. Bryant H, Brasher P. Breast implants and breast cancer–reanalysis of a linkage study. *N Engl J Med.* 1995;332(23): 1535–1539.

   On the basis of the reanalysis in this paper, the incidence of breast cancer among the women who had breast augmentation could not be said to be either significantly higher or lower than that among the general population over the period during which this cohort was followed.

52. Fisher B, Anderson S, Bryant J, et al. Twenty-year follow-up of a randomized trial comparing total

mastectomy, lumpectomy, and lumpectomy plus irradiation for the treatment of invasive breast cancer. *N Engl J Med.* 2002;347(16):1233–1241.

   Lumpectomy followed by breast irradiation continues to be appropriate therapy for women with breast cancer, provided that the margins of resected specimens are free of tumor and an acceptable cosmetic result can be obtained.

53. Clarke M, Collins R, Darby S, et al. Effects of radiotherapy and of differences in the extent of surgery for early breast cancer on local recurrence and 15-year survival: an overview of the randomised trials. *Lancet.* 2005;366(9503):2087–2106.

   In these trials, avoidance of a local recurrence in the conserved breast after BCS and avoidance of a local recurrence elsewhere (e.g., the chest wall or regional nodes) after mastectomy were of comparable relevance to 15-year breast cancer mortality. Differences in local treatment that substantially affect local recurrence rates would, in the hypothetical absence of any other causes of death, avoid about one breast cancer death over the next 15 years for every four local recurrences avoided, and should reduce 15-year overall mortality.

77. Yi M, Kronowitz SJ, Meric-Bernstam F, et al. Local, regional, and systemic recurrence rates in patients undergoing skin-sparing mastectomy compared with conventional mastectomy. *Cancer.* 2011;117(5): 916–924.

   SSM is an acceptable treatment option for patients who are candidates for immediate breast reconstruction.

Local-regional recurrence rates are similar to those of patients undergoing CM.

81. Brachtel EF, Rusby JE, Michaelson JS, et al. Occult nipple involvement in breast cancer: clinicopathologic findings in 316 consecutive mastectomy specimens. *J Clin Oncol.* 2009;27(30):4948–4954.

    Nipple-sparing mastectomy may be suitable for selected cases of breast carcinoma with low probability of nipple involvement by carcinoma and prophylactic procedures. A retroareolar en-face margin may be used to test for occult involvement in patients undergoing nipple-sparing mastectomy.

86. Giuliano AE, Hunt KK, Ballman KV, et al. Axillary dissection vs no axillary dissection in women with invasive breast cancer and sentinel node metastasis: a randomized clinical trial. *JAMA.* 2011;305(6):569–575.

    Among patients with limited SLN metastatic breast cancer treated with breast conservation and systemic therapy, the use of SLND alone compared with ALND did not result in inferior survival.

88. Kronowitz SJ, Hunt KK, Kuerer HM, et al. Delayed-immediate breast reconstruction. *Plast Reconstr Surg.* 2004;113(6):1617–1628.

    Delayed-immediate reconstruction is technically feasible and safe in patients with early-stage breast cancer who may require postmastectomy radiation therapy. With this approach, patients who do not require postmastectomy radiation therapy can achieve aesthetic outcomes essentially the same as those with immediate reconstruction, and patients who require postmastectomy radiation therapy can avoid the aesthetic and radiation-delivery problems that can occur after an immediate breast reconstruction.

90. Motwani SB, Strom EA, Schechter NR, et al. The impact of immediate breast reconstruction on the technical delivery of postmastectomy radiotherapy. *Int J Radiat Oncol Biol Phys.* 2006;66(1):76–82.

    Radiation treatment planning after immediate breast reconstruction was compromised in more than half of the patients (52%), with the largest compromises observed in those with left-sided cancers. For patients with locally advanced breast cancer, the potential for compromised PMRT planning should be considered when deciding between immediate and delayed reconstruction.

11

The oncoplastic approach to partial breast reconstruction

Albert Losken

SYNOPSIS

- Breast conservation therapy increases in popularity, driven by equivalent survival rates, preservation of body image, quality of life and reduced physiological morbidity.
- Poor cosmetic results following BCT are not uncommon and are usually due to breast shape, tumor size, tumor location, and postoperative radiation.
- Partial breast reconstruction is indicated whenever the potential for a poor cosmetic result exists, or patients with tumors in whom a standard lumpectomy would lead to breast deformity or gross asymmetry.

Access the Historical Perspective section online at
http://www.expertconsult.com

Introduction

The term *oncoplastic* is derived from two Greek words "onco" (tumor) and "plastic" (mould). It essentially blends the principles of tumor resection to ensure the best oncological outcome and the principles of plastic surgery, to ensure the best aesthetic outcome. When it is applied to the treatment of breast cancer, it varies in complexity. Although theoretically, the reconstruction of skin sparing mastectomy defects could also be considered oncoplastic, the original description, and focus in the literature and this chapter, is as it applies to breast conservation therapy (BCT).

Disease process

Poor cosmetic results following BCT are not uncommon and are usually due to breast shape, tumor size, tumor location, and postoperative radiation *(Fig. 11.1)*.[13] Traditionally, women with large breasts have been deemed poor candidates for breast conservation surgery, because of reduced effectiveness, increased complications and worse cosmetic outcome. The post-radiation sequela in women with *macromastia* is significantly worse. Radiation-induced fibrosis is thought to be greater in women with larger breasts, late radiation fibrosis is higher, and cosmetic results are also reduced.[14–16] *Tumor location* also plays a role with central or lower quadrant tumors having a worse cosmetic outcome. Lower quadrant tumors give twice as poor cosmetic results as lumpectomies in other quadrants. Central breast tumors close to the areolar have in the past been a contraindication to BCT. The *tumor to breast ratio* is one of the most important factors when predicting the potential for a poor outcome. Studies have shown a decline in cosmetic scores for patients with parenchymal resection greater than 70–100 cm^3, or when the specimen weight to breast volume ratio exceeds 10:1.[17–19] It is important that the reconstructive surgeons

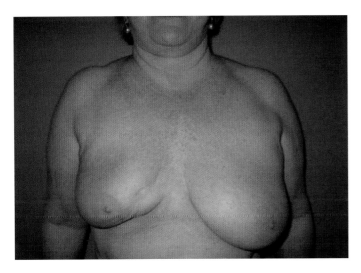

Fig. 11.1 A 42-year-old female who underwent a 20 g resection from the lower inner quadrant. Her resultant BCT deformity demonstrates shape and size distortion 2 years following radiation therapy.

Table 11.1 Terminology		
Partial breast reconstruction		
Timing		**Technique**
Immediate	At the time of resection	
Delayed immediate	1–2 weeks following resection (confirmation of margins status)	Volume displacement Volume replacement
Delayed	Following radiation therapy	

the importance of them being aware of the potential concerns with BCT alone and the various options available for these patients *(Table 11.1)*.

Patient presentation and selection

Partial breast reconstruction is indicated whenever the potential for a poor cosmetic result exists, or patients with tumors in whom a standard lumpectomy would lead to breast deformity or gross asymmetry. Factors in addition to cosmetic reasons as an indication for this approach, include oncologic issues. Important indications include situations where the surgeon is concerned about the potential for negative margins with standard resection, and based on initial pathology or breast imaging studies needs to perform a *wider excision* in order for the patient to be a candidate for breast conserving surgery. Additional indications include women who desire breast conservation, despite potential adverse conditions, as well as older women with large ptotic breasts in whom mastectomy and reconstruction would be difficult.

The initial consideration to partial reconstruction needs to come from the breast surgeon, demonstrating

have an idea on the extent of the resection, whether lumpectomy or quadrantectomy. In general, when more than 20% of the breast is excised with partial mastectomy, the cosmetic result is likely to be unfavorable.

These are all situations where partial breast reconstruction has significantly improved results and broadened the indications for BCT.

Hints and tips

- Consider the oncoplastic approach for patients with a high tumor to breast ratio (>20%), especially in women with small to moderate sized breasts.
- Certain tumor locations (central, inferior, medial) can result in unfavorable aesthetic results with BCT alone.
- Women with macromastia who undergo partial mastectomy are often best treated with a simultaneous reduction procedure.
- The oncoplastic approach will often allow generous resection and can be used when wide excision or quadrantectomy is required or concerns exist about clearing margins.
- Older, obese or high risk patients are poor candidates for SSM and reconstruction and BCT with partial breast reconstruction is often a preferred approach.
- Women with small breasts who desire BCT will often required partial reconstruction to preserve shape and symmetry.

Timing of partial breast reconstruction

In general, partial breast reconstruction, when indicated is best performed at the time of resection (*immediate reconstruction*). This has the benefits of operating on a nonirradiated or surgically scarred defect, resulting in lower complication rates and improved aesthetic results.[7] The main concern with immediate reconstruction is the potential for positive margins. When this concern does exist, the reconstruction can be delayed until final confirmation of negative margins (*delayed-immediate reconstruction*). This then allows the benefits of reconstruction prior to radiation therapy with the luxury of clear margins, although at the expense of a second procedure *(Fig. 11.2)*. Patients at increased risk of positive margins included younger age (<40 years old), extensive DCIS, high grade, history of neoadjuvant chemotherapy, infiltrating lobular carcinoma, Her2/neu positivity.[20–22] The main disadvantage is the need for a secondary procedure, which might be unnecessary in the majority of cases. When a flap reconstruction is required, we prefer to confirm final margin status prior to partial breast reconstruction.

There are situations where poor results are encountered years following radiation therapy, which then require correction (*delayed reconstruction*). Similar techniques are employed in delayed reconstruction, more often requiring flaps such as the latissimus dorsi myocutaneous flap and associated with higher complication rates (42% versus 26%) and worse cosmetic outcome.[7]

Management of margins

The importance of negative margins in BCT cannot be overstated, and has been associated as a factor for increased local recurrence, especially in younger patients.[23] Oncological principles should be applied with equal stringency. This becomes even more critical when reconstructive procedures have been performed since positive margins on final pathology are potentially complicated by altered architecture or elimination of a potential reconstructive option. Careful attention to patient selection and margin status should be performed and every attempt should be made to ensure negative margins. *Preoperative breast imaging* (i.e., MRI, ultrasound or mammography) is helpful in determining the extent of the disease guiding the necessary resection and should be employed judiciously when indicated. An imaging study showed that tumor size was underestimated 14% by mammography, 18% by ultrasound, whereas MRI showed no difference when compared to the pathological specimen.[24] Wire identification

and bracketing wires placed preoperatively will localize the extent of resection.[25] Intraoperative margin assessment requires multidisciplinary, coordination between the surgeons, the pathologist and the radiologist. Multicolored inking kits have proven to be more accurate than traditional stitch markings,[26] especially for the more complex designed oncoplastic specimens. Additional intraoperative confirmatory procedures include gross examination, radiography of the specimen, intraoperative frozen sections for invasive cancer and touch cytology. *Separate cavity margins* sent at the time of lumpectomy significantly reduces the need for re-excision. Cao and co-workers demonstrated that final margin status was negative in 60% of patients with positive margins on initial resection.[27] Rainsbury established a one-stage approach, where bed biopsies are taken from the cavity and subareolar region and sent for frozen section. The entire cavity is then inked and sent as a shave specimen for formal histology.[28] If tumor is still present in the second set of biopsies, then a mastectomy is indicated.

Although actual data is limited, some have proposed that the positive margin rate following oncoplastic resections should be lower, given the ability to perform a generous resection. Oncoplastic resections in some series have been over 200 g compared with institutional norms of about 40–50 g using lumpectomy alone.[22,29] This does not include the additional glandular excisions necessary to achieve symmetry with the reduced contralateral breast in patients with macromastia. Kaur et al. demonstrated an oncological benefit in a comparative study where positive margins were identified in 16% of breast cancer patients who had the oncoplastic approach versus 43% in patients with quadrantectomy.[30] Comparisons in the literature are difficult given the varying institutional definitions of what constitutes a positive margin, however, positive margin rates in most oncoplastic series range from 5–10%[7,22,30] compared with the larger BCT series of 10–15%.[2,3]

Placement of titanium perimeter clips to outline the lumpectomy cavity will guide the radiation therapy with postoperative tumor boost volume during teletherapy (external beam radiation). Communication is necessary between the oncologist and the surgeons especially when glandular remodeling has been performed. These clips will also assist in postoperative surveillance.

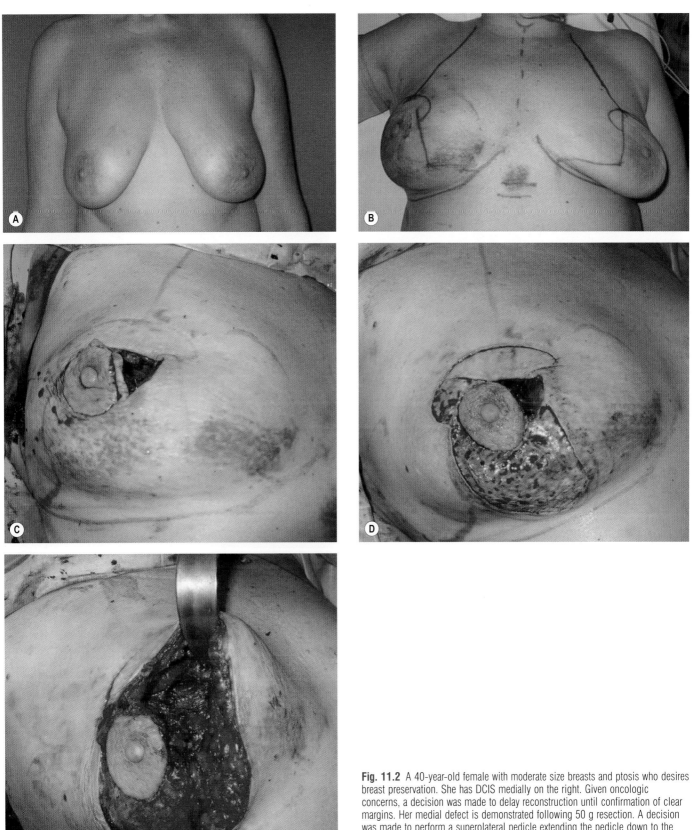

Fig. 11.2 A 40-year-old female with moderate size breasts and ptosis who desires breast preservation. She has DCIS medially on the right. Given oncologic concerns, a decision was made to delay reconstruction until confirmation of clear margins. Her medial defect is demonstrated following 50 g resection. A decision was made to perform a superolateral pedicle extending the pedicle down to the chest wall. This was then rotated into the medial defect and the medial and lateral pillars were plicated. A contralateral symmetry procedure was performed removing 65 g. Her result is shown following radiation therapy with breast edema and size discrepancy. She is then shown 1 year later with good size and symmetry.

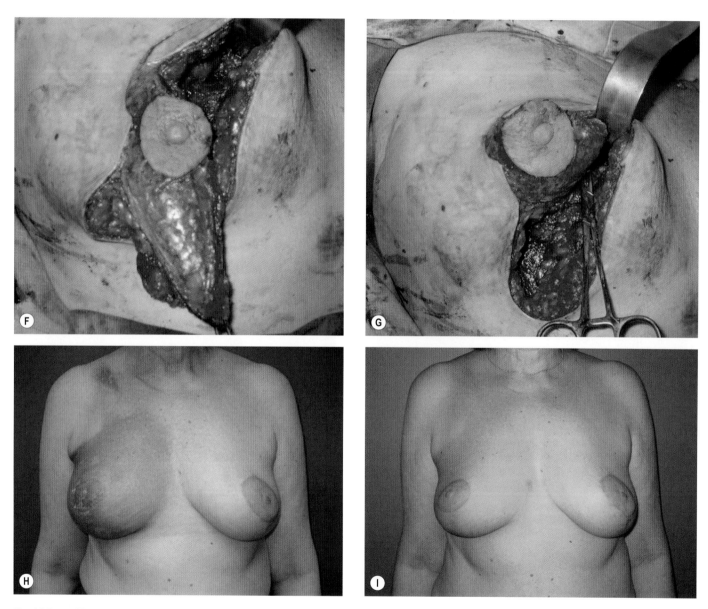

Fig. 11.2, cont'd

Surgical planning

Oncoplastic resection

Although the adverse effects of radiation therapy are often unavoidable, there are principles that can be applied to the resection with or without reconstructive techniques that can be used to minimize the incidence of poor cosmetic results. The oncoplastic approach applies the principles of plastic surgery to the resection as well. A deformity can often be avoided by correctly orienting the breast incisions and parenchymal resection. Neoadjuvant chemotherapy will also downsize the tumor and reduce the required amount of parenchyma resection. Limiting the volume of resection will minimize the incidence of poor cosmetic results. Attention to simple defect closure, including breast advancement flaps and full thickness closures are now commonly performed by most breast surgeons and are ways to improve results. The more complex defects with potential for poor cosmesis will often benefit from partial breast reconstruction.

Treatment algorithm for partial reconstruction

Different algorithms have been described in an attempt to simplify the reconstructive process.[31] There is, unfortunately, a lack of standardization when it comes to partial breast reconstruction, which makes comparative studies difficult. The decision as to which procedure is more appropriate is multifactorial, however, and is ultimately determined by breast size, tumor size, and tumor location. Other factors are also important, including patient risks and desires, tumor biology, and surgeon comfort level with the various techniques. Another way of looking at this is to evaluate the amount of breast tissue that remains following completion of the partial mastectomy, and where that tissue is in relation to the nipple areolar complex, since this will dictate the most appropriate reconstruction option for that particular case. Adhering to strict algorithms is difficult, since every case is different. Being familiar with the various reconstructive tools will allow reconstruction of almost any partial mastectomy defect. It is important to keep in mind that when the defect is extensive with little remaining breast tissue, then completion mastectomy

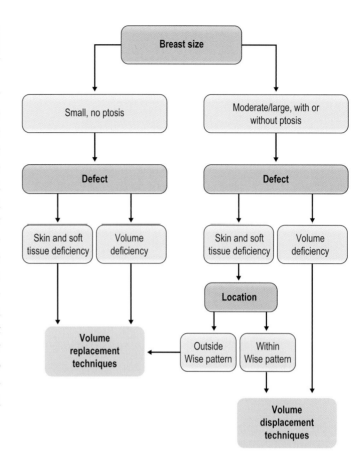

Fig. 11.3 Reconstructive algorithm, based on breast size, shape and tumor location.

and immediate reconstruction is often the more appropriate option. Kronowitz et al. found that most women with medium to large breasts benefit from immediate reconstruction, and that when immediate reconstruction is performed, the preferred technique is local breast tissue – local tissue rearrangement of reduction techniques.[31]

Some simple rules of thumb exist for reconstructing partial mastectomy defects (*Fig. 11.3*). Large or moderate sized breasts, or ptotic breasts with sufficient parenchyma remaining following resection, are amenable to *volume displacement or reshaping procedures.* Quadrantectomy-type resections are possible when within the standard Wise pattern markings. In smaller, or nonptotic breasts, when additional volume is required to match the opposite breast or when skin is required to replace a resection that included parenchyma and skin, then *volume replacement procedures,* including volume and skin are required (*Table 11.2*). Quadrantectomy type

Table 11.2 Partial mastectomy reconstruction techniques

Volume displacement techniques	Volume replacement techniques
"Parenchymal remodeling, volume shrinkage"	"Adjacent or distant tissue transfer, volume preserving"
Primary closure	Implant augmentation – rare
Mirror biopsy/excision Batwing mastopexy	Local flaps Fasciocutaneous
Breast flap advancement technique	Perforator flaps
Nipple areolar centralization	Latissimus dorsi MC flap
Reduction mastopexy techniques	Distant flaps

resections in small breasts, and in the upper or outer quadrant will invariably require a flap reconstruction to preserve shape *(Fig. 11.4)*.

Volume displacement techniques

The breast reshaping procedures all essentially rely on advancement, rotation or transposition of a large area of breast to fill a small or moderate-sized defect. This absorbs the volume loss over a larger area. In its simplest form, it entails mobilizing the breast plate from the area immediately around the defect in a *breast flap advancement technique*.[32] The dissection is over the pectoralis muscle and essentially involves a full-thickness segment of breast fibroglandular tissue advanced to fill the dead space. These procedures are indicated in women with small to medium-sized breasts, where the resection does not lead to any significant volume alteration that might cause breast asymmetry. A contralateral symmetry procedure is typically not required.

Video 1

Perhaps the most popular and versatile breast reshaping options are the *mastopexy or reduction techniques*. The ideal patient is one where the tumor can be excised within the expected breast reduction specimen, in medium to large or ptotic breasts, where sufficient breast parenchyma remains following resection to reshape the mound *(Fig. 11.5)*. Masetti and colleagues describe a four-step design for oncoplastic operations: (1) Planning skin incisions and parenchymal excisions following reduction/mastopexy templates; (2) Parenchymal reshaping following excision;

(3) repositioning the nipple, and (4) correction of the contralateral breast for symmetry.[33] Any moderate to large breast can be reconstructed using these techniques, unless a skin deformity exists beyond the standard Wise pattern.

Plastic surgeons are all familiar with these techniques, making the incorporation of this approach into their reconstructive practice an easy addition. There has been an exponential increase in reports over the last few years describing these techniques. In women with large or ptotic breasts, the numerous reduction patterns or pedicle designs will invariably allow remodeling of a defect in any location and any size, as long as sufficient breast tissue and skin is available. Creative mammaplasty designs can be made for complete removal of the lesion and reshaping of the mound for both lumpectomy and quadrantectomy type defects. *Preoperative markings* are important, and a decision is made on pedicle design, depending on tumor location. Typically if the pedicle points to, or can be rotated into the defect, it can be used. The Wise pattern markings are more versatile, allowing tumor resection in any breast quadrant. Once the resection is performed, the cavity is inspected paying attention to the defect location in relation to the nipple, as well as the remaining breast tissue. The reconstructive goals include: (1) preservation of nipple viability; (2) reshaping of breast mound, and (3) closure of dead space. The nipple and dermatoglandular pedicle is dissected, and the remaining tissue is resected if necessary for completion of the reduction. Occasionally, additional dermatoglandular or glandular pedicles can be created from tissue that might otherwise have been resected, and rotated to autoaugment the defect. The contralateral procedure is performed using a similar technique. The ipsilateral side is typically kept about 10% larger to allow for radiation fibrosis. Additional tissue sampling from the ipsilateral or contralateral breast is also possible using this technique.

Lower quadrant tumors in women with larger breasts are ideally suited for the oncoplastic approach.[34] Quadrantectomy type resections are possible, removing skin and parenchyma form this location, reshaping the breast using a superior or superomedial pedicle *(Fig. 11.5)*. Lower pole tumors in moderate-sized breasts can be excised along with skin as needed in the usual vertical pattern utilizing a superior pedicle followed by

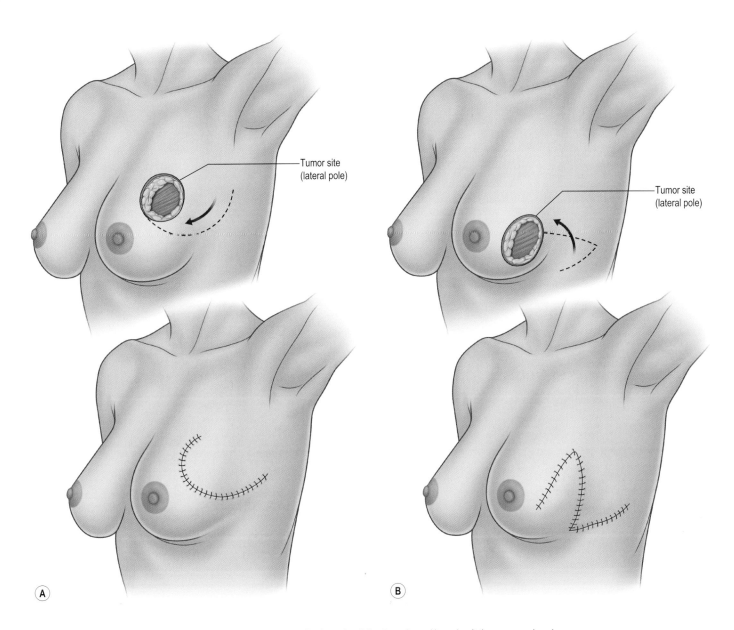

Tumor site
(lateral pole)

Tumor site
(lateral pole)

A

B

Fig. 11.4 (A,B) A lateral quadrantectomy type defect is reconstructed using a local flap to replace skin and soft tissue preserving shape.

plication of the vertical pillars, and vertical reduction on the contralateral side. *Upper quadrant tumors* can be filled as long as the defect is under the skin (lumpectomy type) *(Fig. 11.6)*. Autoaugmentation techniques have become popular to fill the dead space and maintain shape. Inferior or medial pedicles allow for safe excisions in the upper half of the breast without impairing nipple viability and parenchyma is often rearranged when insufficient tissue remains in the upper pole to maintain the desired fullness. When skin is resected in the upper half of the breast, such remodeling techniques

are not possible. *Lateral or upper-outer quadrant* defects allow parenchymal remodeling using the superomedial pedicle. These types of reconstructions become difficult when skin is resected with the specimen and are better suited for the lumpectomy type defects. In women with medium sized ptotic breasts, the superomedial pedicle can be extended down to the inframammary fold as an autoaugmented pedicle. This can then be rotated to fill a lateral volume void. The vertical pillars are then plicated in the usual fashion to maintain shape. If tissue is removed from above the Wise pattern markings, and

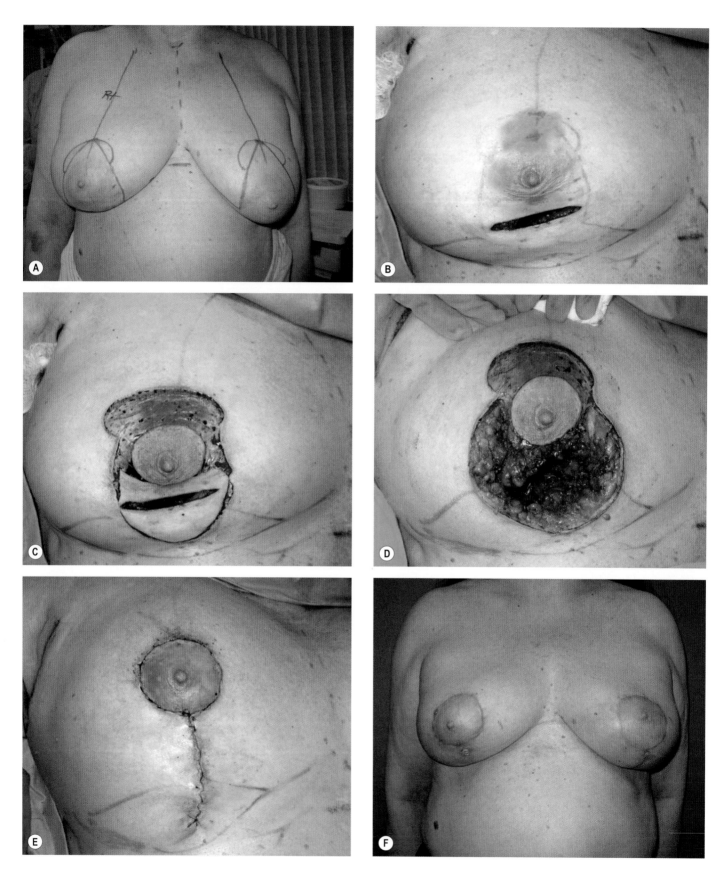

Fig. 11.5 A 53-year-old female with breast asymmetry and a lower pole invasive ductal CA. She underwent a lumpectomy (65 g). The tumor was within the reduction specimen, additional tissue was sent (30 g) and a superior pedicle mastopexy was performed. A similar procedure was performed on the contralateral side removing a total of 110 g. Her early result is shown with improvement of symmetry and shape.

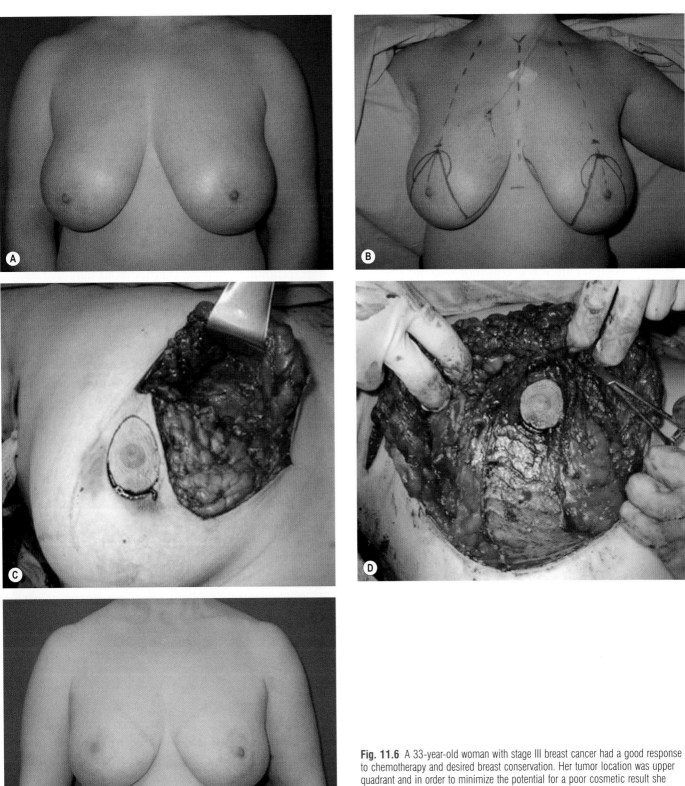

Fig. 11.6 A 33-year-old woman with stage III breast cancer had a good response to chemotherapy and desired breast conservation. Her tumor location was upper quadrant and in order to minimize the potential for a poor cosmetic result she underwent a 100 g lumpectomy with simultaneous bilateral breast reduction. The total volume including specimen on the left was 250 g, and on the right 150 g. An inferior pedicle was used to reposition the nipple and reconstruct the defect. Her result is shown 1 year following completion of right-sided breast irradiation with good symmetry.

flap is often required. In women with macromastia, a reduction can still be performed utilizing the inferior pedicle skin to replace missing breast skin even when above the Wise markings.

Central tumors have in the past been considered relative contraindications to BCT, however, with the oncoplastic approach in women with macromastia, the tumor and nipple areolar complex can be widely excised and reconstructed using a variety of techniques.[35] The mound can be remodeled in the inverted T-closure pattern, similar to breast amputation reduction techniques. The nipple is then reconstructed later using the reconstruction technique of choice. Another option if the tumor is located more superiorly or lateral is to perform a central elliptical excision of skin, nipple and parenchyma, and mirror image contralateral reduction for symmetry. A third option includes creation of a skin island on a dermatoglandular pedicle to rotate into the central defect to allow for shape preservation and nipple reconstruction *(Fig. 11.7)*. The breast is marked preoperatively for an inverted T or a vertical approach depending on breast size, and the skin island is brought in from inferior or medial.

Larger quadrantectomy defects, especially above the nipple can be incorporated into a batwing mastopexy or elliptical type incision and provide preservation or improvement of shape and elevation of the ptotic breast along with the tumor resection. A similar mirror image resection is often performed on the opposite side for symmetry. Additional mastopexy options exist for oncoplastic breast conservation.[32] The *donut mastopexy* allows a breast segment to be removed through a periareolar incision, and is useful for segmentally distributed cancers in the upper or lateral portion of the breast *(Fig. 11.8)*. The *batwing mastopexy* involves a full thickness excision of lesions deep within the breast centrally or adjacent to the nipple-areolar complex *(Fig. 11.9)*. The two similar half-circle incisions with angled wings on either side of the areolar allow advancement of the fibroglandular tissue to close the defect. Since this removes sufficient breast tissue and skin to alter the size of the breast and nipple position, a similar contralateral lift is occasionally required to achieve symmetry. Additionally, if the patient is a candidate for BCT and has multiple areas that need to be resected, as long as sufficient tissue remains, remodeling techniques can be used in a similar fashion.

Volume replacement techniques

Partial mastectomy defects in women with small to medium breasts are often difficult to reconstruct.[36] Women with large tumor to breast ratios and women with small to moderate breasts who have insufficient residual breast tissue for rearrangement require partial reconstruction using nonbreast local or distant flaps. This is now well accepted in the evolution of breast cancer surgery and provides breast symmetry without remodeling the contralateral breast.

Local flaps are often indicated in small or moderate volume breasts with insufficient tissue remains following resection for volume displacement techniques. The usual techniques include: (1) rhomboid flaps; (2) subaxillary flap; (3) superior-based lateral thoracodorsal flap; (4) inferior-based lateral thoracodorsal flap, and (5) the extended lateral thoracodorsal flap *(Fig. 11.10)*. Small lateral defects (<10% of breast size) can be closed with *local flaps*. Clough et al.[37] described using the subaxillary area as a transposition flap, and Munhoz et al. have more recently demonstrated how the lateral thoracodorsal flap (LTDF) is ideal for lateral defects, especially in obese patients.[38] These flaps essentially rotate or transfer skin and subaxillary fat or skin and breast parenchyma into the defect. The same principles can be applied to local flaps taken from outside the breast as described above, or even from within the breast (volume displacement techniques). Attention to flap design is important to ensure flap survival, cosmesis and appropriate conversion to a completion mastectomy if necessary. The latissimus dorsi *musculocutaneous flap* is a common local option for lateral, central, inferior and even medial defects.[28,39,40] It has excellent blood supply and provides both muscle for filling of glandular defects and skin for cutaneous deficiencies. Avoiding a scar on the back can be achieved by harvesting the LD without skin through the lateral breast incision. The use of an endoscope can assist in raising the muscle.[40] A deinnervated and radiated LD will undergo postoperative atrophy. To compensate for the expected loss in muscle volume, a flap much larger than the defect should be harvested, possibly preserving subscarpa's fat on the muscle. A similar skin island to the classical LD musculocutaneous flap can be raised as a *pedicled perforator flap* either from the thoracodorsal or intercostal vessels. Sparing the underlying muscles, or using perforator flaps reduces the

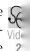

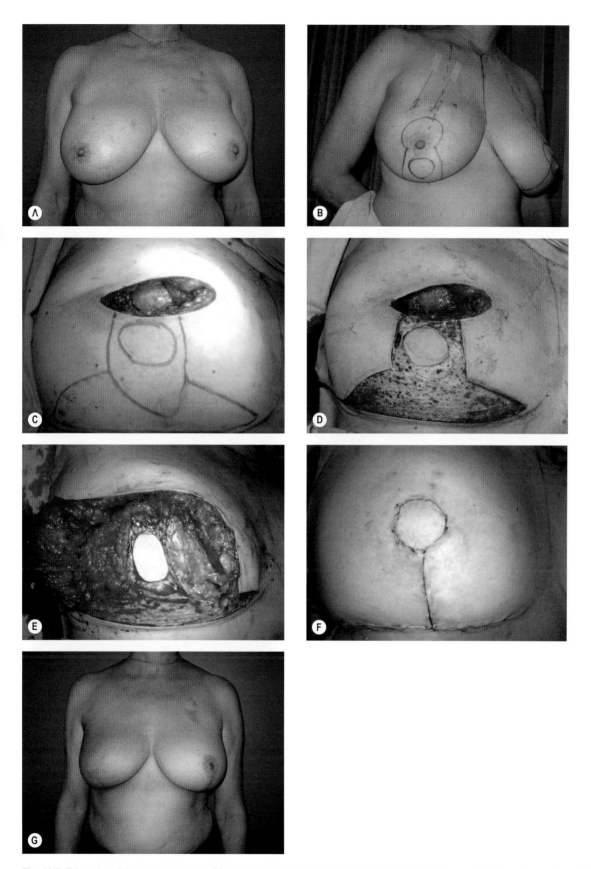

Fig. 11.7 This patient did not want to undergo SSM and reconstruction and despite having a subareolar tumor, elected breast preservation. Given proximity, she had resection of the nipple areolar complex with her partial mastectomy. An inferior pedicle was created leaving a skin island appropriately located for nipple areolar replacement. Her result is shown 9 months following completion of radiation therapy just prior to nipple areolar reconstruction.

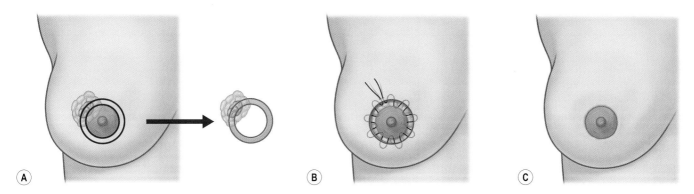

Fig. 11.8 A donut type mastopexy is shown, which repositions the nipple and preserves breast shape by removing a tumor just lateral to the nipple areolar complex followed by reshaping using the mastopexy technique.

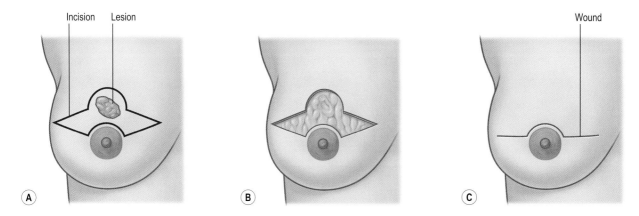

Fig. 11.9 Batwing mastopexy demonstrating removal of a tumor above the nipple, elevation of the nipple areolar complex and breast reshaping.

donor site morbidity to the minimum, with no seroma formation at the donor site.[41,42]

The thoraco-dorsal artery perforator (TDAP) flap can easily reach defects in the lateral, superolateral and central regions of the breast. If no suitable perforators are found, the flap is easily converted to a muscle sparing TDAP or muscle sparing LD flap. *The lateral intercostal artery perforator (LICAP) flap* is another alternative to the TDAP flap for lateral and inferior breast defects. The lateral intercostal artery perforators are found at 2.7–3.5 cm from the anterior border of the LD muscle.[43] *The anterior intercostal artery perforator (AICAP) flap* is similar to the random-designed thoraco-epigastric skin flap; the skin paddle can be harvested as an AICAP flap. The AICAP is based on perforators originating from the intercostal vessels through the rectus abdominis or the external oblique muscles. Since

it has a short pedicle, the AICAP flap is suitable to cover close defects that extend over the inferior or medial quadrants of the breast. *The superior epigastric artery perforator (SEAP) flap* is based on perforators arising from the superior epigastric artery or it superficial branch. It has the same indications as the AICAP flap, however, the SEAP flap has a longer pedicle and therefore it can cover more remote defect in the breast.

Large medial defects are more difficult to reconstruction. The superficial inferior epigastric artery free flap has been described for this location.[44,45] In situations such as this one, or when the partial mastectomy defect is significant with minimal residual breast tissue a decision needs to be made whether to complete the mastectomy and perform total breast reconstruction for both cosmetic and oncological reasons.

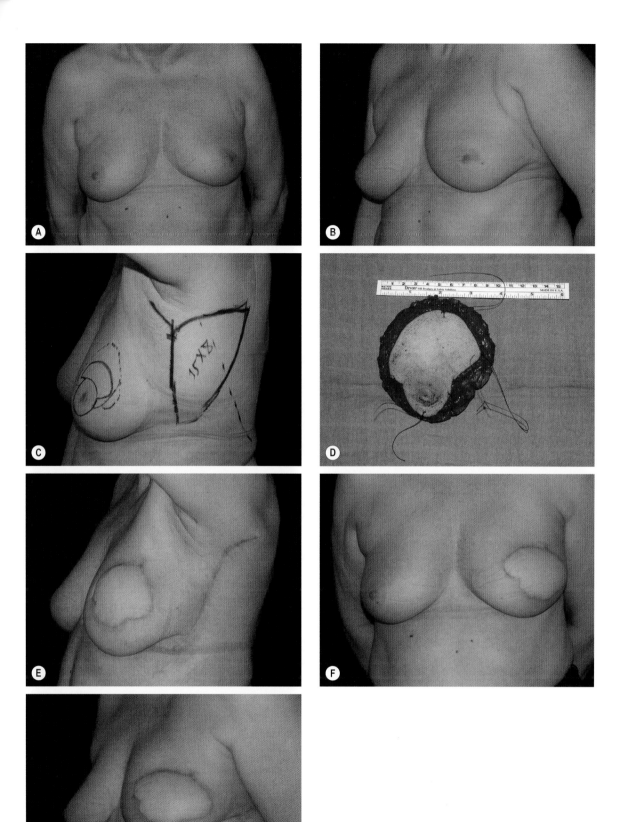

Fig. 11.10 A 46-year-old woman who underwent an immediate partial breast reconstruction with muscle sparing latissimus dorsi (MS LD) flap after quadrantectomy, including the nipple-areola complex and axillary lymph node dissection, for a T2 tumor located at the retro-areolar and the junction of upper quadrants of the left breast. (Courtesy Moustapha Hamdi. Reprinted in Losken A, Hamdi M. Partial breast reconstruction: current perspectives. Plast Reconstr Surg 2009;124(3):722–736.)

Video
3

Various other techniques have been described to fill partial mastectomy defects, however, these are currently less common. They include abdominal adipofascial flaps, omental flaps, and autologous fat injections.[46–49]

Oncologic safety

- Appropriate patient selection
- Preoperative planning (imaging, wires) to assist with resection
- Confirm negative margins in high risk patients (DCIS, age <40)
- Consider confirmation of negative margins when performing flap reconstruction
- Intraoperative margin assessment (multidisciplinary approach)
- Separate cavity sampling
- Clip cavity for radiation planning and surveillance
- Appropriate postoperative surveillance protocols.

Postoperative care

One main concern with partial breast reconstruction is that it might impair the ability to screen and detect recurrent breast cancer. Some fear that glandular re-arrangement, additional scarring and the disruption of architecture might alter the potential patterns of local recurrence of the ability to screen and detect these lesions. Although this is a valid concern, adherence to appropriate surveillance and cross specialty communication will reduce this as an issue. The three main tools when it comes to postoperative surveillance include the physical examination, radiologic imaging, and tissue sampling. It is important that all members of the team are aware of the various surgical components, since differences in presentation might exist, depending on the type and technique of reconstruction. We recently demonstrated that mammography following partial breast reconstruction using reduction techniques was just as sensitive as a screening tool when compared to patients with BCT alone.[50] Although the qualitative mammographic findings were similar in the two groups over the average 6-year follow-up, there was a slight trend towards longer times to mammographic stability in the oncoplastic reduction group (25.6 months versus 21.2 months in the BCT alone group). This means that it might take the oncoplastic reduction patients slightly

longer to reach the point where any change in mammographic findings might be suspicious for malignancy. An accurate interpretation requires familiarity with these temporal changes and mammograms should be compared over time. These data need to be taken into consideration when designing the most appropriate surveillance programs for these patients. Mammographic findings following myocutaneous flap reconstructions typically show areas of radiolucency consistent with a fibrofatty component in most flaps. Microcalcifications and areas of fat necrosis are easily identified, and no interference in postoperative surveillance has been demonstrated. Other imaging techniques such as ultrasound and MRI will likely become more popular as technology improves. Although routine tissue sampling is not recommended for screening, any clinical concern necessitates fine needle aspiration, core needle biopsy, or surgical biopsy, to rule out malignancy. Patients who undergo partial breast reconstruction are expected to have an increase in the amount of tissue sampling requirements, as demonstrated in our series (53% in the oncoplastic group compared with 18% in the BCT alone group over an average of 7 years).[50] Although these are typically benign, additional scarring from the reconstruction might raise clinical suspicion, which is why more biopsies are expected in patients who undergo partial breast reconstruction.

Outcomes and secondary procedures

It is important that complications resulting from oncoplastic techniques do not interfere with the initiation of adjuvant therapy. Careful selection of surgical technique, appropriate patient selection and meticulous execution will minimize the incidence of postoperative complications. Additional procedures will invariably increase complications, however, most of these are minor. Some larger series with volume displacement techniques report complications such as delayed wound healing (3–15%), fat necrosis (3–10%), and infection (1–5%).[7,20,51] Overall complications following volume replacement techniques are slightly higher (range 2–77%) and this is likely due to the addition of donor site complications and potential flap loss issues.[28,39,40] Delayed complications with the oncoplastic approach include breast fibrosis and asymmetry. Although the goal of partial breast reconstruction is to prevent the unfavorable cosmetic result, this approach cannot prevent or reverse the effects of radiation therapy. Since these effects will persist, the assessment of shape and symmetry needs to be made in the context of long term. However, with partial reconstruction shape is typically preserved and it is easier to adjust the contralateral side secondarily if necessary than reconstruct a radiated BCT deformity. Asgeirsson reviewed numerous series with intermediate follow-up and demonstrated cosmetic failure rates of 0–18%.[52] BCT alone has a poor aesthetic result in 20–30 patients,[6] however, with the incorporation of oncoplastic breast surgery techniques, this can be dropped to below 7% at 2 years.[53] *Local recurrence* is another important outcome that needs to be evaluated in the oncoplastic patient. Most reviews in the literature are of intermediate follow-up (up to 4.5 years), with local recurrence rates varying from 0–1.8 % per year.[52] Actuarial 5-year local recurrence rates range from 8.5% to 9.4%. Longer term studies are required.

Secondary procedures are not common, and usually for size of shape changes long term. Although this approach minimizes the potential for poor aesthetic results, the effects of radiation therapy persist and can contribute to changes over time. It is better to wait at least a year following completion of radiation therapy to discuss revisional procedures. Even with resolution of acute radiation changes and tissue edema, it is

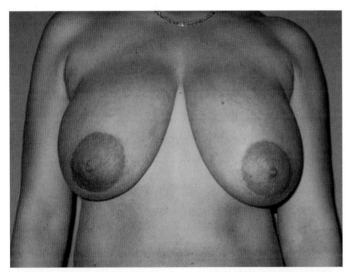

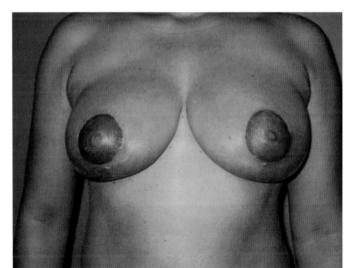

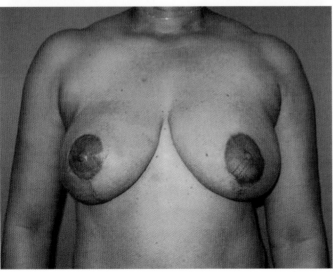

Fig. 11.11 A 43-year-old female with right-sided breast cancer who underwent partial reconstruction using the oncoplastic reduction approach. Her lumpectomy margins were clear, however DCIS was identified in the additional tissue removed during the right reduction. A decision was made to perform a right skin sparing mastectomy and she underwent a latissimus dorsi reconstruction with implant.

Table 11.3 **Partial mastectomy reconstruction using reduction techniques**

Author	Cases (n)	Partial mastectomy Specimen weight (g)	Complications (%)	Cosmetic result/ patient satisfaction (good–excellent)	Local recurrence (%)	Follow-up (months)
Losken et al. 2007.[20]	63	236	22	95	2	40
Clough et al. 2003.[29]	101	222	20	88	7	46
Munhoz et al. 2006.[51]	74		17	93	0	22
Goffman et al. 2005.[54]	55	NR	NR	72	13[a]	18
Chang et al. 2004.[55]	37	NR	19	70	0	

[a]High percentage of T3,T4 tumors. NR, not reported.

important to respect tissue planes and blood supply and if possible keep any revisions to a minimal since it is still an irradiated breast and carries the associated risks. Perhaps the largest series of 540 consecutive cases from the Institut Curie demonstrated that in patients with high tumor-to-breast volume ratios, use of the oncoplastic approach provides good outcomes.[50] The 5-year local recurrence (6.8%) and overall survival rates (92.9%) were acceptable with low complication rates (16%) and good aesthetic results at 1 year (97.7%) and at 5 years (90.3%).

When completion mastectomy and reconstruction is required following oncoplastic reduction techniques the disadvantages of this approach are minimal *(Table 11.3)*.[56] All reconstructive options are still available, the contralateral symmetry procedure has already been performed, and then it is easier to reconstruct a smaller breast *(Fig. 11.11)*.

Conclusion

The benefits of using the oncoplastic approach with breast conservation therapy have been well demonstrated, and will continue to gain popularity and acceptance in the future. The options for women with breast cancer are numerous, and this provides an additional, often favorable one. We need to critically evaluate results measuring functional, oncological and aesthetic outcomes in an attempt to establish safe and effective practice guidelines to maximize oncological safety.

 Access the complete reference list online at **http://www.expertconsult.com**

6. Clough KB, Cuminet J, Fitoussi A, et al. Cosmetic sequelae after conservative treatment for breast cancer: classification and results of surgical correction. *Ann Plast Surg.* 1998;41:471–481.

7. Kronowitz SJ, Feledy JA, Hunt KK, et al. Determining the optimal approach to breast reconstruction after partial mastectomy. *Plast Reconstr Surg.* 2006;117(1):1–11.

8. Losken A, Hamdi M. Partial breast reconstruction: current perspectives. *Plast Reconstr Surg.* 2009;124(3): 722–736.

12. Munhoz AM, Aldrighi CM, Ferreira MC. Paradigms in oncoplastic breast surgery: a careful assessment of the oncological need and esthetic objective. *Breast J.* 2007;13(3):326–327.

20. Losken A, Styblo TM, Carlson GW, et al. Management Algorithm And Outcome Evaluation of Partial Mastectomy Defects Treated Using Reduction or Mastopexy Techniques. *Ann Plast Surg.* 2007; 59(3):235–242.

This paper presents a treatment algorithm using reduction techniques to correct partial mastectomy defects based on tumor location. It is a safe approach with limited morbidity. Margins status is discussed and it is felt that younger patients, extensive DCIS and lobular pathology are at increased risk of positive margins. Their reconstruction is deferred until confirmation of clear margins. Completion mastectomy and reconstruction following oncoplastic reduction techniques is still possible if disease persists.

29. Clough KB, Lewis JS, Couturaud B, et al. Oncoplastic techniques allow extensive resections for breast-conserving therapy of breast cancer. *Ann Surg.* 2003;237(1):26–34.

This paper discusses the beneficial role of oncoplastic reduction techniques in terms of broadening the indications for breast conservation therapy. The mean resection weight in the series was 221 g. The authors feel that without this technique such large resections would not have been possible while preserving breast shape.

31. Kronowitz SJ, Kuerer HM, Buchholz TA. A management algorithm and practical oncoplastic surgery techniques for repairing partial mastectomy defects. *Plast Reconstr Surg.* 2008;122(6):1631.

    A management algorithm is designed based on certain clinical parameters to help decide on the breast approach to reconstruct a partial mastectomy defect. Breast size plays a major role in the decision process. The timing of reconstruction is either immediate, Complications are higher when reconstructions are performed following completion of radiation therapy, and the technique is more likely to be a flap reconstruction. The role of a multidisciplinary team is discussed.

43. Hamdi M, Spano A, Van Landuyt K, et al. The lateral intercostal artery perforators: anatomical study and clinical application in breast surgery. *Plast Reconstr Surg.* 2008;121:389–396.

51. Munhoz AM, Montag E, Arruda EG, et al. Critical analysis of reduction mammaplasty techniques in combination with conservative breast surgery for early breast cancer treatment. *Plast Reconstr Surg.* 2006;117(4):1091–1107.

56. Munhoz AM, Montag E, Arruda E, et al. Assessment of immediate conservative breast reconstruction: A classification system of defects revisited and an algorithm for selecting the appropriate technique. *Plast Reconstr Surg.* 2008;121:716–727.

    A classification system is proposed based on breast size in relation to tumor location and the extent of the resection. The indications for flap techniques, and reduction techniques are discussed. Good results are possible regardless of defect if appropriately selected.

12

Patient-centered health communication

Gary L. Freed, Alice Andrews, and E. Dale Collins Vidal

SYNOPSIS

- Healthcare decisions, particularly preference-sensitive decisions, are complicated because they involve trade-offs between benefits and harms.
- Patients may have different values regarding the potential benefits and harms when compared with providers, and similar patients may make different decisions even under similar circumstances.
- Research evaluating unwarranted geographic variation suggests that physician preference may trump patient preference, even though informed patient decision-making can improve efficiency and outcomes.
- Two-way patient communication is complicated by a lack of evidence for many procedures and the difficulty of communicating risk.
- Shared decision-making and decision aids improve patient knowledge and engage patients in the decision-making process.
- The legal standard for preference-sensitive care should move away from informed consent and towards informed patient choice.

Healthcare decisions

Plastic surgery often involves choices between options. For example, should a breast cancer patient receive an implant or have autologous reconstruction? Should it be pedicled or free tissue transfer? No reconstruction at all? Each of these options entails some downsides, such as donor site morbidity or the risks of additional surgery.

For each person, this choice is highly individual and should be dictated by personal preferences and a decision about which trade-offs between benefits and harms are most acceptable to the individual.

Yet how are these decisions made in practice? Do physicians and patients generally share the decision-making process? Patient-centeredness is one of the six dimensions identified by the Institute of Medicine for improving quality of care[1,2] and an integral part of the "Triple-Aim:" improving the care experience, improving the health of populations, and reducing costs.[1] However, patient involvement is not always observed in practice. In many types of medical treatment decisions, physician preference determines the choice.[3,4] For example, if surgeons are experienced in or prefer a particular technique, this knowledge will influence their conversations with patients about available reconstruction options. Providers may not be aware of this bias, or may not be cognizant of the fact that patients have different values regarding the potential benefits and harms of treatment. Consider two women with stage I breast cancer who have been informed that chemotherapy will reduce their chance of recurrence by 1–2%. These women may feel differently about whether that risk reduction is worth exposure to the potential harms of chemotherapy. To some women, that 1–2% risk reduction will sound very large, while to others, it will feel small and worth foregoing additional treatment.

Unwarranted variation in medical practice

These physician preferences may be observable by examining practice patterns across geographic regions. Dr Jack Wennberg developed a methodology (see the Dartmouth Atlas Project at: www.dartmouthatlas.org) enabling the comparison of procedure rates and the identification of regional variation across hospital systems and localities. This methodology segments the United States into 3436 Hospital Service Areas (HSAs) representing local healthcare markets. These HSAs are then aggregated to 306 Hospital Referral Regions (HRRs), each of which is a market for tertiary care. All HRRs contain at least one city where both cardiovascular and neurosurgery are performed (for additional information about these regions, see http://www.dartmouthatlas.org/data/region/).

Dr Wennberg's research determined that dramatic geographic variation exists across these regions of the United States in terms of the number of hospital and doctor visits, surgical procedures, and other treatments. Some of this variation is unexplained, in that it persists even after adjusting for factors such as case mix and physician payment systems. This variation instead may reflect the general consensus of the local medical community.[3,5,6] Rates of surgical procedures alone show up to 10-fold differences in procedure rates.[7] This variation in surgical procedures has been termed a "surgical signature".[8,9] When this unexplained variation is due to factors other than patient preference, one can argue that it represents *unwarranted variation*.

Categories of variation and preference-sensitive decisions

Dr Wennberg characterized this unwarranted variation into three types: the *underuse of effective care*, the *overuse of supply-sensitive care*, and the *misuse of preference-sensitive care*.[4] Effective care is defined as those interventions where evidence would routinely support their use; underuse of this type of care often is a patient safety issue. For example, the use of a beta-blocker in a patient with a myocardial event is considered standard of care. Underuse would occur if a beta-blocker is indicated but not prescribed for one of these patients.

Supply-sensitive care refers to care driven by an oversupply of resources such as specialists or hospital beds, and these excess resources result in an overuse of services. An example is the management of chronic illness. Variation exists because medical evidence is lacking to determine the appropriate use of resources, such as number of return visits or whether patients should be hospitalized or referred to specialists. Excess capacity will be filled in these situations. Finally, preference-sensitive care involves situations where treatment choices include multiple options with trade-offs between risks and benefits. Under these conditions, the choice of treatment should belong to the patient[4] or the patient may receive treatment they neither need nor want. For example, a Canadian study of patients with hip and knee arthritis showed that only 8–15% of patients eligible for arthroplasty definitely wanted to undergo the procedure.[10] As such, unwarranted variation in preference-sensitive care is considered a "misuse" of medical resources.

Variation in surgical decisions

Many surgical decisions fall into the category of preference-sensitive care. The amount of variation in these procedures can be more clearly illustrated with Medicare data collected in the Dartmouth Atlas Project. *Figure 12.1* displays what are called "turnip plots." These plots show rates of surgical procedures for hip fracture, knee replacement, hip replacement, and back surgery relative to the US average for Part A Medicare enrollees in 2007. Each dot on the plot represents one of the 306 HRRs. The scale on the y-axis ranges from 0.1 to 10.0. A dot at 3.0 would be an HRR that has three times the rate of surgeries as the US average; a dot at 1.0 would represent an HRR equal to the US average; and a dot at 0.5 would correspond to an HRR with a rate that is 50% *lower* than the national average. Variation increases as the plots become taller and narrower.

The turnip plot for hip fractures shows the least variation in procedure rates across the United States. The HRRs are tightly clustered together, with a coefficient of variation equal to 14.4. The coefficient of variation is the standard deviation (SD) divided by the mean, and commonly is used to represent the amount of variation within a particular measure or variable.[11] In comparison

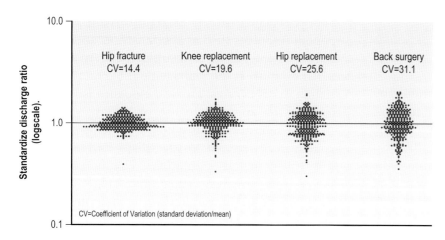

Fig. 12.1 "Turnip" plots showing rates of surgical procedures hip fracture, knee replacement, hip replacement and back surgery for Part A Medicare enrollees during 2007. Each dot represents the rate at one of the 306 Hospital Referral Regions (HRRs) relative to the US average (an average HRR would have a value of 1.0). The coefficient of variation is the standard deviation divided by the mean, used to represent variation within a particular measure or variable. (Data from the Dartmouth Atlas Project.)

with hip fracture, the coefficients of variation for knee replacement, hip replacement, and back surgery are 19.6, 25.6, and 31.1, respectively. Variation is lowest for hip fracture because surgical management of hip fracture is an accepted standard of care (or *effective care*). With effective care, preferences of the surgeon and the patient are closely matched. In contrast, surgical necessity for procedures like knee replacement, hip replacement, and back surgery is less well defined. This variability is reflected in the procedure rates.[8]

Plastic surgery is no exception. Postmastectomy reconstruction rates vary both across countries and within the United States.[12,13] In an analysis of 81 479 cancers, Polednak observed rates varying from 3.3% in Hawaii to 16% in Atlanta, even after adjusting for factors such as stage at diagnosis.[12]

These differences may be driven by regional opinion about whether or when these procedures are indicated. Or they may result from provider experience, preference, or personal opinion about which techniques provide the best outcome. Misinformation or lack of knowledge on the part of the referring provider also may cause variation in postmastectomy reconstruction rates.[14] Note, however, that all of these reasons revolve around the provider, not the patient. If reconstruction decisions were made based on patient-centric factors (all options made available to patients, and all risks and benefits clearly defined), we would expect to observe similar rates of each procedure across regions given a fixed patient profile.

One area of debate regarding physician and patient preference involves whether women with early stage breast cancer should be treated with breast conservation or mastectomy. Some authors believe high rates of mastectomy suggest that women are unaware that breast conservation is an option. Others believe that patient preference is being trumped by physician preference or by nonclinical factors such as the availability of radiation therapy required for breast conserving surgery.[15,16] High rates of breast conservation have been suggested as a quality measure. However, Collins *et al.*[17] showed that approximately 35% of well-informed women choose mastectomy, even when breast conservation surgery was an option. Therefore, high rates of breast conservation may not reflect patient preference. No-one can really say which rate is right. However, in situations where practice patterns differ and the choice will not affect survival, we should ask whether the patient was adequately and appropriately involved in the decision-making process.

When surgical procedures show an exceptionally high degree of variation, we need to evaluate how clinical decisions are made and determine whether patients have adequate knowledge and input to make an informed choice. Although the physician traditionally has directed healthcare decision-making, it is the patient who must live with the outcome. For preference-sensitive decisions, where multiple treatment options exist, patients should have the opportunity to decide on the best choice for them.

What about evidence?

Another reason for variation in preference-sensitive care is that even when there is a single best option, doctors may not be aware of it. There is a nearly endless array of medical evidence accumulating, and everyone in every specialty is challenged to keep up. In 1991, the Pew Health Commission estimated that if a conscientious health professional were to read two articles every day, in 1 year, he or she would be over 800 years behind in the literature.[18]

Worse than not knowing, clinicians may have strong evidence to dictate practice and be well aware of that evidence – yet still fail to act on it. The Rand Corporation conducted a study revealing that only 45% of adults presenting with an acute myocardial infarction received beta-blockers and only 39% of adults with pneumonia received the recommended care (Pneumovax, influenza vaccine, and antibiotics).[19]

Making matters even more complicated, medical evidence can be inconclusive, contradictory, or just plain wrong. John Ioannidis, a meta-researcher and expert on the credibility of medical research, estimates as much as 90% of published research is flawed. Why? In addition to the normal flaws inherent to medical research, at every step, there is an opportunity to conflate results and a clear intellectual conflict of interest to do so. In the "publish or perish" world of academic medicine, it is the eye-catching findings that get into top journals. Using a mathematical model that builds in even modest amounts of bias, Ioannidis predicted rates of incorrect findings at the rate they were later refuted at 80% for nonrandomized trials and 25% of randomized controlled trials.[20]

Risk communication

Even when we get the evidence right, clinicians are not well equipped to communicate risks and benefits of treatment choices effectively to patients. Risk communication is critically important to effective patient-centered communication, but the challenge begins at the most basic level. Individuals lack knowledge about health risks; even the risk of heart attack and stroke.[21] Being a patient does not necessarily improve one's knowledge either. A New Zealand study showed that patients' perceived risk of having a future heart attack was unrelated to age, sex, family history of MI, diabetes, smoking, or several other known heart attack risk factors.[22]

Risk language

However, improving risk communication requires more than just handing information to patients about risk factors. Edwards et al.[23] note the importance of moving beyond the traditional one-way dissemination of information from clinician to patient. They define risk communication as "the open two way exchange of information and opinion about risk, leading to better understanding and better decisions about clinical management". The "two way" portion is critically important, yet extremely challenging to do in practice.

One factor underlying this challenge is that many people (clinicians and patients alike) have low "statistical literacy" (sometimes referred to as low "numeracy"). This term refers to an inability to reason with or understand numbers and other mathematical concepts.[24,25] In an attempt to avoid the problems inherent in communicating statistical evidence, qualitative terms often are used. For example, "The risk of infection is 'rare' or 'unlikely'." But what does "rare" or "unlikely" mean? These terms are "elastic," in that they convey different meanings to different people under different circumstances.[23]

Figure 12.2 illustrates the problem with using this qualitative terminology. A group of doctors and administrators were asked the following question: "If you learn that the risk of a side effect from this medication is either rare, unlikely, probable, or very likely, what do you think is the probability (percentage chance) that it will occur? For example, if 'the risk of a side effect from this medication is certain,' you might enter 100%." The figure shows the distribution and range of responses to each of these qualitative terms. Although the lines trend towards more frequent events being assigned higher probabilities, the overlap across categories is considerable even among this very knowledgeable audience. Thus, simplifying language to avoid numbers actually may result in greater miscommunication.

While using real numbers avoids some confusion presented by qualitative terminology, *which* numbers to present provides enormous challenges as well. Medical evidence is described using terminology that could rightfully be labeled "jargon." Statistics such as *relative risk* or *number needed to treat* are unfamiliar to most individuals. It is important to translate these terms to

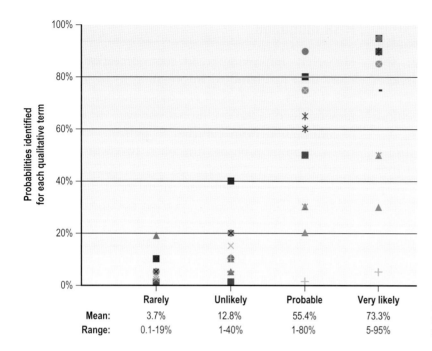

Fig. 12.2 Probabilities associated with qualitative terminology. Each data point is an individual response indicating the probability associated with each term (e.g., 'rarely').

	Rarely	Unlikely	Probable	Very likely
Mean:	3.7%	12.8%	55.4%	73.3%
Range:	0.1-19%	1-40%	1-80%	5-95%

language that is understandable by both the patient and physician.

Schwartz *et al.*[26] developed a numeracy scale with three questions to test the statistical literacy of individuals. The three questions involved converting a percentage to a proportion (1% to 10 in 1000); converting a proportion to a percentage (1 in 1000 to 0.1%); and basic probability ("How many heads in 1000 coin flips?"). In a representative sample of US adults aged 35–70, only 25% of the population (and only 27% of individuals with post-graduate degrees) could convert "1 in 1000" to 0.1%.[26] The other two questions had a higher percentage of correct answers, but these still ranged from just 60–86%, depending on the respondent's education. Schwartz *et al.* expanded this exercise to include other measures such as whether people could make comparisons (the Medical Data Interpretation Test).[27]

Absolute versus relative risk

Further complicating the situation is that medical results often are reported in relative terms. Relative risks are useful for making comparisons, but they tend to make effects appear larger than they would be if presented as absolute numbers. Woloshin and colleagues[28] present the example of an advertisement

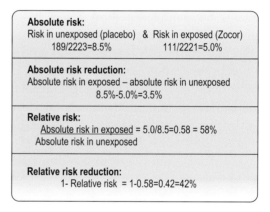

Fig. 12.3 Four statistics describing the effect of Zocor on heart attack deaths. (Data from Woloshin S, Schwartz LM, Welch HG. Know your chances: understanding health statistics. Berkeley: University of California Press; 2009.)

for the drug Zocor. The advertisement states that the drug provides a "42% reduction in heart attack death compared to a placebo." This effect sounds very large, but further inquiry shows that the 42% is a relative risk reduction. *Figure 12.3* shows how different statistics can be used to make the effect appear large or small.

The top box in *Figure 12.3* shows the absolute risk, or the effect of the drug in each group. According to the advertisement, among 2221 people in the study who took Zocor, 111 died of a heart attack, or 5%. The risk of heart attack death in the placebo group was 8.5%. Absolute risks include a *base rate*, or the overall *number* of people who were in each group. Absolute numbers make it easier to judge the true benefit of the drug because you can clearly determine the effect in each group. Note that these numbers (8.5% and 5.0%, and their *absolute risk reduction*, 3.5%) both sound much smaller than 42%.

Relative risks compare the effect of one treatment to another. If the risk is equal in both groups, the relative risk is equal to the number 1. In our example, the relative risk of heart attack death in the Zocor group compared with the placebo group is 5.0%/8.5% or 58%. If you subtract the relative risk from the number one, the result is 42% (1.00−0.58=0.42). This number is termed a *relative risk reduction*, and it describes how much *lower* the risk of heart attack death is in the Zocor group than it would be if the risks in the two groups were comparable. Woloshin *et al.*[28] compare these numbers to a sale at a store. A 50% discount on an item may sound very large, but whether it is worth buying depends on the base rate. For example, a 50% discount on a flat screen television is much different than a 50% discount on a tube of toothpaste in terms of the absolute dollars saved. The *base rate* matters.

Relative risks are useful and may be the only available statistic if the base rate is unknown (as in a case–control study). Relative risks also are useful for comparing treatments in a head to head trial. However, in much of medical writing and advertising, benefits are reported as relative risks and harms are reported as absolute risks. This bias in reporting results in patients overestimating benefits and underestimating the risk of harms. How widespread is this problem? A 2007 study found that one in three articles in the BMJ, Lancet and JAMA had mismatched framing of relative versus absolute risks for benefits and harms.[29] Even the United States Preventive Task Force's Guidelines for sigmoidoscopy use relative risks to describe benefits and absolute risk to describe potential harms.

Better data presentation

Visual aids

To avoid bias in presenting risk information and to improve patient decision-making, physicians need to understand the statistics and be able to present them in a transparent manner to patients. One helpful technique is to provide pictures rather than numbers to illustrate risk. *Figure 12.4* shows four types of graphs used to display information about a woman's lifetime risk of a breast cancer diagnosis.[30] The top left picture shows 100 figures of women. Nine of these figures, representing the overall lifetime risk of breast cancer, are colored in gray. This type of display provides information both on the number of people who get the disease and the number of people who do NOT get the disease. The bottom left picture shows a simple percentage (9% out of 100%). The top right compares the risk of breast cancer to the risk of getting other diseases. Comparing risks to some other baseline is a helpful way to put a risk into perspective. The 9% may sound quite large, but it is very small compared to the risk of heart disease. The chart in the bottom right is similar to the first chart. A total of 100 boxes are drawn, and nine of them (representing the 9%) are colored in. However, the colored boxes are *randomly* distributed throughout the full set of 100 boxes. This type of display is useful for conveying the chance nature of developing a disease, but it is not as useful for helping individuals judge the magnitude of the risk.

Balanced framing

An important aspect of both the top left and bottom right pictures is that both allow for visualization of who avoids developing a disease. Presenting data in this manner is referred to *balanced framing*. Balanced framing is important because framing decisions in only a positive or a negative frame will change the individual's perception of the size of the risk. For example, patients who were told a procedure was 99% safe greatly preferred it over a procedure that had a 1% risk of complications, even though these are exactly the same data.[25] In general, it is most effective to give your patients risk information in both positive and negative terms. For example, say "The risk of death from this procedure is 1 in 1000. This means that 1 out of every 1000 people who have this procedure will die, and 999 out of every 1000 people who have this procedure will survive."

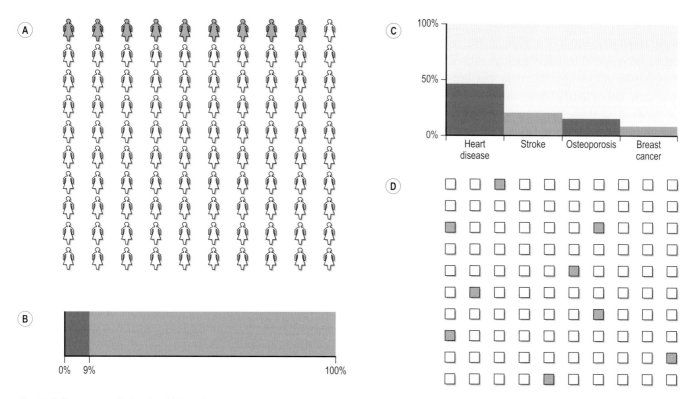

Fig. 12.4 Four ways to display visual information about a woman's lifetime risk of breast cancer. (With permission from Apter AJ, Paasche-Orlow MK, Remillard JT, *et al.* Numeracy and communication with patients: they are counting on us. J Gen Intern Med 2008; 23(12):2117–2124.)

Teach-back method

Finally, when presenting risk data it is useful to build in a method to check that the person you are communicating with understands what you have told them. Employing a "teach-back" (or "show-me") method can help clinicians determine whether the patient's perceptions match the clinician's.[31] Ask patients to say what they will tell a family member about the clinical conversation. This exercise can help reveal areas where communication still is unclear.

Creating a high quality decision

Understanding variation in practice and the challenges of risk communication is important, because actively involving patients in decision-making results in better decision quality. Helping patients achieve high quality decisions for preference-sensitive conditions requires that they have adequate decision-specific knowledge and an understanding of their personal values so that their treatment choice is consistent with those values.[32]

One way to achieve these goals is through *decision aids*. Good decision aids move beyond dissemination of information; they provide both the requisite knowledge and also engage patients in a values-clarification process. A Cochrane Collaboration meta-analysis of available randomized controlled trials[33] defined the aims of decision aids as *providing evidence-based information*; helping patients *recognize and clarify the values-sensitive nature of the decision*; and *providing structured guidance in making a decision and communicating* with others involved in the decision (e.g., clinician, family, friends).

This same study found evidence for the efficacy of decision aids. Overall, decision aids *increased patient involvement* in the decision. They *reduced decisional conflict associated with feeling uninformed, decisional conflict related to personal values*, and *conflict related to the decision after the intervention*. For some elective invasive surgical procedures, decision aids decreased the rate of surgery without affecting health outcomes or patient satisfaction.

Decision aids that are evidence-based

Standards have been adopted for assessing whether decision aids meet stringent criteria. The International Patient Decision Aid Standards (IPDAS) group was established by a set of interested experts, stakeholders and practitioners (see http://ipdas.ohri.ca/resources.html). They developed a checklist of criteria to assess and ensure the quality of decision aids. These include:

1. Systematic development process
2. Decision aid acceptability and balance
3. Up-to-date evidence
4. Disclosure of interests
5. Plain language
6. Internet delivery guidelines
7. Information about options
8. Risk communication
9. Values clarification
10. Structured guidance in deliberation and communication
11. Balanced display
12. Decision process.

Decision aids that meet IPDAS standards inform patients about treatment options and accurately specify benefits and risks in understandable terms. An inventory of decision aids, including a generic decision aid called the "Ottawa Personal Inventory Guide," is available on the University of Ottawa website (http://www.ohri.ca/DecisionAid/). It is important to note that decision aids serve as a guide in patient discussions with their clinicians and other interested parties, such as family members. But decision aids are designed to be adjunct to counseling. They support, rather than replace, the patient–provider conversation.

Shared decision-making

Evidence, risk communication, and decision aids are designed to help foster shared decision-making (SDM), which puts this knowledge into practice. Shared decision-making is defined as decisions that are shared by clinicians and patients, informed by the best evidence, and weighted according to the preferences and values of the patient.[34] It has been argued that SDM can reduce unwarranted variation in preference-sensitive care.[34,35] How does the shared decision-making process work in practice? SDM can be implemented in numerous ways; we describe how shared decision is used for breast cancer treatment at one academic medical center.[36]

A shared decision-making process

Figure 12.5 shows a flowchart of the process a woman goes through when diagnosed with early stage breast cancer at this institution. The process generally begins after an image guided needle biopsy by the radiologist. The radiologist generally informs the patient of the diagnosis, and often a social worker is present during that conversation. If not, the social worker will call the patient to provide support and answer questions. The social worker helps the patient understand the steps that will occur through the treatment process. The social worker also coordinates with the surgical schedulers to set-up the patient's necessary appointments, the first of which usually is with a surgical oncologist.

Once the diagnosis is made, a decision aid entitled "Early stage breast cancer: Choosing your surgery" (Health Dialog©, 2002–2009) automatically is sent to a patient's home. Decision aids about reconstruction and chemotherapy also may be sent if applicable. For example, the reconstruction DVD contains questions like: Do you want reconstruction? When to have a reconstruction? What type of reconstruction do you want? This preparation is useful because it gives the patient time before meeting with a surgeon to think about the options, to review the material, and to integrate the information they have just heard. They can watch the DVD or read the pamphlet with family members. These decision aids are updated regularly so that they provide the most current state of the evidence, and where uncertainty exists, it is explained. Patients get a more realistic view of what benefits their treatments might provide.

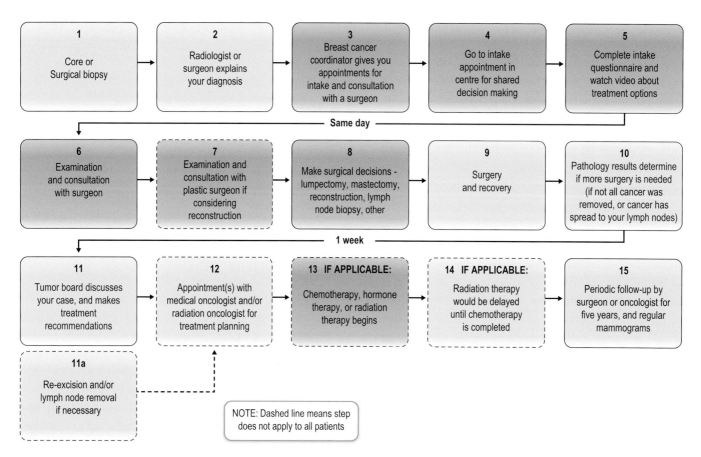

Fig. 12.5 Algorithm showing the treatment process for a patient with early stage breast cancer. Orange boxes show where shared decision-making is involved or decision aids are or can be used.

Decision quality reports

When patients meet with their surgeon after viewing a decision aid, their questions are focused specifically on the issues that are of most concern to them. The surgeon's time is used more effectively, because the surgeon does not have to review all details of every option. The surgeon's role is to help patients weigh the options, answer questions, and guide the patient towards the best decision for that individual. In some cases, a "Decision Quality Report" is provided to the surgeon ahead of time. Along with some general patient data, this report contains the results of the knowledge and values questions contained in the decision aid.

The decision quality report can identify a mismatch between what the patient is communicating and what they really feel. The decision quality report example in

Figure 12.6 is based on a real patient seen by the senior author (DC). This woman had chosen mastectomy and was being seen to discuss reconstruction options. She placed a high value on keeping her breast and avoiding reconstruction, and a low value on removing her breast for peace of mind. The report also indicated that she did not understand the knowledge questions on recurrence and survival. This revealed that she did not have the facts needed to make an informed decision. So, rather than discuss treatment choices for reconstruction, the discussion focused on surgical options for early stage breast cancer. This patient ultimately went on to choose breast conservation over mastectomy. Without the decision quality report, her surgeon would have been unaware that the patient had basic misunderstandings about the options and the conversation would have likely focused on reconstructive options only *(Box 12.1)*.

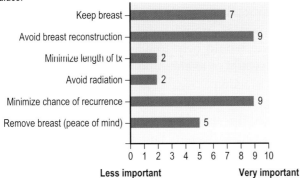

Decision Making
Leaning toward: Mastectomy and reconstruction
Sure about choice: Unsure

Knowledge:
 Understands:

☐ survival rates
☐ recurrence rates

Values:

Fig. 12.6 Decision quality report showing a treatment choice that is uninformed and inconsistent with the woman's personal values.

Box 12.1 Patient case study

Dr Collins was seeing a patient in consultation for breast reconstruction. The patient had already met with a surgical breast oncologist and she indicated that she was having a mastectomy. She was very quiet, offering little about her preferences. She confirmed that she had watched a video-based decision aid on breast reconstruction, but had not reached any conclusion about which option she would prefer. As Dr Collins went on to probe, she noted the decision quality report on the choice for mastectomy versus breast conservation *(Fig. 12.6)*. The surgeon noticed that she had scored highly the values questions that would typically predict a choice of breast conservation ("Keep breast" and "Avoid breast reconstruction,") and low on the option that is most associated with mastectomy ("Remove breast for peace of mind") had a low score. In addition, the patient did not understand the key knowledge questions (the boxes are not checked) about the equivalence of survival and the similar rates of recurrence associated with each option. Dr Collins then realized the patient may not have a sufficient understanding of her surgical options for breast cancer. So, rather than continue to discuss options for reconstruction, the plastic surgeon reviewed the surgical options for early stage breast cancer. The patient went on to choose breast conservation.

The value proposition for shared decision-making

There is an ongoing push for greater clinical efficiency in order to maintain revenues at the *status quo*. At the same time, clinicians must evaluate and inform patients about increasingly complex treatment options – often in situations where the evidence may be lacking or inadequate. The end result is that there is less time for meaningful interactions between clinicians and patients, while the need for discussion is greater than ever. The experience at this and other medical centers that have implemented shared decision-making indicates that incorporating evidence-based decision aids can improve the quality and efficiency of the clinical encounter.

Patients' perception of SDM

In our medical center example, patients are highly satisfied with the decision aids and with the SDM process. Patients surveyed after using decision aids felt their understanding of options was improved. Several patients noted they were more comfortable with their treatment decision and experienced less decisional conflict after using decision aids. Patients also felt the process improved relationships with their providers.[17]

Surgeons' acceptance of shared decision-making

Surgeons need to feel that shared decision-making will improve the care they give in order to adopt the practice. Orthopedic surgeons treating patients with knee and hip osteoarthritis were surveyed to evaluate their attitudes towards the shared decision-making process.[37] These surgeons gave high ratings to the use of decision aids in the treatment of their patients. The decision aids were noted to be helpful in educating patients about surgical and nonsurgical options and helped to identify patients' preferences in developing a treatment plan. Similar acceptance was noted among back surgeons.

However, even with these gains, implementing decision aids is challenging. Despite both patient and surgeon acceptance of decision aids, there is still a low level of utilization of the decision aids in many clinical services where they could be used. The greatest uptake has occurred where these tools automatically are given or sent to patients diagnosed with a specific condition (as with breast cancer patients). Further implementation of shared decision-making will require greater education and training on the part of both physicians and patients.

Looking forward: informed consent versus informed choice

O'Connor and others argue that implementation of decision aids will occur once a "tipping point" is reached, and when informed patient choice becomes the standard of practice.[3,35] They contend that informed patient choice could replace the legal standard of informed consent for preference-sensitive care. Informed consent in different states is divided into a patient-based standard and physician-based standard.[38] In the physician-based standard, the physician must inform the patient of risks, benefits and alternatives that would be considered standard for a practitioner in that field. A patient-based standard involves also informing the patient of all of the above risks, benefits and alternatives, but is based on what a *patient* would find significant.[38]

Is informed consent merely the time when we obtain a signature on a consent form? The consent process should include time spent communicating with the patient about the risks and benefits of a given procedure. How we go about this process revolves around the legal considerations. Most valuable to the patient is actually defining the important issues, such as whether or not a treatment or procedure is worth the potential or likely undesirable outcomes, or whether that individual will experience the benefits. Implicit in defining whether or not the patient will accept the potential risks is determining the patient's values in making a decision.

Krumholz[39] suggests a way to standardize consent for elective procedures in order to facilitate an informed decision making process. He advocates for a patient-centered approach that would provide "core information" written by experts and given to patients at least 1 day before treatment. The document would look quite different from the common consent form we currently are accustomed to because it would include details about all available options. Krumholz notes five critical elements needed for this form: information about risks, benefits, alternatives, experience, and cost. His editorial proposes a standardized consent form for percutaneous coronary intervention and provides an example.

This form would help ensure that the patient is driving the decision. It would foster patient-centered communication by requiring a standard conversation to occur between the provider and the patient. Ideally, this conversation would help to alleviate issues associated with unexpected outcomes and would improve overall patient satisfaction.

This type of consent form does have limitations. The authors note the challenge of individualizing the form – providers may be reluctant to share data on their experience or the data simply may not be available, and the evidence related to the patient's own risk might not be known. Yet true patient-centered communication requires an attempt at this type of transparency.

Summary

Health decisions, particularly preference-sensitive decisions, are complicated. Individuals differentially value trade-offs between benefits and harms and these values should be incorporated into the patient–provider interaction. Taking time to include the patient and to make sure he or she understands all available options with their associated benefits and risks may sound time consuming and contrary to today's efforts to do more with less. However, shared decision-making has been shown to improve both the quality of care and the efficiency of the patient–provider interaction. Its goal is to avoid a misuse of services, and to achieve the "right rate" of surgical treatments and procedures based on the patients' informed choice.

 Access the complete references list online at **http://www.expertconsult.com**

1. Berwick DM, Nolan TW, Whittington J. The triple aim: care, health, and cost. *Health Aff (Millwood)*. 2008;27(3): 759–769.
   This paper from the Institute for Healthcare Improvement (IHI) proposes an agenda for providing the best care for the entire population at the lowest cost. The second aim is to enhance the patient care experience. This would include patient-centered health communication, providing the patient has the knowledge and authority to make decisions about their medical care.

3. Wennberg JE, O'Connor AM, Collins ED, et al. Extending the P4P agenda, Part 1: How Medicare can

improve patient decision making and reduce unnecessary care. *Health Aff (Millwood)*. 2007;26(6):1564–1574.

A seminal paper on variation in medical practice. This work defines population-based rates using hospital referral regions. This was the first paper in the USA to describe marked geographic variation in practice.

6. Wennberg JE, Fisher ES, Skinner JS, et al. Extending the P4P agenda, Part 2: How Medicare can reduce waste and improve the care of the chronically ill. *Health Aff (Millwood)*. 2007;26(6):1575–1585.

10. Hawker GA, Wright JG, Coyte PC, et al. Determining the need for hip and knee arthroplasty: the role of clinical severity and patients' preferences. *Med Care*. 2001;39(3):206–216.

23. Edwards A, Elwyn G, Mulley A. Explaining risks: turning numerical data into meaningful pictures. *Br Med J*. 2002;324(7341):827–830.

24. Gigerenzer G, Gaissmaier W, Kurz-Milcke E, et al. Helping doctors and patients make sense of health statistics. *Psycholog Sci Public Int*. 2008;8(2):53–96.

This paper outlines the challenges and presents strategies for communicating health statistics to patients, clinicians, and the general public. Exposes common practices that make it difficult to convey numeric information in an easily understood form.

28. Woloshin S, Schwartz LM, Welch HG. *Know your chances: Understanding health statistics*. Berkeley: University of California Press; 2009.

29. Sedrakyan A, Shih C. Improving depiction of benefits and harms: analyses of studies of well-known therapeutics and review of high-impact medical journals. *Med Care*. 2007;45(10 Suppl 2):S23–S28.

32. Sepucha KR, Fowler FJ Jr, Mulley AG Jr. Policy support for patient-centered care: the need for measurable improvements in decision quality. *Health Aff (Millwood)*. 2004;(Suppl Web Exclusives):VAR54–VAR62.

38. King JS, Moulton BW. Rethinking informed consent: the case for shared medical decision-making. *Am J Law Med*. 2006;32(4):429–501.

These lawyers make the legal case for shared decision-making and informed patient choice.

39. Krumholz HM. Informed consent to promote patient-centered care. *JAMA*. 2010;303(12):1190–1191.

Harlan Krumholz suggests a reworking of the informed consent document to include elements not currently included in routine practice. These include alternative treatments with associated risks and benefits, cost of treatment, and practice volume.

13

Imaging in reconstructive breast surgery

Jaume Masia, Carmen Navarro, and Juan A. Clavero

SYNOPSIS

- DIEP is the the most used flap for an autologous breast reconstruction.
- Perforator vessels arising from the deep inferior epigastric system are anatomically highly variable regarding their number, location, caliber and relationships with surrounding structures.
- The ideal perforator should have a large caliber, a short intramuscular course, the easiest dissection, a suitable location within the flap and subcutaneous branching with intra-flap axiality.
- Nowadays Imaging techniques (DMCT and MRI) have become the favorite techniques for the preoperative study of these patientes.
- Imaging techniques provide anatomical images that allow us not only to locate the dominant perforator but also extra information about the vessels and donor area.
- It is essential to have a good assesment protocol of the images to select the most suitable perforator.

Access the Historical Perspective section online at
http://www.expertconsult.com

Introduction

Surgical techniques for breast reconstruction have been greatly refined in last decades and important landmarks have been achieved. Autologous reconstruction with microsurgical flaps marked a before and after in breast reconstruction because the aesthetic outcome is improved, a prosthesis is not needed and long-term results are good. Different types of flaps have been used to create a new breast with similar characteristics in shape, size, contour and position to the contralateral one. The preferred donor site for this purpose is the abdominal wall. The skin and subcutaneous fatty tissues of the lower abdomen provide tissue that has a soft texture that is perfect for breast reconstruction and donor site morbidity is minimal.[1-3] In function of these advantages the DIEP flap has become the "gold standard" for breast reconstruction in many hospitals.[4]

Abdominal perforator vessels vary greatly in size and distribution from one patient to another, and, even from one hemi-abdomen to the other in the same patient. As the anatomy of these vessels is not constant, it is helpful to have a preoperative method that provides an overall view of the distribution of the abdominal vascular anatomy. In the search for refinements in planning perforator flaps, several techniques have been described for the preoperative evaluation of donor areas. Although most of them were initially described to study the abdominal area, they are useful for preoperative evaluation of other flaps, such as the SGAP. Imaging techniques have led to a revolution in preoperative mapping of donor areas in breast reconstruction patients. Multidetector-row computed tomography (MDCT) and magnetic resonance imaging (MRI) can provide anatomical images with detailed information about the caliber, location and course of the main vessels and their perforators and can therefore play a vital role in the preoperative investigation of perforating vessels.

Defining the ideal perforator vessel

The two flaps most commonly used for autologous breast reconstruction are DIEP and SGAP. In both cases, perforator vessels arising from the source vessels are extremely variable and it is hard to predict how many are present, what their caliber is, where they pierce the fascia, and what course they take within the muscle. Therefore it is very useful to have a reliable preoperative method to locate the best supplying perforator. Several factors must be taken into account when we are selecting this best perforator. The ideal perforator should have a large caliber, a short intramuscular course, the easiest dissection, a suitable location within the flap and subcutaneous branching with intra-flap axiality. In some cases of DIEP, we can find paramuscular vessels that initially follow a retromuscular plane before piercing the muscular fascia in the exact abdominal midline. Many of these perforators have a good caliber and good arborization in the subcutaneous tissue and could be considered to be the ideal perforators because their course facilitates the surgical dissection (*Figs 13.1, 13.2*).[19]

In view of the difficulties in finding the best perforator in the donor areas, it is of great help to dispose of a technique that locates the individual perforating vessels and allows qualitative preoperative evaluation. This is possible with imaging techniques. MDCT and MRI provide anatomical images that delineate the main vessels, their course and their relationship with the surrounding structures. Studying all this information before surgery, surgeons can decide in advance which perforator they are to center the flap on or which hemi-abdomen or buttock should be used.

Conventional preoperative mapping methods in perforator flaps

Before imaging techniques were described for the study of abdominal perforators, the two most widely used approaches were hand-held Doppler ultrasound and color Doppler imaging. Below is a brief summary of these techniques.

Hand-held Doppler ultrasound

Hand-held Doppler ultrasound was the first method described for the study of perforators. It is still the most widely used method to locate a perforator, due to its low cost and simplicity of use. The information it offers, however, is limited. It does not distinguish between perforating vessels and main axial vessels. Furthermore, the relationship between acoustic signal and vessel size is unreliable and fails to determine the size of the vessel. Besides, this technique has shown an unacceptable

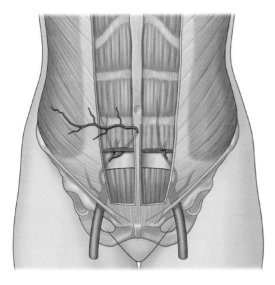

Fig. 13.1 Paramuscular perforator of the deep epigastric vessels with its medial location.

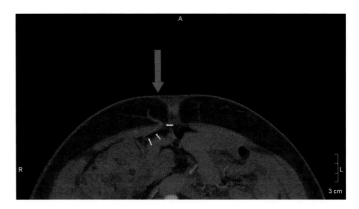

Fig. 13.2 Axial MDCT image of a paramuscular perforator of the deep epigastric vessels with its branching in the subcutaneous tissue. Yellow arrows indicate the course of the paramuscular perforator. Magenta arrow indicates the point in which the perforator arises from the fascia.

number of false positives and tiny vessels can be confused acoustically with a good perforator.[7,8] But despite these drawbacks, hand-held Doppler ultrasound remains useful in our daily practice and can still be useful for specific indications, such as to assess the location and the course of the superficial epigastric vessels.

Color Doppler imaging

Color Doppler imaging of the donor area provides much more reliable information than Doppler sonography.[9] It can identify and locate the dominant perforators. It is very sensitive and it provides information about the caliber and blood flow of the main vessels and perforators. It provides dynamic information on vessel flow, but flow rates may not always reflect the absolute size of the perforator. Vessel damage caused by atherosclerosis, previous surgery or blood vessel disorders and congenital abnormalities or anatomical variants can be diagnosed. However, this method also has some significant drawbacks. It is a long test, possibly lasting up to an hour, and this can be uncomfortable for patients as they have to remain in the same position during the procedure. In addition it is technician-dependent and the radiologist who performs the technique must have a sound knowledge of perforator surgery.

Imaging techniques in breast reconstruction

Imaging techniques have revolutionized the preoperative mapping of abdominal perforators. The first studies on their application were published in the preoperative evaluation of breast reconstruction patients,[10] and since then, MRI and MDCT have become the preferred technique for the study of these patients.[12]

With the incorporation of imaging techniques for mapping the abdominal vascularization, we are not only able to locate the dominant perforators but we also receive extra information about the vessels and the donor area, thanks to the anatomical images that these methods provide. The two imaging techniques used are the MDCT and, more recently, the MRI. Both of them have shown they are highly reliable methods for the preoperative study of the abdominal perforators. By providing anatomical images, they inform us about the

number of perforators, their location, their intramuscular course and their distribution inside the subcutaneous tissue. They have 100% sensitivity and specificity at the time of locating the dominant perforator, and they are also technically reproducible. This last characteristic is especially handy, as it means we can record the information on a CD or pen-drive and have it at our disposition at the moment of surgery. Besides, the increased spatial resolution offered by MDCT and MRI allows highly accurate multiplanar and 3D reconstructed images, creating a 3-dimensional map of the perforating vessels. Another advantage is the fact that they provide an anatomical reference of the area. This is particularly useful in patients who have had previous surgeries because it identifies any possible changes that may have taken place in the vascularization or surrounding tissues. They have also reduced surgery time and the number of complications.[10,11]

It should also be mentioned that MDCT is very fast to perform and a considerable number of thin sliced CT images are obtained in a short time. The quality of the images is superior to MRI, especially in the capacity of three-dimensional reconstruction *(Fig. 13.3)*. In spite of all its advantages, the MDCT has two clear drawbacks. The first is the radiation the patient receives when the test is performed (effective dose is 5.6 mSv, similar to conventional abdominal CT-scan). However, the effective dose of radiation used with this technique is 5.6 mSv, which is less than that used for an opaque enema or a conventional abdominal CT scan. The second drawback of the MDCT is the need to administer an intravenous

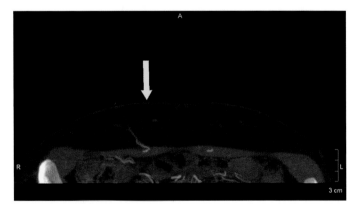

Fig. 13.3 Axial MDCT image of an intramuscular perforator of the deep epigastric vessels with its branching. Yellow arrow indicates the point in which the perforator pierces the fascia.

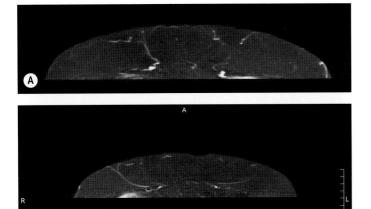

Fig. 13.4 (A,B) Axial non contrast-MRI images showing the course of some intramuscular perforators arising from the deep epigastric vessels.

medium; this is uncomfortable for the patient and can cause allergic reactions.

On the other hand, although the quality of the images is not so good, with the MRI, we avoid the unnecessary radiation to the patient. And more recently, with the noncontrast MRI, we can obtain good quality images avoiding the administration of intravenous contrast (see *Fig. 13.4*).[18]

Radiological protocol of the acquisition sequence

MDCT

The machine the authors use in our practice today is a 64 or 320 crown multidetector-row CT scanner (Aquilion 16; Toshiba Medical, Tokyo, Japanthe). However, a scanner of 16 crowns is sufficient to acquire the necessary information for an adequate perforator mapping. The study is conducted according to the following parameters: 120 kVp; 80–120 mAs (0.4 s gantry rotation period); detector configuration 64 × 0.5 mm; 54-mm table travel per rotation; 512 × 512 matrix; and a 180–240 field of view. To conduct the test, it is necessary to use 100 mL i.v. nonionic iodinated contrast medium with a concentration of 300 mg L/mL (Xenetix 300 [iobitridol]; laboratories Guerbet, Paris, France).

It should be emphasized that when performing the MDCT, patients must be positioned in the same position they will be placed for surgery. Patients for a reconstruction with a DIEP flap are placed supine. If an SGAP is to be performed, however, the patient is placed prone or lateral, according to surgeon preference. In the study of the abdominal area, images are obtained from 5 cm above the umbilicus to the lesser trochanter of the hip during a single breath-hold of approximately 10–12 s. When the study is done in the gluteal area, the sections are obtained from the lower back to below the infragluteal crease. The technique is fast to perform and the acquisition time is about 3–4 s. The whole procedure does not thus exceed 10 min and it is well tolerated by the patients. The volumetric data acquired are then used to reconstruct images with a slice width of 1 mm and a reconstruction interval of 0.8 mm. The set of reconstructed images is then automatically transferred to a computer workstation (Vitrea version 4.0.1, Vital Images, Plymouth, MN). Next, the reformatted images are generated on multiple planes (coronal, axial, sagittal and oblique) and in three-dimensional volume rendered images. The captured images can be stored on a CD or pen-drive and for later viewing on a conventional computer.[20]

Noncontrast MRI

Images are obtained with the patient positioned as for surgery. Unlike MDCT during this test, the patient does not require intravenous contrast administration, so there is no need for fasting. We use high speed parallel imaging (speeder technology) to obtain accelerated scan times. In a first step, sagittal scouts are acquired to delimit the study zone. After this, a sequence phase 3D+5_FSfbi is implemented in the anterior coronal plane, using the following parameters: TR: 2694, TE:80, slice thickness 1.5 mm, number of slices: 50, number of acquisitions: one, 512 × 512 matrix, field of view 380 × 380 mm, TI:160 and resp + ECG gate. A sequence phase 3D+5_FSfbi is then performed in the axial plane using the following parameters: TR:2900, TE:78, slice thickness 3 mm, number of slices: 56, number of acquisition: one, 704 × 704 matrix, field of view 380 × 380 mm, TI:160 and resp + ECG gate. This technique takes longer than MDCT, lasting between 10 and 20 min. Multiplanar formatted images and 3D volume rendered images are regenerated on a Vitrea computer workstation (Vitrea version 4.0.1. Vital Images, Plymouth, MN).[18]

How to select the most suitable perforator

The images obtained after the study are assessed jointly by the radiologist and plastic surgeon. When choosing the best perforator several factors must be considered. It is important to assess the size of the vessels. Obviously, the higher the caliber, the more preferred the perforator. It is important to assess the caliber of the vessel at the suprafascial level. Its location must also be considered; those in a medial position are preferred. We also evaluate the course of the perforator, and a paramuscular route is more desirable than an intramuscular one. In the case of intramuscular perforators, it is preferable that the course within the associated muscle be as short as possible. It is also important to assess the arborization of the perforator in the subcutaneous tissue. We then choose the most suitable perforator for irrigating the flap.

The DIEP flap is the most commonly used flap for autologous breast reconstruction and a series of steps should be followed to assess the images. The first step is to select the most suitable perforator. This will allow us to establish x/y coordinates centered on the umbilicus. With MDCT and MRI, the images are obtained in axial, sagittal and coronal views. Axial and sagittal views are extremely useful for evaluating the characteristics of the different perforators, their relationship with the muscle and the level at which they pierce the fascia. With the images of the study, we can also assess the relationship of the perforator with the deep epigastric and the superficial systems. Extrapolating all this information, we can mark the skin of the patient at the exact point where the selected perforator pierces the fascia and enters in the subcutaneous tissue.

Images are evaluated in the following order:

Step 1: Study of the images in an axial view. The first point to assess is the characteristics of deep and superficial epigastric systems from their origin to 5 cm cranial to the umbilicus. In function of their caliber we identify the best perforator vessels on each side. Once the best are selected, we study their relation with the muscle and their distribution in the subcutaneous tissue. In the axial cuts, we also assess the superficial epigastric system. We consider that the artery is a good gauge when its diameter is greater than 0.6 mm and that is when we consider the possibility of a superficial inferior epigastric

artery flap *(Fig. 13.5)*. When we find the best perforator, we mark an arrow at the exact point where it pierces the fascia. This arrow remains as we assess all the images, allowing us to measure the distance from the arrow to the midline. The value

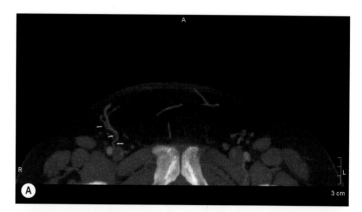

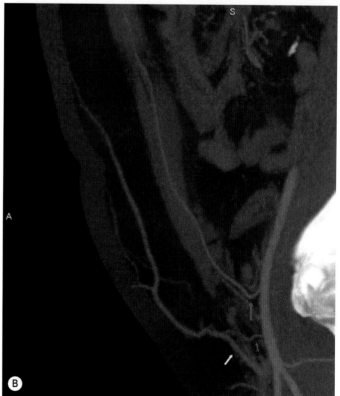

Fig. 13.5 Images showing a good superficial inferior epigastric system. **(A)** Axial MDCT image showing the superficial inferior epigastric artery arising from the femoral artery and its branching in the subcutaneous tissue. Yellow arrows indicate the origin and course of the superficial inferior epigastric artery. **(B)** Sagittal view MDCT image of the same patient showing both superficial and deep epigastric systems and their connections. Magenta arrows indicate the origin of the deep and superficial inferior epigastric arteries. Yellow arrow indicates the origin of the superficial vein.

obtained is the "x" used in the coordinate system centered on the umbilicus.

Step 2: Study of the images in a sagittal view. After studying axial images, we value the best perforators in the sagittal view. We measure the distance from the output of the selected perforator to the level of the umbilicus, thus obtaining the "y" value of our coordinate axis. With the sagittal view we also appreciate the connections between the superficial and deep epigastric systems.

Step 3: A three-dimensional reconstruction of the abdomen. Next we perform a 3D reconstruction of the abdomen to precisely locate the points on the skin surface where the best perforators emerge from the fascia of the rectus abdominis muscle. Using a virtual coordinate system with the umbilicus at the centre, all information is transferred to a data form sheet so that the perforators are mapped in a format that allows us to transpose their position preoperatively onto the patient's abdomen *(Fig. 13.6)*.

Step 4: Study of the images in a coronal view. To complete the assessment we look at the coronal cuts. This allows us to visualize the arborization in the subcutaneous tissue of the superficial epigastric system and its connections with the deep system *(Fig. 13.7)*.

Therefore, depending on the findings of the images provided by the MDCT or the MRI, we will decide which vessel is going to nourish the flap. The first point to check is the superficial system. If the superficial vessels have a good caliber, i.e., more than 0.6 mm, and a medial distribution in the abdomen, a SIEA flap could be performed. When there is not a good superficial system, we will consider the deep epigastric system. The second aspect is to search for a good paramuscular perforator. If we find a suitable one, we will center the flap on it, as its dissection is easier and faster. If we do not find a good paramuscular perforator, we will choose an intramuscular one. Several factors must be taken into account when we are selecting the perforator that is going to nourish the flap. Whenever possible a direct branch from the deep inferior epigastric artery and the one with the shortest intramuscular course will be selected as our perforator. The location of the perforator should be as central as possible within the flap and it should have a good intraflap axiality and subcutaneous branching.

To evaluate images in patients, candidates for a SGAP flap, the coordinate axis, will be centered on the coccyx at the beginning of the intergluteal fold *(Fig. 13.8)*.

Conclusion

The popularity of perforator flap surgery for breast reconstruction has grown rapidly over the last few years. Locating perforating vessels so as to raise these flaps is a difficult task and much effort has been devoted to finding preoperative methods that can guide us about their location in each patient.

Since the first reports on MDCT appeared, many centers have focused on developing and improving this technique. MDCT today is considered the technique of choice in the preoperative evaluation of patients who are candidates for autologous breast reconstruction. In the continuing search for the ideal technique and to minimize the disadvantages of MDCT, many eyes are presently on MRI and results to date seem promising.

With MDCT and MRI we have achieved a breakthrough in the preoperative evaluation of the perforator surgery. Compared with the hand-held Doppler and color Doppler imaging, the advantages are multiple. They have clearly proven to be a reliable method for the vascular mapping of the abdominal wall, and they do not show false negatives and false positives. They delineate the dominant perforator, its intramuscular course, and its relationship with the surrounding structures, thereby reducing the duration of surgery and postoperative complications. In addition, they are reproducible, allowing us to check the information at the time of the surgery. They are fast to perform and well tolerated by patients. Another advantage is that surgeon stress is lower because they enable preoperative planning of the surgery.

As part of breast reconstruction, over the last few years, we have begun to incorporate lymphatic surgery, so as to minimize the consequences of the oncological breast surgery. We combine two techniques: lymphovenous anastomosis and lymph node transfer. For both techniques, we use imaging techniques in a preoperative study. To prepare the lymph node transfer, we use MDCT to locate the superficial epigastric lymph nodes and

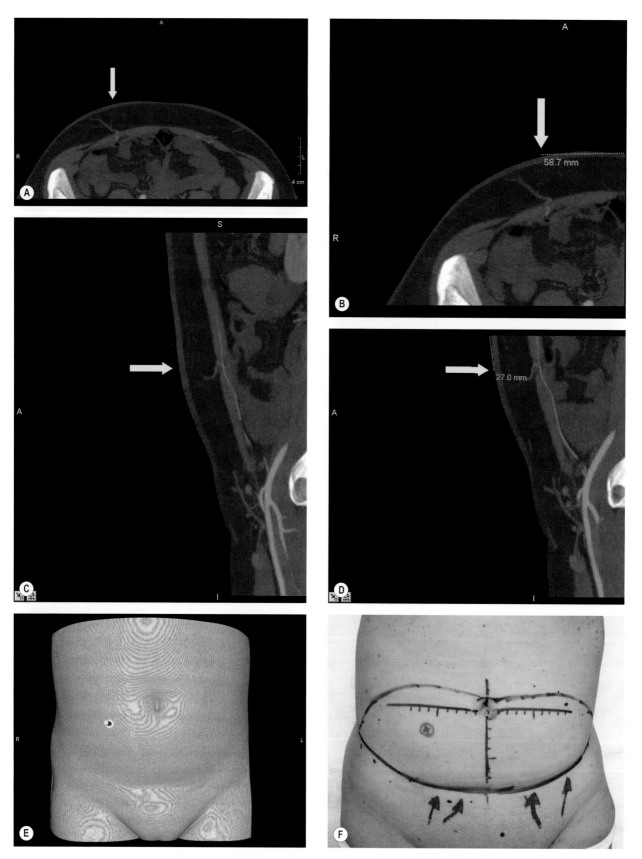

Fig. 13.6 Protocol for images assessment. **(A)** Axial MDCT image showing the most suitable abdominal perforator in this patient. The yellow arrow indicates the point where the perforator arises from the muscle. **(B)** We measure the distance from the midline to the perforator in the axial view, and this is given the value of "x". **(C)** Sagittal MDCT image showing the perforator. The yellow arrow indicates the point where the perforator pierces the fascia. **(D)** The second measure is done in the sagittal view measuring from the umbilicus level to the exit of the perforator. This will be the "y" value. **(E)** MDTC 3-D reconstruction for the same patient. The yellow arrow indicates the exactly point where the perforator pierces the fascia. **(F)** Preoperative markings in the patient with the dominant perforator located.

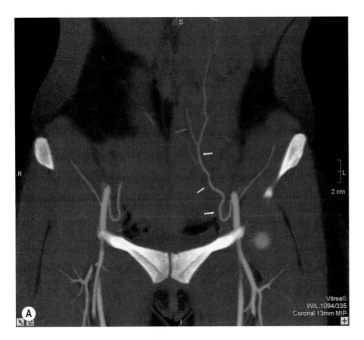

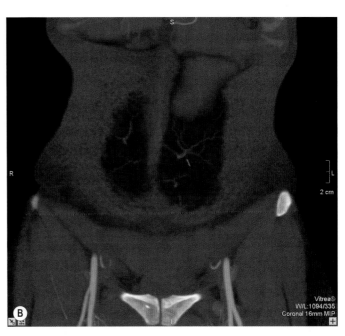

Fig. 13.7 (A) Deep level: Coronal image showing the course of the deep epigastric vessels (yellow arrows) and the origin of the main perforator (magenta arrow). **(B)** Superficial level: Coronal image showing the perforator connecting with the superficial vascular network. Magenta arrow marks the same perforator.

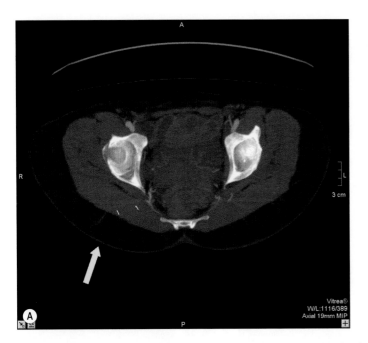

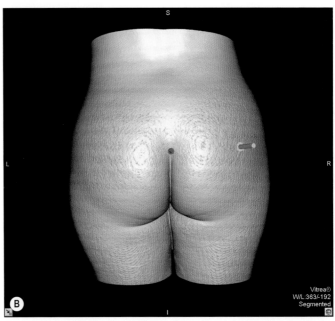

Fig. 13.8 (A) Axial MDCT image of an intramuscular perforator of the superior gluteal artery in a patient candidate for a reconstruction with a SGAP flap. The yellow arrow indicates the point where the perforator pierces the fascia. The small arrows indicate its intramuscular course. **(B)** MDTC 3-D reconstruction for the same patient. Yellow arrow indicates the exactly point where the perforator pierces the fascia. Magenta arrow indicates the coccyx at the beginning of the intergluteal fold which is the center of our coordinate axis.

assess their vascularization *(Fig. 13.9)*. To prepare lymphovenous anastomosis, in addition to the infrared camera with green dye indomethacin, we perform a new protocol with lympho-MRI injecting gadolinium intradermally. This is a new technique that we are validating and we hope to be able to assess the functionality of the lymphatic channels at the subcutaneous tissue and the interconnections between the deep and superficial lymphatic systems *(Fig. 13.10)*. In coming years it seems clear that we will see a significant improvement in the results of lymphatic surgery, and this will be due, at least in part, to imaging techniques.

Considerable discussion remains concerning whether MDCT or noncontrast-MRI is the more ideal method for the preoperative study of perforators. Which of the two is more suitable will depend on the facilities at each center, but if we know that we can achieve the same information with both techniques, we should use that which has less morbidity for the patient, MRI. In our practice, we use MDCT in two main situations: (1) when we can take advantage of the extension study requested by the oncologist in cases of delayed reconstruction and (2) in cases when we need to study a large extension of the body to rule out anatomical abnormalities.

Day-to-day progress is being made in the quality of images and radiological equipment. The ideal preoperative method will be that which offers the best quality

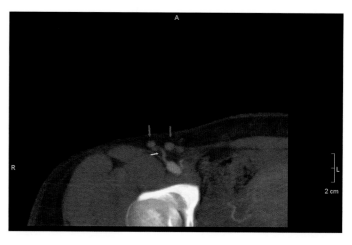

Fig. 13.9 Axial MDCT image showing the superficial inferior epigastric artery arising from the femoral artery and its course through the superficial epigastric lymph nodes. The yellow arrow indicates the origin and course of the superficial inferior epigastric artery. The magenta arrows indicate the lymph nodes.

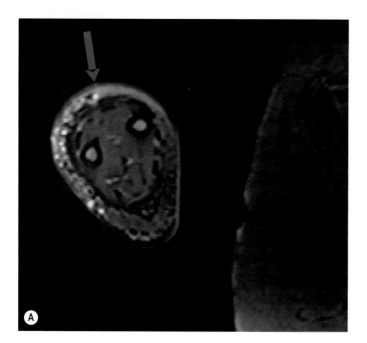

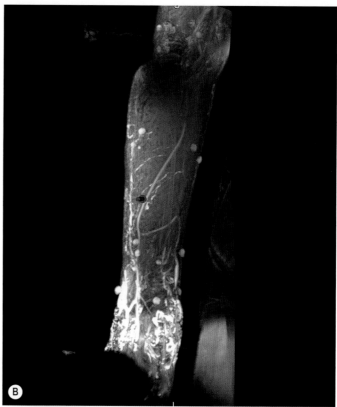

Fig. 13.10 Images of lympho-MRI for a preoperative study of lymphovenous anastomosis in a patient with lymphedema. **(A)** Axial lympho-MRI view. Magenta arrow indicates the lymphatic vessel filling of contrast and the vein attached with signal void. **(B)** 3-D MIP reconstruction of the same patient. Magenta arrow indicates the point where is the lymphatic vessel.

images with minimal inconvenience to the patient. MDCT and MRI are clearly the best tools available as yet to make a complete preoperative study prior to breast reconstruction. With the application of increasingly sophisticated, faster and less invasive, methods, we are getting closer to a virtual dissection of the perforator before surgery. There is still a long road ahead but we have undoubtedly come a long way.

Access the complete reference list online at **http://www.expertconsult.com**

10. Masia J, Clavero JA, Larrañaga JR, et al. Multidetector-row computed tomography in the planning of abdominal perforator flaps. *J Plast Reconstr Aesthet Surg.* 2006;59:594–599.

   The authors describe a new method for the preoperative study of abdominal perforator flaps. They validate the technique presenting a study in which they compare the images obtained with the operatory findings, not encountering any false positive and negative. They also describe the main advantages of MDCT, such as reduction of operating time and complications. They conclude that MDCT provides valuable information and anatomical images before surgery about the perforators and main vessels of the inferior abdominal wall.

11. Uppal RS, Casaer B, Van Landuyt K, et al. The efficacy of preoperative mapping of perforators in reducing operative times and complications in perforator flap breast reconstruction. *J Plast Reconstr Aesthet Surg.* 2009;62(7):859–864.

12. Mathes DW, Neligan PC. Preoperative imaging techniques for perforator selection in abdomen-based microsurgical breast reconstruction. *Clin Plast Surg.* 2010;37(4):581–591.

   This is a review article and the authors describe different techniques for the preoperative study in microsurgical breast reconstruction. They emphasize the advantages of imaging techniques over classical techniques. They conclude that CTA seems to be the gold standard in the preoperative evaluation, but that MRI is increasingly achieving better results. They also provide a nice review of recent publications associated with imaging techniques.

13. Hijjawi JB, Blondeel PN. Advancing deep inferior epigastric artery perforator flap breast reconstruction through multidetector row computed tomography: an evolution in preoperative imaging. *J Reconstr Microsurg.* 2010;26(1):11–20.

   The authors describe the many advantages of the MDCT versus duplex imaging. They conclude that MDCT is currently the technique of choice in the preoperative mapping of abdominal perforators, emphasizing that this method contribute significantly to the reliability, speed, and minimal donor site morbidity of these procedures.

14. Hamdi M, Van Landuyt K, Hedent EV, et al. Advances in autogenous breast reconstruction. The role of preoperative perforator mapping. *Ann Plast Surg.* 2007;58:18–26.

   This is a review article and the authors describe different techniques for the preoperative study in microsurgical breast reconstruction. They emphasize the advantages of imaging techniques over classical techniques. They conclude that CTA seems to be the gold standard in the preoperative evaluation, but that MRI is increasingly achieving better results. They also provide a nice review of recent publications associated with imaging techniques.

15. Rozen WM, Ashton MW, Grinsell D, et al. Establishing the case for CT angiography in the preoperative imaging of abdominal wall perforators. *Microsurgery.* 2008;28(5):306–313.

16. Rozen WM, Stella DL, Bowden J, et al. Advances in the pre-operative planning of deep inferior epigastric artery perforator flaps: magnetic resonance angiography. *Microsurgery.* 2009;29:119–123.

18. Masia J, Kosuotic D, Cervelli D, et al. In search of the ideal method in perforator mapping: noncontrast magnetic resonance imaging. *J Reconstr Microsurg.* 2010;26(1):29–35.

   To minimize the drawbacks of MDCT in abdominal wall free flap reconstruction, the authors present good results with noncontrast MRI. They validate the technique comparing the images with the operative findings. They emphasize the advantages of nonradiation for the patient and elimination of the need for intravenous medium as compared to MDCT.

19. Masia J, Larrañaga J, Clavero JA, et al. The value of the multidetector row computed tomography for the preoperative planning of deep inferior epigastric artery perforator flap: our experience in 162 cases. *Ann Plast Surg.* 2008;60:29–36.

   This study evaluates the utility of MDCT in planning abdominal perforator surgery for breast reconstruction in 162 patients who had undergone mastectomy and were reconstructed with DIEP or SIEA flaps. Also the authors perform a comparative study between 100 cases using MDCT and 100 cases without imaging technique preoperatively. In conclusion they claim that MDCT enables accurate identification of the most suitable dominant perforator vessel. Also the use of MDCT has been shown to decrease surgical time and postoperative complications, therefore making surgical perforator flap procedures for breast reconstruction faster and safer.

20. Clavero JA, Masia J, Larrañaga J, et al. MDCT in the preoperative planning of abdominal perforator surgery for postmastectomy breast reconstruction. *Am J Roentgenol.* 2008;191:670–676.

14

Expander-implants breast reconstructions

Maurizio B. Nava, Giuseppe Catanuto, Angela Pennati, Valentina Visintini Cividin, and Andrea Spano

SYNOPSIS

- Implant-based breast reconstructions can be employed in all patients, provided that they have not been previously irradiated.
- Medium size anatomically-shaped permanent silicone implants can be employed to reconstruct virtually all breasts, irrespective of shape and size.
- A contralateral adjustment should be part of the reconstructive project.
- Breast reconstruction in the large breast can be accomplished in one stage ("skin reducing mastectomy").

 Access the Historical Perspective section online at
http://www.expertconsult.com

Introduction

Implant-based breast reconstructions can be employed in all patients, provided that they have not been previously irradiated. Medium size anatomically shaped permanent silicone implant can be employed to reconstruct virtually all breasts, irrespective of shape and size. A contralateral adjustment should be part of the reconstructive project. Breast reconstruction in the large breast can be accomplished in one stage ("Skin reducing mastectomy").

Basic science

Basic science in the field of breast implants, no differently from other branches of plastic surgery, is affected by a generalized lack of evidence. Most of the researches currently published in international journals are based on very empirical observations and rely mainly on expert opinions or on small retrospective series. A recent systematic review on the assessment of health-related quality of life included[2] a total of 34 papers and most of them appeared to be compromised by poor statistics, lack of reproducibility due to the use of generic instruments of evaluation, reliance on single center's observations and no unequivocal reports on complications. Furthermore, among the 34 examined papers, only two were based on level 1 evidence and 11 on level 2. The authors conclude that there is an urgent need for standardized instruments for outcome evaluation to provide a reliable guidance for further research.

Basic research on implants is strictly tightened to breast shape assessment. A quantitative analysis of breast shape and of its modifications over times is not possible, the few tools proposed in literature have been tested by our group with very disappointing results. A more precise geometrical language should be available and estimates from geometry of curved surfaces should replace currents linear measurements that are unable to assess complex round territories like the female breast.[3]

Capsular contracture cannot be assessed without such estimates. A three-dimensional representation of the mammary appearance allows an objective evaluation of breast changes following cosmetic and reconstructive surgery.

Research efforts should also be made to analyze the breast deformation during walking or with the movements of the trunk and of the arms. In fact, the breast is not a static object and capsular contracture mainly affects breast softness and plasticity.[4,5]

Capsular contracture has been widely investigated as the major trade-off of prosthetic reconstructions. Several explanations have been proposed according to endogenous or exogenous hypothesis and capsular contracture appears to be a multifactorial clinical condition related to surgical technique, implant manufacturing, anatomical plane of implantation, etc. Infections can be the leading cause generating this condition.[6,7] This theory gives explanations for asymmetric contractures and for effective reduction using implants in association with topic antibiotics or iodopovidone,[7] and is supported by studies that demonstrate a much higher percentage of positive culture rates in severely contracted capsules (89.5% vs 10.5% in grades I and II).[8]

Any convincing theory for capsular contracture is tightly related to an upregulated response to foreign bodies. Several logistic mediators, together with fibroblasts, macrophages and CD4 are involved in this process, and it has been argued that a good treatment could be related to topic or systemic administration of anti-inflammatory drugs. Leukotrienes such as zafirlukast have been investigated with positive results.[9]

In this series of 37 patients who underwent primary submuscular breast augmentation with saline-filled, smooth implants, were evaluated by independent observers and rated for capsular contracture using a modification of the Baker classification. Patients who suffered capsular contracture were offered zafirlukast 20 mg for 3 or 6 months. A total of 41 breasts in this series (55.0%) were found to have early, mild capsular contracture. Favorable results with complete or partial response to treatment were seen in a statistically significant proportion of the treated breasts (75.7%, $p<0.05$). This response lasted in the long term (mean follow-up of 16.5 months).

Our research group confirmed this observation in an experimental study,[10] in which we evaluated the effectiveness of zafirlukast. Disks of textured implant material were placed dorsally into each of the subcutaneous tissues of 40 rats that were subdivided into two groups: 20 rats treated with zafirlukast and 20 controls. At autopsy 77 days after treatment, each implant with its surrounding collagenic tissue was excised, and the macroscopic measure of the membrane thickness was compared with the pathology reports, to definitely assess the foreign body reaction. The mean total thickness of the capsule around the implants was 161.97 μm in the zafirlukast-treated group compared with 345.98 μm in the control group ($p<0.001$). Outstandingly, the collagen fibres and fibroblast layer were reduced in the zafirlukast-treated group compared with the controls. Our study confirms the effectiveness of this compound in preventing fibrosis and reducing the extent of collagen reaction when a capsule has been formed.

Several clinical investigations of the effects of shell texturization in preventing capsular contracture were conducted. Barnsley[11] performed a meta-analysis of seven trials[12–20] comparing smooth and textured implants; only three of these studies demonstrated significantly lower rates with the use of textured implants. However, a pooled analysis of all seven studies demonstrated an odds ratio (OR) of 0.19 indicating a protective effect for surface texturing on the rate of capsular contracture. The only subgroup who did not benefit from texturization was the one belonging to a single trial, in which the implants were put in a submuscular position.

A further meta-analysis of trials of subglandular breast augmentation by Chin-Ho Wong[21] reported similar results, although several limitations were correctly pointed out by the authors. Although in the presence of clinical trials with a robust design (prospective controlled randomized), the outcome evaluation is substantially biased by subjective and non-reproducible observations, as capsular contracture was assessed according to the subjective Baker scale. The authors correctly stated that clinically important contractures (Baker III and IV) were defined as capsular contracture in all studies and that two or more observer independent examiners were employed for patient evaluation and that discordant opinions were solved by consensus. Moreover, other limitations arise from the lack of standardization of surgical techniques and incision approaches, the short-term follow-up (only two studies with a follow-up longer than 1 year), with several patients lost to follow-up and consequently data deterioration after the first year of observation. Notwithstanding the efforts in providing a higher level of evidence, more objective and quantitative tools for assessment of the outcome of plastic surgery of the breast should be provided.

The use of human acellular dermal matrix has been reported as a possible tool for prevention of capsular contracture. A study by Basu and colleagues[22] on 20 patients who underwent two stage breast reconstruction, investigated the histopathologic characteristics of the capsule in the bio-integrated area and in the native subpectoral capsule. A semi-quantitative analysis was performed, the scores were statistically analyzed and significant differences were observed in favor of the acellular dermis. The acellular dermal matrix facilitates breast reconstruction, avoiding the harvesting of the serratus muscle; it also provides a good definition to the lower pole of the breast and a more natural ptosis. However, in this study it is demonstrated that the acellular dermal sheet, consisting in a biological matrix deprived of cells, allows the implantation of cells and vessels from the host, establishing a physiological matrix cell interaction. For this reason, host cells are able to revitalize the exogenous matrix, also containing extracellular matrix proteins (such as hyaluronic acid, fibronectin, collagen, and fibronectin), facilitating normal wound healing and avoiding chronic inflammatory changes and foreign body giant cell formation.[23–25]

The beneficial effects of the acellular dermal matrix in the prevention of long-term complications such as capsular contracture or poor morphological results may be hindered by a higher percentage of short-term severe complications.

The largest series on this device reports on two groups of patients who underwent breast reconstruction either using the acellular device or not. The seroma and infection rates were higher in the acellular dermal matrix group (14.1% vs 2.7%, $p=0.0003$, for seroma; 8.9% vs 2.1%, $p=0.0328$, for infection) and acellular dermal matrix and body mass index were statistically significant risk factors for developing seroma and infection. The authors concluded that although the acellular dermal matrix enhances final results, a higher short-term complication rate is awaited (OR seroma 4.24 times, $p=0.018$ and infection 5.37 times, $p=0.006$).[26]

Similar conclusions are report by Newman et al.[27] in a recent meta-analysis, in which they concluded that the incidence of short-term complications with human acellular matrices is approximately 12%.

Breast reconstruction with tissue expansion and permanent implants

Factors including the type of mastectomy, timing of reconstruction, tissue expansion, and implant design have made expander-implant techniques an important method for breast reconstruction. Tissue expansion was first reported by Neumann in 1957, for coverage of a subauricular defect.

Although Neumann's[28] report appeared in *Plastic and Reconstructive Surgery* and demonstrated the feasibility of the procedure, major interest in tissue expansion did not occur for another 20 years. Working independently, Radovan[29] and Austad[30] developed silicone tissue expanders and published their findings in 1982. Radovan performed his first tissue expansion in 1976. Austad developed a self-inflating silicone prosthesis and investigated the histologic effects of tissue expansion. Subsequent to this early work, tissue expansion has been investigated thoroughly and gained widespread acceptance on the basis of its proven safety and efficacy.

The silicone implant was initially incorporated into breast reconstruction as a device to provide a safe and stable breast mound. At the time of its inception, the radical mastectomy and modified radical mastectomy were routinely used to extirpate breast cancer. The implant could rarely be used under the preserved skin envelope because of existing scar tissue and inadequate and often unstable skin coverage at the mastectomy site. Therefore, the implant was used in conjunction with a flap for coverage. With the evolution of mastectomy techniques and diagnosis of breast cancer at an earlier stage, more conservative approaches to mastectomy, including skin-preserving and skin-sparing mastectomy, have been used. With increasing recognition of the value of immediate reconstruction for the mastectomy patient, the option of expander-implant became more practical for incorporation into techniques for reconstruction.

With the development of the concept of tissue expansion, a deflated implant can be inserted beneath the mastectomy skin that will not adversely affect mastectomy skin survival. The expander can subsequently undergo inflation both to stretch the dimensions of the retained skin envelope and to avoid wound contraction during the process of wound maturation after the mastectomy. With improvement in the design of tissue expanders, the port is now incorporated into the surface of the implant, eliminating the dissection distant to the mastectomy site to place the valve for later expander inflation. With the use of a textured expander, the expander will not migrate away from the area of greatest skin tightness (usually the inferior half of the preserved breast skin envelope) and will maintain a well-defined inframammary line, despite the mastectomy dissection. These innovations have made the expander-implant for breast reconstruction a reliable technique to restore form at the site of mastectomy. The process of reconstruction with the use of an expander-implant is generally a two-stage procedure.

The first stage is insertion of the expander either at the time of mastectomy or delayed until the patient is referred or presents for reconstruction. If the first stage is not performed at the time of the mastectomy, it is preferable to delay reconstruction a minimum of 3 months and until adjuvant treatments are completed.

The *advantages* of the expander-implant technique for breast reconstruction include the following:

- Minimal morbidity
- Reduced operative time. Although there are usually two procedures, each is short in the range of 1–1.5 h and requires only one night in hospital. The second stage may be performed on an outpatient basis according to the preference of the patient and the surgeon
- No donor site morbidity, unlike in flap procedures, when the patient will have an additional scar at the flap harvest site
- If the patient becomes dissatisfied with the result, all pre-existing flaps are still available, and the expander-implant maintains the breast space if the flap is later incorporated into a secondary reconstruction

The *disadvantages* related to expander-implant use include the following:

- Complications inherent to implant use, including implant deflation or malfunction, capsular contracture, and fear of adverse interactions between the patient's immune system and the device
- Contour irregularities visible on skin surface due to underlying implant. Again, because the implant is gradually encapsulated with scar, the adhesions of the scar to the implant and skin may result in unnatural appearance
- The implant will not behave like normal vascularized tissue. It will remain cooler than adjacent body parts when ambient temperature is low, and the reconstructed breast will not develop natural ptosis with advancing age because of scar attachment between implant and chest wall and overlying skin envelope as opposed to the contralateral breast

Certain general criteria are required before a patient represents an appropriate candidate for implant-expander reconstruction

- The patient must have an adequate skin envelope to support the expander-implant. In delayed reconstruction, irradiated skin represents a relative contraindication to the expander-implant because implant exposure may occur and the skin envelope will usually not respond to the expansion process. If the patient is a smoker or is being treated for scleroderma, use of an expander-implant is a relative contraindication.
- Cessation of smoking for 6 weeks may be acceptable to proceed with the expander-implant, although skin circulation may still be adversely affected. The patient must agree to delayed surgery of the opposite breast to establish symmetry with the reconstructed breast mound (reduction mammaplasty or mastopexy, augmentation).

The patient must be well informed about all options for breast reconstruction. In general, autogenous breast reconstruction will provide a more natural breast but will require more complex surgery and additional donor site scars. The patient must be willing to accept the use of a permanent prosthesis. At present, both the silicone gel- and saline-filled implants are approved by the Food and Drug Administration (FDA) for breast reconstruction.[31]

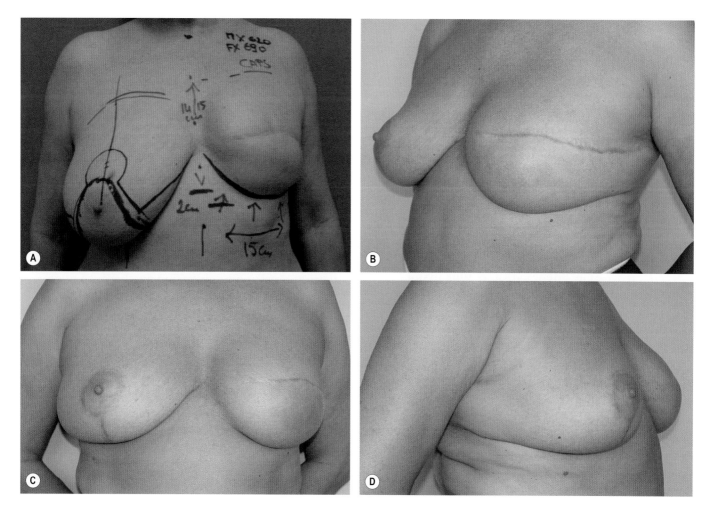

Fig. 14.1 Two-stage expander-implant breast reconstruction.

The technique for expander-implant use generally requires two stages. Each stage is discussed in regard to marking, position, dissection, closure, dressing, and postoperative care. Special considerations, including single-stage expander-implant reconstruction, techniques for expander-implant muscle coverage, alternative approaches for expander-implant use in patients with an inadequate skin envelope, and outcomes, are also reviewed.

The expander-implant breast reconstructions have evolved during the last few years *(Fig. 14.1)*. In the past, prostheses were mainly employed to reconstruct small breasts; nowadays, thanks to the modern anatomical devices, it possible to reconstruct a cosmetic medium-sized bosom (with contralateral adjustment) for all patients, independently from the original breast shape. We contraindicate this technique only to previously radio-treated patients.

We validated a modern surgical model for two stage reconstructions and we expanded the indication to one stage reconstruction with a new technique called "Skin reducing mastectomy" *(Fig. 14.2)*. This technique is currently under development at our institution and it allows one stage reconstruction in women with large breasts with contralateral symmetrical scarring. Implant reconstruction can be performed either in the same surgical time of the mastectomy or as a delayed procedure *(Fig. 14.3)*. ⊛ FIGS **14.2**, **14.3** APPEAR ONLINE ONLY

Reconstructive paradigms and surgical strategy

An established paradigm for breast reconstructions to rebuild, after mastectomy, an identical and possibly symmetrical breast mound is required. Autologous

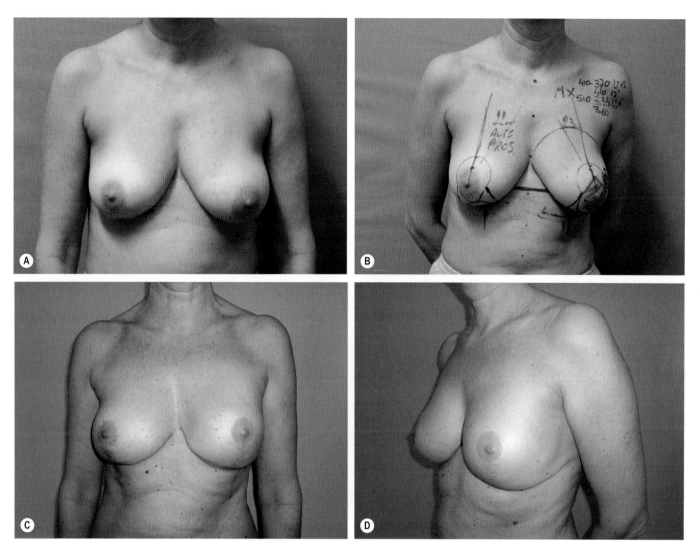

Fig. 14.2 Left one stage skin reducing mastectomy. **(A)** Frontal view. **(B)** Frontal view of skin reducing mastectomy contralateral mastopexy and auto-prosthesis preoperative project. **(C)** Frontal and **(D)** lateral views showing the postoperative results.

flaps were favored in the reconstruction of large and ptotic breasts due to their ability to reproduce a natural symmetry even with a contralateral ptotic gland. Reconstructions with sub-pectoral implants were indicated mainly for small and medium-sized glands with a moderate degree of ptosis. Operations on the healthy breast in search of symmetry were considered undesirable, as they were expected to compromise surveillance on contralateral disease.[32,33]

Extra-projection devices gave us the chance to modify this reconstructive predicament *(Figs 14.4, 14.5)*. Modern anatomically-shaped implants can be employed for breast reconstruction and can spare women from complex operations that, as far as myocutaneous flaps

are concerned, can generate severe biomechanical complications.

Extra-projection prostheses filled with highly cohesive gel can yield not only a rewarding cosmetic outcome but a safe surgical approach *(Fig. 14.6)*.[34,35] ⊛ FIG **14.6** APPEARS ONLINE ONLY

In the authors' experience, breast reconstructive surgery aims to create, for all women, a bilateral cosmetic medium-sized breast (400–500 cc), highly projected, with little to moderate ptosis, rather than a ptotic gland exactly matching the contralateral. This is demonstrated by the medium volume of implanted prosthesis in comparison to the contralateral adjustment technique; this ranges from 397 cc for women with small

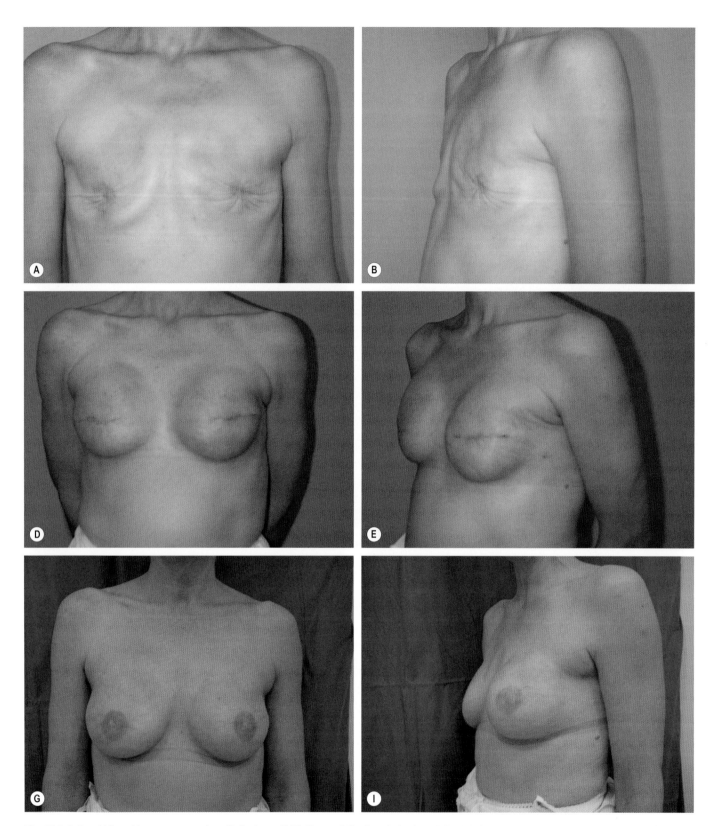

Fig. 14.3 Delayed bilateral breast reconstruction with implants. **(A,B)** Chest wall flat (frontal view-lateral views) before delayed bilateral breast reconstruction. **(D,E)** Tissue expansion (frontal and lateral views). **(G,I)** Final results (frontal and lateral views).

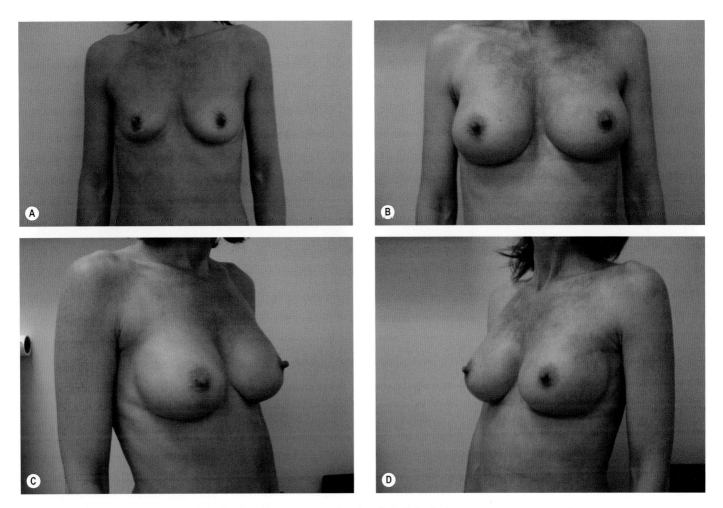

Fig. 14.4 Indications and contraindications in implant based breast reconstructions in radio-treated patients.

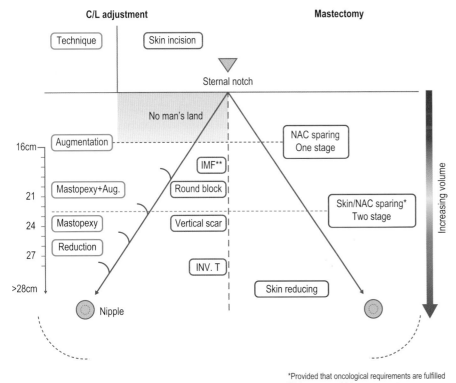

C/L adjustment

Mastectomy

Technique   Skin incision

Sternal notch

No man's land

16cm   Augmentation   NAC sparing
                            One stage

                    IMF**

21   Mastopexy+Aug.   Round block   Skin/NAC sparing*
                                        Two stage

24   Mastopexy   Vertical scar

27   Reduction

                    INV. T

>28cm   Skin reducing

        Nipple

Increasing volume

*Provided that oncological requirements are fulfilled
**Inframammary fold

Fig. 14.5 Mastectomy techniques and contralateral adjustment according to breast measurements and morphology.

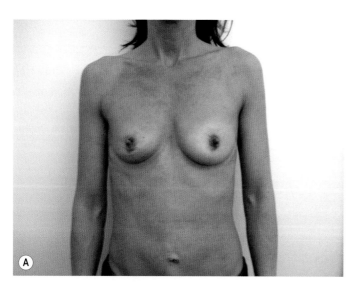
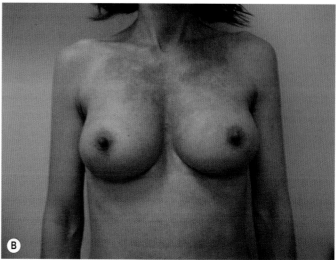

Fig. 14.6 Cosmetic breast reconstruction with extra-projection implants. **(A)** Right breast cancer in patient with small breasts: preoperative view. **(B)** Final results after two stage right nipple sparing mastectomy and contralateral augmentation: frontal and lateral views.

breasts who received an augmentation, to 533 cc for those whose healthy side required reduction surgery.[36]

Our approach substantially differs from that reported by Losken *et al.*[33] in one of the largest series on breast reconstructions. In this work, one-third of patients who underwent breast reconstruction did not receive contralateral adjustment, whereas this incidence in our experience does not exceed one case out of ten.

The reconstruction of the large breast can be easily accomplished also using implants, coupling it with a contralateral reduction. A modification of "Wise pattern" mastectomies that we called "Skin reducing mastectomy" may allow one stage reconstructions with symmetrical inverted T scarring. Also small and very small breasts can be reconstructed in a single stage.

The observation of sub-groups stratified according to operations on the opposite site demonstrated that the cosmetic and reconstructive purpose of this methodology is emphasized when implants are used also contralaterally *(Fig. 14.7)*. A higher satisfaction rate is reported in this case, while on the other hand ptotic breasts treated only by mastopexy tend to recur over years *(Fig. 14.8)*. We are aware that women who have developed breast cancer are at a higher risk of a second malignancy in the contralateral breast;[37] for this reason contralateral augmentations in this setting are still debatable. ✤ FIG **14.8** APPEARS ONLINE ONLY

In healthy women, it is well known that despite the diminished sensitivity of mammography with implants,

augmented and nonaugmented patients are diagnosed at a similar stage and have a comparable prognosis.[36] Much longer follow-up in this study and the increased role of MRI will probably also clarify this aspect.[38]

The adjunct value of contralateral reduction relies on the possibility to identify contralateral occult breast carcinomas. The incidence of occult cancer in the histology specimen as previously reported, after reduction mammoplasty is not high, but still needs to be taken into consideration. The postoperative specimen should be marked as for common excisions and if any incidental lesion is postoperatively discovered, this will require an axillary evaluation in a second surgical stage. Positive margins can be occasionally re-excised, although in some cases a mastectomy could be the best option for optimal local control. All patients scheduled to undergo a contralateral adjustment should be preoperatively assessed with clinical examination, mammography and if required, ultrasound. Any suspicious condition needs to be reported and investigated. The follow-up should not be different from that commonly done for breast cancer patients.

Diagnosis and patient presentation

According to our reconstructive strategy, the choice for implant-based reconstructions should not be driven only by dimensional considerations.

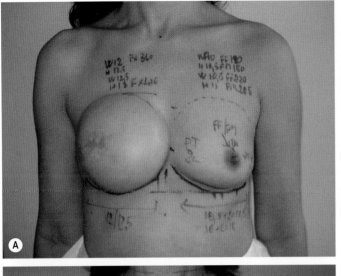

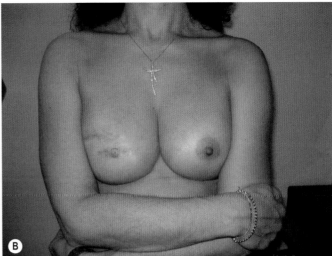

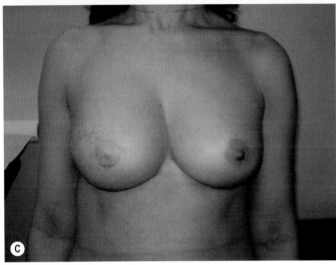

Fig. 14.7 Cosmetic breast reconstruction with extra-projection implants and contralateral augmentation. **(A)** After tissue expansion: a larger expander in place to match the symmetry after contralateral augmentation. **(B)** Postoperative results after right nipple sparing mastectomy, contralateral augmentation and refinements with fat grafting. **(C)** The reconstructed breast.

Exclusion criteria

Prosthesis for reconstructions can be employed in all women undergoing immediate or delayed breast reconstructions that did not receive previous radiation. Several studies demonstrated a higher complication rate after implant positioning in a radio-treated field.[39–41] Similar observations are reported for the reconstructed breast receiving radiotherapy on temporary expanders. For this reason, patients preoperatively scheduled to undergo radiotherapy for locally advanced breast cancer are discouraged to undergo an immediate reconstruction and a delayed flap-based reconstruction is recommended *(Fig. 14.9)*. FIG **14.9** APPEARS ONLINE ONLY

Radiation therapy determinates a progressive change of the skin surface that originates in an inflammatory chronic condition. We can observe early effects and long-term effects. The first occur within 90 days of treatment and include dryness, epilation, pigmentation changes, and erythema.[42] After 90 days, a chronic logistic condition may appear with progressive induration of the skin, fibrosis, and oedema. The ultrastructural analysis of this condition reveals clear signs of ischemia, with capillary vessels reduced in number and exhibiting duplication of the basal membrane, ectatic lumen cytoplasmic activation of endothelial cells.[43] Any attempt to perform alloplastic reconstruction in this setting of chronic ischemia has demonstrated to yield an unacceptable rate of severe complications with implant extrusion, capsular contracture or implant displacement.[39,44] A trial is ongoing in our institution for patients whose indication for radiation is not known before mastectomy. In such cases we perform an immediate two-stage breast reconstruction. Patients undergo tissue expansion during postoperative chemotherapy and once the second stage of the reconstruction has been accomplished, they receive radiation on the permanent implant. According to preliminary results, this strategy has extended the indications for implant-based reconstruction also to women requiring post-mastectomy radiotherapy. This strategy allows reduction of the complication and extrusion rates, especially in comparison with patients who receive radiation on tissue expanders. The capsular contracture rate of irradiated breast reconstruction is clearly higher and in accordance with that reported by other authors.[45] However, we observed satisfaction rates not particularly different from that reported by patients who did not received radiation.

Women who received neoadjuvant chemotherapy for large nonadvanced tumors that still require a mastectomy are expected to complete their treatment with radiation before change of temporary expanders with permanent implants. In these cases, due to the high complication rate, it is advisable to warn the patients about the risk of extrusion and make them aware of the possible need to change to a "flap-based" reconstruction strategy.

Fat grafting to treat radio-induced damages of soft tissue is being widely employed in the field of breast reconstruction with prosthesis (*Fig. 14.10*). This simple procedure, commonly performed under local anesthesia, has changed the fate of reconstructions at high risk of complications. Since the first report from Rigotti *et al.*,[43] who described the effectiveness of transplantation of lipo-aspirates to treat radio-induced inflammation, other authors have confirmed the effectiveness of this technique. Serra-Renom *et al.*[46] for instance, recently demonstrated that in mastectomized patients who received radiotherapy, fat grafting in addition to traditional tissue expander and implant breast reconstruction will lead to better reconstructive outcomes with the creation of new subcutaneous tissue, accompanied by improved skin quality of the reconstructed breast without capsular contracture.

Inclusion criteria according to dimensional considerations

All non previously radio-treated patients can be candidates to immediate or delayed reconstructions and are subdivided into three subgroups according to breast shape and size. As demonstrated by our report, contralateral adjustment plays a major role in implant-based breast reconstructions.

Patients with small breasts

These patients can be candidates for immediate one stage reconstructions. If a delayed reconstruction is required, this will certainly require two stages (*Fig. 14.11*).

Patients with medium-sizes breasts

This is the largest subgroup of patients in our experience; a two-stage immediate or delayed expander-implant procedure provides the best results (*Fig. 14.12*).

Patients with large breasts

Immediate reconstruction for these patients can be accomplished with skin reducing mastectomy in one stage. A delayed reconstruction will be based on a two-stage technique. (*Fig. 14.13*). ⊛ FIG **14.13** APPEARS ONLINE ONLY

Surgical technique

Breast reconstruction with implants does not require complex operations. However, final results are strictly dependent on personal experience and the ability to correctly estimate the final postoperative results to be achieved.

The comprehensive preoperative project

The preoperative project is currently made the day before the operation (*Fig. 14.14*). If an immediate breast reconstruction has to be performed, we accurately evaluate the biologic properties of the disease, its local extend and the nipple-areola complex involvement. On the reconstructive side, we estimate characteristic

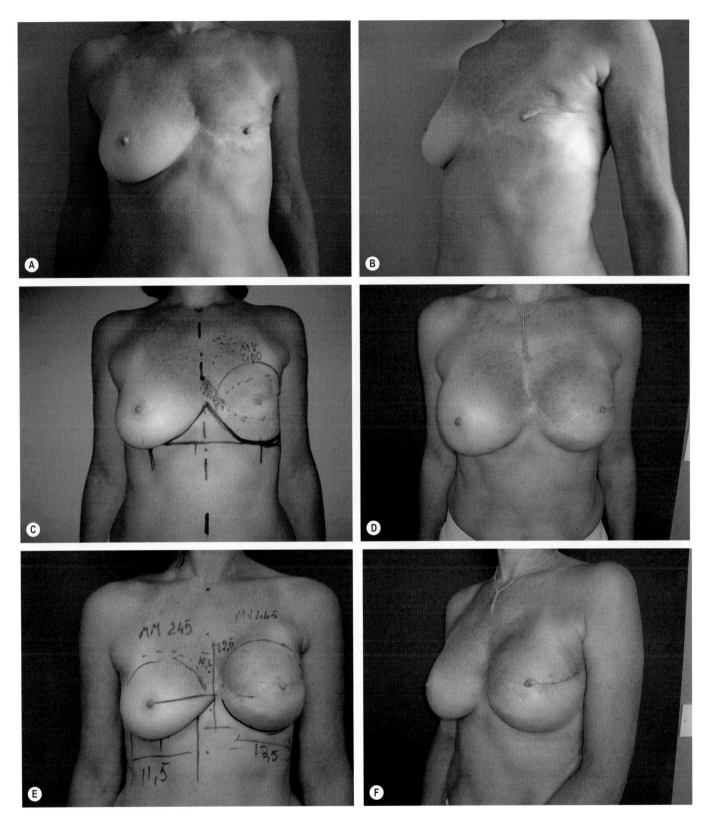

Fig. 14.10 Unexpected favorable results in radio-treated patients treated by three preoperative fat graftings **(A–C)** and one fat grafting at the time of expander positioning **(D–F)**. Electric diathermy was not employed to preserve blood supply.

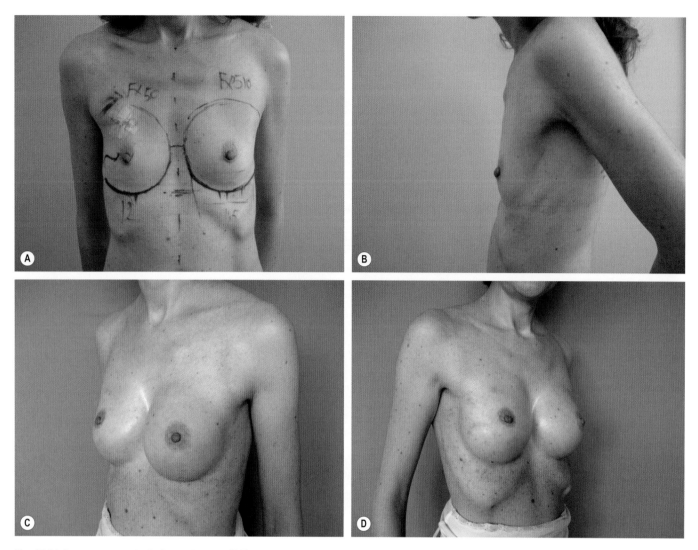

Fig. 14.11 Breast reconstruction in the small breast. **(A,B)** A two-stage+ contralateral augmentation preoperative project and view. **(C,D)** Three years after nipple sparing mastectomy and reconstruction with implants; conservative surgery was not possible due to small size of the gland.

distances such as the nipple to sternal notch distance, the areola to inframammary fold distance and the breast width. All these data will be combined to determine breast size and ptosis degree. Skin thickness is also evaluated using a caliper and performing a "pinch test". Skin elasticity and quality has to be accurately assessed. Poor quality may compromise the final result of the breast reconstruction with implants, and can increase ischemic complications. The contralateral breast is then gently compressed against the chest wall to demarcate the boundaries of the upper pole. This estimate will be determinant for the selection of the implant to be employed.

During this step, photographs of the patient are taken, either before or after marking her with preoperative draws, including the surgical access for breast removal.

Once the objective evaluation of disease and reconstructive needs have been performed we discuss all the possible reconstructive options. The patient–surgeon interaction is a crucial step of reconstructive workflow. According to our survey, we can discuss a delayed or an immediate reconstruction (especially if it is likely that post-mastectomy has to be performed), whether one stage or two stages, and possible cosmetic wishes (augmentation, reduction, mastopexy or no-intervention

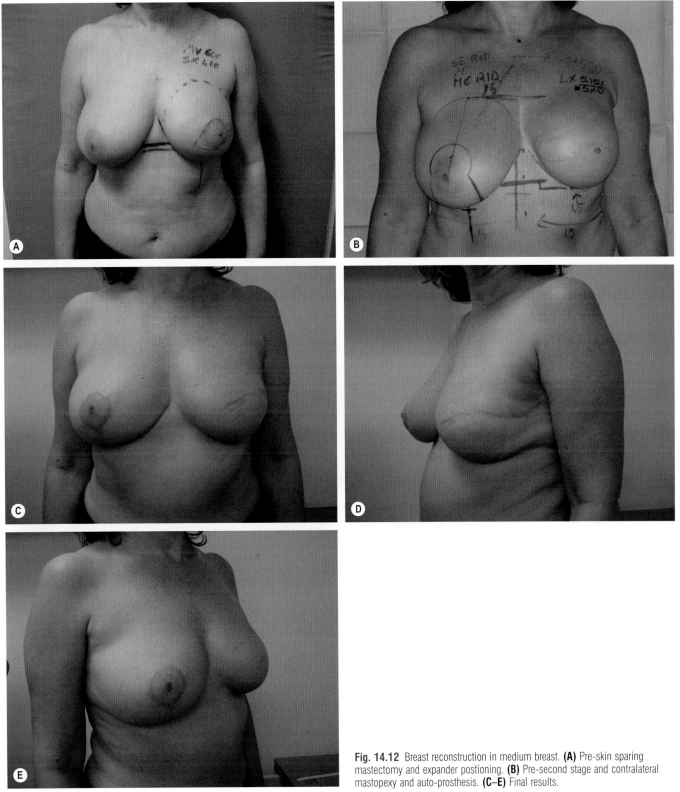

Fig. 14.12 Breast reconstruction in medium breast. **(A)** Pre-skin sparing mastectomy and expander postioning. **(B)** Pre-second stage and contralateral mastopexy and auto-prosthesis. **(C–E)** Final results.

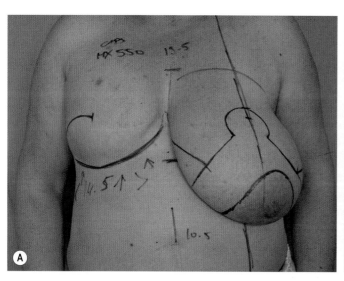 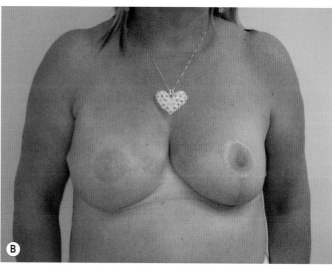

Fig. 14.13 Breast reconstruction in large breast. **(A)** Large pendulous breast on the left side before second stage; in a previous era, a large discrepancy between the two sides as in this case would have required flap-based surgery. **(B)** Modern implants allow fair results with contralateral reduction (inferior pedicle) and extra-projection implants.

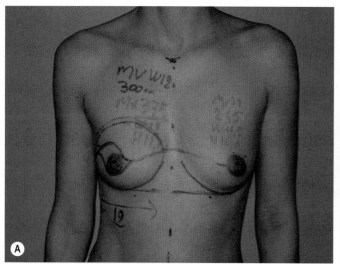 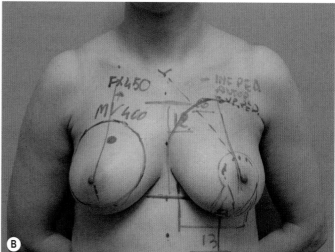

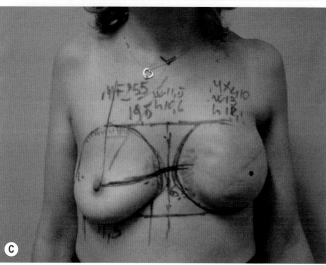

Fig. 14.14 Preoperative projects. **(A)** Preoperative project in a patient who has small breasts scheduled to undergo mastectomy and CL augmentation. **(B)** Preoperative project in a patient who has medium breasts scheduled to undergo mastectomy and CL mastopexy. The templates provided by the manufacturer assist the surgeon in the correct selection of the implants. The whole reconstructive program needs to be planned before the mastectomy. **(C)** A re-evaluation before the second stage is, however required.

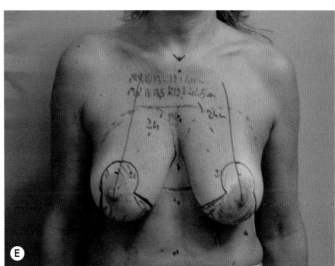

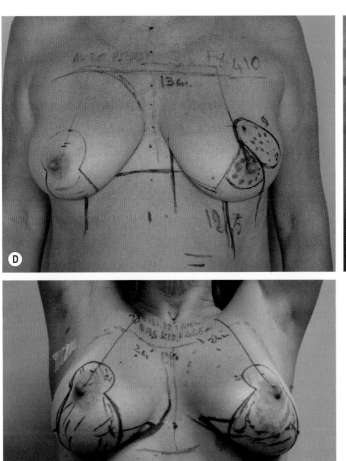

Fig. 14.14, cont'd **(D–F)** Preoperative project of skin reducing mastectomy and contralateral adjustment. **(F)** Skin reducing mastectomy with raised arms. Inferior pole.

on the contralateral side.) Once a final agreement has been reached, we proceed with the selection of the temporary expander or implant that we are going to utilize.

The size of the device is based on breast width, size and the shape of the contralateral breast but it must take into account the patient's wishes on contralateral technique. For instance if a contralateral augmentation is required, a larger tissue expander has to be employed in order to match a proper symmetry at the final stage with the opposite augmented breast.

On the other side, if reconstruction is performed for very large breasts, it is not advisable to use expanders >15 cm. This is the maximum size that can be usually allocated without compromising the mobility of the

ipsilateral arm. Moreover, a contralateral reduction will decrease the width of the opposite breast.

The expander should be usually the same height of the contralateral breast; we would recommend avoiding very low expanders (that will not expand the upper pole of the breast sufficiently) or too high expanders (that could create an excessive pouch with possible rotation or malpositioning of the permanent implant).

The projection of tissue expanders is normally variable and depends on the level of inflation. However, some producers have delivered on the market, expanders with very full projection that can be helpful, especially in skin sparing mastectomies, as they normally allow an easy allocation of full and extra-projection permanent implants. Very full projection tissue expanders used in the setting of nipple sparing mastectomies require a very accurate positioning and an accurate check of nipple positioning during tissue expansion as the artificial projection of the expander cannot be coincident with the actual position of the preserved nipple areola complex. Partial inflation or expanders with low projection can be helpful in this event.

Evolution of prosthetic implants

Modern prosthetic devices have evolved into shape, shell, and filler materials.

Shape (Fig. 14.15)

Breast implants up to the late 1990s were mainly round-shaped to prevent alteration of breast shape due to rotation of the device. Although already present on the market, anatomical teardrop prostheses became popular when highly cohesive silicone gel and textured shells were developed to prevent malpositioning.

The original teardrop-shaped permanent implants evolved with delivery on the market of large combinations of sizes, based on three dimensions (implant width, height and projection); more recently, a variation of the shape of the superior contour has been introduced. Round implants are still available and we prevalently employ them for minimal contralateral augmentations.

Round temporary expanders partially filled with saline solution and silicone gel (Becker's) have been abandoned in our current practice. Anatomically-shaped permanent expanders can be considered for selected cases.

Shell (Fig. 14.16)

Breast implants are made up of a silicone shell; originally this was a monolayer sheet with a smooth surface. Currently, the most advanced devices have a triple layer and a textured surface to prevent gel migration and capsular reaction to foreign body. FIG **14.16** APPEARS ONLINE ONLY

Filler materials (Fig. 14.17)

The large majority of prostheses are currently filled with silicone gel, saline solution or both in various percentages. The authors only use implants with a very dense silicone gel ("highly cohesive"). The firmness of the filler material prevents capsular contracture and preserves the original shape of the implant. Temporary tissue expanders are filled with saline solution that can be injected through an integrated injection port, which does not require an additional procedure for removal. The most recent implants can be filled with gels at different levels of cohesion to enhance the extra-projection at the tip of the breast. FIG **14.17A** APPEARS ONLINE ONLY

Dimensions

Anatomically-shaped prostheses from the major manufacturers are based on three dimensions (width, height, and projection). The implant volume in no longer considered a determinant size. We normally employ full and extra projection prostheses on the reconstruction

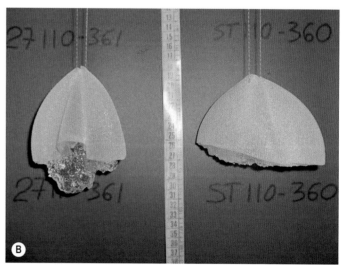

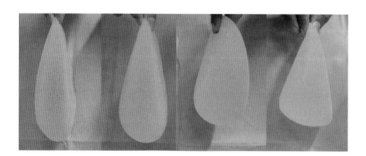

Fig. **14.15** Modern anatomical implants: multiple shapes.

Fig. **14.17** **(B)** The high cohesive gel does not drop.

side. They give to the new breast the aspect of a pleasant breast; on the contralateral side, if an augmentation is required, we use implants with a lower projection.

The selected implant width is commonly based on the width of the breast footprint we are going to replace; the height is usually based on the height of the contralateral breast estimated as previously described.

A good reconstruction always starts with a good mastectomy
(Figs 14.18, 14.19)

An accurate preservation of blood supply is a mandatory part of a correct breast reconstruction. Bearing in mind the oncological principles of breast removal, it is advisable to avoid aggressive dissections of skin flaps that do not add much to curative intents. The type of incision and amount of skin that has to be resected at the time of mastectomy should be preoperatively planned according to breast volume and degree of ptosis. ⊛ FIGS **14.18**, **14.19** APPEAR ONLINE ONLY

They have to be planned at this stage in order to be symmetrical, with any contralateral adjustment at the final surgical step. Preservation of the inframammary fold can be safely performed because breast parenchymal tissue rarely lies distal to this level. This region is a specialized part of the superficial fascial system, being composed of two subcutaneous layers and one superficial fascial layer.

Nonetheless, if this structure has to be sacrificed, a new inframammary fold can be restored at the time of reconstruction, or during any subsequent surgical revision. A further surgical landmark is the fascia overlying the pectoralis muscle. We would suggest avoiding removal to prevent weakening of the covering muscle. Minor disruptions of the pectoralis major muscle should not interfere with any planned breast reconstruction. However, tears in the muscle must be closed with soluble sutures (preferably before insertion of an implant to avoid inadvertent needle puncture). If the nipple areola complex can be preserved a double biopsy of retro-areola ducts (on the mastectomy flap and on the specimen) can confirm the absence of residual neoplastic disease.

The total amount of residual skin after a radical modified mastectomy needs to be estimated; there must be sufficient skin to allow primary closure without tension following insertion of the implant. If a tissue expander is used, minimal inflation is carried out at the time of initial placement to avoid excessive tension either within the skin and subcutaneous tissues or the pectoral muscles.

Immediate breast reconstruction after mastectomy (first stage)

Once glandular removal has been completed, it is possible to start an immediate reconstruction.

Video 1

The surface markings of the sub-pectoral pocket can be outlined on the chest wall using the templates provided by the manufactures. The lower border of the pocket should lie just below the sub-mammary crease but not by more than 1 cm, allowing for upward shift of the lower edge with inflation of the expander. The sub-muscular pocket will have the same dimensions of the selected expander and will reflect the base width and height of the contralateral breast.

The patient must be correctly positioned on the operating table: initially she will lay in the supine position with the arm of the mastectomy side at abducted at 90° to allow axillary surgery, soon after the mastectomy the arm should be adducted at 60° to obtain a complete relaxation of pectoralis major so to facilitate blunt dissection of the pouch *(Fig. 14.20)*. ⊛ FIG **14.20** APPEARS ONLINE ONLY

The contralateral breast has to be visible because is a natural guide for the correct positioning of the implant. The total amount of skin and the quality of the pectoralis major muscle, together with the definition of the inframammary fold and fascial attachments should be re-evaluated. The lower limit of the sub-pectoral pocket is marked and the transverse and vertical diameters re-estimated to confirm the size of the expander that has been preoperatively selected expander.

Surgical steps for insertion of expander

The dissection starts from the lateral border of the pectoralis major muscle and it follows underneath the pectoralis major muscle superiorly, medially, and inferiorly. Inferolaterally, it exposes the aponeurosis of the anterior rectus muscle and of the external oblique; then the sternal attachments of the pectoralis major are detached from the second intercostal space to the inferior edge of

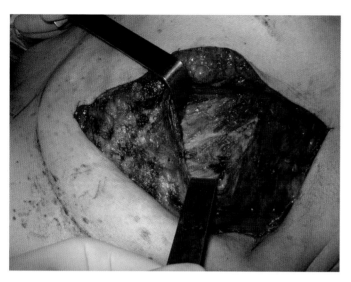

Fig. 14.22 The totally submuscular pouch is made up of pectoralis major and serratus.

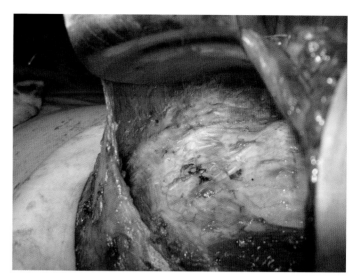

Fig. 14.24 Final aspect of the pouch.

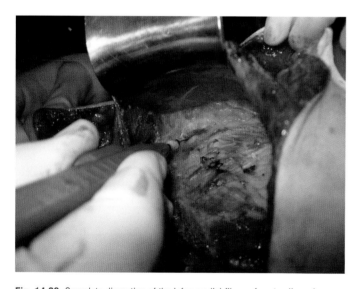

Fig. 14.23 Complete dissection of the inferomedial fibres of pectoralis major.

the pocket *(Fig. 14.21)*. The pocket should be completely sub-muscular except at the inframammary fold where, if this has been correctly preserved, it should extend into the deep fascial layer avoiding direct continuity with the mastectomy site *(Figs 14.22–14.24)*. 🔘 FIG **14.21** APPEARS ONLINE ONLY

We normally evacuate the tissue expander from any retained air; we then partially inflate the prosthesis with saline to ensure there is no leakage; a small amount of saline (up to 20–30% of final volume) facilitates the insertion. The prosthesis is then immersed in povidone iodine solution or in antibiotics. Drains should be placed in the submuscular pocket in the mastectomy cavity (and in the axilla if an axillary dissection has been performed), before the expander is introduced and correctly orientated *(Figs 14.25, 14.26)*. At this stage we can sit the patient up to check the correct expansion of the lower pole of the breast. The sub-muscular pouch is then closed with re-absorbable interrupted stitches. Afterwards, we can inflate the expander up to around 50% of the overall volume *(Fig. 14.27)*. Initial expansion is desirable provided there is no skin tension. 🔘 FIGS **14.25–14.27** APPEAR ONLINE ONLY

Skin reducing mastectomy

Immediate breast reconstruction in one stage for large and ptotic glands

Mastectomies with skin or nipple preservation for large and ptotic glands can become challenging due to a large discrepancy between the cutaneous envelope and the sub-muscular pouch. An alternative technique that we named "skin reducing mastectomy" is currently under development in our unit. The glandular removal is commonly performed through a Wise pattern access *(Fig. 14.28)*. An inferior dermal flap is de-epithelialized and the mastectomy then follows with special care in preservation of subdermal vascularity of the cutaneous flaps. Once the glandular removal has been completed the pectoralis major muscle is dissected from its infero-lateral attachments; the serratus anterior (or its superficial fascia) is dissected no differently from a conventional technique. Both the two structures are then sutured with the dermal-adipose inferior flap and a large combined pouch is finally harvested *(Fig. 14.28)*. After drain insertion we can position a large implant and close the pouch laterally. Afterwards we suture the skin flaps with the final inverted T scar *(Fig. 14.29)*.

The authors usually perform a breast reduction on the contralateral breast. We normally employ a supero-medial pedicle technique or an inferior pedicle technique, depending on the distance of the nipple areola complex from the sterna notch. The final aspect of a skin reducing mastectomy as far as scarring is concerned, is not very different from that of a bilateral breast reduction with inverted T scars *(Fig. 14.30)*. Although the skin reducing mastectomy provides extremely satisfactory cosmetic results with a natural ptosis in one stage and symmetrical scarring, it is a challenging technique with quite a high complication rate. This can be due to the creation of very long and angular flaps that can generate necrosis of the T junction. This occurrence may dramatically change the fate of the

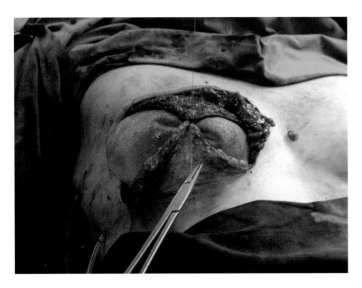

Fig. 14.28 Closure of the pouch.

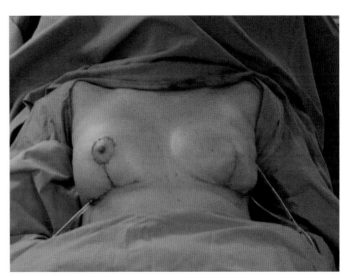

Fig. 14.30 Sit-up position and final results of skin reducing mastectomy.

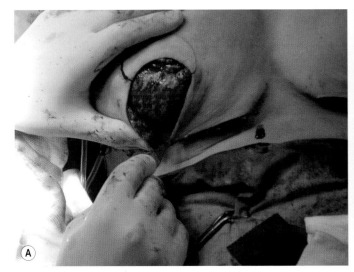

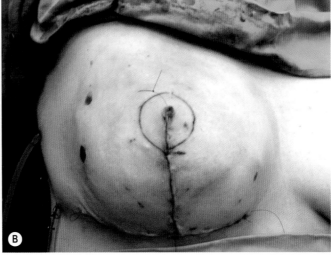

Fig. 14.29 (A,B) Skin closure and inverted T-scar.

reconstruction with implant extrusion and delays in further reconstructive procedures and oncological treatments. An accurate selection of patient candidate to this technique is mandatory, as well as an extremely meticulous dissection of the inferior dermal flaps. This should aim to preserve an accurate vascularity of the flaps without compromising oncological safety and complete glandular dissection.

For all these reasons, the technique should be contraindicated in heavy smokers and in patients with skin of poor quality. All conditions affecting vascularity may challenge the final results of this technique. Alternative techniques have been proposed by other authors (also in cooperation with our research group), this can include permanent expanders or temporary expanders. The first have proven to effectively reduce complication rates although cosmetic results seem poorer due to the moderate expansion that can be provided to the lower pole. There are no scientific reports to date on the use of temporary tissue expanders as an effective tool to prevent complications in skin reducing mastectomies.

Second stage of immediate two stage reconstructions

The second stage is commonly performed 6 months after the end of tissue expansion. This delay allows tissue stretching and provides an initial degree of ptosis to the reconstructed breast; completion of adjuvant therapies is also allowed. The expander is removed and replaced by a permanent anatomical implant. A total capsulectomy has to be performed to let the permanent prosthesis perfectly accommodate in the pouch preventing rotation and displacement. Furthermore, minor refinements to the reconstructed breast can be undertaken such as enlargement of the pocket and contouring of the breast.

Width and height of the permanent anatomical implant should be already calculated at the time of the first surgical stage and are normally very similar to those of the temporary expander to those of the temporary expander. Small variations can be decided intraoperatively and are related to the final degree of ptosis also. Disposable intraoperative sizers are available on the market by the largest manufacturers to assist low experienced surgeons.

We would advise consideration of the third parameter (i.e., projection) as a constant and to employ only prosthesis with a high projection. Contralateral breast must be accurately re-assessed. Its width and height are crucial parameters in planning the final contralateral procedure. On the healthy side, a breast reduction or a mastopexy are required procedures for large or ptotic breast; the shape of a small breast is very difficult to match without augmentation on the healthy side. The operative field should be arranged to let both breasts to be visible within the operative field; the level of both inframammary folds has to be marked.

Surgical steps for prosthesis insertion

The mastectomy scar is normally removed and a new access is created in the same place (*Fig. 14.31*). The subcutaneous layer is then dissected from the muscular fibers that are incised alongside its anatomical direction.

Capsulectomy is normally performed with cutting diathermy with the expander still in place (*Fig. 14.32*). Once the capsule is almost entirely dissected from the pectoralis major, we remove the expander and we complete the capsulectomy. Following capsulectomy, the superficial fascia is divided at the level of the inframammary fold, which is marked by needles inserted into the pouch through the skin. The lower edge of the superficial fascia is sutured to the chest wall musculature using continuous sutures of strong absorbable material (1/0). Before implantation, we normally put one drain in the pouch (*Fig. 14.33*). The selected prosthesis is then inserted and the final result is checked with the patient in the sitting position (*Fig. 14.34*). The wound is closed in two layers using absorbable sutures material. We normally perform the second stage of breast reconstruction in a double equip. Two surgeons operate on the mastectomy side, while a second team works on the healthy side. We use all the techniques of cosmetic surgery of the breast for reshaping of the contralateral breast. The final result should resemble the reconstructed breast. ⊛ FIGS **14.32, 14.34** APPEAR ONLINE ONLY

Contralateral adjustment

Patients with small breasts

A contralateral breast augmentation is advisable in this cohort of patients. We prefer to put the implant in a

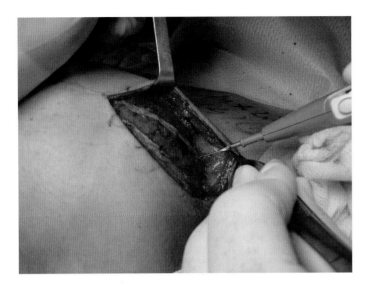

Fig. 14.31 Second stage; change of tissue expander for permanent implant. Incision along the previous mastectomy scar.

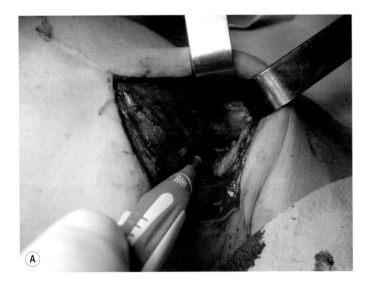

Fig. 14.32 (A) Total capsulectomy is always performed with cutting diathermy or using fingers.

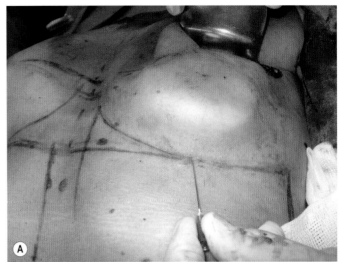

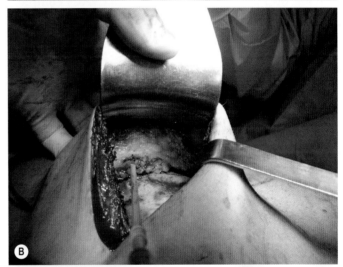

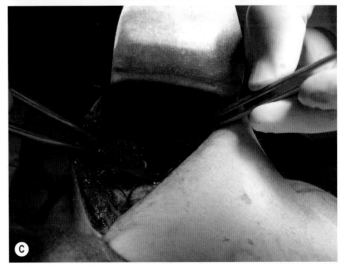

Fig. 14.33 Reconstruction of the inframammary fold. **(A)** Needle insertion to mark the fold from outside. **(B)** The superficial fascia is harvested and ready for suturing. **(C)** Strong absorbable material is used is used for running suturing.

sub-fascial place to obtain a natural final result with an appropriate degree of ptosis. The implant can be also placed totally sub-muscularly or in a dual plane with muscular coverage for the upper pole and with the lower pole in sub-glandular position. The reconstruction can be sorted in one stage.

Patients with medium size breasts

This subset of patients mainly benefits from a con-tralateral mastopexy that we call "autho-prosthesis".

Using a usual incision (Wise pattern), we harvest a superior flap bearing the nipple areola-complex (NAC) and an inferior dermal adipose flap that can be put underneath the nipple to over project it. The excessive skin in this way can be reduced and the cutaneous envelope is reshaped with repositioning of the NAC at a proper distance from the sternal notch. Implants can also be employed if an augmentation is required.

Women with >22 cm from sternal notch (SN) to nipple (N) or with a ptotic breast or a long inferior pole are good candidates for this technique. The distance between the SN and N is not a determinant parameter, it is possible to use a superior or a medial pedicle for moving up the nipple-areola complex (NAC) complex, This choice depends also on the consistency of the glandular tissue, although the authors prefer the superior pedicle to move up the NAC no more than 6–8 cm and the medial pedicle when this distance is higher.

Patients with large breasts

Women with large breasts can benefit from breast reductions. We usually perform reductions employing a supero-medial or an inferior pedicle. This technique warrants proper cosmetic results and can be safely performed. In selected cases for larger reduction, an inferior pedicle reduction can be employed. Also in this case, a second surgical step can be avoided. Using a skin reducing mastectomy, the breast reduction can be accomplished in one stage with the mastectomy.

Delayed reconstruction

A delayed breast reconstruction is performed for several reasons: uncertainty regarding the need for postoperative radiotherapy; patient's decision for psychological reasons; mastectomy performed by surgeons not prepared for breast reconstructions. Delayed reconstructions need a careful preoperative assessment to reach good final results. The patient's oncological status should be updated to avoid operating in the presence of local or metastatic recurrent disease. Contralateral mammography is mandatory if not performed within 6 months before the operation.

The tissues of the chest wall must be carefully examined with attention to the quality of skin, scars, and pectoralis major muscle. If the chest wall musculature is severely atrophic and associated with thin, tight skin, implant insertion is contraindicated. Fat injection may be advisable in such cases or alternatively, a myocutaneous pedicled or free flap may be considered. In order to get satisfactory results in delayed reconstruction, the pectoralis major muscle, together with skin and subcutaneous tissue, must be adequately preserved following elevation from the chest wall. The muscle may be deficient inferiorly where prosthesis coverage is constituted of skin and subcutaneous layers only. As for immediate reconstruction, width and height of the contralateral breast guide the selection of an appropriately sized expander. If the contralateral breast has marked ptosis and there is adequate skin, a larger expander can be chosen in order to generate over expansion. All other steps as well as the contralateral adjustment are not different from immediate breast reconstructions.

Postoperative care

Implant-based reconstructions do not require special postoperative care. Prophylactic antibiotics with activity against staphylococcal bacteria should be routinely administered and therefore postoperative administration is not required without clinical signs of infection. Postoperative pain and discomfort is generally of short duration with this form of reconstruction and can be controlled with routine analgesia.

Applying bandaging can help enhance the inframammary fold, but only surgical correction will create a durable fold in the long term. A well-fitting sports bra should be worn following reconstruction and contralateral surgery. Intensive exercise should be avoided for 2–3 weeks, although arm and shoulder mobilization is important following formal axillary dissection. Inflation of the prosthesis should be carried out weekly and ideally performed in a designated outpatient area. After surgery, the dressing is changed on the first postoperative day and the wound is cleaned with iodopovidone solution.

If no complications occur and the drainage fluids are not hematic, the patient can be discharged on the second postoperative day. We do not remove the drain until it reaches 30–40 ml per day and we send the patient home with prescription of oral antibiotic therapy.

At 3–4 days after discharge, the patient is seen in the outpatient clinic for drain removal and renewal of the dressing that will be removed 10–12 days after surgery. During the first stage of a two-stage procedure, we normally insert a pre-filled temporary expander at 30–40% of its final volume and carry on fillings for a couple of weeks afterwards. We normally inject 60–100 cc of saline solution every 3 weeks (on the day before chemotherapy if this has to be performed). We complete the expansion in 2 months but 6 months at least are required to let the tissues relax before replacing the temporary expander with a permanent prosthesis. No special care is required in the interim. According to a study protocol currently ongoing in our institution, we perform the expansion phase in a very short time in all women scheduled to undergo post-mastectomy radiotherapy; the change for a permanent implant has to be performed before starting radiation.

In normal conditions, the second stage can be performed 6–12 months later. After the second operation, the management of the prosthesis does not require special follow-up. An ultrasound scan on clinical indication can be diagnostic in case of implant ruptures. The MRI scan is of course the "gold standard" to diagnose shell ruptures. This does not need to be performed on a regular basis.

Outcomes and complications

Hematoma

This usually shows up in the first or second postoperative day. If bleeding occurs and the drain is working properly, the patient has to be referred back to theatre to reduce the risk of systemic complications (*Fig. 14.35*). Large clots may stop suction and may accumulate in the pocket; even in this case, it is advisable to take the patient back to theatre for surgical revision of the pouch. Bleeding complications may appear also on the contralateral side. In this case, the treatment will vary according to the technique employed for symmetrization: usually small stable hematomas after breast pexy/reduction do not need any treatment and they resolve completely after a couple of weeks; it can be useful to use heparin cream, however, if an augmentation has been performed, even a small hematoma

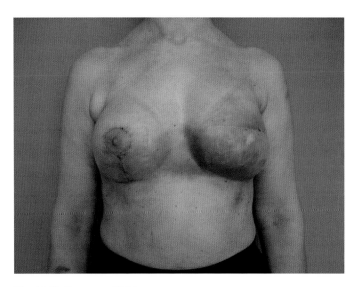

Fig. 14.35 Hematoma of left breast.

inside the pocket around the implant needs to be evacuated because they can compromise the overall long-term result, producing a very high rate of capsular contracture.

Before taking the patient back to theatre, the radiologist can attempt to evacuate the bleeding using ultrasonography. It is also possible to attempt to replace the drain already blocked by clots; even in this case, if the maneuver is performed on US-scan guidance, the risk of implant rupturing can be minimized. Large clots however, do not leave any alternative to surgical evacuation.

Erythema and cellulitis

Erythema (*Fig. 14.36*) is a frequent response of the skin to dissection and it will resolve spontaneously. If erythema is associated with symptoms of infection (malaise, fever, or an increase in drainage through the suction catheters), intravenous antibiotic therapy either on an inpatient basis or via a home-care service, should be provided. Failure of cellulitis to resolve indicates peri-implant infection. Expander removal is required with a repeat of stage 1, in 3–6 months.

Persistent serous drainage through suction catheter

After 10 days, wound contamination at the drain exit site becomes a real risk. Drain removal and aspiration

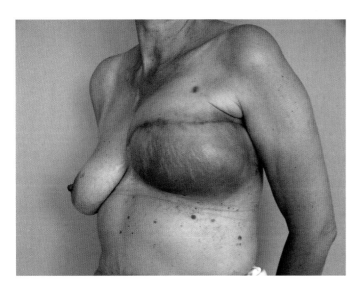

Fig. 14.36 Skin cellulitis inflammation.

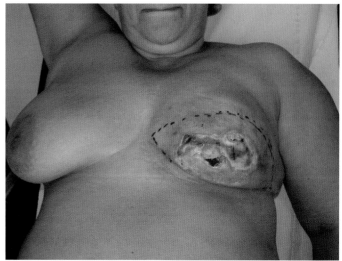

Fig. 14.37 Skin necrosis and implant exposure.

of fluid lateral to the anterior axillary line are feasible because implant migration lateral to the anterior axillary line is avoided by the pectoralis major muscle flap. If serous accumulation is extensive, reoperation with culture of the expanders, irrigation of the space, and insertion of new drains are appropriate.

Partial or complete skin necrosis

Minimal epidermolysis at the wound edges may be observed after removal of dressing. In our experience, this is not going to compromise the implant stability but it may reduce the overall cosmetic results.

If partial or complete skin necrosis at the suture line is observed, muscle coverage of the expander in this region is generally provided by the pectoralis major muscle or a segmental rectus muscle flap. For small areas of necrosis, the use of topical antibiotics and local wound care are generally adequate. We normally apply "Hydrogel" dressing; however, the main point is to identify the deepness of the necrosis without removing the superficial necrotized layer too quickly. In cases of evident deep skin necrosis, we start with a moderate curettage of the superficial layer every 2 days, combined with advanced wound dressing to help the deep layers to heal. Is difficult to solve big areas of skin necrosis and often implant removal may become unavailable. Small defects can be washed with antibiotic solution (amikacin) and a salvage multiple layers suture can be performed.

When necrotic complications occur, the expansion process has to be delayed pending healing of areas of partial or complete skin loss.

If there is concern about impending expander exposure, options include:

1. Excision of the area of skin necrosis and advancement of the remaining envelope for closure and implant closure and implant coverage
2. Use of a distant flap
3. Expander removal with plans for delayed reconstruction.

In general, if the skin necrosis is extensive, expander removal with a plan for delayed reconstruction is preferred. If the implant-expander is exposed with peri-implant purulent drainage, expander removal is also recommended. With implant removal, culture-specific antibiotic therapy on an outpatient basis will resolve the infection. Expander-implant reinsertion can be scheduled after a minimum of 3–6 months, depending on the status of the overlying skin envelope.

Expander failure or malfunction

Expander failure or malfunction (*Figs 14.37, 14.38*) may occur if the expander will not retain saline injections because of loss of expander wall integrity. In this instance, expander replacement as an operative procedure is required. The position of the expander port should be confirmed both at the time of the

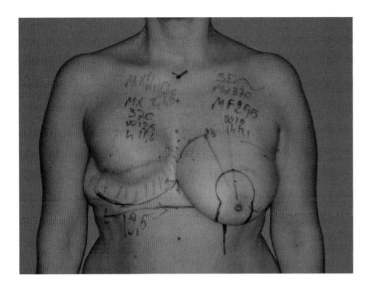

Fig. 14.38 Expander malpositioning and rotation.

expander insertion (intraoperative position) and immediately before inflation of the expander (outpatient facility). Position of the expander port may be determined by a combination of palpation and use of an appropriate port locater, based on the manufacturer's recommendations.

If the expander or a distant port has been placed upside down or rotated during the postoperative period, the position must be altered to allow inflation with saline. If attempts to manipulate the expander or port fail, the patient will require intraoperative relocation of the device to allow sequential inflation. This problem can usually be avoided if the port location and access are confirmed after wound closure while the patient is still under anesthesia.

Infection

If an infection occurs, there can be systemic and local temperature increase as well as and pain and redness of the soft tissues covering the prosthesis. If this phenomenon appears during a short course of postoperative oral amoxicillin and in absence of exudates for microbiology culture, we prescribe levofloxacin or other broad spectrum antibiotics. A correct choice of antibiotics may positively prevent tissue erosion and implant extrusion.

Complications occur in the perioperative period, early (3–6 weeks), and late. Studies investigating complications common to expander-implant reconstruction show great variability in reported rates.[47]

Perioperative complications include hematoma, seroma, and infection. Hematoma requires reoperation and ranges from 0% to 5.8%. Seroma is usually avoided with a closed suction system, but if it is extensive, it may require open drainage. Infection rates range from 0% to 15%. Antibiotic therapy for early cellulites may be effective. Perioperative antibiotics in immediate reconstruction are recommended. Early complications usually involve skin envelope necrosis, infection, and expander-implant malfunction. Skin envelope necrosis may occur in the range of 0% to 21%.[47] A rate exceeding 10% may represent a relative contraindication to immediate reconstruction, particularly in skin-sparing mastectomy. Usually, a small segment of skin at the incision site may be vulnerable to ischemic necrosis. With muscle coverage of the expander-implant, local wound care, and topical antibiotics, healing should occur without jeopardy to the implant. When skin necrosis is more extensive, unless the implant is well covered with muscle, implant exposure may occur, and subsequent removal may become necessary. When infection occurs in the implant space, implant removal is necessary with delayed secondary reconstruction after wound healing and scar maturation are achieved. Tenderness, late seroma development, low-grade fever, and leukocytosis usually indicate implant space infection.

Malfunction of the expander-implant in the early postoperative period should be rare. Proper placement of the expander and confirmation of port patency after skin closure during the operative procedure should avoid problems. Confirmation with devices to locate the port during early expansion will avoid inadvertent puncture of the expander. If malfunction occurs in the early postoperative period, re-exploration is required with replacement of the nonfunctional expander-implant.

Late complications related to expander-implant reconstruction extend throughout the life of the patient. Delayed implant deflations and rupture represent the greatest concern for the patient. Deflation and rupture rates are difficult to determine because the design of both saline- and gel-filled implants is constantly changing. The risk, however, does increase with implant age. A minimum of 15% of modern implants can be expected to rupture 3–10 years after implantation. This observation is based on a study of 271 women who had received breast implants at least 3 years before their evaluation by sequential magnetic resonance imaging. Long-term saline implant deflation rates are reported in the 5–6% range.[48,49] The diagnosis of saline implant failure is easily made because of implant deflation and loss of breast volume. Exploration and implant exchange are required. With the silicone gel implant, it is difficult to diagnose implant rupture.

The breast size and shape will not necessarily change because the silicone remains in the breast pocket, and a mammogram will not always detect implant rupture. Magnetic resonance imaging can help confirm diagnosis of a ruptured silicone gel implant with a reported sensitivity for detection of implant rupture of 86.7%, with a specificity of 88.5%.[38]

The Baker classification continues to be the most common rating system for capsular contracture *(Table 14.1, Fig. 14.31)*. Capsular contracture occurs at a variable rate ranging from 1–38%. The capsular contracture rate is similar after reconstruction with either saline or silicone gel implants and appears to be in the 16–30% range (Baker III/IV), based on implant studies reported at FDA hearings for the major implant manufacturers.[50] The most common reason for reoperation in the expander-implant patient is for correction of capsular contracture or implant shell failure with rupture or leak. Wrinkling is another long-term problem observed with implants and may be observed in the range of 20–25% of patients (www.fda.gov).

Sub-muscular positioning of the implant will avoid adherence of the skin envelope to the implant and resultant distortion of the skin overlying the implant. The use of a textured implant shell may prevent symptomatic capsular contracture but seems to increase the rate of wrinkling due to adhesions of the skin envelope to the implant shell. Since 1980, there has been concern about the possible association between silicone gel implants and autoimmune diseases. In the Institute of Medicine study of Safety of Silicone Implants report, it was noted that there is no plausible evidence of a novel autoimmune disease because of silicone gel implants. Similar observations reviewed by large meta-analyses have concluded that there is no association between implants and autoimmune diseases (e.g., rheumatoid arthritis, systemic lupus erythematosus, and scleroderma).

Table 14.1 Baker classification of capsular contracture

Grade	Description
I	Soft
II	Less soft, but implant not visible
III	Moderate firmness, implant can be palpated or distortion can be seen
IV	Very firm, hard, tender, painful, and cold

(Reproduced with permission from Baker JL Jr. Classification of spherical contractures. Paper presented at the Aesthetic Breast Symposium, Scottsdale, AZ, 1975.)

Several clinical studies have been conducted by the largest manufacturer to determine the most common complications, as well as the benefits of their implants. Allergan for instance conducted several clinical studies to test its saline-filled breast implants, including the Large Simple Trial (LST), the 1995 Reconstruction Study (R95) (and augmentation cohort, A95), and the Post Approval Survey Study.[47,51] The LST was designed to determine the 1-year rates of capsular contracture, infection, implant leakage or deflation, and implant replacement or removal.[52,53] There were 2333 patients enrolled for augmentation, 225 for reconstruction, and 317 for revision (replacement of existing implants). Of these enrolled patients, 62% returned for their 1-year follow-up visit. The R95 and A95 studies were designed to assess all complications as well as the patient's satisfaction, body image, body esteem, and self-concept during the initial 5 years after breast reconstruction. Patients were observed annually, and data through 3 years (with partial 4-year data) were presented to the FDA for pre-market device approval. The most common complications reported were asymmetry and capsular contracture *(Table 14.2)*. During the 5 years reviewed by the study, there were 70 devices removed in 62 patients. Of these 70 devices, 49 were replaced and 21 were not. The most common reason for implant removal through 5 years was capsular contracture (31% of the 70 implants removed).

After premarket approval, Allergan transitioned data collection to a post-approval study. The Post Approval Survey Study (PASS) was designed to collect long-term safety data from patients 6–10 years after implant placement. The patients receive surveys each year. The PASS data are shown for both the R95 (reconstructive) cohorts.

Table 14.2 Complications reported for reconstruction patients (INAMED R95 study)

Complications (n=237 patients)	3-year complication rate (%)[a]	5-year complication rate (%)
Additional operation (reoperation)	39	45
Asymmetry[b]	33	39
Capsular contracture	25	36
Implant replacement or removal for any reason	23	28
Wrinkling[b]	23	25
Implant palpability or visibility[b]	20	27
Breast pain[b]	15	18
Loss of nipple sensation[b]	12	18
Implant malposition[b]	12	17
Irritation or inflammation[b]	7	7
Leakage or deflation	6	8
Intense skin sensation[b]	6	6
Scarring complications	6	6
Infection	5	6
Capsule calcification[b]	5	5
Seroma	4	4
Skin or tissue necrosis	4	4
Delayed wound healing[b]	3	3
Implant extrusion	3	3
Rash	3	3
Hematoma	1	1

[a]As reported in original premarket approval submission. [b]These complications were assessed with severity ratings. Only the rates for moderate, severe, and very severe (excludes mild and very mild ratings) are shown in this table.
(Reproduced with permission from INAMED. Making an informed decision (patient brochure). Santa Barbara: INAMED Aesthetics; January 2005.)

Table 14.3 Complications (INAMED pass study)

Complication (n=237 patients)	7-year complication rate (%)
Reoperation	49
Capsular contracture	43
Implant removal	31
Breast pain	26
Implant deflation	12

(Reproduced with permission from INAMED. Making an informed decision (patient brochure). Santa Barbara: INAMED Aesthetics; January 2005.)

Table 14.4 Primary reason for implant removal (INAMED pass study)

Primary reason for implant removal (n=81)	Implants removed through 7 years (%)
Implant deflation	25
Capsular contracture	25
Patient choice	24
Infection	9
Implant extrusion	5
Other[a]	5
Implant malposition	4
Wrinkling	3
Asymmetry	3
Total	100

[a]Other reasons, as reported by the physician, were recurrent carcinoma (n=1); abnormality on computed tomographic scan at mastectomy site (n=1); poor tissue expansion due to irradiation (n=1); and second stage breast reconstruction (n=1).
(Reproduced with permission from INAMED. Making an informed decision (patient brochure). Santa Barbara: INAMED Aesthetics; January 2005.).

The data presented through 7 years include earlier data shown in the tables with new information added *(Tables 14.3, 14.4)*. Of the patients who provided satisfaction scores at 7 years after implant placement, 88% indicated that they were satisfied with their implants.

Outcomes of breast reconstruction with implants

In a study comparing three consecutive study groups, there was no significant difference in major and minor complication rates between autogenous and non-autogenous reconstruction.[54] Similarly, in the Michigan Breast Reconstruction Outcome Study, total complication rates between the expander-implant reconstructive groups and the combined TRAM flap groups showed no significant difference *(Table 14.5)*. When the operative time is compared, the total time for expander-implant procedures remains much less than for flap procedures, but the average number of procedures is greater *(Table 14.6)*.

Thus, the patient's choice, the status of the mastectomy site, and the status of the contralateral breast will

Table 14.5 Frequency of complications by type of reconstruction

Complication	Implants n	Implants (%)	Pedicle TRAM flaps n	Pedicle TRAM flaps (%)	Free TRAM flaps n	Free TRAM flaps (%)
Back pain	1	1.3	4	2.2	4	6.0
Hernia/abdominal wall laxity	–	14	7	8	8	11.9
Lymphedema	33	8	10	5.6	3	4.5
Capsular contracture	12	15.2	–		–	
Implant shift	1	1.3	–		–	
Wound dehiscence	3	3.8	10	5.6	1	1.5
Partial flap loss (fat necrosis)	5	6.3	29	16	2 10	14.9
Total flap loss	0		2	1.1	1	1.5
Anastomotic thrombosis	–		–		4	6.0
Implant failure	3	3.8	–		–	
Infection	28	35.4	21	11.7	12	17.9
Clostridium difficile colitis	0		1	0.5	0	
Hematoma/seroma of the breast	4	5.1	7	3.9	6	9.0
Hematoma/seroma of the abdomen	–		7	3.9	3	4.5
Abdominal wall necrosis	–		3	1.7	0	
Cardiac/pulmonary complications	1	1.3	6	3.4	6	9.0

(Reproduced with permission from Wilkins EG, Cederna PS, Lowery JC, *et al*. Prospective analysis of psychosocial outcomes in breast reconstruction: one-year postoperative results from the Michigan Breast Reconstruction Outcome study. Plast Reconstr Surg 2000; 106:1014–1027.)

Table 14.6 Average operative time for each technique and average number of procedures for final result

	Average operative time by technique (h)	Average number of procedures[a] on reconstructed breast by technique
Implant (n=82)	1.2	1.8
Staged tissue expander-implant (n=142)	3.2	2.4
Latissimus dorsi implant (n=107)	3.8	1.7
TRAM flap (n=106)	5.5	1.2
Free flap (n=12)	9.0	1.2

Operative techniques have improved with experience, and time required for free flaps has been reduced by 3 h on average. [a]Does not include nipple-areola reconstruction. (Reproduced with permission from Trabulsy PP, Anthony JP, Mathes SJ. Changing trends in postmastectomy breast reconstruction: a 13-year experience. Plast Reconstr Surg 1994; 93:1418–1427.)

determine which procedure offers the best outcome for the individual patient. Because of decreased technique complexity, no additional donor site scar and potential complications, and shorter recovery time, many patients will select nonautogenous expander-implant reconstruction. The choice in breast reconstruction primarily centers on nonautogenous versus autogenous. Nonautogenous reconstruction encompasses a wide range of techniques, including implant alone, postoperative adjustable implant, staged expander-implant, and flaps incorporating an implant for breast mound volume (e.g., latissimus dorsi muscle, TRAM, abdominal advancement). Similarly, there is a wide variety of autogenous reconstruction techniques, including pedicled TRAM flap, free TRAM flap, perforator flaps, and latissimus dorsi musculocutaneous flaps. It is therefore difficult to compare outcome results because each surgeon and breast care center emphasize different procedures on the basis of experience and confidence, with specific techniques. Implant-expander techniques are widely used throughout the world, providing safe and reliable breast reconstruction. The Michigan Breast Reconstruction Outcome Study[55] demonstrated greater aesthetic and general satisfaction of patients undergoing reconstruction by pedicled and free TRAM flaps compared with patients undergoing expander-implant reconstruction. However, pedicled or free TRAM flap procedures are more complex and require longer hospitalization and outpatient recovery time. Post-reconstruction satisfaction rates vary for expander-implants, but in most studies, they range from 78%[56] to 61%.[57] Clough[58] noted a decline in aesthetic satisfaction from an initial rate of 86% at 2 years to 54% at 5 years after implant reconstruction. The linear decrease in satisfaction is multifactorial but may be a result of long-term complications, such as capsular contracture and asymmetric contralateral ptosis.

Experience of the authors

We demonstrated that implant based two stage breast reconstruction generates high satisfaction rates in patients' and surgeons' opinion.[59] A three-step evaluation scale was employed in our study (medium good bad); a large majority (66%) of patients with a good opinion of the reconstruction was demonstrated. The surgeons' rate regarding the shape of the reconstructed breast was rated as good in 75.2% of cases. The Achilles' heel of this strategy is the difficulty in reaching a satisfactory symmetry. However, even in this case, the large majority of cases received a good rate (54.8%) and only a residual subgroup was rated as "bad".

Patients with bilateral prosthesis (contralateral augmentation) reached the best scores (79.2% good results; no bad results). This observation demonstrated the cosmetic purpose of our reconstructive strategy. The best results are obtained when a significantly improved appearance of breast shape is attained.

The complication in the setting of nonirradiated patients is very low (8% overall) as well as the extrusion rate. No Baker III and IV were observed in our series although the observation period was quite short. On the contrary, a high secondary replacement rate has been reported (7.7%); this can be an effect of our attempt to pursue effective cosmetic results.

A higher complication rate is demonstrated in "skin reducing mastectomies". Long and angulated residual flaps may become easily ischemic and the larger the breast we are going to remove, the higher is the risk of flap necrosis. Alteration of shape may also be due to implant rotation and malpositioning; inframammary fold malposition can also be possible.

Secondary procedures

Although a low complication rate is demonstrated, in our experience secondary procedures can be required in selected patients.

Revision for cosmetic purposes

An implant replacement only for cosmetic purposes *(Fig. 14.39)* can be justified in view of the low invasiveness of the procedure. A fine adjustment can improve the results in terms of symmetry, still the real limitation of this strategy *(Fig. 14.32)*. In such cases, implant removal can be indicated only when it creates difficulties in dressing up or in wearing a bra and could be interfering with the activities of everyday life.

At the time of revision, it is also possible to discuss with the patient a synchronous revision of contralateral surgery. Sometimes an implant may be required to regain a good projection. We would also suggest a total capsulectomy be performed, to prevent rotation and malpositioning.

Fat injection

The substitution rate has been recently lowered by the advent of fat injection *(Fig. 14.40)* for cosmetic and regenerative purposes. The Coleman technique can be employed to graft adipose tissue and fill areas of partial defects due to excessively aggressive mastectomies or mistakes in survey and projecting. FIG 14.40 APPEARS ONLINE ONLY

Fat can be harvested from the hips and abdomen and then grafted into the subcutaneous- layer of the reconstructed breast. The liposuction can further increase the cosmetic effectiveness of this reconstructive strategy.

Nipple reconstruction

The nipple areola complex, when not preserved, is reconstructed in a second stage with a local flaps

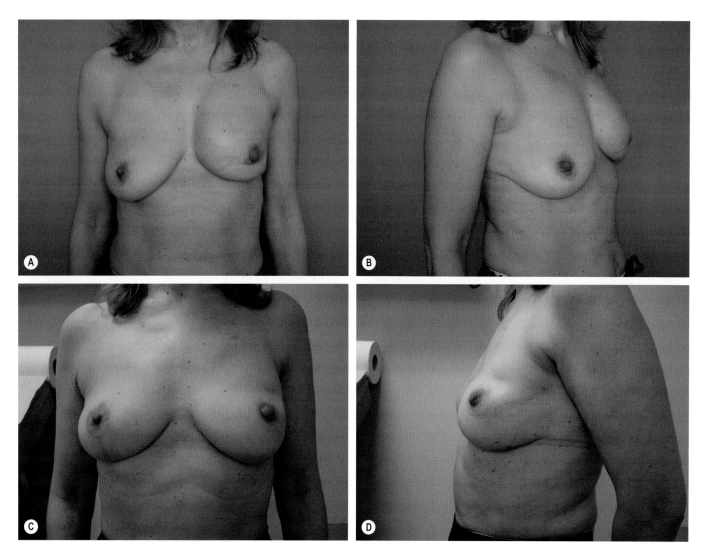

Fig. 14.39 Revision for cosmetic purposes. **(A)** Frontal view after the second stage. **(B)** Lateral view: dislocation; **(C,D)** Cosmetic results after 6 years from mastectomy.

technique 6 months after the second surgical stage. A tattoo is performed to replace the hyperchromic areolar tissue.

Other reconstructive techniques involving implants and/or tissue expansions

Adjustable, permanent expander-implant (Fig. 14.41)

Although this is not the authors' recommended method of reconstruction, and we employ it in a minimal percentage of cases, we would like to briefly describe breast reconstructions in one stage with permanent expanders. In 1984, Hilton Becker designed the first adjustable, permanent implant-expander with a detachable reservoir to allow the device to be left in place as a permanent implant. In 1992, about 14% of reconstructions with implants were estimated to be permanent expander-implants.[60] The original Becker-type design of expander implant has a silicone gel-filled outer lumen (25% or 50% overall volume) that surrounds an expandable saline inner lumen. The newer Mentor Spectrum implant is saline filled and more widely used because of the FDA restrictions placed on silicone gel-filled implants in 1992.[31] Improvements made as a result of early experience include a textured surface (to mitigate both capsular contracture and implant migration) and the availability of anatomically shaped devices. FIG **14.41** APPEARS ONLINE ONLY

The obvious advantages of the adjustable, permanent expander-implant include the single-stage procedure and ability to adjust the size of the implant postoperatively. Patients with smaller breasts can undergo skin-sparing mastectomy with immediate permanent tissue expanders placement with nominal saline fill volumes.

Addition of a latissimus dorsi musculocutaneous flap to this approach provides a small skin island to fill the areola defect. With preservation of the complete skin envelope and the addition of latissimus muscle coverage of the implant, a breast mound can be established with the adjustable implant without limitations resulting from closure of the areola excision site.

A disadvantage of a single-stage implant-based reconstruction is the inability to adjust the breast (and contralateral breast) aesthetically at a second procedure. Immediate reconstruction with the permanent implant-expander is also a relative contraindication in patients requiring postoperative radiotherapy. Furthermore, the permanent expanders do not allow a proper degree of expansion to the lower pole and at without a second surgical stage there is no chance for inframammary fold reshape.

Disadvantages are also related to the increased complications, such as capsular contracture, rupture, hematoma, wound infection, wound seroma, extrusion of implant, migration of implant, leakage of implant, chronic pain, skin or fat necrosis, and wound dehiscence.[47,51,61–64] Gui et al.[47] reported on immediate breast reconstruction with bio-dimensional anatomic permanent expander-implants. They found that this one-stage procedure with anatomically shaped implants gave good results. The implant was filled to 50% with saline intraoperatively, after placement and closure of the sub-muscular and sub-cutaneous pockets. Final implant filling was usually achieved in one or two outpatient visits, as opposed to the multiple visits most often reported. Although no information about capsule formation was reported because of the short-term follow-up of patients, early complication rates were moderate to low, including infection (5.2%), hematoma (1.6%), seroma (0%), skin necrosis (3%), implant loss or extrusion (3.9%), and deflation (0%). The results of a questionnaire, to which 96 of the 107 patients studied responded, indicated that 88% of patients were satisfied with their reconstructive outcome.

Despite the reported complications, 89% of women expressed satisfaction during follow-up, to the plastic surgeon. With the popularity of the skin-sparing mastectomy, when immediate single-stage reconstruction is planned with use of a permanent adjustable implant, the closure of the defect at the site of the resection of the NAC is difficult to accomplish without some distortion of the preserved skin envelope. Direct closure usually requires extension of the incision laterally to avoid unnatural appearance of the retained skin in proximity to the areola defect closure.

Expander-implant use in association with flaps

A flap is often used for breast reconstruction to avoid a staged procedure, which is required when an implant is used. However, there are instances in which an implant used in association with a flap will enhance or even enable the reconstructive process. A permanent prosthesis may be used in conjunction with an immediate flap after failed breast reconstruction in which skin necrosis led to implant exposure. In such cases, there may be a lack of healthy tissue to provide a good coverage.

In this condition, we prefer to use a latissimus dorsi muscle flap although we must admit that its role for secondary reconstruction is even more restricted to patients that are not suitable for fat grafting and delayed breast reconstructions.

Breast envelope preservation for staged flap reconstruction

When use of a flap is anticipated for immediate breast reconstruction, there may be concern about tumor margins or requirements for radiation therapy based on pathologic examination of the permanent specimen.

Temporary use of an expander allows preservation of the skin envelope, particularly after skin-sparing mastectomy. If radiation therapy is required, flap reconstruction can be delayed until after therapy is completed to avoid damage to an autogenous flap. During the process of radiation therapy, the expander will preserve the skin envelope and reduce the requirement for skin replacement at the second-stage reconstruction. There is still an ongoing discussion of the value of immediate flap reconstruction with irradiation of the flap versus delay in the flap until the radiation therapy is completed.

Developments

The development of fat injection techniques to refine the results of implant-based breast reconstructions is changing the outcome of this surgery. On the discovery of this new tool, it is possible that in a few years implants will disappear and that fat injection will permanently take their place. In our opinion however, this is not going to be immediate. As happens in other fields, a new technology replaces the old one only after a variable period of coexistence. This is the reason why the authors are currently developing and validating a transition surgical model that we have named "hybrid breast reconstructions".

This new system encompasses prosthesis and fat grafting as integrated tools to improve the final reconstructive outcome. Fat grafting in this view is not only employed for refinements or to treat radio-induced damages but is a preoperatively planned part of the reconstruction. The final volume we want to achieve will be made up of fat and implants in a variable percentage according to body contour and breast morphology. For instance, a thin lady who has no fat will be likely to receive a reconstruction whose volume will be made of implants nearly at 100%. On the other hand, a woman with fatty hips and small breasts could obtain a full fat breast reconstruction.

The large majority of patients, either in the first surgical stage or in the second one, may require a temporary or permanent implant to mold the shape of the new breast. A total replacement of prosthesis with fat is not realistic at this moment. The use of implants will be required unless new technologies of regenerative medicine are discovered to stabilize the shape of a full-fat reconstructed breast.

Concerns are still present regarding the safety of inducing tissue regeneration and neo-angiogenesis in areas that previously hosted a neoplasm.

 Bonus images for this chapter can be found online at **http://www.expertconsult.com**

28. Neumann CG. The expansion of an area of skin by progressive distention of a subcutaneous balloon. *Plast Reconstr Surg.* 1957;19:124.

An historical study on tissue expansion.

29. Radovan C. Breast reconstruction after mastectomy using the temporary expander. *Plast Reconstr Surg.* 1982;69:195.

32. Carlson GW, Bostwick 3rd J, Styblo TM, et al. Skin-sparing mastectomy. Oncologic and reconstructive considerations. *Ann Surg.* 1997;225:570–575.

This study introduced the basic concepts of skin preservation. Skin incisions for removal of glandular tissue are subdivided into four groups.

33. Losken A, Carlson GW, Bostwick 3rd J, et al. Trends in unilateral breast reconstruction and management of the contralateral breast: The Emory experience. *Plast Reconstr Surg.* 2002;110:89–97.

36. Handel N, Silverstein MJ. Breast cancer diagnosis and prognosis in augmented women. *Plast Reconstr Surg.* 2006;118(3):587–596.

38. Herborn CU, Marincek B, Ermann D, et al. Breast augmentation and reconstructive surgery: MR imaging of implant rupture and malignancy. *Eur Radiol.* 2002;12:2198–2206.

39. Krueger EA, Wilkins EG, Strawderman M. Complications and patient satisfaction following expander/implant breast reconstruction with and without radiotherapy. *Int J Radiat Oncol Biol Phys.* 2001;49:713–721.

45. Cordeiro PG, Pusic AL, Disa JJ, et al. Irradiation after immediate tissue expander/implant breast reconstruction: outcomes, complications, aesthetic results, and satisfaction among 156 patients. *Plast Reconstr Surg.* 2004;113(3):877–881.

The impact of radiation in implant-based reconstruction is investigated in this study. The authors would support this technique as a proper alternative to flap-based reconstructions.

46. Serra-Renom JM, Muñoz-Olmo JL, Serra-Mestre JM. Fat grafting in postmastectomy breast reconstruction with expanders and prostheses in patients who have received radiotherapy: formation of new subcutaneous tissue. *Plast Reconstr Surg.* 2010;125(1):12–18.

This study investigates the effects of fat grafting in the treatment of radio-induced dermatitis. This is the largest series currently available in literature.

59. Nava MB, Spano A, Cadenelli P, et al. Extra-projected implants as an alternative surgical model for breast reconstruction. Implantation strategy and early results. *Breast.* 2008;17(4):361–366.

A new reconstructive paradigm is introduced in this paper. Breast reconstructions aim to rebuild a bilateral breast mound of a medium size, with extra-projection and cosmetically pleasant.

15

Latissimus dorsi flap breast reconstruction

Scott L. Spear and Mark W. Clemens

SYNOPSIS

- The latissimus flap includes a large well-vascularized flat muscle that is well suited for dealing with poorly-vascularized or radiated defects, contour deformities following breast conservation therapy, or for covering an implant.
- Placement of a tissue expander under the latissimus muscle allows postoperative adjustment of breast volume and ultimately better symmetry with the opposite breast.
- Complete mobilization to reach medial breast defects may require the partial release (90%) of the latissimus dorsi insertion. This helps avoid the displeasing bulge in the low axilla, however care must be taken to protect the thoracodorsal vessels.
- The extended latissimus dorsi flap is a reliable method for totally autologous breast reconstruction and can be considered a primary choice for breast reconstruction, particularly in women who otherwise are at high risk for a TRAM flap or an implant procedure.

 Access the Historical Perspective section online at
http://www.expertconsult.com

Introduction

In 2009, the National Cancer Institute reported nearly 200 000 new diagnoses of invasive breast cancer among women, as well as an additional 60 000 cases of *in situ* breast cancer.[1] Progressively more of these women are receiving adjunctive radiation and may not be candidates for implant alone reconstructions. The main workhorses of autologous reconstructions are abdominal based flaps, however the latissimus dorsi myocutaneous flap is an essential reconstructive option. A renewed interest has developed in the latissimus dorsi flap for breast reconstruction due to its reliability, ease of dissection, versatility, and minimal donor site morbidity.

Anatomy

The latissimus dorsi muscle is a large, flat, triangular muscle measuring approximately 25×35 cm and covering the posterior inferior half of the trunk. The major part of its outer surface is subcutaneous. Its superomedial fibers are deep to the trapezius muscle. The remainder of the muscle is superficial to the serratus anterior and posterior muscles, a portion of the external oblique muscle, and the erector spinae.

The muscle originates from the iliac crest, the posterior layer of the thoracolumbar fascia, the lower six thoracic spines, and the lower third to fourth ribs laterally, where it is closely associated with some origins of the external oblique muscle. As the muscle passes toward the axilla, near the tip of the scapula, it converges in a spiral fashion and joins with fibers of the teres major to form the posterior axillary fold. The latissimus dorsi insertion is through a 3 cm-broad tendon attached to the intertubercular groove of the humerus.

At the level of the tenth to eleventh rib, there is a firm, thick aponeurotic attachment between the serratus anterior and the latissimus. These aponeurotic attachments correspond to the lower border of the serratus anterior; they must be divided during latissimus dorsi flap elevation to prevent inadvertent elevation of the serratus anterior muscle along with the latissimus dorsi flap.

The pattern of circulation of the latissimus dorsi muscle is type V according to the Mathes and Nahai classification.[13,14] The dominant pedicle is composed of the thoracodorsal artery, two veins, and the thoracodorsal nerve. The length of the thoracodorsal artery is 8 cm with a diameter of 2.5 mm. This vessel's relatively large diameter, predictability, and minimal anatomic variation along with the large musculocutaneous unit it supplies make the latissimus dorsi flap a highly reliable donor site as a transposition or free flap for breast reconstruction.

The thoracodorsal artery, along with the circumflex scapular artery, is a branch of the subscapular artery arising from the axillary artery. The thoracodorsal artery gives off a branch to the serratus muscle shortly after entering the underside of the latissimus muscle in the posterior axilla 10 cm inferior to the muscle insertion into the humerus *(Fig. 15.1)*. Understanding of the anatomy in this area is important. In patients with previous axillary dissection, when the thoracodorsal pedicle has been divided, a reversal of flow through the serratus branch can provide adequate blood flow to the flap, allowing the use of the latissimus dorsi muscle as a transposition flap based on its dominant vascular pedicle.[11] Once it is in the muscle, the vascular pedicle bifurcates into a large lateral descending branch and a smaller transverse branch. These branches arborize within the muscle to produce extensive intramuscular collateralization.[15–17] A precise knowledge of the internal vascular anatomy of the muscle makes it possible to split it for use as a double flap or to preserve half of the muscle to maintain function.

Secondary segmental pedicles enter the underside of the muscle through the lateral perforators row off the posterior intercostal arteries 5 cm from the posterior midline and through the medial perforators row off the lumbar artery adjacent to the site of muscle origin. These perforators allow the use of the latissimus dorsi as a foldover flap to cover midback defects.[18,19]

Numerous musculocutaneous perforators extend from this rich intramuscular vascular network into the

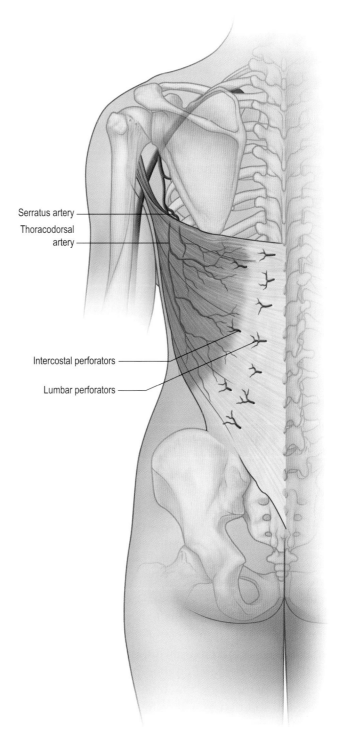

Serratus artery

Thoracodorsal artery

Intercostal perforators

Lumbar perforators

Fig. 15.1 The blood supply to the latissimus dorsi muscle.

overlying skin and subcutaneous tissue, allowing skin islands to be safely designed anywhere within the margin of the muscle. The largest perforators branch from the lateral branch of the thoracodorsal artery, making safest the skin island located in a lateral vertical orientation.[15–17]

The latissimus dorsi muscle adducts, extends, and rotates the humerus medially. It also assists in securing the tip of the scapula against the posterior chest wall. It is an expendable muscle because function is preserved by the remaining synergistic shoulder girdle muscles. Transposition of this muscle anteriorly has been shown to be well tolerated by patients and results in only a minimal functional deficit,[20,21] although dynamic weakness in shoulder extension and adduction may occur.[22]

Patient presentation

A preoperative consultation should gather detailed information about the patient's medical history, the state of local tissues, the condition of the breast, the possible donor sites, and the patient's wishes. Preoperative consultation should also address with the patient the advantages and disadvantages of an immediate versus a delayed reconstruction.

There remain some significant advantages to immediate reconstruction, including the plastic surgeon's help in design of the pattern of skin excision. When the skin defect can be limited to the areola, this allows a reconstruction with no visible scar on the breast. Scars are limited to the areolar skin island, where a small portion of flap skin is transposed to replace the areola. Immediate reconstruction has other benefits to the patient, including psychological as well as those of economies of time, money, and discomfort.

Nevertheless, there are advantages to delayed reconstruction too. Most notably, the final pathologic process will be known and all or most of the cancer treatment will have been completed, including the mastectomy, chemotherapy, and radiation therapy. In the context of delayed reconstruction, the breast skin, chest wall muscles, and soft tissues will be healed, and any resulting defects or problems should be apparent. The risk of infection, hematoma, and, most important, mastectomy flap necrosis should also be less.

In patients who will undergo immediate breast reconstruction, the planning requires an estimate of how much skin and breast tissue will be removed. Particular attention is given to the amount of skin and subcutaneous tissue obtainable in the dorsal region. A good indication is given by pinching the lateral dorsal pad to estimate the thickness of the adipose layer. It is vital to compare the mass available with that which will be needed to achieve a suitable breast size.

It is also important preoperatively to assess the function of the latissimus dorsi muscle. Denervated and nonfunctional muscle after an axillary dissection increases the risk of damaged thoracodorsal vessels or inadequate circulation. In this instance, the latissimus dorsi must then be elevated on an intact serratus collateral pedicle. Functioning muscle is most often a favorable sign for the integrity of the pedicle; however, it does not guarantee intact thoracodorsal vessels.

Arteriography is not ordinarily thought to be necessary to obtain information about the status of the thoracodorsal artery when there is good muscle function. The flap's nearly perfect reliability when the serratus collateral is preserved makes arteriography and electromyography virtually unnecessary.

Patient selection/indications

The decision to select the latissimus flap reconstruction must take into account the patient's motivations, the anatomy of the breast as well as of the back, the nature of underlying breast disease, and the competency of the surgical team.

The latissimus dorsi is helpful for breast reconstruction after a skin-sparing mastectomy when a breast prosthesis is part of the plan. The latissimus dorsi skin can be used to replace the missing skin at the site of the nipple-areola, and the muscle can be used to provide improved soft tissue coverage of the breast implant or expander *(Fig. 15.2)*. Placement of a tissue expander under the latissimus muscle allows postoperative adjustment of breast volume and ultimately better symmetry with the opposite breast *(Fig. 15.3)*. Use of the autogenous latissimus dorsi alone without a prosthesis does not allow as much range in the size of the reconstructed breast. In either instance, it is difficult to assess

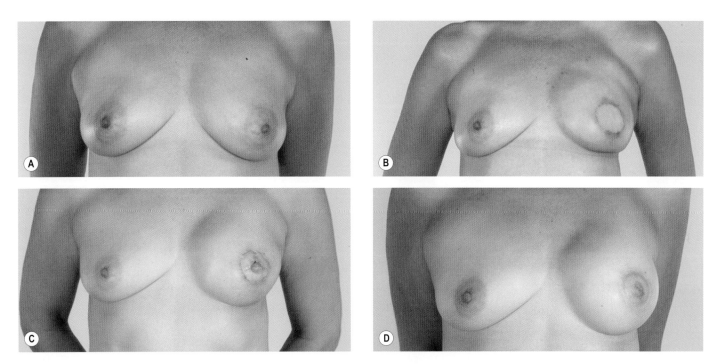

Fig. 15.2 **(A)** Preoperative appearance of a 48-year-old female with left breast cancer following breast conservation therapy and radiation. **(B)** Postoperative; patient is 2 months post-left mastectomy with reconstruction with a left latissimus dorsi flap and expander. **(C)** Postoperative; patient is 3 months post-left nipple construction and exchange of expander to silicone implant. **(D)** 1-year postoperatively.

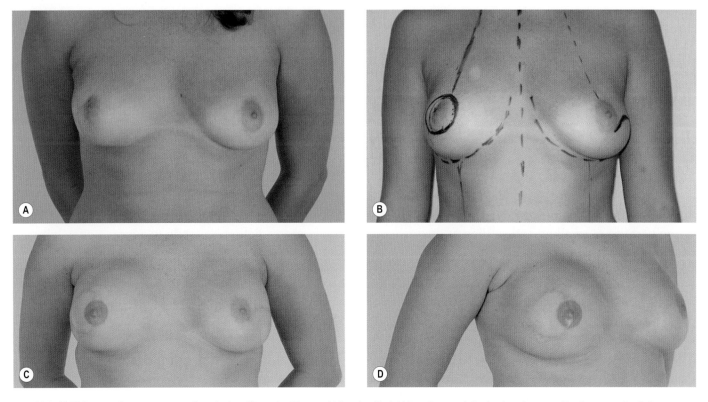

Fig. 15.3 **(A,B)** Preoperative appearance and surgical markings of a 30-year-old female with right breast cancer following breast conservation therapy and radiation. **(C,D)** Postoperative; patient is 5 months post-right simple mastectomy and left nipple-sparing mastectomy, right breast reconstruction with latissimus dorsi and implant and left breast reconstruction with expanders. In a separate procedure, she received right nipple construction and left exchange to silicone implant.

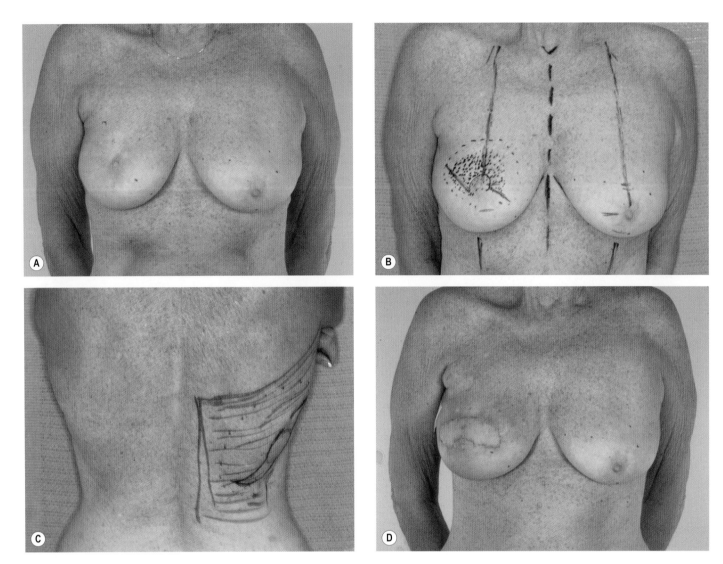

Fig. 15.4 (A) Preoperative appearance of a 62-year-old female with history of right breast cancer who received lumpectomy and radiation. This resulted in significant distortion, concavity, and asymmetry. **(B,C)** Surgical markings. **(D)** Postoperative; patient is 6 months post-right latissimus dorsi flap reconstruction.

the final volume of the reconstructed breast at the initial setting because of swelling and settling of the breast in the postoperative course.

Primary reconstruction can still be accomplished without an implant, especially for women with a small to medium-sized breast.[23] An extended latissimus dorsi musculocutaneous flap without an implant could even be used for a larger breast, especially in patients with at least 2 cm of pinch thickness of back fat.[24–28] The texture of the breast and the absence of an implant are major advantages of the purely autogenous breast reconstruction.[29] Finally, the latissimus dorsi flap is particularly useful for reconstruction of partial mastectomy

or lumpectomy deformities *(Fig. 15.4)*. In such patients, in whom irradiation is certain to aggravate the lumpectomy deformity, the latissimus flap can replace some or all of the missing tissue and thus mitigate the eventual damage.

Specific indications

Patients who are not candidates for a TRAM flap

Some women who need supplementary autologous tissue for a satisfactory breast reconstruction or who

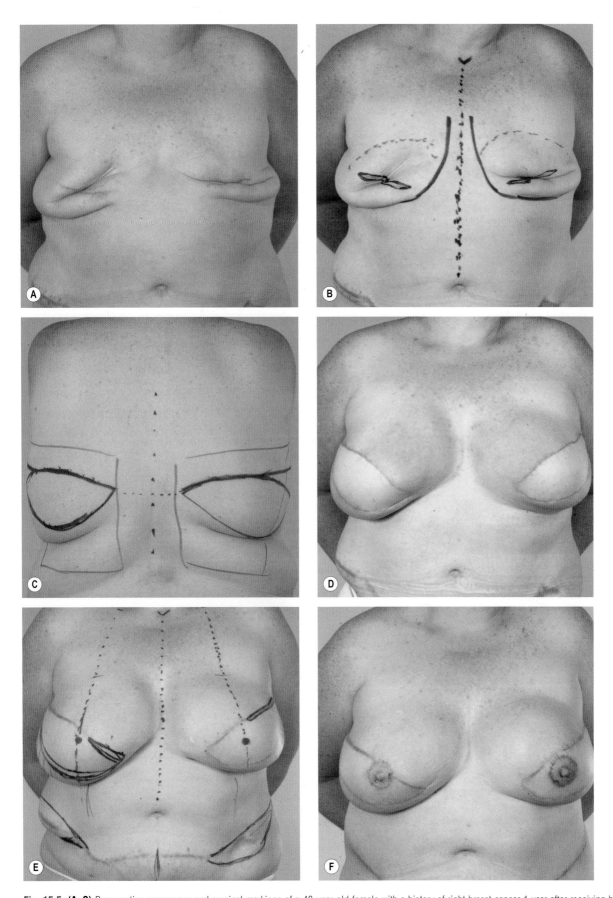

Fig. 15.5 (A–C) Preoperative appearance and surgical markings of a 48-year-old female with a history of right breast cancer 1 year after receiving bilateral mastectomy. Patient had previously undergone a panniculectomy. **(D)** Postoperative; patient is 4 months post-delayed bilateral latissimus dorsi flap reconstruction with expanders. **(E)** Surgical markings at revision. **(F)** Postoperative; 5 months after bilateral exchange to silicone implants and nipple construction.

wish to have purely autogenous breast reconstruction may not be candidates for the TRAM flap.[30] This includes women who have had a previous abdominoplasty or TRAM flap, and it may also include women with insufficient abdominal skin or fat *(Fig. 15.5)*. Women who smoke, have diabetes, or are obese may be considered to be too high risk to undergo a TRAM flap. Some women may choose not to undergo on operation as extensive and lengthy as a TRAM flap, particularly in light of the time required for recuperation. When a TRAM flap is not available or advisable, the latissimus flap becomes an obvious option. Aside from being an alternative when a TRAM flap is not the right choice, the latissimus flap has certain attributes and advantages that may make it a better choice. The latissimus flap includes a large well-vascularized flat muscle that may be better suited for dealing with poorly vascularized defects or for covering an implant. In patients with small defects, particularly laterally, the latissimus may be the best choice.

Previous irradiation during breast conservative therapy

Several papers have discussed the detrimental effects radiation has on tissues and breast reconstruction. Contracture, wound healing problems, implant exposure, infection, skin necrosis and pigmentary changes are all commonly associated with radiation therapy *(Figs 15.6, 15.7)*. If the consultation takes place after

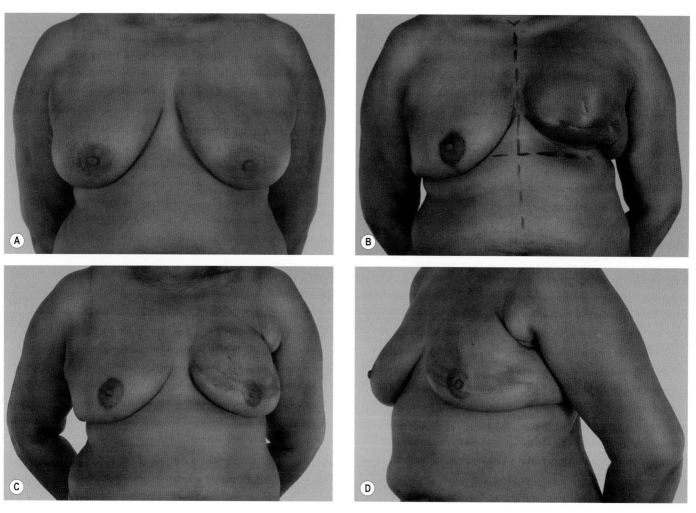

Fig. 15.6 (A) Preoperative appearance of a 61-year-old female with history of left breast cancer who received a modified radical mastectomy, immediate reconstruction with expander and acellular dermal matrix, and right breast reduction for symmetry. **(B)** Postoperatively, she received chemotherapy and left breast radiation and subsequently developed a scarred and abnormal contour of the left breast. **(C,D)** Postoperative; patient is 1 year post-left latissimus dorsi flap breast reconstruction with expander followed by exchange to implant and nipple construction.

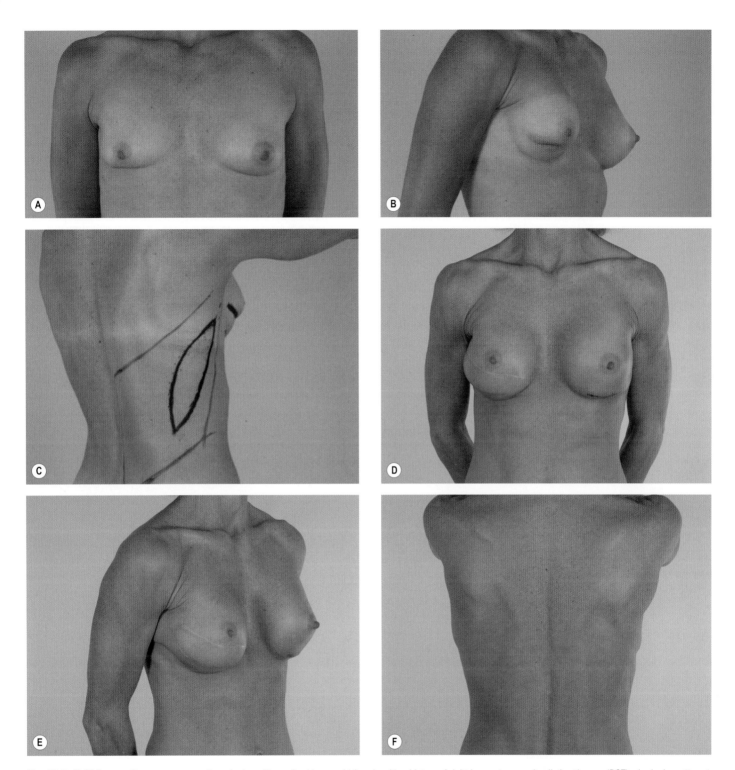

Fig. 15.7 (A,B) Preoperative appearance and surgical markings of a 44-year-old female with a history of right lumpectomy and radiation therapy (BCT) who had an attempt at correction of her lumpectomy deformity with an implant that became encapsulated. **(C)** Plan for a Latissimus flap in an addition to the existing implant for correction of her partial breast deformity. **(D–F)** Postoperative; patient is 1 year post-right latissimus dorsi flap reconstruction with implant and a left breast augmentation to address ptosis and projection.

radiation therapy, it is important to determine the indications for the radiation, the dose and site of the radiation, and most important, the quality of the remaining tissues. The presence of radiation damage is significant because reconstructions in irradiated tissues, regardless of the method, always lead to a diminished result and a higher rate of complications. Large doses of radiation, as high as 10 000 cGy, typically leave the tissues feeling inelastic, tight, and thickened.[31] This is especially troublesome when the radiation is given during the reconstruction when a tissue expander is already in place. In any case, reconstruction with an implant alone may not be possible and may result in significant complications or, at the very least, a disappointing result. Reconstruction with the help of autologous tissue may be critical because it brings well-vascularized tissue to the ischemic chest wall. The pedicled latissimus flap provides a moderately sized skin island as well as a large amount of well-vascularized muscle. It is a hardy flap that can be used despite irradiation to the axilla.

The skin flaps of a previously irradiated breast are unreliable from a circulatory point of view and inelastic from a tissue expansion perspective. If no radiation therapy is anticipated, the addition of a latissimus musculocutaneous flap at the time of an immediate postmastectomy reconstruction makes the operation safer and improves the odds that the ultimate result will be satisfactory.[32] Adding a latissimus flap to the inferior pole of the breast (as opposed to opening the mastectomy scar and placing the skin paddle mid-breast) has helped in creating a favorable contour for the breast when combined with an implant. Critical to this concept is that the latissimus flap be added only after radiation therapy has occurred. Adding the latissimus skin paddle to the inferior pole is critical in releasing the non-compliant radiated skin and soft tissue that prevents the implant from creating the normal breast contour and ptosis *(Fig. 15.8)*. In a review of consecutive patients over 5 years at our institution, 15% received radiation following immediate reconstruction.[31] It was found that for patients with expander based reconstructions, the majority went on to successful two-stage device-only reconstructions (60%). For the remaining 40%, the addition of a latissimus dorsi flap to the lower pole provided adequate release of constricted lower mastectomy flaps with an improved cosmetic appearance.

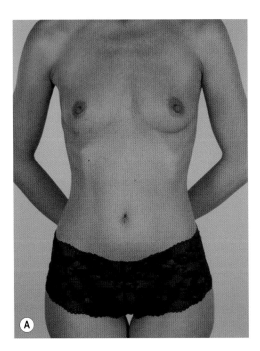
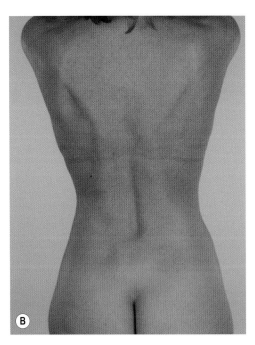

Fig. 15.8 (A–D) Preoperative appearance and surgical markings of a 38-year-old female with a history of right breast cancer who received a right simple mastectomy, left nipple sparing mastectomy, and immediate reconstruction with expanders followed by implants. She received right breast radiation and subsequently developed capsular contracture and right superior implant malposition.

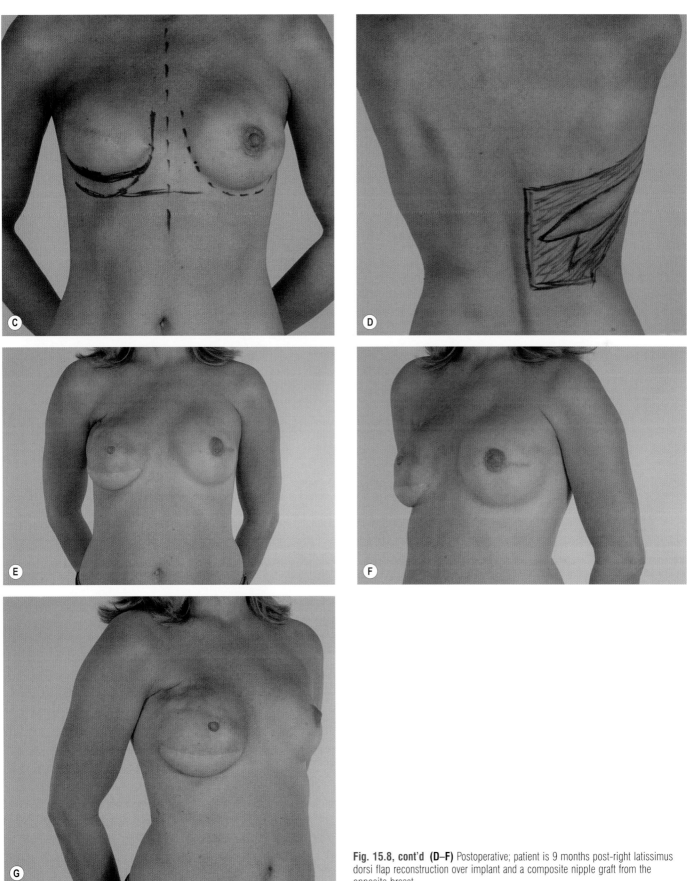

Fig. 15.8, cont'd (D–F) Postoperative; patient is 9 months post-right latissimus dorsi flap reconstruction over implant and a composite nipple graft from the opposite breast.

Partial mastectomy defects

In women in whom a lumpectomy would establish an undesirable defect, the latissimus flap can replace or make up for the missing tissue.[33]

Excessively thin or unreliable skin flaps over an implant

The latissimus dorsi flap can provide additional skin cover and soft tissue padding to properly cover an implant or expander *(Fig. 15.9)*.[34,35]

After a previous mastopexy or reduction

The skin flaps in these patients may be unreliable. A skin-sparing mastectomy approach to these patients makes them good candidates for the latissimus flap over a prosthesis to provide safe cover if flap necrosis should develop.

Augmented breasts

Women who have had breast augmentation previously may select a skin-sparing mastectomy with a latissimus flap over their breast prosthesis to have the greatest likelihood of symmetry and an attractive result from their reconstruction.[36]

Large ptotic breasts

Generally speaking, as the breast gets larger or more ptotic, it becomes more difficult to reconstruct the breast

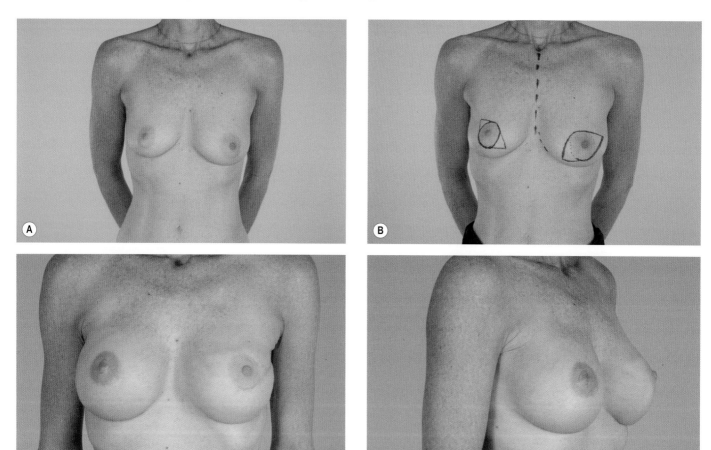

Fig. 15.9 (A,B) Preoperative appearance and surgical markings of a 48-year-old female with right breast cancer requiring radiation. **(C,D)** Postoperative; patient is 11 months post-bilateral mastectomies with expander reconstruction, then radiation followed by right breast reconstruction with latissimus dorsi and implant and left breast reconstruction with expander. In a separate procedure, she received right nipple construction.

with an implant alone. There is frequently a need for a larger prosthesis associated with longer and frequently thinner skin flaps. A common solution is to reduce or to lift (mastopexy) the opposite side, thus allowing the reconstruction of a smaller or less ptotic breast. However, for a number of reasons, either aesthetic or personal, the decision may be made to reconstruct the breast to a large size or with a significant amount of ptosis. The latissimus musculocutaneous flap allows greater support of the implant by virtue of the muscle. It can also augment the soft tissue cover by interposing the latissimus muscle and perhaps some of its overlying fat between the native breast skin and chest wall muscles. Finally, the availability of a significant skin island (up to 10×30 cm) provides the possibility of true breast ptosis and the placement of an implant substantially larger than otherwise would be possible.

Prophylactic mastectomy

For some women, particularly younger women undergoing prophylactic mastectomy, the ultimate cosmetic results can be important. The latissimus flap can be used in these women to maximize the aesthetic results, including retention of the nipple as a skin graft or as a nipple sparing mastectomy with placement of the latissimus skin paddle inferiorly.

Contraindications

The main contraindication to use of the latissimus dorsi flap is a previous posterolateral thoracotomy in which the latissimus muscle had been divided. This makes the dorsal donor site unavailable for ipsilateral breast reconstruction. A relative contraindication is an atrophic latissimus dorsi muscle after division of the thoracodorsal nerve during an axillary dissection. The volume of the latissimus dorsi muscle is decreased by denervation atrophy. This may not provide enough tissue to permit breast reconstruction or to achieve symmetry, especially in planning total autogenous reconstruction. Moreover, the risk of damaged thoracodorsal vessels is increased in a nonfunctioning latissimus muscle, necessitating an intact serratus collateral pedicle to elevate the flap.

Finally, the use of the latissimus flap electively with skin-sparing mastectomy before radiation therapy is probably unwise. The immediate use of the latissimus dorsi muscle would result in the needless irradiation of the flap and the likely corresponding damage to it. In such circumstances, it is a safer and more predictable strategy to postpone the latissimus flap reconstruction until after the mastectomy and subsequent radiation therapy.[37] Skin-sparing mastectomy with a latissimus flap thus should be reserved for patients unlikely to undergo postmastectomy adjuvant radiation therapy.

Techniques

If performing an immediate reconstruction, the plastic surgeon and general surgeon can work together to preserve important landmarks, such as the inframammary fold and the native unaffected breast skin envelope, which define the unique shape of a woman's breast. This preservation allows the reconstructed breast to assume a more natural and symmetric shape once the volume is restored. The quantity of skin excised during mastectomy dictates the skin requirement for breast restoration. Knowing the exact skin requirement and replacing it facilitate the reconstruction. When the latissimus flap is planned, the nipple-areola can be removed as the aesthetic unit of a circle, rather than as an ellipse as is typically done with a standard mastectomy.[38] When a biopsy has been performed previously or the tumor is close to the skin, that skin too should be marked for excision. This additional skin to be removed may be excised as a separate ellipse or as a piece contiguous to the areola, thus requiring a larger patch for its replacement. An axillary incision, when it is considered, is usually done through a separate incision, which should be closed primarily. After the likely skin requirement resulting from the mastectomy has been determined, consideration can be given to planning of the latissimus flap itself. Some thought should also be given to how much muscle may be needed as well as where it may be needed and in what relationship to the skin island.

In a delayed reconstruction, marking of the anterior chest wall should begin with the inframammary fold of the contralateral breast, the midsternal line, and the mastectomy scar. These are used to determine the appropriate position of the mastectomy site inframammary line. If the patient has undergone previous bilateral mastectomies, the inframammary fold can often still be visualized in the sixth intercostal space. If this location is not appropriate for the new construction, the new fold can be determined intraoperatively. The radical mastectomy has long since fallen out of favor. However, the rare patient may have an absent pectoralis major muscle. In this case, the planned position of the latissimus muscle may be outlined to simulate the position of the contralateral pectoralis major muscle.

The preoperative planning and markings are done with the patient in the upright position. The planned skin excision, midline, and inframammary folds are marked first. Before designing the flap itself, examine the patient's back and mark the lateral margin of the latissimus dorsi muscle along the posterior axillary line down to the posterior iliac crest by supporting the patient's abducted arm and palpating the muscle laterally as the patient pushes downward *(Fig. 15.10)*. The superior margin of the flap is identified by locating the tip of the scapula, with the patient's arms at the sides *(Fig. 15.11)*.

The skin island may be designed laterally, obliquely in a natural skin line along the lower midback, or transversely where the scar can be hidden within the confines of the bra straps. Even though the latissimus flap may be designed to replace the circular aesthetic unit of the areola, the skin pattern of the latissimus flap itself is ultimately closed always as an ellipse leaving a linear scar at the donor site.[38] Bailey and colleagues reported that scar location is an important consideration when performing breast reconstruction using the latissimus dorsi flap.[39] In a survey of 250 women, the authors demonstrated that the low transverse incision (below the level of the inframammary fold) was preferred in 54% of women. This was in contrast to the middle transverse incision (at the level of the inframammary fold), which was preferred in 22%; and the upper transverse incision (above the level of the inframammary fold), which was preferred in 13%. Vertical and oblique incisions were the least preferred (3% and 9%, respectively). These findings were similar in women with and without breast cancer, and no association was found to patient age, clothing preferences, body mass index, or body image. While this data is compelling, it must be balanced against the needs of the breast reconstruction. The skin paddle of the latissimus dorsi should be designed keeping in mind patient preference, nature of any lipodystrophy, the resting skin tension lines, and

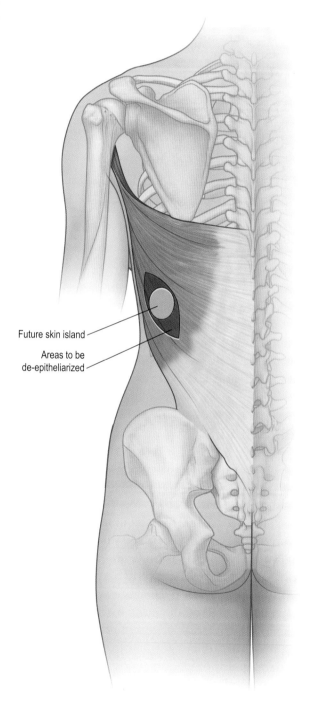

Future skin island

Areas to be de-epitheliarized

Fig. 15.10 Common placement of the skin island in planning of latissimus dorsi flap reconstruction with a prosthesis.

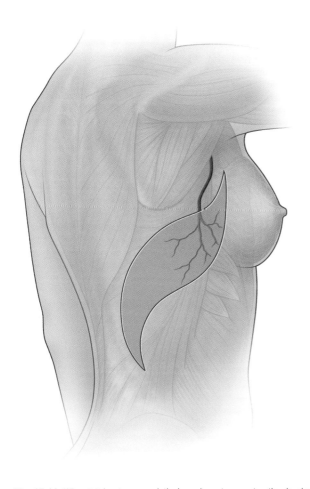

Fig. 15.11 When total autogenous latissimus breast reconstruction is planned, the skin island is designed to include all available excess back skin and fat.

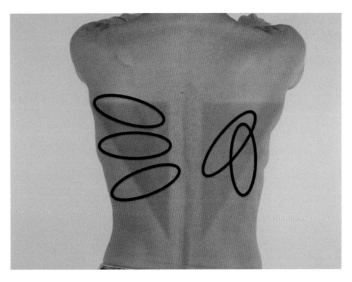

Fig. 15.12 The latissimus dorsi skin paddle may be designed transversely (lower, middle, and upper), obliquely, or vertically. Each design has distinct advantages and disadvantages to dissection exposure, amount of harvestable tissue, and final scar contour and location.

the vascular perfusion. In some instances, a larger volume skin paddle may be harvested based on anatomy rather than location *(Fig. 15.12)*. Skin paddle design and resultant scar location have advantages and disadvantages. A high transverse scar, above the level of the inframammary fold, allows for excellent dissection exposure as well as the ability to incorporate additional periscapular tissue into the design. Note over-resection of parascapular tissue can create a contour deformity of the back. The middle transverse scar, at the level of the inframammary fold, similarly affords excellent exposure and the final scar may hide within a bra line though is not hidden within an open-back dress. The low transverse scar, below the level of the inframammary fold, affords less than ideal dissection exposure but is more readily concealed within clothing. This low transverse skin paddle also best

addresses skin role redundancy and back contour. Hand-held Doppler exam or intraoperative fluorescein angiography may be beneficial to ensure recruitment of perforators within the low lumbar region *(Fig. 15.13)*. The vertical and oblique donor-site locations enable wide exposure of the flap harvest and pedicle, however this orientation has been criticized for running perpendicular natural skin tension lines.

Latissimus flap elevation is performed in the lateral decubitus position *(Fig. 15.14)*. To begin with, the skin island is incised. When an autologous latissimus dorsi flap reconstruction without an implant is planned, dissection is carried out just beneath the superficial fascia, leaving the deep fat attached to the surface of the muscle *(Fig. 15.15)*. The fascia superficialis is a useful guide for this procedure because it ensures that a consistent thickness of fat is kept on the cutaneous flaps, thus helping avoid any secondary dorsal irregularities or, worse, flap loss. The fat left attached to the surface of the muscle is well vascularized by the perforators coming from the muscle itself. The entire surface of the muscle to be used is exposed in this same plane. The dissection then proceeds laterally to identify the lateral border of the latissimus dorsi muscle. The latissimus dorsi muscle is separated from the serratus anterior, and the flap is elevated along its lateral edge. The lumbosacral fascia is divided at the level of the posterior

Video 1

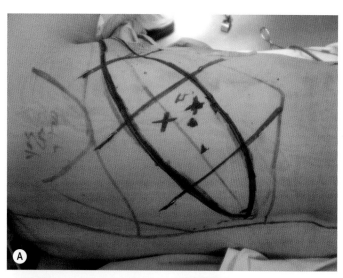

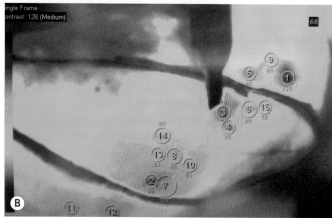

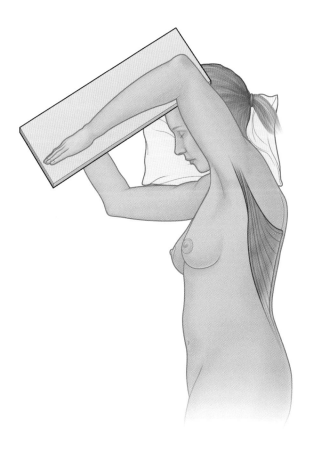

Fig. 15.14 The patient is positioned in the lateral decubitus position for latissimus flap elevation. This allows easy access to the entire muscle and its insertion.

Fig. 15.13 **(A)** A large obliquely designed latissimus dorsi skin paddle was designed based centered over Dopplerable perforators. **(B)** Preoperative fluorescein angiography (SPY system; Novadaq Technologies Inc, Concord, ON, Canada) evaluation determined that perfusion was instead greater with a low horizontally oriented skin paddle. Note the area of greatest perfusion is outside of the planned markings. Because of the large skin requirements, the skin paddle design was reoriented prior to incision.

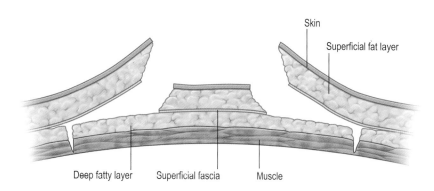

Skin

Superficial fat layer

Deep fatty layer   Superficial fascia   Muscle

Fig. 15.15 In the autogenous latissimus flap, the deep fat is left attached to the muscle as the dissection is carried out just beneath the fascia superficialis. This ensures adequate volume for reconstruction and preservation of the dorsal skin flaps.

axillary line, then the latissimus fibers of origin are separated from the paraspinous muscle fascia. Care must be taken to avoid incising through the paraspinous fascia because this makes identification of the proper plane of dissection difficult. The remaining fibers of origin are divided medially from the vertebral column. In dividing these fascial attachments, large intercostal perforating vessels should be carefully controlled to prevent bleeding and postoperative hematoma formation. Superomedially, the covering fibers of the trapezius muscle are identified and elevated away from the underlying latissimus muscle. After the superior border of the latissimus is identified, dissection is carried out laterally toward the axilla, separating away the fibers of the teres major muscle that diffuse with those of the latissimus. The entire muscle flap is then elevated toward the axilla *(Fig. 15.16A)*. The thoracodorsal artery and vein are identified at the point of entrance into muscle. The serratus branch is easily

identified and may be left intact, especially if the patient had axillary dissection in which the thoracodorsal artery may have been injured. The additional blood inflow through the serratus branch may be critical. It is desirable in most patients to divide the latissimus dorsi muscle near its insertion at its attachment to the humerus. Release of the insertions helps avoid the displeasing bulge in the low axilla that is sometimes seen when the insertion is left intact.[40] Care must be taken during this step to preserve the thoracodorsal vessels. A small cuff of muscle, 10 20%, may be preserved to help protect from traction on the pedicle. The flap is then transferred to the mastectomy defect through a subcutaneous tunnel high in the axilla to further prevent an unnatural lateral bulge and to fill the axilla *(Fig. 15.16B)*. Suturing of the muscle at the anterior axillary line should be performed to prevent lateral migration of the flap and implant and to protect the pedicle from tension.

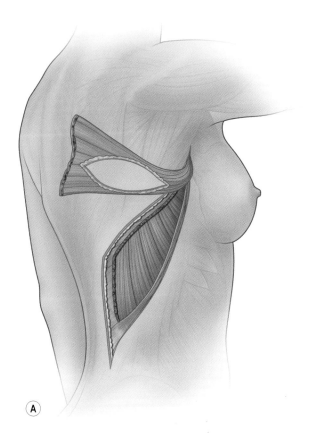 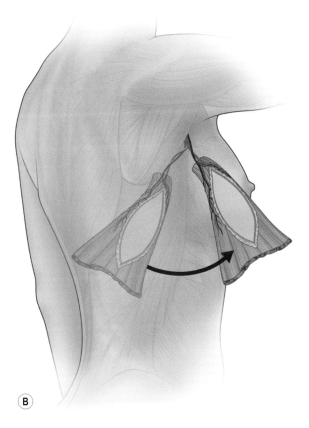

Fig. 15.16 (A) Elevation of the latissimus dorsi musculocutaneous flap and the underlying anatomy. **(B)** After division of the muscle insertion, the latissimus flap is transposed anteriorly to the mastectomy defect through a subcutaneous tunnel high in the axilla.

The back incision is first temporarily stapled; closed over a suction drainage tube. When fibrin glue is used, several transverse lines of approximation are then marked with a pen, and the staples are removed. Fibrin sealant adhesive, in appropriate concentrations, may be used to encourage the adherence of the superficial skin flaps to the underlying deep tissues. The fibrin sealant is sprayed, and the patient is then stapled again as previously marked. The spray is applied in less than 60 s so that the fibrin does not set up before the closure has occurred. Pressure is then maintained on the skin flap for 4 or 5 min to promote a good fibrin bond. The donor site is then closed over the previously inserted suction drain in layers including 2-0 polydioxanone to the fascia superficialis followed by interrupted and running intradermal 3-0 Monocryl to the dermis.

The patient is then placed in a supine position for insetting of the flap. The placement of the flap depends on the particular circumstances of the reconstruction.

For immediate reconstruction after a modified radical mastectomy, the skin paddle is positioned at the site of the skin excision. After a skin-sparing mastectomy in which only the areola is excised, only an areolar size disk of back skin over the latissimus is preserved; the rest of the dorsal cutaneous paddle is de-epithelialized. In prophylactic skin-sparing mastectomy, the nipple-areola may be preserved as a full-thickness skin graft and sutured back in place on top of the de-epithelialized latissimus skin island.

When reconstruction is planned with use of the latissimus flap over an expander, it is easier and quicker to leave the pectoralis major muscle intact and to place the expander between the latissimus and pectoralis major muscles *(Fig. 15.17)*. The latissimus muscle is inset just beneath the upper mastectomy skin flap. This position helps achieve some soft tissue filling of the upper pole of the reconstructed breast. The latissimus dorsi muscle is sutured medially and inferiorly to the underlying

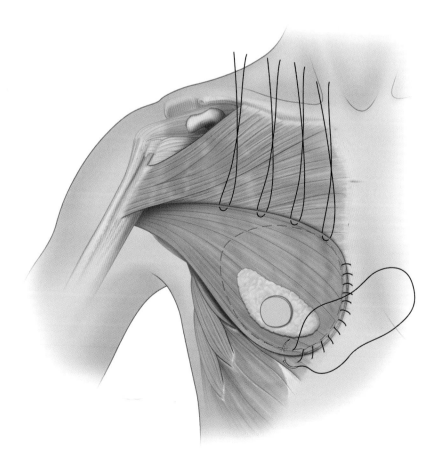

Fig. 15.17 When immediate latissimus flap reconstruction is planned with a prosthesis for skin-sparing mastectomy, the skin pattern is designed as a discrete small island. After transposition of the flap, the expander is placed between the latissimus and pectoralis major muscles.

muscle and fascia in such a way as to help establish those borders of the breast. Superiorly, marionette half-mattress sutures are used between the overlying breast skin and the edge of the latissimus muscle to help cover the entire mastectomy defect with the latissimus muscle. Not tying these sutures provides access for placement of the expander.

For delayed reconstruction, the latissimus flap is used both for inferior pole fullness and to cover an expander or implant. In most cases, an incision is made at or just above the predetermined inframammary fold along a line from the lateral sternal border to the anterior axillary line. The superior chest wall skin flap is elevated, usually in the subcutaneous plane, and the latissimus flap is brought through the tunnel and into the defect. Suturing of the muscle at or near the anterior axillary line should be performed to prevent lateral migration of the flap and implant and to protect the pedicle from tension. The best projection is achieved when the pectoralis major muscle is left intact and the expander or prosthesis is placed between the latissimus and pectoralis major muscles. The latissimus dorsi muscle is sutured medially and inferiorly to the underlying muscle and fascia in such a way as to help form those borders of the breast. Superiorly, three to five marionette, half-mattress 3-0 Prolene sutures are placed between the overlying breast skin and the edge of the latissimus muscle to help cover the entire mastectomy defect with the latissimus muscle. The expander is inserted from above and may be filled with several hundred milliliters of saline because there is generally no tightness to the sub-latissimus pocket. Postoperatively, the tissue expander is further inflated until the desired volume is achieved, starting 2 weeks postoperatively or once the wound is healed. The second stage of the reconstruction is typically performed after 4–8 months, allowing adequate healing and settling of the soft tissue. An implant of appropriate size and shape is then inserted through the previous incision after the expander is removed. Symmetry can be improved by correction of any soft tissue or contour deformity as well as by correction of the inframammary fold. The nipple and areola are usually reconstructed at the same procedure.

When reconstruction is planned with use of the total autogenous latissimus dorsi flap, the cutaneous paddle is molded in the form of an asymmetric U *(Fig. 15.18)*.

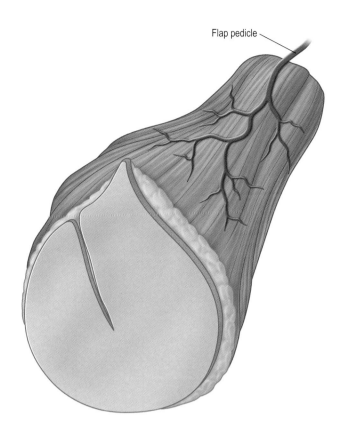

Fig. 15.18 For total autogenous latissimus reconstruction, the flap is folded into a cone shape to increase the volume and projection of the reconstructed breast.

The curved base of the U gives the apex of the breast. The distal part of the muscle and its underlying fat are folded under this breast cone to increase the volume and the projection of the breast. Various moldings can be tried until one arrives at a satisfactory shape for the rebuilt breast. This procedure of molding is crucial to the final quality of the result, and one must understand how to achieve the different arrangements necessary for a good morphologic result.

Main surgical variants

Several surgical variations of the latissimus dorsi have been described based on anatomy, which include split latissimus dorsi,[41] extended latissimus dorsi, and muscle-sparing latissimus dorsi.

Particularly large breast defects requiring completely autogenous reconstruction may benefit from an extended latissimus dorsi design variant. The extended

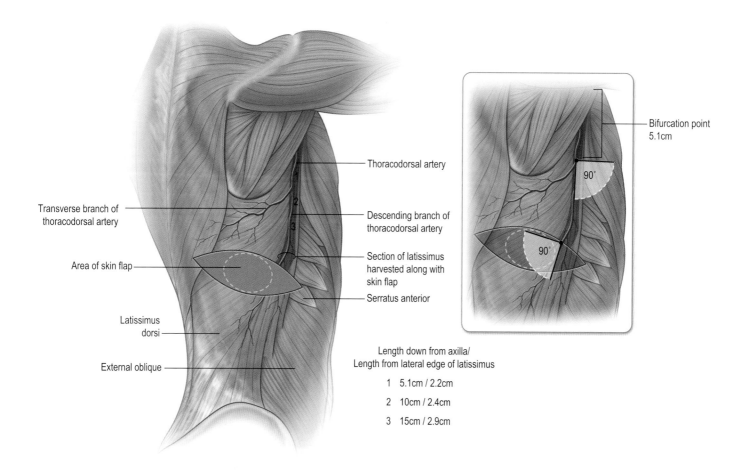

Transverse branch of
thoracodorsal artery

Area of skin flap

Latissimus
dorsi

External oblique

Thoracodorsal artery

Descending branch of
thoracodorsal artery

Section of latissimus
harvested along with
skin flap

Serratus anterior

Bifurcation point
5.1cm

90°

90°

Length down from axilla/
Length from lateral edge of latissimus

1   5.1cm / 2.2cm

2   10cm / 2.4cm

3   15cm / 2.9cm

Fig. 15.19 Relevant anatomy and design of the muscle-sparing latissimus dorsi muscle flap based on the descending branch of the thoracodorsal artery. Limited undermining of skin flaps is used to minimize seroma formation and limit donor-site morbidity. (Redrawn from Saint-Cyr M, Nagarkar P, Schaverien M, et al. The pedicled descending branch muscle-sparing latissimus dorsi flap for breast reconstruction. *Plast Reconstr Surg.* 2009;123(1):13–24.)

latissimus dorsi flap can provide 300–400 mL or more of soft tissue volume for breast reconstruction. Postoperative muscle atrophy of 20–25% should be taken into consideration during the insetting and sizing of the flap. A fleur-de-lis skin island may be used resulting in an inverted T-shaped scar. Up to 7 cm wings may be designed which can increase the amount of skin and subcutaneous fat available for breast reconstruction. The latissimus dorsi flap harvest may also be extended to include the parascapular tissue from the teres major down to the iliac crest subcutaneous tissue and fascia. Chang et al demonstrated excellent outcomes with this technique though noted a significantly higher rate of donor-site complications within the obese patient population.[42]

Thoracodorsal artery perforator flaps and muscle sparing flap designs have been introduced in an attempt to reduce donor site morbidity. The muscle sparing latissimus dorsi flap is based on the descending branch of the thoracodorsal vessels and the skin paddle may be oriented vertically or horizontally.[43] In this technique, dissection begins caudally and the latissimus dorsi muscle is split vertically along its natural muscle fiber orientation staying 1–2 cm medial to the descending branch of the thoracodorsal vessels (*Fig. 15.19*). Dissection continues superiorly to the level of the lateral mammary fold just before the bifurcation of the descending and transverse branches. This bifurcation can be found an average 5.1 cm from the posterior axillary fold (range, 2.1–7.5 cm) and a mean of 2.2 cm (range, 1.3–3.1 cm) from the lateral edge of the latissimus dorsi muscle.[44] The width of the latissimus dorsi muscle harvested is between 3 to 4 cm. Utilizing this technique in twenty patients, Saint-Cyr reported zero seromas, no significant loss of muscle strength, and high patient satisfaction scores.[43]

Secondary procedures

Secondary procedures after latissimus dorsi flap reconstruction are performed after three months. These include expander implant exchange, contralateral procedures to improve breast symmetry, and nipple areolar reconstruction. Further surgery is performed after the completion of any adjuvant chemotherapy.

Exchange of expander to implant

For staged reconstruction with latissimus dorsi and a tissue expander, expansion begins once incisions show adequate signs of healing, usually by the second postoperative visit, or 2 weeks postoperatively. Serial expansions (on average 2–3) continue at intervals of 2 weeks. The expander is exchanged for a permanent implant (either saline or silicone) 4–6 weeks after the last expansion. The surgical approach to the expander usually proceeds through the previous mastectomy incision. Dissection is carried down to the muscle and the mastectomy flaps are elevated 1–2 cm circumferentially to facilitate a layered closure. To avoid vascular compromise, the latissimus dorsi muscle is split parallel to fiber orientation. Fold modification, capsule adjustment, and implant pocket revisions may be performed during this stage. A latissimus skin paddle placed mid-breast may be reduced to the diameter of a planned areola to better adhere to aesthetic subunits.

Secondary thoracodorsal nerve ligation

Some surgeons think that the intact thoracodorsal nerve may help preserve maximum volume of the flap in the long term and therefore advocate not dividing the thoracodorsal nerve when the flap is used in this fashion. They also argue that because the latissimus dorsi muscle is fixed to the chest wall in a relaxed manner, little contraction is noticed in the flap postoperatively when the nerve is left intact. On the other hand, when the muscle is used over an expander, postoperative voluntary muscle contraction can be significant when the thoracodorsal nerve is left intact. Secondary thoracodorsal

nerve ligation may be performed through an anterior approach to the axilla with the patient placed supine. The thoracodorsal nerve is a branch from the posterior cord of the brachial plexus and joins the thoracodorsal vascular pedicle approximately 3–4 cm prior to entering the lateral edge of the muscle. A nerve stimulator may facilitate dissection through heavy scar or previously irradiated tissue. The thoracodorsal nerve is identified proximally with care taken to prevent injury to the vascular pedicle.

Postoperative care

At the conclusion of the operation, antibiotic ointment and standard dressings are applied to breast and back incisions. Patients will have two back drains and one to two breast drains. A loose circumferential dressing or surgical bra may be used with placement axillary gauze for padding however care should be taken to avoid any direct compression over the vessels in the axilla. Dressings are removed in 24–48 h and which point patients may shower. Appropriate antiembolic prophylaxis is utilized, and early ambulation with aggressive pulmonary toilet is encouraged. Length of hospitalization is on average three days and patients can expect to return to normal work function from 3–6 weeks. Suction drains will remain in place until output is <30 mL/day, with back drains in place up to 3–4 weeks. Patients may benefit from consult with physical therapy and physical activity is limited for 3–4 weeks. Upper extremity strengthening and range-of-motion exercises are begun 2 weeks postoperatively assuming sufficient progression of healing.

Outcomes and complications

Breast reconstruction with the latissimus dorsi musculocutaneous flap has been associated with significant patient satisfaction. Moore reviewed their experience in 170 patients and found a 90% patient satisfaction.[45] Within this same study, disease recurrence was not delayed or masked by this type of reconstruction. Delay reported outcomes in 50 women reconstructed with a latissimus dorsi flap and found that at after an average follow-up of 27 months, patients results were comparable or superior to other published outcomes on autologous reconstruction such as the TRAM flap.[46] A total of 56% of patients had fine or very fine sensitivity, though 70% deemed this sensitivity to be less than that of the opposite breast. The superior medial part of the breast had the greatest sensitivity, both objectively and subjectively. Some 94% of patients perceived the reconstructed breast as integral to their body image.

Flap necrosis

The latissimus dorsi flap is a hardy flap that has an excellent and reliable circulation. There is a minimal risk of flap necrosis even in smokers and diabetics. Significant flap necrosis is unusual and nearly always associated with injury to the vascular pedicle. The pedicle can be injured either directly during the dissection around the pedicle or indirectly by twisting or thrombosis from tension on the pedicle by the weight of the flap, especially if the flap is not properly secured to the chest wall.

Partial flap necrosis has been noted in up to 7% of patients but is more common when an extended flap has been elevated.[47] On the other hand, necrosis of the mastectomy skin flaps is a more common complication.

Donor site morbidity

By far the most common complication is seroma at the back donor site.[48] The rate of dorsal seroma may be increased when an extended flap is performed.[49,42]

Dorsal skin flap necrosis also occurs, especially with large skin paddles, resulting in excessive tension on the back closure. Dissection in too superficial a plane in trying to leave subcutaneous fat on the flap also puts the skin flaps at greater risk. Other possible donor site problems are loss of shoulder mobility, shoulder weakness, winging of the scapula, and dorsal hernia.[50]

A complication related to the use of prosthetic devices in conjunction with the latissimus flap is migration of the expander or implant through the axilla and into the back.[51] This should be avoidable by secure suturing of the latissimus muscle to the lateral chest wall. Other implant-related complications include capsular contracture,[52,53] device failure, periprosthetic infection, and device extrusion. Fortunately, the incidence of all of these is fairly low.

Conclusion

Breast reconstruction and conservation have become an integral part of breast cancer treatment, and more and more patients are benefiting from reconstruction after mastectomy. Not only is the combination of a latissimus flap and implant a good option for breast reconstruction in cases such as a skin-sparing mastectomy, it is also a highly effective tool in dealing with the many difficult situations seen in the radiated breast. This flap is reliable, and its elevation is technically straightforward. Outstanding results can be obtained over and above those obtained with tissue expanders and implants alone. Complications are few and results are predictable, especially in appropriately selected patients.

It is frequently combined with tissue expansion or an implant to enhance symmetry and to reduce capsular contracture. It is useful for supplementing other techniques, for filling in contour deformities after breast conservation surgery, and for autogenous tissue reconstruction for women who have excess lateral back tissue.

The extended latissimus dorsi flap is a reliable method for totally autologous breast reconstruction and can be considered a primary choice for breast reconstruction, particularly in women who otherwise are at high risk for a TRAM flap or an implant procedure.

Financial disclosure

Dr Spear is a paid consultant to Lifecell, Ethicon, and Allergan corporations. This study was conducted without any funding. Dr Clemens has no disclosures.

Access the complete reference list online at **http://www.expertconsult.com**

6. Schneider WJ, Hill HL, Brown RG. Latissimus dorsi myocutaneous flap for breast reconstruction. *Br J Plast Surg.* 1977;30:277.

20. Laitung JKG, Peck F. Shoulder function following the loss of the latissimus dorsi muscle. *Br J Plast Surg.* 1985;38:375.

21. Russell RC, Pribaz J, Zook EG, et al. Functional evaluation of latissimus dorsi donor site. *Plast Reconstr Surg.* 1986;78:336.

22. Fraulin FOG, Louie G, Zorrilla L, et al. Functional evaluation of the shoulder following latissimus dorsi muscle transfer. *Ann Plast Surg.* 1995;35:349.

Fraulin et al. looked at the functional effects of latissimus dorsi muscle harvest on shoulder strength and mobility. This was a study of 26 patients (10 males, 16 females) who underwent a pedicled or free vascularized latissimus dorsi muscle transfer. Muscle testing was performed using a Kinetic Communicator machine (Kin Com) and the Baltimore therapeutic equipment (BTE) work simulator. The female unilateral pedicle group (n = 13) showed a significant difference between operated and nonoperated shoulders for both peak torque (power) and work (endurance) measurements of shoulder adduction and extension (mean ratios operated/nonoperated shoulders, 55–69%). The male free vascularized group (n = 10) similarly showed a significant deficit of both peak torque and work for shoulder extension and adduction (mean ratios, 74–84%). The paper concluded that dynamic muscle tests demonstrate a deficit of muscle power and endurance of shoulder extension and adduction following latissimus dorsi muscle transfer.

23. McCraw JB, Papp C, Edwards A, et al. The autogenous latissimus breast reconstruction. *Clin Plast Surg.* 1994;21:279.

24. Papp C, McCraw JB. Autogenous latissimus breast reconstruction. *Clin Plast Surg.* 1998;25:261.

29. Delay E, Gounot N, Bouillot A. Autologous latissimus breast reconstruction: a 3 year clinical experience with 100 patients. *Plast Reconstr Surg.* 1998;102:1461.

Delay et al. presented their technique of autologous breast reconstruction using the latissimus dorsi flap and studied the results that can be expected. A consecutive sample of 100 patients was studied (average follow-up 20 months). Supplementary volume of the latissimus dorsi was obtained from five fatty zones: fat on the cutaneous paddle, fat taken from the surface of the muscle, the scapular fat pad, the anterior fatty zone, and the supra-iliac fat pad. The authors found the following complications: 1% partial necrosis; 1% total necrosis of the flap, and seroma 79%, most regularly in obese patients. The level of patient satisfaction was high. Indications for this technique include, when one can bury the cutaneous paddle: cases of skin-sparing mastectomy and cases of conversion of implant reconstruction to an autologous reconstruction.

31. Spear SL, Clemens MW, Boehmler J. Latissimus dorsi flap in reconstruction of the radiated breast. In: Spear SL, ed. *Surgery of the Breast: Principles and Art,* 3rd ed. Amsterdam: Wolters Kluwer; 2010.

The authors reviewed their experience with the latissimus dorsi flap and a prosthesis in reconstruction of the previously irradiated breast. Twenty-eight patients all had soft breasts at follow-up, with no evidence of capsular contracture. Donor-site complications included five donor-site seromas. The majority of patients (65%) underwent a planned two-stage reconstruction, and the majority of the revision operations were for exchanges to smaller implants. The overall satisfaction rating was 8.8 of 10. The authors concluded that although purely autologous reconstructions may be the best choice for many irradiated breasts, it has been shown in this study that a cosmetically acceptable reconstruction with manageable risk can be performed using a prosthesis combined with a latissimus dorsi flap.

38. Hammond DC. Latissimus dorsi musculocutaneous flap. *Plast Reconstr Surg.* 2009;124:4.

The author presents his extensive experience with the latissimus dorsi musculocutaneous flap in both immediate and delayed breast reconstruction. Five technical modifications in surgical technique are introduced including orientation of the skin island along the relaxed skin tension lines, harvesting the deep layer of fat with the flap, cutting the thoracodorsal nerve, partially dividing the insertion of the muscle, and using a staged expander/implant sequence. These principles result in a thin line and smooth donor-site scar. The flap advances completely to the breast because of the partial release of the insertion of the muscle, and the volume provided by the flap is increased by keeping the deep layer of fat attached to the flap. Breast animation is minimized as a result of sectioning of the thoracodorsal nerve, and the consistency and quality of the result are improved by using a staged tissue expander/implant strategy. The study concluded that with advancements in surgical technique and improvements in tissue expander and implant design, outstanding results can be obtained using the latissimus dorsi flap in breast reconstruction.

39. Bailey S, Saint-Cyr M, Zhang K, et al. Breast reconstruction with latissimus dorsi flap: Women's preference for scar location. *Plast Reconstr Surg.* 2010;126:358–365.

41. Tobin GR, Moberg AW, DuBou RH, et al. The split latissimus dorsi myocutaneous flap. *Ann Plast Surg.* 1981;7:272–280.

42. Chang DW, Youssef A, Cha S, et al. Autologous breast reconstruction with the extended latissimus dorsi flap. *Plast Reconstr Surg.* 2002;110:751.

The authors present their experience with the extended latissimus dorsi myocutaneous flap for replacement of breast volume without an implant. A total of 75 extended latissimus dorsi flap breast reconstructions were performed in 67 patients (mean age 51.5 years). Flap complications developed in 21 of 75 flaps (28.0%), and donor-site complications developed in 29 of 75 donor sites (38.7%). Mastectomy skin flap necrosis (17.3%) and donor-site seroma (25.3%) were found to be the most common complications. There were no flap losses. The study concluded that patients who are obese are at higher risk of developing donor-site complications.

43. Saint-Cyr M, Nagarkar P, Schaverien M, et al. The pedicled descending branch muscle-sparing latissimus dorsi flap for breast reconstruction. *Plast Reconstr Surg.* 2009;123(1):13–24.

44. Schwabegger AH, Harpf C, Rainer C. Muscle-sparing latissimus dorsi myocutaneous flap with maintenance of muscle innervation, function, and aesthetic appearance of the donor site. *Plast Reconstr Surg.* 2003;111:1407–1411.

45. Moore TS, Farrell LD. Latissimus dorsi myocutaneous flap for breast reconstruction: long term results. *Plast Reconstr Surg.* 1992;89(4):666–672.

46. Delay E, Jorquera F, Lucas R. Sensitivity of breasts reconstructed with the autologous latissimus dorsi flap. *Plast Reconstr Surg.* 2000;106: 302–309.

16

The bilateral pedicled TRAM flap

L. Franklyn Elliott, John D. Symbas, and Hunter R. Moyer

SYNOPSIS

- The pedicled TRAM flap is still the most popular way of transferring abdominal tissue to the breast.
- This technique, introduced by Dr Carl Hartrampf, is consistently successful if it is performed properly.
- The muscle and fascial sparing technique ensures abundant vascularity to the TRAM flap, while allowing secure and complication free closure of the abdominal wall.
- The shaping of the breast using the pedicled TRAM flap is enormously simplified in the immediate reconstructive setting.
- We recommend utilizing the pedicled TRAM flap for bilateral reconstruction and the free TRAM flap for unilateral reconstruction.

Access the Historical Perspective section online at
http://www.expertconsult.com

Introduction

The TRAM flap is now thirty years old. After much thought, study and late night cadaver dissections the first TRAM was successfully performed on September 9, 1980. The vascular anatomy of the rectus muscle and the direction of the blood flow at the junction of the superior and inferior deep epigastric vessels was unknown at this time.

Therefore, the first TRAM and my early experience was with an upper abdominal flap based on isolated superior deep epigastric vessels. This is a very safe procedure with very little chance of post-op hernia. The only drawbacks are a residual mid-abdominal scar, and the operation is a bit challenging for the surgeon.

My early lower abdominal TRAMs were performed after a delay by ligating the inferior deep epigastric vessels. My next stage in the development of the TRAM was an un-delayed lower abdominal flap, with special attention given to including the peri-umbilical perforators. From that time on I never employed a delaying procedure. My flaps were healthy, and I never felt the need for a delay.

During these early days it became obvious to me the adverse affects smoking will have on the healing of the patient's tissues. Cigarette smoking, current or past, is a contraindication to the performance of the pedicled TRAM flap.

Breast reconstructions using the pedicled TRAM are now frequently performed procedures in the U.S. and worldwide.

The rest is history…"

(Carl R. Hartrampf Jr., M.D.)

The pedicled TRAM (transverse rectus abdominus myocutaneous) flap is a well-established procedure that continues to be the most popular technique utilized by plastic surgeons in North America for transferring abdominal tissue to the breast for reconstruction. While the free technique utilizing the inferior epigastric vessels undoubtedly provides additional blood flow to the transferred abdominal tissue, it carries with it the need for advanced microsurgical training and, in most hands, a significantly longer operative time. In bilateral reconstruction, the pedicled TRAM is preferred over the free technique, unless the patient is at high risk for flap loss. The muscle and fascial sparing technique, when performed as described, leaves an abdominal defect that can be closed primarily in the vast majority of cases. Abdominal closure is facilitated by simultaneous closure of both abdominal defects so that the stress is distributed all the way across the abdominal wall. Additionally, the muscle and fascial sparing technique allows the surgeon to create a relatively small tunnel for the flap and thus, results in a relatively crisp inframammary fold postoperatively. It is not uncommon to see some venous congestion of a pedicled flap either on the table or in the immediate postoperative setting as the choke vessels in the flap's pedicle open up. Lastly, loosely tied internal tacking sutures from the flap to the chest wall help to stabilize the flap in an aesthetically pleasing manner.

Basic science/anatomy

The TRAM flap is based on the blood supply from the perforating vessels through the rectus abdominis muscle and the deep epigastric system *(Fig. 16.1)*. These perforating vessels are supplied primarily as branches from the deep inferior epigastric artery but can also be supplied by the adjacent territory of the superior epigastric artery. The anatomy of the perforating vessels is somewhat variable and may be predominantly along the lateral third of the muscle, in the central third of the muscle, or even in the medial third. The concept of the epigastric artery as the pedicle source was originally described by Mathes.[2] The vascular anatomy of the epigastric arteries as they relate to the TRAM flap was described by Moon and Taylor.[3] They described three basic arterial schemata. In a type I pattern, a single intramuscular vessel extends from the superior epigastric artery to the deep inferior epigastric artery. The

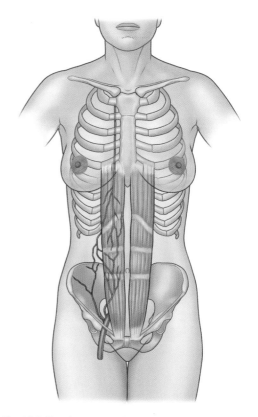

Fig. 16.1 Vascular anatomy of the deep epigastric system.

majority of patients in their study exhibited a type II system, in which the inferior epigastric artery branches into two vessels at the arcuate line and communicates with the superior epigastric through anastomosing choke vessels. Patients with a type III pattern exhibited three branches of the inferior epigastric at the arcuate line. These patients, on average, showed an even greater number of anastomoses with the superior epigastric artery. Only 2% of patients showed symmetry between their rectus muscles; most showed different vascular patterns on each side. The epigastric vessels send perforators through the rectus muscle that cross the anterior rectus sheath generally in two rows, one medial and one lateral. The rectus abdominis muscle is a type III muscle, as described by Mathes[2] and has, in addition to the superior and inferior epigastric vessels, circulation from branches of the 8th, 9th, 10th, 11th, and 12th intercostals vessels. These vessels enter the rectus muscle after anastomosis with the superior and deep inferior epigastric vessels posterior to the muscle. They penetrate the posterior rectus sheath just medial to the linea semilunaris. The rectus abdominis muscles also derive

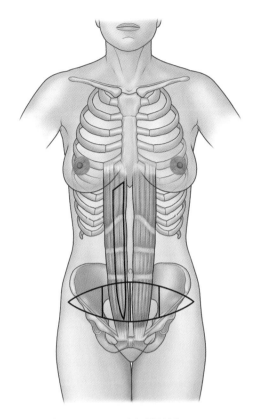

Fig. 16.2 Circulatory zones of the TRAM flap.

their motor innervations from the intercostals nerves T8 through T12.

The primary blood supply to the lower rectus muscle is from the deep inferior epigastric artery. Hence, the blood supply with the use of the inferior epigastric artery for the free TRAM flap or perforator flap is substantially richer than the blood supply available from the superior epigastric artery.[4]

The circulation from either rectus muscle across the lower abdomen is divided into four zones *(Fig. 16.2)* Zone I is the zone immediately overlying the rectus muscle. Zone II is described as a zone immediately across the midline. Zone III is the ipsilateral zone just lateral to the rectus muscle border, and zone IV is the contralateral zone lateral to the contralateral rectus border. The circulation is best in zone I, somewhat variable in zones II and III, and usually poor in zone IV, particularly with a pedicled TRAM flap. In each of these zones, the blood supply is improved to some degree by use of the perforator flap, free flap, or pedicled flap after a delay procedure.

Patient selection

The aims of breast reconstruction are to form a breast with natural appearance and feel, comfortable and in harmony with the contralateral breast. Additional aims include leaving the abdominal donor site undamaged and, if possible, improved in appearance. In order to accomplish these goals, several factors should be considered. These include the size and shape of the opposite breast, the plans for altering the opposite breast, the nature of the mastectomy defect, the pathologic stage of the breast cancer, the likelihood of postmastectomy irradiation, the general health of the patient, the availability of donor tissue, the lifestyle of the patient, and finally the patient's goals and expectations. Once the factors are all taken into consideration, the reconstructive surgeon has a wide variety of options from which to choose, including prosthetic techniques, autologous techniques, and combined autologous tissue and implant techniques. In addition, a number of matching procedures are available for the contralateral breast to help with symmetry.[5]

If a TRAM flap is to be chosen, there are a number of options available. Surgeons generally choose these options based on the presence or absence of risk factors which significantly increase the risk of complications to both the TRAM flap and the donor site. These risk factors are obesity, smoking, diabetes, hypertension, collagen vascular disease, and other significant systemic illnesses (such as pulmonary, renal, or cardiac disease). In terms of circulation, the single-pedicled TRAM flap has its best application in patients who do not have any of these risk factors and who have enough tissue in the lower abdomen for reconstruction of the breast to the desired shape and size. Generally speaking, with the unilateral pedicled TRAM, approximately 50% of the lower abdominal tissue typically removed in an abdominoplasty procedure will be available in most patients without risk factors to provide tissue for breast reconstruction. Patients who have risk factors or who need more tissue than 50% of the lower abdomen need a TRAM flap with a more robust circulation. This moves them into the category of patients who would benefit from a free TRAM flap, a TRAM with a preliminary delay procedure of the deep inferior epigastric vessels, or a double pedicled TRAM flap.[6,7] There is also the option of performing a single-pedicled TRAM flap with the addition of a prosthesis in patients who have no risk factors but who need more volume than the TRAM flap alone will provide. The deep inferior epigastric artery perforator (DIEP) flap is a free flap based on one, two, or more perforating vessels, but it does not carry the whole, most, or, in some circumstances, any of the lower rectus abdominis muscle. This procedure provides an enhanced circulation compared with a single-pedicled TRAM flap, but it is most likely not as hardy or as simple to harvest as a free TRAM flap, which carries most of the perforators and a small corresponding segment of rectus abdominis muscle.[8]

Although, at present, it is likely that the majority of TRAM flaps done in North America are single-pedicled procedures, in the senior author's opinion, the free techniques utilizing the inferior epigastric vessels do supply additional blood flow to the TRAM flap and also create less of an abdominal wall defect. Therefore, the free TRAM is preferred over the pedicled TRAM. This is true especially for unilateral breast reconstruction since the added time for a single sided free TRAM is not significantly increased as opposed to the bilateral free TRAM which can take significantly longer than the bilateral pedicled TRAM. Furthermore, the additional muscle and fascial harvest required in the bilateral pedicled TRAM technique is located in the upper abdomen where abdominal wall problems are rarely encountered. In addition, the bilateral TRAM technique necessarily only requires a hemi-flap for fat perfusion, decreasing the requirements for perfusion of the overlying fat of the TRAM flap. Because each hemiflap is smaller than that of a unilateral technique, which may incorporate contralateral skin and fat, the tunnel through the inframammary fold does not have to be as large, which results in a crisper and more aesthetically pleasing IMF postoperatively. For all of these reasons, in the normal risk patient, the bilateral pedicled TRAM is preferred over the bilateral free TRAM. On the other hand, the unilateral free TRAM is preferred over the unilateral pedicle TRAM mostly for perfusion pressure reasons.

In the higher risk patients, though it is probably still a good idea to use the bilateral free TRAM technique for bilateral breast reconstruction. Higher risks patients include those who are smoking or have recently smoked, are overweight, have certain scars on the abdomen, have diabetes, and/or have had previous radiation to the chest. In all of these cases, the free microvascular technique is preferred.

Treatment/surgical technique

Preoperative considerations

The patient is admitted the day of surgery and marked in the preoperative room. Markings are limited to the chest area in the preoperative room. Skin sparing mastectomies are routinely employed in immediate reconstruction, and an agreement between the oncologic surgeon and the plastic surgeon is made as to how much and in what location skin is to be removed on the breast. A commonly employed incision for a skin sparing mastectomy is a circumareolar incision only. While this is a very safe oncologic procedure and is attractive aesthetically, the small skin defect does make it more difficult for the surgeon to resect the breast and for the plastic surgeon to shape the TRAM on the chest wall. Because of this, we prefer a small transverse incision laterally from the circumareolar incision. This leaves a scar that is similar to a breast biopsy. Because the surgical oncologist has a larger incision, there is increased visibility for the resection and probably less trauma to the native skin flaps due to retraction.

Once the breast incisions are agreed upon, the patient is moved to the operating room. Patients are not routinely typed and crossed for transfusion even in the face of bilateral mastectomies and bilateral reconstruction in the more obese patient. From time to time, blood transfusions are required but they are rare. In our series, the incidence is <5%. Patients are given 250 mg of methylprednisolone as well as IV antibiotics in the preoperative area. Compression garments are used on the lower extremities prior to induction of anesthesia and during the operation.

Operative procedure

The surgical procedures, resection of the breast and subsequent reconstruction are done sequentially. While it is certainly possible to elevate the TRAM flap while the mastectomies are being performed, we have chosen not to pursue that approach. We have found that while technically it is feasible to have two operating teams

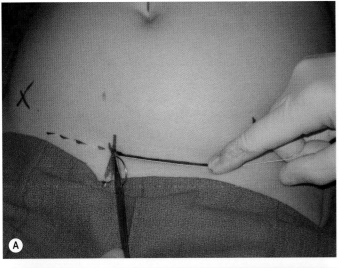

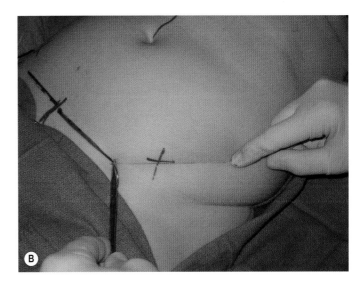

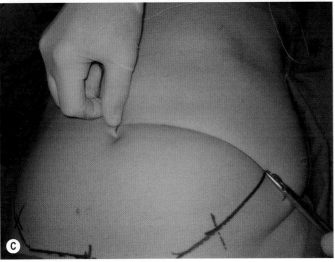

Fig. 16.3 (A–C) Abdominal markings.

working at once, we have found it more efficient to let the surgical oncologist complete his job and leave the reconstructive team with access to the entire operating field.

The abdominal flap is designed at this time. The lower transverse incision is located two fingerbreadths above the pubic symphysis. The upper incision is usually just at the upper border of the umbilicus. The lower incision extends out laterally and crosses over the anterior superior iliac spine and angles cephalad. The upper incision is essentially level extending laterally until it meets the rising lower incision. The suture technique is useful for ensuring that each line is equal *(Fig. 16.3)*.

Hints and tips

- If the upper incision is straight across, the resulting scar will curve upward. If the upper incision is curved down laterally the resulting scar will be straight across.
- The inframammary lines drawn preoperatively are reinforced and the tunnel positions on the right and the left are also drawn in place.

These tunnel positions are at the 5- and 7-o'clock positions on the right and the left respectively *(Fig. 16.4)*. These tunnel locations necessarily violate part of the medial portions of the inframammary lines bilaterally. However, the tunnels will only ultimately contain

Video 1

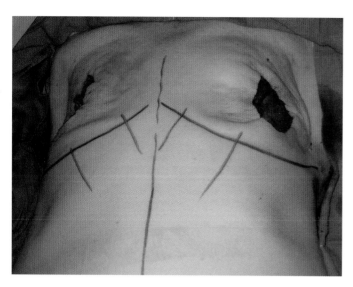

Fig. 16.4 Tunnel locations.

a small segment of muscle thus avoiding significant bulk at the inframammary line if the muscle and fascial sparing technique (described below) is employed. In addition, the most medial aspect of the inframammary lines bilaterally is left intact. This small portion medially, along with the inframammary line left intact laterally, is enough to create a very distinct inframammary line even immediately postoperatively (see *Fig. 16.19*).

Hints and tips

Make the tunnel slightly smaller than you think the flap will need for easy passage. By rocking the flap medially and laterally, the flap will pass through a smaller tunnel than one may predict.

Contrary to the thinking in the early 1980s, it is not a good idea to dissect over the lower sternum and xiphoid for the tunnels to the chest. This often leaves bulk in an area which is unattractive and dissection of an area that will not always scar back down in an aesthetically pleasing fashion. Thus, the combination of precise tunnel location as well as only leaving small amounts of muscle in the tunnel combine in most cases to yield crisp distinct inframammary lines in both the early and late postoperative periods.

The superior skin incision is made and the dissection continues with the cautery. The cautery is set on a blend of coagulation and cutting which allows the dissection to continue rapidly through the fat with a minimum of bleeding. The superior incision through the fat is beveled superiorly to recruit additional fat into the flap. One must exaggerate this beveling somewhat to enjoy the fruits of additional fat harvest and the possible recruitment of additional perforators in the superior periumbilical region. Once the fascia is reached, the upper abdominal flap is elevated up to and over the costal margins bilaterally for about 2 cm. The dissection in the midline continues up to the xiphoid. The tunnels are then created on the right and the left to the chest dissection area, usually with the aid of a large Deaver or Harrington retractor. Normally, a cautery extender or lighted retractor is not necessary but certainly could be utilized if one desired.

Once a connection has been made between the abdominal dissection and chest dissection areas, the tunnel can be carefully widened. This is usually done bluntly using the fingers or the hand to very gradually dilate the tunnels. It is a good idea to leave the tunnels slightly smaller than one thinks is necessary as they can always be made slightly larger if necessary. On average, each tunnel needs to accommodate approximately four fingers to allow passage of each hemiflap. These tunnels can be an aggravating source of bleeding and must be inspected carefully to be sure all bleeding points are controlled.

The lower incision is then made. No attempt is made to bevel inferiorly as the fat in the pre-pubic region is probably not as reliable based on the superior epigastric system as we would like to think. Thus, the incision inferiorly should be relatively straight down to the underlying fascia. The umbilicus is circumscribed and left in position with some surrounding fat and the flap is split in the midline down to the deep fascia. This dissection is continued from medial to lateral on each side until the medial row of perforators is encountered *(Fig. 16.5)*.

Proposed markings of the boundaries of the left and right rectus sheaths, as well as the costal margin are now made in the superior epigastrium using methylene blue. One must carefully observe the degree of the diastasis recti, which is present, as well as the change from the rectus sheath to the oblique musculature laterally. This can be seen through the epimysium and external fascia if one is careful to observe this *(Fig. 16.6A)*.

The sterile Doppler is now used to locate the position of the superior epigastric artery as it passes from deep

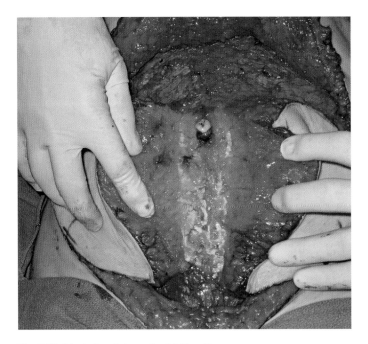

Fig. 16.5 Extent of medial suprafascial dissection.

to the costal margin. This location is important as it should become the center of the muscle portion that is harvested superiorly *(Fig. 16.6B)*.

The proposed muscle and fascial harvest is drawn in using methylene blue incorporating the emanation of the superior epigastric vessels superiorly and harvesting approximately one-third to one-half of the central rectus fascia as the proposed muscle and fascial flap pedicle.

We also continue this proposed flap harvest drawing down over the skin islands bilaterally. It is important to draw both of these proposed harvest outlines prior to beginning the harvest of either muscle *(Fig. 16.6C)*. Once one flap has been elevated the closure of the fascia distorts the opposite side and can disorient the surgeon if one is not extremely careful. That is the reason for making the drawings on both sides prior to harvesting either of the flaps (see *Fig. 16.14*).

Dissection begins at the costal margin laterally and extends through the fascia for 2–3 cm caudal to the costal margin. At this point, the anterior fascia is elevated laterally to confirm the position in the muscle relative to its lateral border. We try to leave 1–2 cm of muscle and, more importantly, fascia laterally. One must confirm though that the dissection is not too far lateral or too far medial high up before the dissection continues inferiorly *(Fig. 16.7A)*.

The dissection then continues using the cautery on the blend setting. It is important to be sure that the patient has complete muscular paralysis during this intramuscular dissection.

The dissection can then continue expeditiously through the overlying fascia and underlying muscle down to and below the level of the umbilicus. Small oblique vessels will be noted but are only perineural vessels accompanying the lower abdominal wall nerves to the rectus segments reminiscent of intercostal nerves more cephalad. The location of the inferior epigastric vessels is in a relatively constant position two thirds of the way caudad from the umbilicus to the pubic symphysis. Once one is near that location, dissection continues more cautiously with the use of a dissecting clamp and the cautery. Dissection through the muscle proceeds more cautiously until the inferior epigastric vessels are located *(Fig. 16.7B)*.

The muscle can also be elevated from lateral to medial and the vascular hilum of the inferior epigastric vessels entering into the muscle might be noted prior to seeing the inferior epigastric vessels inferiorly *(Fig. 16.7C,D)*.

As the central segment of the muscle is elevated out of its bed inferiorly it can also be elevated superiorly and the superior epigastric vessels can also be visibly identified. The muscle is now well mobilized, and the inferior epigastric vessels are identified. They are clipped and transected with a medium clip applier, specifically the Ethicon Ligaclip MCA titanium.

The medial dissection on the fascia and muscle can now be performed. With one hand behind the muscle, one can establish the location of the medial border of the muscle. Once again, we shift laterally for 1–2 cm where an incision in the fascia and underlying muscle is made. This is usually first performed at the level of the umbilicus *(Fig. 16.8)*.

Dissection then continues vertically inferiorly and is curved just below the level of the inferior epigastric vessels to meet the lateral dissection. The muscle and overlying flap must be controlled at all times by the

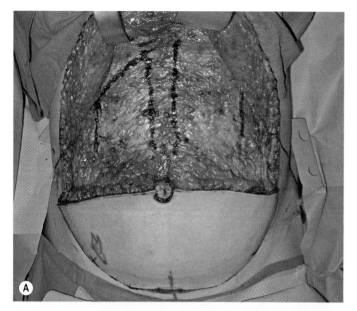

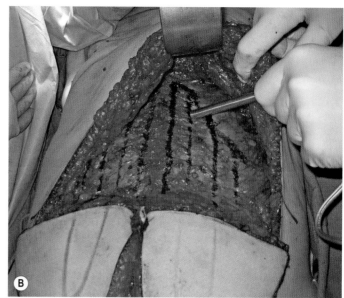

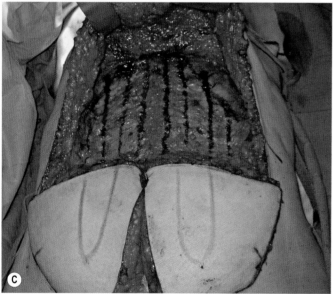

Fig. 16.6 (A) Marking extent of recti. **(B)** Proposed fascial strip centered over SEA signal. **(C)** Final markings of fascial and muscle strip.

surgeon as he conducts the fascial and muscle dissection *(Fig. 16.9)*. At this point, the flap is freed up inferiorly essentially up to the level of the umbilicus.

The superior dissection medially is now completed by a vertical incision up towards the costal margin. The superior epigastric vessels have been visualized as well as located using the sterile Doppler so this dissection continues up without threat of injury to these vessels. This intramuscular dissection is facilitated by controlling the muscle and fascial pedicle with one hand, placing hemostats on the medial fascia for counter-

traction and performing the medial intramuscular dissection with cautery *(Fig. 16.10)*.

The incision in the fascia continues up over the costal margin and meets the original lateral incision in the fascia; however, muscle is left intact for about 1–2 cm caudal to the costal margin medially. This thins the muscle proximally at the costal margin to 1–2 cm in width. However, this is safe because the presence and location of the superior epigastric pedicle is confirmed with the sterile Doppler, direct vision, and/or palpability. I This creates a muscular-fascial pedicle

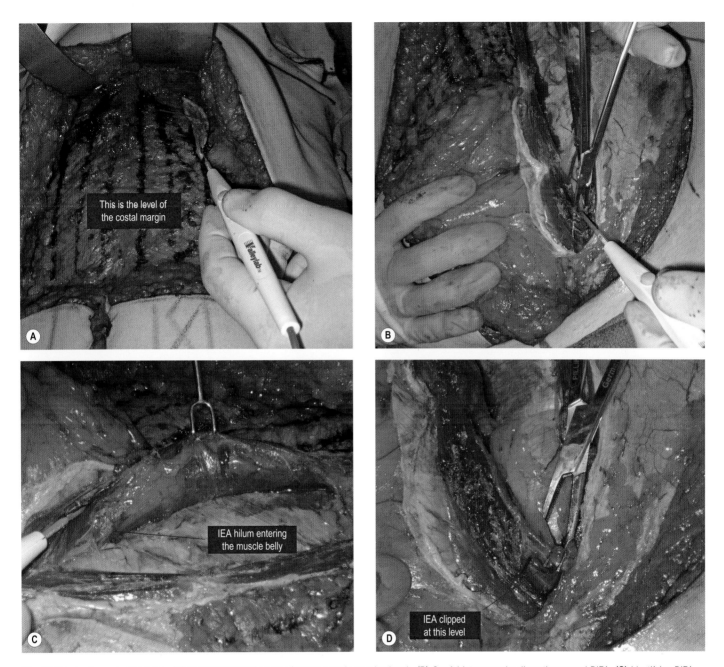

Fig. 16.7 Lateral muscle dissection. **(A)** Identifying lateral extent of rectus muscle as a landmark. **(B)** Careful intramuscular dissection around DIEA. **(C)** Identifying DIEA hilum entering inferolateral edge of muscle. **(D)** Clipping the DIEA.

length of usually ≥8–9 cm. In addition, the superior epigastric pedicle is found deep to the costal margin, so by meeting the lateral and medial fascial incisions up high over the costal margin, the pedicle remains safe *(Fig. 16.11)*.

It is important to remember that the distance from the costal margin to the inframammary line of the breast is only about 5–6 cm, so 8–9 cm is more than an adequate length of muscle pedicle to easily reach the chest area *(Figs 16.11B, 16.12)*.

The flap is generally weighed using the sterile fish scale. The flap skin is moistened and the flap is gently passed ipsilaterally through the tunnel. We use ipsilateral transfer because this avoids crossing the pedicles in

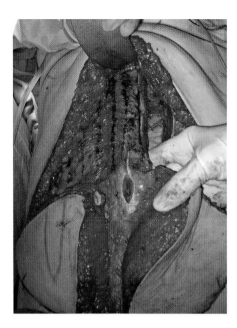

Fig. 16.8 Medial dissection maintaining control of flap at all times with opposite hand.

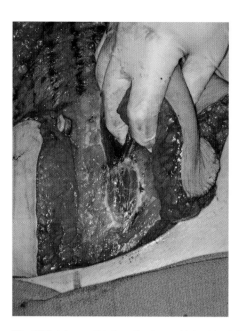

Fig. 16.9 Inferomedial dissection to meet inferolateral dissection.

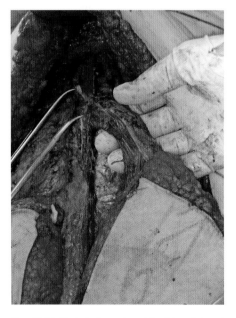

Fig. 16.10 Control of muscle and fascial pedicle and use of countertraction on the fascia in during superomedial dissection.

the inferior corner first through the tunnel, the other corner then follows easily. Once the flap is in the chest pocket the pedicle is carefully adjusted at the costal margin so that it turns around the costal margin and does not flip over the costal margin.

If the pedicle flips over the costal margin it then has to flip back for the flap to be oriented properly on the chest wall. This causes two major twists in the pedicle which are unnecessary if the gentle turning of the pedicle is instead employed *(Fig. 16.13)*. The flap is stabilized in the chest pocket by stapling the skin and the abdominal fascia is approximated using a skin stapler temporarily. Approximating the abdominal fascia at this point prevents lateral retraction while the contralateral side is elevated, thus easing fascial closure once both flaps are elevated.

The opposite flap is now elevated in a similar manner. The methylene blue lines are reinforced if necessary and the distortion from the closure on the opposite side is evident *(Fig. 16.14)*.

The dissection continues in an identical manner beginning again laterally at the costal margin and continuing inferiorly on the lateral side. The inferior epigastric vessels are divided, and the medial dissection is completed as described above. The flap is passed as mentioned, and the pedicle is carefully adjusted at the

the midline. However, it is probably safe to use either technique.

It is helpful to use a towel clip on the lateral tip of the TRAM flap which passes through the tunnel first. It is also helpful then to either work the superior corner or

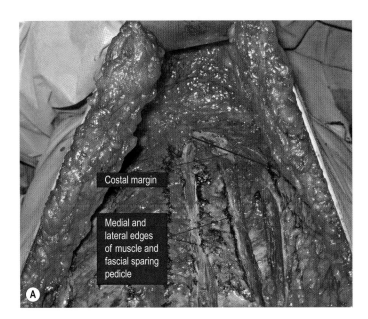

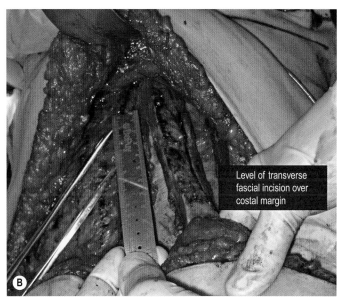

Fig. 16.11 **(A,B)** Demonstrating width and length of fascial and muscle strip and extent of dissection up over costal margin.

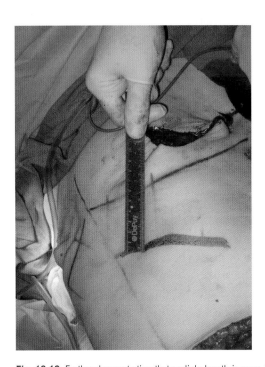

Fig. 16.12 Further demonstrating that pedicle length is more than adequate to reach chest wall defect.

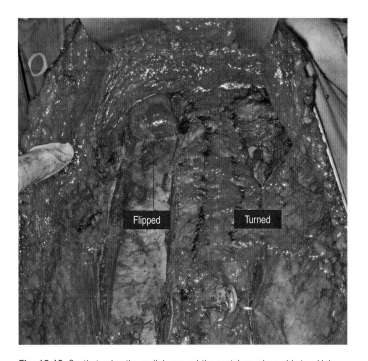

Fig. 16.13 Gently turning the pedicle around the costal margin avoids two kinks which result if the pedicle is flipped.

costal margin to be sure it is not flipped up over on itself. The abdominal fascia is again closed temporarily using skin staples *(Fig. 16.15)*.

The abdominal wall closure is facilitated by the fascial sparing TRAM harvest. That is, if fascia is left medially

and laterally in 1–2 cm segments, the closure is relatively straightforward. Additionally, closing both fascial defects simultaneously is a technical maneuver which makes the abdominal wall closure easier *(Fig. 16.16)*. One must have an assistant who is very well trained in

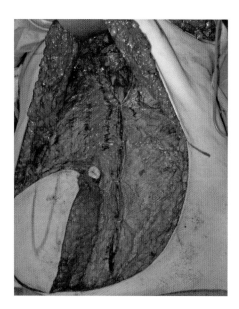

Fig. 16.14 Note the distortion of the lines towards the side of closure.

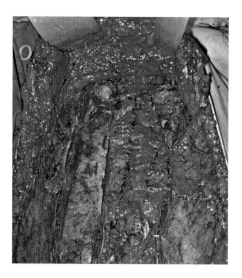

Fig. 16.15 Seen here on one side only, staples were used identically on the contralateral side. Also note the turning of the pedicle around the costal margin.

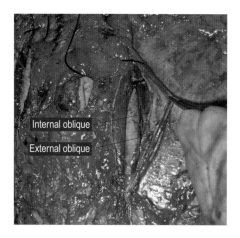

Internal oblique

External oblique

Fig. 16.16 Both the external and internal oblique components of the rectus fascia must be incorporated into the abdominal closure.

abdominal wall closure to ensure that the closure is sound. If both sides are closed simultaneously the stress is distributed all the way across the abdominal wall as the closure is conducted.

The closure begins superiorly using double stranded 0-nylon sutures. The double stranded suture is looped and avoids a knot superiorly. Though not routinely kept on shelf in the operating room, we prefer to use 0 Ethilon, 72 inches, looped, on a tapered XLH needle (lot #D5854). The closure then proceeds inferiorly in tandem

being careful to include both the external and internal oblique components of the anterior rectus sheath. These two components become very obvious at and below the level of the umbilicus *(Fig. 16.17)*.

It is extremely important to include both of these components, particularly the internal layer which probably accounts for the most important strength of the closure. It is our belief that if this internal component is not included, or "slips out" in the early postoperative period, weakness of the abdominal wall could be observed later. This is usually not a "hernia" but a weakness or eventration of the abdominal wall probably caused by the fact that the external component of the anterior rectus fascia is intact but the internal has slid back. The most difficult part of this closure is below the umbilicus and attention to detail must be stressed here to be sure that the closure is sound. Each bite is at least 1 cm back on the fascia, and each bite advances 1–2 cm inferiorly on the fascia. The closure is completed with the double stranded suture, and fascial staples are added on both sides over the suture line for additional support.

If there is any concern about the abdominal wall closure, Prolene mesh support is added over the closure once it is completed. However, the intention is to provide as anatomic and sound a closure as possible using the nylon prior to adding Prolene mesh, which is used as an overlay and for additional support. Mesh is rarely, if

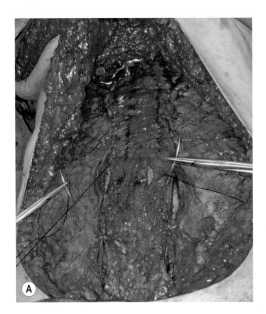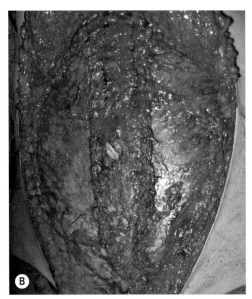

Fig. 16.17 (A,B) Simultaneous fascial closure distributes tension across the abdomen and aides in primarily closing the fascial defects.

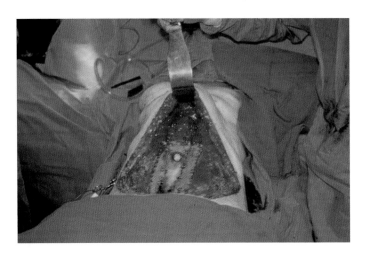

Fig. 16.18 Double layer prolene mesh.

ever, used or needed for replacement of abdominal wall structure but instead used over an anatomic abdominal wall closure as additional overlay support.

The Prolene mesh, if used, is used in a double layer and is sutured in place using 0-Prolene in a running and interrupted manner *(Fig. 16.18)*. Prolene mesh is used in approximately 30% of our bilateral patients.

The abdominal wall is then closed over two closed suction drains after the abdominal wall is irrigated. We feel it is very important to irrigate prior to closure as this reduces the incidence of postoperative infection. The closure is done in two layers using a barbed suture deep in Scarpa's fascia and one in the deep intracuticular layer. A site for the umbilicus is cut out and it is inset in the appropriate position.

Shaping of the TRAM flap breast reconstruction

Once the flaps are on the chest, the pedicles have been checked to be in the proper orientation and the abdominal wall has been closed; the breasts are shaped. This gives some intervening time between the passage of the flaps to the chest wall and the final shaping for any vascular compromise to occur and to be observed. The flaps should have good pink color at this time. If any duskiness is noted one may release the clips on one or both inferior epigastric veins. The flap usually pinks up immediately after this maneuver. Additionally, one can look for large veins just above Scarpa's fascia. Releasing these veins directly decompresses the superficial fat and skin. Thus, by the time the flap is deepithelialized, red healthy bleeding should be observed from the dermis. If not, the pedicle should be examined visibly for undue twisting and with the sterile Doppler for arterial inflow. It is not uncommon at this point in the pedicled TRAM procedure for there to be some venous imbalance probably due to the need for the choke vessels to open up fully. Release of these larger veins can "relieve" the flap as this process is occurring. Additionally, one may find that the patient's blood pressure may be relatively low since the patient has been completely paralyzed for the muscle dissection and abdominal wall closure. Furthermore, the patient has not been stimulated greatly during the abdominal skin closure – this contributes also to a lower blood pressure at this point in the operation. However, if a good arterial Doppler signal is detected, one can be assured that as the patient wakes up, the blood pressure will attain a more normal level and perfusion to the TRAM tissues will be more than adequate.

Shaping of the TRAMs in the immediate setting is significantly assisted by the presence of native skin on the chest. While there are many variations of remaining skin after skin sparing mastectomies, the idea is to leave a remaining skin envelope which will cover the TRAM flaps with mild but not undo tension. The TRAM flaps are sutured internally in the pocket medially, superiorly and laterally to stabilize the TRAM flaps on the chest wall so that the skin closure will effect the final shaping. It is important to adequately fill any deficit in the infra-clavicular location, as this is an extremely important aesthetic subunit of the breast because it is frequently seen. Superior sutures in the pocket will secure filling in this area. Laterally, the TRAM flap should be tacked to the chest wall to define the lateral contour of the breast as sharply as possible. However, any sutures placed through TRAM tissue for positioning purposes should be tied down relatively loosely to avoid localized areas of fat necrosis. Shaping of the breast becomes more difficult during secondary procedures; therefore every effort should be made at the time of initial reconstruction to obtain the very best shape. A vision of the final shape of the breast should be in mind even at the beginning of the operation, as maneuvers early on can affect the final product. As mentioned early in the chapter, the tunnels used to pass the TRAM flaps onto the chest wall should be large enough to pass the flaps safely, but should leave a small portion of the IMF intact medially, and a larger portion left intact laterally so that the IMF is crisp even immediately postop *(Fig. 16.19)*. Drains are placed laterally and sutured in place.

Attention to detail throughout the operative procedure will give the patient a long lasting and natural looking result. *Figures 16.20–16.23* are pre- and postoperative photographs of four patients who underwent bilateral pedicled TRAMs. In each of these four examples, the senior author has achieved good shape,

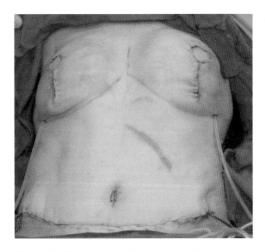

Fig. 16.19 Note the distinct inframammary lines immediately postoperative.

symmetry, and natural appearance, while also improving their abdominal contours.

Postoperative care

All of these procedures are performed as inpatient procedures. Patients generally spend 2–4 days in the hospital after the operation, with the average being 3 days. The patient is allowed to shower on postoperative day 3 and simply changes the dressings around the drains, and leaves all skin tapes in place. Skin tapes are the only dressings used for the incisions and these are changed at the first postoperative visit and then weekly by the patient as instructed. The tape is 1.0 inch paper tape, sterile in the operating room but not sterile as the patient changes the tape. We prefer to have the patient continue taping the incision for 6 weeks after the operation as scar treatment. We feel that this improves and flattens the scar and compares favorably to other methods of scar treatment. It is also inexpensive and there are very few side-effects. If the patient becomes sensitive to the tape, it is discontinued and vitamin-E or aloe is suggested.

Patients are encouraged to increase their activities immediately after surgery in terms of ambulation and trying to stand as straight as possible. Usually, patients are able to drive within the first 2–3 weeks after surgery, but are instructed not to do so as long as they are on pain medication. Other more extensive exercises are limited until the patient is 4–6 weeks postoperative.

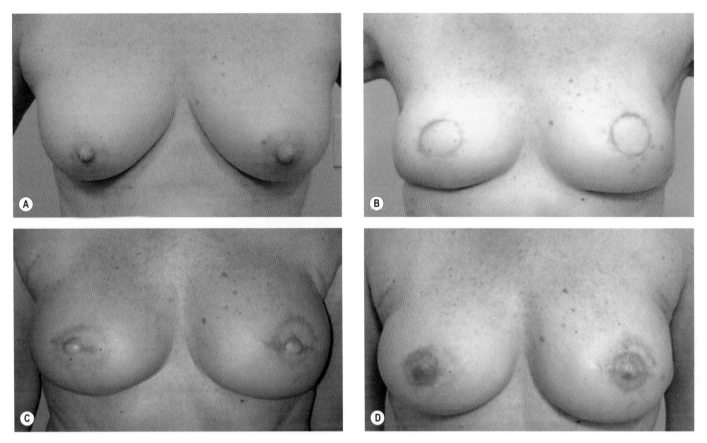

Fig. 16.20 (A) Preoperative photograph for bilateral mastectomies in a 48-year-old patient. **(B)** Three months status after the bilateral pedicle TRAM. **(C)** Two months after nipple reconstruction. **(D)** Two months after areolar tattoo.

Outcomes, prognosis, complications

The outcomes and, indeed, the prognosis after this operation are affected significantly by the preoperative risks of each patient, as well as postoperative motivation, desires, and even personality. Certainly, preoperative risks such as smoking, radiation, and obesity can significantly increase the chance of postoperative complications. However, it is also true that postoperative patient motivation and desires can affect the speed of recovery and their acceptance of their new breasts. Ultimately, the patient's acceptance of her new breasts is the most telling indicator of success. Acceptance of cancer by the patient can also affect the patient's outcome. If the patient cannot accept that she has cancer, this may also relate to the patient's acceptance of the reconstruction. A healthy relationship with the diagnosis and prognosis seems to be directly related to the patient's postoperative recovery.

The most common complications of this type of reconstruction include loss of native breast skin, small areas of fat necrosis, dog ears of the abdomen, peri-flap depressions as well as other contour deformities secondary to the extent of the mastectomy, and, rarely, seromas. Significant flap loss and even total flap loss is exceedingly rare with the technique as described above. Our incidence of fat necrosis (<10% of the flap) is 9% and flap loss or necrosis (>25%) is <1%. The number one goal is symmetry and is readily achieved with bilateral pedicled TRAM flaps *(Figs 16.20–16.23)*.

The incidence of loss of native skin of the breast can be reduced with the use of dye techniques such as fluorescein or the new SPY technique.[9,10] Both of these techniques utilize dyes to visualize the degree of perfusion to the mastectomy skin. These techniques are particularly helpful in pigmented patients. However, if native skin loss is encountered in the early postoperative period, it is probably best treated with early excision and closure. This reduces the patient's healing time and

Fig. 16.21 (A,B) Preoperative photographs of a 45-year-old patient. **(C,D)** Three months after a bilateral pedicle TRAM. **(E,F)** Three months after nipple reconstruction and one mont after an areolar tattoo.

avoids the unpleasant dressing changes that accompany treatment of an open wound postoperatively. However, secondary excision and closure may affect the breast shape. If this is the case, this can be adjusted at the time of the secondary revision and nipple reconstruction.

If small areas of fat necrosis exist, they are best treated by excision because they create concern for cancer recurrence by any subsequent examining physician. Usually these excisions do not lead to any type of breast deformity; however, if they do, small areas of depression can be treated with fat injections. Autologous fat transfers

(AFTs) have become an important part of the secondary breast reconstruction. Fat can be easily transferred from one part of the body to another using syringe techniques and Telfa purification of the fat to yield purified fat cells that predictably have a 45–50% chance of survival. AFTs can then be used to treat any residual deformities in the superior pole of the breast where they are most commonly found. This location is common because there can be a subcutaneous gap between the superior border of the TRAM flap and the extent of the mastectomy. The superior-medial aspect of the breast is arguably the

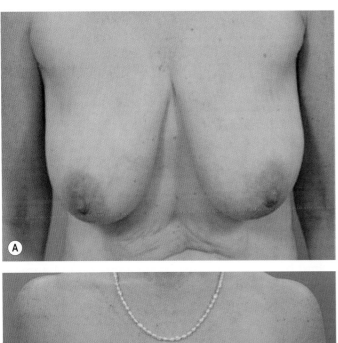

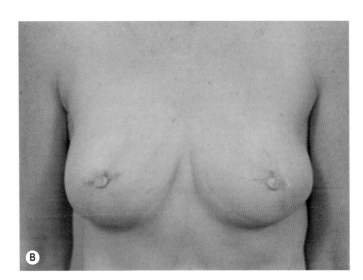

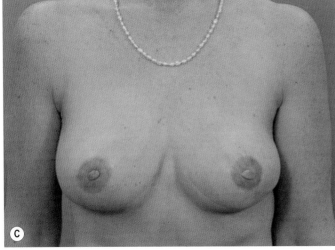

Fig. 16.22 (A) Preoperative photographs of a 58-year-old patient. **(B)** Six months after bilateral pedicle TRAM, and two months after nipple reconstruction. **(C)** Six months after areolar tattoo.

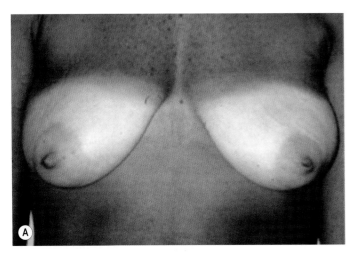

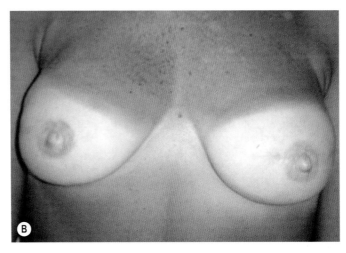

Fig. 16.23 (A) Preoperative photograph of a 42-year-old patient. **(B)** One year after reconstruction with bilateral pedicle TRAMS.

most important aesthetic subunit because it is readily visible in many types of clothing. AFTs provide good correction of postoperative deformities in this area known as the décolletage.

Persistent seromas after drain removal can occur but are less frequent today. If seromas occur after drain removal, re-aspiration is tried for 1–2 weeks. If the seroma continues to recur, a second drain is placed and this generally resolves the problem. Patients never like drains, either the first or the second time; therefore, we try to avoid any reinsertion of a drain.

Secondary procedures

We prefer to wait 2–3 months after the initial procedure to perform a secondary and, hopefully, final procedure. This timeframe may be delayed further if chemotherapy and/or radiation are necessary postoperatively. If radiation is required postoperatively we prefer to wait at least 6 months after the radiation has been completed before performing any secondary procedures. On the other hand, with chemotherapy, we wait only until the patient's blood counts have returned to normal before performing the secondary procedure. This generally is only a month or so after chemotherapy has been completed.

Secondary procedures often include nipple/areolar reconstruction and autologous fat transfer around the breast to improve any persistent contour deformities. If any areas of fat necrosis are present these are removed.

Occasionally, there are larger areas of fat necrosis that would incur a deformity of the breast if completely removed. In this situation, it is occasionally necessary to use an inferior thoracoepigastric flap to fill in inferior deformities of the breast or to use a latissimus myocutaneous flap to fill in lateral or superior deformities of the breast that are larger than 25% of the breast.

"Dog-ear" deformities are always removed if present on the abdominal wall at this time as well. In the past we have suctioned these areas, but have not found that this technique adequately resolves the prominence of the "dog-ears". For that reason, we excise these in essentially every case. Deformities of breast contour along the lateral breast or along the inframammary fold are rare because these areas are established at the time of breast shaping at the initial operation. In addition, any bulges along the medial inframammary fold are rare because of the small size of the muscle-sparing pedicle, as well as the location where the pedicle is passed. As mentioned, we prefer to pass the pedicle at the 5-o'clock position on the patient's left and the 7-o'clock position on the right, thus avoiding disruption of the skin overlying the lower sternum and xiphoid.

Nipple/areolar reconstruction is performed using a Star flap, which is a modification of the Skate technique. The nipple is essentially a flap raised up and based inferiorly with healthy underlying fat since the tissue is taken from a healthy TRAM flap. Finally, the areola is recreated by tattooing 2–3 months after the nipple/areolar reconstruction has been performed.

Access the complete references list online at **http://www.expertconsult.com**

1. Hartrampf CR, Scheflan M, Black PW. Breast reconstruction with a transverse abdominal island flap. *Plast Reconstr Surg.* 1982;69:216–224.
   The seminal article on TRAM flaps.
2. Mathes SJ. A rectus abdominis myocutaneous flap to reconstruct abdominal wall defects. *Br J Plast Surg.* 1977;30:282–283.
   Originally described the epigastric artery as the pedicle source.
3. Moon HK, Taylor GI. The vascular anatomy of rectus abdominis musculocutaneous flaps based on the deep superior epigastric system. *Plast Reconstr Surg.* 1988;82:815–831.

   Describes the epigastric arteries as they relate to the TRAM flap.
4. Mathes SJ, Logan SE. The use of a rectus abdominis myocutaneous flap to reconstruct a groin defect. *Br J Plast Surg.* 1984;37:351–353.
5. Spear SL. *Surgery of the breast: principles and art.* Philadelphia: Lippincott-Raven; 1997.
   Describes matching procedures that are available for the contralateral breast to help with symmetry.
8. Baldwin BJ, Schusterman MA, Miller MJ, et al. Bilateral breast reconstruction: conventional versus free TRAM. *Plast Reconstr Surg.* 1994;93:1410–1416.
   Pedicle versus Free TRAMs and differences in perfusion.

17

Free TRAM breast reconstruction

Joshua Fosnot and Joseph M. Serletti

SYNOPSIS

- The free TRAM is one tool in an entire armamentarium used for breast reconstruction.
- Although controversial, the free TRAM likely limits donor site morbidity and ischemic complications when compared with the pedicled TRAM.
- Free TRAM reconstruction can be performed safely in an immediate or delayed fashion.
- For the most part, radiation therapy after reconstruction yields more unpredictable results than radiation before reconstruction.
- Free TRAM flap breast reconstruction requires intraoperative attention to detail and postoperative vigilance.
- Although revision is not uncommon, the free TRAM provides for excellent, predictable aesthetic results with a high degree of patient satisfaction.

 Access the Historical Perspective section online at
http://www.expertconsult.com

Introduction

Although the pedicled transverse rectus abdominis myocutaneous (TRAM) flap provided a foundation for the burgeoning field of breast reconstruction, the overall contemporary trend has focused on approaches which provide improved aesthetic outcomes while minimizing complications and donor site morbidity. Advances in microsurgical technique have thus led the field toward the utilization of free flaps, which benefit from a more profound blood supply while sacrificing less of the abdominal wall. A spectrum exists, which includes the free TRAM, muscle sparing free TRAM, deep inferior epigastric perforator (DIEP) flap and superficial inferior epigastric artery (SIEA) flaps, all of which utilize the same transverse island of lower abdominal wall skin and soft tissue for the recreation of a breast mound with varying degrees of abdominal wall intrusion. The purpose of this chapter is to discuss in detail the most common and perhaps the least technically demanding of these procedures, the free TRAM.

Basic science/disease process

One out of every eight women in the United States will develop breast cancer at some point in their lifetime. In total, roughly 2.5 million women in the United States are survivors of breast cancer, with this number expected to increase dramatically over the next decade.[9] Given that mastectomy plays a major role in the treatment algorithm of breast cancer, it is not infrequent that women are faced with the decision of whether to have a breast mound reconstructed. In most cases, mastectomy offers the chance for cure and reconstruction provides a woman a better aesthetic result. In some cases however, even patients who have advanced metastatic cancer may be candidates for reconstruction, such as for radiation ulcers or nonhealing wounds.[10] In addition, with the advent of genetic testing for BRCA I and II for risk stratification, an increasing number of women are electing to undergo prophylactic mastectomy.[11] Likewise, the frequency of contralateral prophylactic mastectomy is increasing dramatically in patients who have undergone mastectomy for DCIS.[12] As a whole, more and more reconstructive procedures are being performed annually in the United States.

The mastectomy defect can be devastating both physically and psychologically. Numerous studies have documented the significant improvement in self confidence and mental health following breast reconstruction.[13–15] Autologous reconstruction in particular, has the benefit of replacing "like with like", which in turn contributes to an improved feeling of restoration of the self after this devastating injury.[16]

Although breast cancer is by far the leading source of a thoracic defect requiring autologous reconstruction, it should not be forgotten that free TRAM reconstruction may also be used for defects such as chest wall sarcomas or lung cancer invading the chest wall where soft tissue coverage is needed after resection.[17,18]

Anatomy and physiology

The anatomy of the abdominal wall is critical to a complete understanding of the differences between various forms of abdominal based breast reconstruction such as the pedicled TRAM, free TRAM, deep inferior epigastric perforator (DIEP), and superficial inferior epigastric artery (SIEA) flaps. The rectus abdominis muscles run in parallel on either side of the midline (*Fig. 17.1*). The origin is the symphysis pubis, whereas the insertion is the subcostal margin of ribs 5–7 and the xiphoid process. The recti are separated in the midline by the linea alba and crossed transversely by fibrous bands called tendinous inscriptions. The rectus muscles rest within the rectus sheath, a confluence of the aponeuroses of the external and internal oblique muscles, as well as the transversus abdominis. The arcuate line, a transverse line roughly one-third the distance between the umbilicus and the pubic symphysis, marks a transition in the composition of the rectus sheath. Above this line,

the anterior rectus sheath is comprised of the external oblique and a portion of the internal oblique; whereas, the posterior sheath is comprised of a portion of the internal oblique and the transversus abdominis. Below the arcuate line, the posterior rectus sheath disappears and all three components of the aponeurosis pass anterior to the recti. Perhaps more importantly for the discussion of TRAM reconstruction, the arcuate line also marks the point where the inferior epigastric vessels perforate the rectus muscles.

The blood supply of the lower anterior abdominal wall comes from both the superior and inferior deep epigastric arteries which connect to one another via "choke" vessels in the mid-abdomen (*Fig. 17.1*). The arteries send perforating vessels through the rectus muscle to the soft tissue and skin of the abdominal wall. Having two dominant pedicles, this rectus is a Mathes and Nahai type III muscle.[19] The typical TRAM flap utilizes skin and soft tissue from infra-umbilical redundancy; therefore, when harvesting a pedicled TRAM flap, the survival of the flap island is dependent on the choke vessels at the end of the superior epigastric artery. As a result, the flap runs the risk of ischemia. A free TRAM has the benefit of a more robust blood supply because the perforators off of the inferior epigastric artery offer a more direct route of blood flow. In addition, because these perforators can often times be visualized, some of the rectus muscle may be salvaged.

The superior and inferior epigastric arteries originate from the subclavian arteries via the internal mammary arteries and the external iliacs respectively. To allow for adequate pedicle length, the inferior epigastric artery dissection is usually carried down to the external iliac artery immediately above the inguinal ligament.

The function of the rectus muscles includes flexion of the trunk and lumbar vertebrae. It plays a key role in overall posture, acting as a counterbalance to the muscles of the back and is also responsible for creating intraabdominal pressure for urination and defecation. The rectus acts in concert with the external oblique, internal oblique and transversus abdominus muscles. The innervation of the rectus muscle enters laterally from the intercostal nerve bundles. Preservation of some of these nerves allows for the possibility of residual functional ability of any remaining rectus muscle postoperatively.

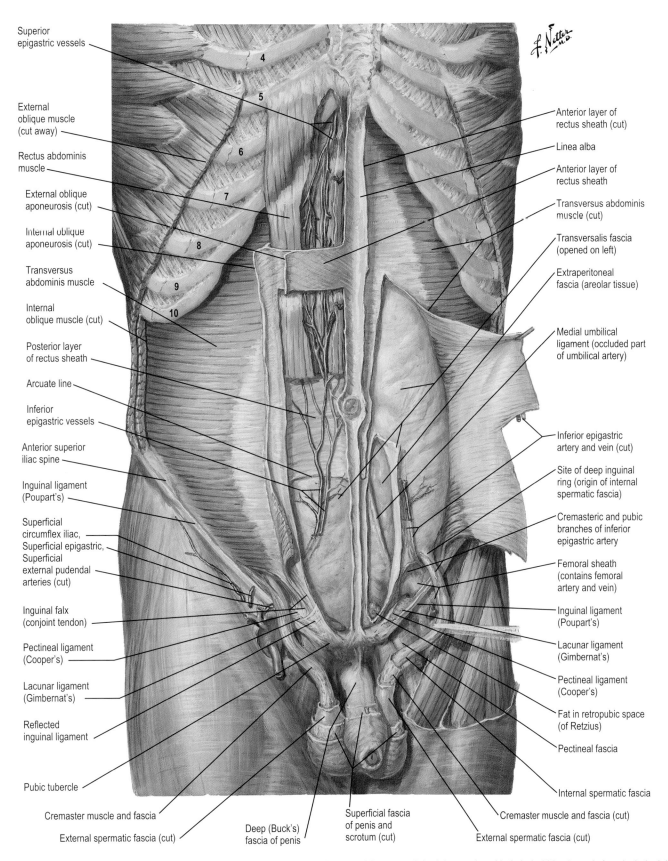

Superior epigastric vessels

External oblique muscle (cut away)

Rectus abdominis muscle

External oblique aponeurosis (cut)

Internal oblique aponeurosis (cut)

Transversus abdominis muscle

Internal oblique muscle (cut)

Posterior layer of rectus sheath

Arcuate line

Inferior epigastric vessels

Anterior superior iliac spine

Inguinal ligament (Poupart's)

Superficial circumflex iliac, Superficial epigastric, Superficial external pudendal arteries (cut)

Inguinal falx (conjoint tendon)

Pectineal ligament (Cooper's)

Lacunar ligament (Gimbernat's)

Reflected inguinal ligament

Pubic tubercle

Cremaster muscle and fascia

External spermatic fascia (cut)

4

5

6

7

8

9

10

Anterior layer of rectus sheath (cut)

Linea alba

Anterior layer of rectus sheath

Transversus abdominis muscle (cut)

Transversalis fascia (opened on left)

Extraperitoneal fascia (areolar tissue)

Medial umbilical ligament (occluded part of umbilical artery)

Inferior epigastric artery and vein (cut)

Site of deep inguinal ring (origin of internal spermatic fascia)

Cremasteric and pubic branches of inferior epigastric artery

Femoral sheath (contains femoral artery and vein)

Inguinal ligament (Poupart's)

Lacunar ligament (Gimbernat's)

Pectineal ligament (Cooper's)

Fat in retropubic space (of Retzius)

Pectineal fascia

Internal spermatic fascia

Cremaster muscle and fascia (cut)

External spermatic fascia (cut)

Deep (Buck's) fascia of penis

Superficial fascia of penis and scrotum (cut)

Fig. 17.1 The anatomy of the abdominal wall. In particular, note the parallel nature of the rectus abdominis muscles with their dual blood supply from both the inferior and superior epigastric vessels. Multiple layers of muscle and fascia contribute to the overall strength of the abdominal wall. (Netter illustration from www.netterimages.com. ©Elsevier Inc. All rights reserved.)

Diagnosis/patient presentation

Occasionally, patients may present to the plastic surgeon de novo; however, more commonly patients present as referrals from their surgical oncologist or general surgeon. Unfortunately, many cancer patients are never referred to a plastic surgeon to discuss reconstruction options. In one survey, only 24% of general surgeons referred greater than 75% of their patients for reconstruction.[20] In addition, once referred, the best outcomes are ensured by an open dialogue between the oncologic and plastic surgeon with regards to incision planning and skin flap creation. As a result, the overall approach to breast cancer and subsequent reconstruction to ensure excellent results and patient satisfaction should be multidisciplinary. That being said, patients present to the office in various stages of their cancer treatment and one must be aware of the implications, most notably timing of reconstruction with respect to mastectomy and radiation therapy.

Timing: delayed versus immediate reconstruction

Free TRAM reconstruction can be safely performed in either an immediate or delayed fashion with respect to the mastectomy. Immediate reconstruction has several advantages. Most notably, patients benefit from only needing one operation. In addition, most surgeons find that immediate reconstruction is easier to perform and the mastectomy skin flap envelope is more predictable. In conjunction with the oncologic surgeon, skin sparing or nipple sparing mastectomy techniques are options in some patients to minimize the loss of the native envelope. This in turn makes symmetry easier to obtain. Mastectomy planning will be discussed later in this chapter.

Many patients present in a delayed fashion, either because they did not undergo any reconstruction at the time of mastectomy or because they had prosthetic reconstruction which subsequently failed. Generally speaking, delayed reconstruction should not be undertaken sooner than 6 months following mastectomy due to immature scar formation; however, there is no temporal limit. Delayed reconstruction requires re-elevation of the skin flaps which are often times scarred and less compliant. The mastectomy scar should be completely excised and if radiation injury is evident, this should be excised as well. Scarred or radiated skin can result in inadequate ptosis and poor symmetry over time. The contralateral breast is used as a template for defining the limits of dissection.

The pedicled versus free TRAM

The main issues at stake when comparing these two techniques are: the technical aspects of the operation, the long term results, and the donor site morbidity. The pedicled TRAM requires complete dissection of the rectus muscle up to the level of the xiphoid (see Ch. 15). The pedicle and flap are then transposed through a tunnel in the most medial aspect of the inframammary fold. Because the flap and pedicle are turned over, there is the risk of twisting; thus, the insetting of the flap itself can be quite challenging. It is also not unusual to have contour irregularities along the inferomedial mammary fold and symmetry may be more difficult to achieve.[21,22] The free TRAM on the other hand requires the additional expertise of a microanastomosis; however, once the pedicle is created, the insetting of the flap tends to be less problematic.

Aside from the technical aspects of the two operations, one must compare the long term results weighed against the donor site morbidity. Due to the reliance on "choke" vessels for flap survival in the pedicle TRAM, there is a theoretical increased risk of ischemic complications such as partial or total flap loss and fat necrosis. This theory has been put to the test in multiple studies, but results are conflicting. Andrades et al. compared 147 pedicled TRAMs to 154 free TRAMs of various muscle sparing (MS) iterations. MS0 connotes complete transection of the muscle; whereas, MS1 involves transection of most of the muscle, MS2 only the central portion and MS3 (DIEP) none. This showed a significant increase in mild and severe fat necrosis in pedicled TRAMs compared to MS0 free TRAMs. Interestingly, evaluation of MS1 and MS2 flaps suggest that as the degree of muscle sparing increases, so does the rate of fat necrosis. In fact, there does not seem to be a significant difference in flap necrosis between pedicled TRAM and MS2 free TRAM. There was no significant difference in partial or total flap loss.[23] Alderman et al. prospectively followed patients who underwent expander/implant, pedicle

TRAM and free TRAM over a 2-year period. They showed no significant differences in complication rates between pedicled and free TRAM.[24]

Although sacrificing the rectus muscle will not leave a patient completely disabled, patients may notice a considerable difference in flexion strength and abdominal contour when the rectus muscles are sacrificed. Research on abdominal wall strength comparing pedicled to free TRAM has been conflicting. Objective measures of abdominal wall strength after pedicled or free TRAM reconstruction have consistently shown a deficit in strength which may persist long term. Following pedicled TRAM, one study has shown that patients may experience on average up to a 23% deficit in trunk flexion, but this may be as high as 40% in bilateral reconstruction. In unilateral free TRAM, this deficit may be up to 18%.[25] However, multiple studies have tried to evaluate pedicled versus free TRAM head to head and none have been able to show a significant difference in long term abdominal wall function.[26,27] This is likely due to the fact that during a standard free TRAM, the entire width of the lower rectus muscle is sacrificed. Further studies are needed to differentiate long term abdominal wall function comparing MS0, MS1, MS2 and DIEP flaps.

In summary, although there may be subtle differences in outcomes between pedicled and free TRAM, major differences in outcomes have yet to be proven in large prospective studies. Although not proven in a large trial, the literature would suggest that bilateral reconstruction in particular would likely benefit from some form of muscle sparing procedure. Free TRAM has become increasingly popular at academic institutions; however, pedicled TRAM is still a safe and predictable option and in fact may be more preferable at hospitals where microsurgical techniques and rigorous postoperative monitoring may not be available. In the end, surgeon familiarity and experience with either procedure likely is the most important predictor of a good outcome.

Other options available for breast reconstruction include tissue expander/implant, latissimus dorsi, DIEP, SIEA, Ruben's, transverse upper gracilis flap (TUG), and inferior or superior gluteal artery flaps. The gluteal flaps may be harvested as perforator flaps as well (SGAP, IGAP). These flaps are discussed in other chapters in this book; however, knowledge of them is necessary to a complete understanding of surgical options, especially in cases where inadequate abdominal tissue is available for transfer, or previous abdominal operations make a free TRAM flap technically impossible.

Radiation therapy

Radiation therapy is a component of multimodality therapy for many types of cancers. Current guidelines support using radiation therapy for breast cancer in the adjuvant setting following lumpectomy for DCIS, with the possible exception of small tumors with a focus of low grade tumor that has been resected with wide margins. In patients with early stage (T1–2) invasive cancer undergoing breast conservation, radiation therapy decreases the risk of local recurrence in patients who are node negative or positive; therefore, it is offered to patients who are node negative with the exception of those individuals over the age of 70 and are hormone receptor positive. Patients with four or more positive lymph nodes benefit from irradiation to the remaining nodal basin as well.[28] Aside from its use in breast conservation therapy, radiation therapy is also used as adjuvant therapy following mastectomy. In this setting, patients who have close surgical margins, four or more positive lymph nodes or are clinical stage III or IV benefit from radiation therapy.[29] Traditionally, radiation therapy has been used to decrease local recurrence. Although this remains its primary benefit, recent studies have suggested a modest albeit, improved survival benefit with radiation in both breast conservation and mastectomy patients.[30] In addition, studies have suggested that one to three positive lymph nodes may be an indication for radiation therapy in certain patients and as such, radiation is increasingly being utilized. More studies are needed for a consensus on management of these patients.[31] Taken as whole, more and more patients are currently being offered radiation therapy making knowledge of its effects paramount to the reconstructive plastic surgeon.

Unfortunately, radiation therapy is fraught with side-effects not only to native tissue, but also to any form of reconstruction. Short term side effects of radiation therapy include skin excoriation or sloughing, pain and erythema. Long-term, late toxic effects of radiation therapy include lymphedema, radiation pneumonitis, cardiac injury, loss of skin compliancy, brachial plexopathy and places the patient at risk for delayed secondary malignancy.

In the reconstructed breast, radiation may play havoc, especially following tissue expansion/implant reconstruction which is prone to capsular contracture and asymmetry. Aside from poor aesthetic outcomes, contracture can be so severe, patients are at risk for chronic pain and implant extrusion. Autologous reconstruction, although significantly better than prosthetic reconstruction when faced with irradiation, still is at higher risk of complications when compared to non-irradiated patients.[32,33]

Nevertheless, patients will continue to need irradiation and until a less invasive but effective treatment alternative surfaces, the main question will remain: does the timing of radiation therapy in relation to reconstruction matter? The answer to this question deals with two topics. First, and perhaps most importantly, reconstruction should at no point compromise the treatment of the breast cancer, nor sacrifice the efficacy of the radiation therapy itself. Retrospective studies have found acceptable outcomes following immediate reconstruction followed by irradiation; however, no large prospective study has ever attempted to answer this question.[34] Although the local recurrence rate has never been shown to be higher, the ideal radiation field may be compromised following immediate reconstruction.[35] Motwani et al. were able to show that autologous breast reconstruction did compromise radiation delivery in 52% of immediate reconstruction patients, this in comparison to 7% of age matched controls.[36] Although the radiation field design required changes, the clinical significance of this remains unknown.

Second, one must consider the effects that radiation has on complications and long term aesthetics. Most articles suggest that post reconstruction radiation increases the risk of volume loss, fat necrosis, contracture and asymmetry. Taken all together, at this time, most centers prefer to offer patients delayed reconstruction when postoperative radiation is expected; however, this must be balanced with the patient's wishes to avoid a secondary major operation. One must always take the time to understand the patient's perspective – in the setting of the diagnosis of cancer, a mastectomy, chemotherapy and radiation, the prospect of then having to undergo another major operation for reconstruction should not be minimized.

An alternative to immediate reconstruction followed by radiation is the so-called "delayed-immediate" breast reconstruction.[37,38] The postoperative plan for adjuvant therapy is often unknown prior to mastectomy as it is ultimately based upon the tumor characteristics and node status of the final pathology. However, patients who definitely will need post mastectomy radiation therapy are ideal candidates for this option. In this method, patients undergo a mastectomy immediately followed by subpectoral tissue expander placement. The tissue expander is partially inflated in the operating room and further postoperatively in an effort to maintain the volume of the native breast skin envelope. The expander is deflated in order to undergo radiation without a compromised field and subsequently reinflated after radiation in complete. Several weeks after radiation, when the effects of the radiation have matured, the patient returns to the operating room for removal of the tissue expander and definitive reconstruction with autologous tissue. Although this method is increasingly being used at several medical centers, the overall benefits of this option have yet to be fully elucidated.

Patient selection

Risk factors

From the SEER database, the peak incidence of breast cancer in the United States is age 61, with almost 60% of all cases of breast cancer under age 65.[39] The significance of this is that the majority of women tend to be fairly young and without major co-morbidities. As a result, it is exceedingly rare for a woman to be considered too high risk for surgery; rather, understanding the predictors of poor outcomes consequently has more to do with proper patient education for expectations and to modify risk wherever possible.

In a review of 500 free flaps, Selber et al. were able to demonstrate an increased risk of wound infection, mastectomy flap necrosis, abdominal flap necrosis and fat necrosis in smokers. In addition, obese patients are more likely to experience wound related complications including mastectomy flap necrosis. Peripheral vascular disease was identified as a risk factor for wound infection.[40] Greco et al., in a similar review, did not corroborate the smoking data; however, they too found obesity to play a major role in wound related complications.[41] Although not definitively shown in the breast free flap literature, smoking cessation preoperatively has been shown to decrease wound related complications following surgical procedures in general. Although, adequate soft tissue is necessary to be able to use the transverse island of tissue for reconstruction, the obesity end of the spectrum demonstrates that too much of a good thing clearly leads to poor outcomes. Patients undergoing breast reconstruction are usually either confined by the timing of their mastectomy or eager for reconstruction making the prospect of preoperative weight loss to improve outcomes unlikely. Although diabetes mellitus has long been looked at as a harbinger of surgical complications, in free flap reconstruction, it has not been shown to increase risk of poor outcomes. Miller et al., in their review of 893 free flaps, failed to show a significant difference in outcomes when comparing type I, type II and nondiabetic patients.[42] That being said, there is a substantial bit of literature suggesting that tight glucose control in the postoperative period decreases wound related complications.[43] Although it is unclear if this is generalizable to free flap reconstruction, given the body of literature, attention should be paid to this detail in the postoperative period.

Prior abdominal operations have been shown to increase the risk of complications associated with TRAM flap reconstruction.[44] Most importantly, prior transversely oriented incisions might be an indicator that the epigastric vessels have been sacrificed. Techniques for minimizing risk include skewing the abdominal flap away from the previous scar, using hemiflaps, minimizing flap undermining, and supercharging.[45] Similarly, a prior abdominoplasty is generally considered an absolute contraindication to TRAM flap reconstruction because the prior skin flap sacrifices all perforating vessels. Although there are reports of successful TRAM following abdominoplasty, this should not be attempted without considerable expertise and a complete analysis of other options.[46] A thorough knowledge of abdominal wall vascular anatomy, the likely effects of prior standard abdominal incisions as well as the proposed surgery all contribute to an overall successful endeavor.

From a psychosocial perspective, many studies have demonstrated the benefit of breast reconstruction on patients' well being following treatment for breast cancer. An important component of this is proper patient education. Patients should not only be made aware of the inherent risks of the surgery including the possibility of complications, they should be educated as to the limitations of reconstructions as well. For instance, it is helpful to point out asymmetries preoperatively to demonstrate living with variability. One of the goals of breast reconstruction is to recreate a breast mound which looks natural under clothing. Scarring is an unfortunate phenomenon of which patients should have expectations postoperatively. Similarly, patients should be told of the likelihood of significant sensory loss – although some sensation may return most women never achieve a fully sensate mound. Patients who do not appear to understand these concepts preoperatively should be approached with patience as a brief dialogue preoperatively will go a long way toward improved patient satisfaction and the avoidance of perceived poor outcomes.

Procedure selection

Reconstruction of a breast mound using autologous tissue can be performed using multiple techniques, but there is no one perfect flap which can be used in all circumstances. The free TRAM has become a workhorse of autologous breast reconstruction. Ultimately, deciding whether to use a pedicled versus a free TRAM mostly has to do with surgeon training, preference and hospital resources such as an operating microscope and microsurgical instruments; however, there are certain circumstances where the free TRAM should be considered superior. As mentioned before, the free TRAM has a more robust blood supply. Under routine circumstances the clinical significance of this may be difficult to discern. Under additional strain however, this difference may become more apparent. Smoking, as we have discussed, increases the risk of wound related complications and fat necrosis. Smoking likely augments the discrepancy of outcomes between the pedicled and free TRAM. Therefore, smokers (even if they quit) should probably be offered a free rather than pedicled TRAM. Likewise, when a larger volume flap is needed for reconstruction, this pushes the vascular supply of the pedicled TRAM to its limits. As a result, if a larger volume is needed for reconstruction, the free TRAM is likely the better choice. In addition, any previous upper abdominal surgery which may have created a scar in the rectus sheath or destroyed the superior epigastrics should be offered a free TRAM preferentially.

Of course, the free TRAM is not the end all and be all of breast reconstruction. Often times, there is not adequate lower abdominal tissue sufficient for reconstruction in thin women. In these cases, an inferior gluteal flap, TUG flap or prosthetic reconstruction remain better options. The DIEP and SIEA remain excellent options utilizing the same lower abdominal island of tissue – the benefits being less abdominal wall invasion and resultant long term abdominal wall function. The downside of course is the more tenuous blood supply. These techniques and their advantages are discussed more completely in other chapters in this text.

Treatment/surgical technique

The patient should be met in the preoperative holding area for marking in an upright position before the induction of anaesthesia. This will ensure the best attempt at symmetry. If undergoing unilateral delayed reconstruction, the contralateral infra-mammary fold should be used as a guide. Even in immediate reconstruction, often times this landmark is less appreciable on the side of reconstruction following completion of the mastectomy; therefore, this should be marked preoperatively. In bilateral delayed reconstruction, a brassiere may be used as a guide for placement of the inframammary fold. If the patient is undergoing a contralateral mastopexy or reduction, measurements and planning should be performed at this time as well. Next, the transverse flap island is marked. The apices of the flap, whenever possible, should be placed in a concavity to help minimize dog-ears upon closure. The upper border of the flap is typically 1–2 cm above the umbilicus, the lower border close to the pubic hairline; however, this border should go no lower than the point of adequate subcutaneous soft tissue. If a Pfannenstiel incision is present, the inferior margin is typically drawn to excise the scar. Typically, the resultant flap is a standard ellipse; however, in thinner women, this may be modified to a more trapezoidal pattern. The height

of the flap should be estimated to allow for abdominal closure which will not be subject to too much tension. Sometimes it is helpful to assess the degree of abdominal tissue by having the patient flex at the waist preoperatively. In addition, palpation of the native breast preoperatively should be compared to the volume of the planned flap to aid in proper flap design. The overall plan of this flap is broken down into four zones *(Fig. 17.2)*. Zone IV is typically discarded prior to insetting due to lack of reliable perfusion. Lastly, the midline should be marked from sternum to pubis to aid in symmetrical closure.

The patient is placed in a supine position with arms abducted and undergoes general anaesthesia. A Foley should be placed to allow for adequate recording of urinary output intra-and postoperatively. Enough room around the table should be present to allow for two simultaneous teams working on the abdominal and chest components of the procedure. After prepping the patient from neck to pubis and laterally to the table, the patient is draped. The inframammary folds are additionally marked with either sutures or skin clips to ensure this orientation is not washed off during the course of the procedure. Prophylactic antibiotics should

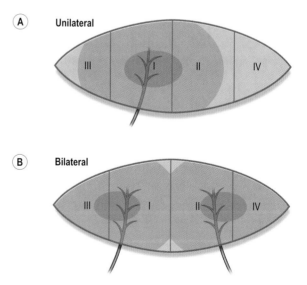

Fig. 17.2 The standard elliptical design of a TRAM flap with Zones I through IV. **(A)** Zone I lies directly over the vascular pedicle and is the most reliable. Zones II and III are generally reliable; however, zone IV should be approached with caution due to its distance from the vascular pedicle. **(B)** In bilateral reconstruction, the majority of each hemiflap is used.

be administered prior to incision. Due to the length of bilateral procedures, an additional dose may be warranted prior to completion of the operation.

Mastectomy planning

Traditionally, the modified radical mastectomy with a large transverse or obliquely oriented elliptical skin incision was always employed for treatment of breast cancer. Over the years, oncologic surgeons have steered away from this invasive option, toward procedures which spare more of the native skin envelope. Skin sparing mastectomy includes a circumareolar incision, a circumareolar incision plus a lateral extension or a small ellipse. In addition, a Wise or vertical reduction pattern mastectomy can be performed which places all scars around and inferior to the nipple areolar complex. This plan is helpful in cases of large ptotic breasts preoperatively where the reconstruction serves as a simultaneous lift or reduction *(Fig. 17.3)*.

The nipple areolar complex has historically always been included in a mastectomy; however, more recently there has been a trend toward more specific therapies depending on tumor characteristics that are designed to be less debilitating. One of these areas of interest has been an emerging utilization of nipple sparing mastectomy. The major benefits of nipple sparing mastectomy include less surgery, obviating the need for nipple areolar reconstruction (NAR). Perhaps more importantly however is a more natural cosmetic appearance as NAR often times cannot satisfactorily mimic proper projection, texture and tone. In addition, there is also the possibility of retention of some sensation which should not be discounted.[47] There are some reports that suggest the loss of the NAC is more detrimental psychologically to a women then loss of the mound itself. It should be noted that as high as 11% of women will experience NAC necrosis following nipple sparing mastectomy.[48] Although the indications for its use are likely to broaden, currently, the use of nipple conservation is limited to prophylactic mastectomy and perhaps well selected pathologic small lesions, remote from the NAC and of favorable histology.[49,50] Large, ptotic breasts should be considered a relative contraindication due to the difficulty of complete mastectomy, reliability of the skin envelope, and NAC viability after dissection.

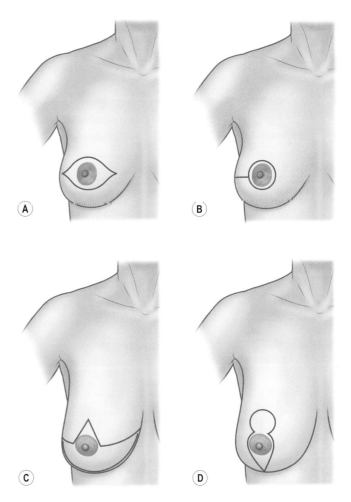

Fig. 17.3 Mastectomy planning. **(A)** A standard mastectomy incision via an ellipse that is oriented either obliquely or transversely. **(B)** A skin sparing mastectomy via periareolar incision which may be supplemented with an extension for better access to the tail and axilla. **(C)** A Wise pattern mastectomy or **(D)** vertical reduction pattern – both are useful for macromastia in which the reconstruction will be smaller than the preoperative state.

Flap dissection

The dissection of the TRAM flap begins with an incision over the upper border of the skin island *(Fig. 17.4)*. In addition, the umbilicus is circumscribed using a 15 blade and the stalk is dissected out with scissors down to the level of the fascia. The flap incision is carried down to the abdominal wall fascia using electrocautery and this is followed by undermining of the upper abdominal skin and subcutaneous tissue up to the level of the costal margins and xiphoid. Every attempt at preserving the perforators in the subcostal regions bilaterally should be made to ensure viability of the remaining skin and subcutaneous tissue for abdominal wound

 Video 1

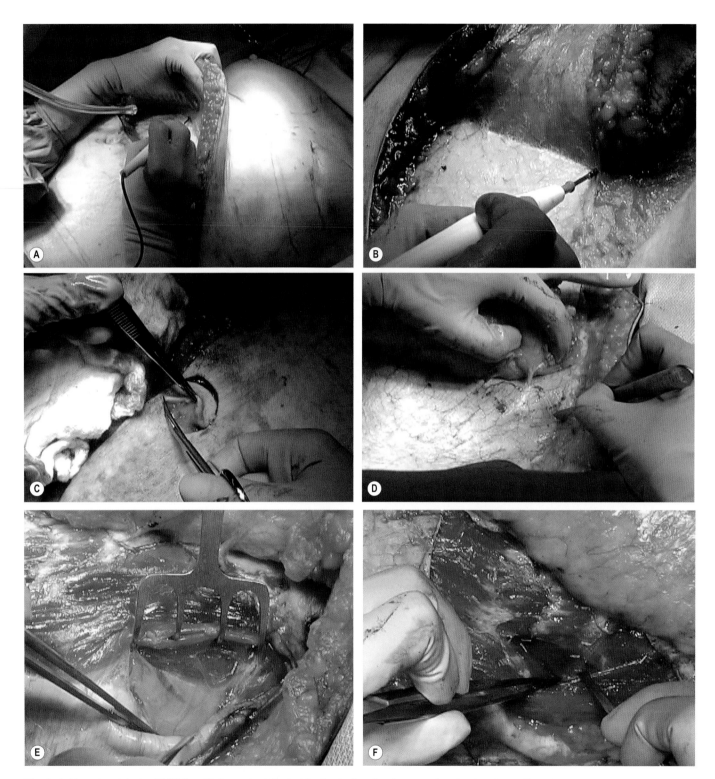

Fig. 17.4 Dissection of the free TRAM flap. **(A)** A superior abdominal flap is raised to allow for eventual tension free closure. The height of the TRAM flap is dependent on the mobility of this flap. **(B)** The lateral flaps of the TRAM are raised to the point of the lateral perforators. **(C)** The umbilicus is preserved. **(D)** An anterior rectus sheath fasciotomy is made above and below the perforators. **(E)** Within the rectus sheath, the muscle is reflected medially to allow for visualization and dissection of the inferior epigastric vessels. **(F)** The perforators are identified and preserved as they traverse the muscle. This allows for preservation of at least the lateral aspect of the rectus muscle for a muscle sparing free TRAM.

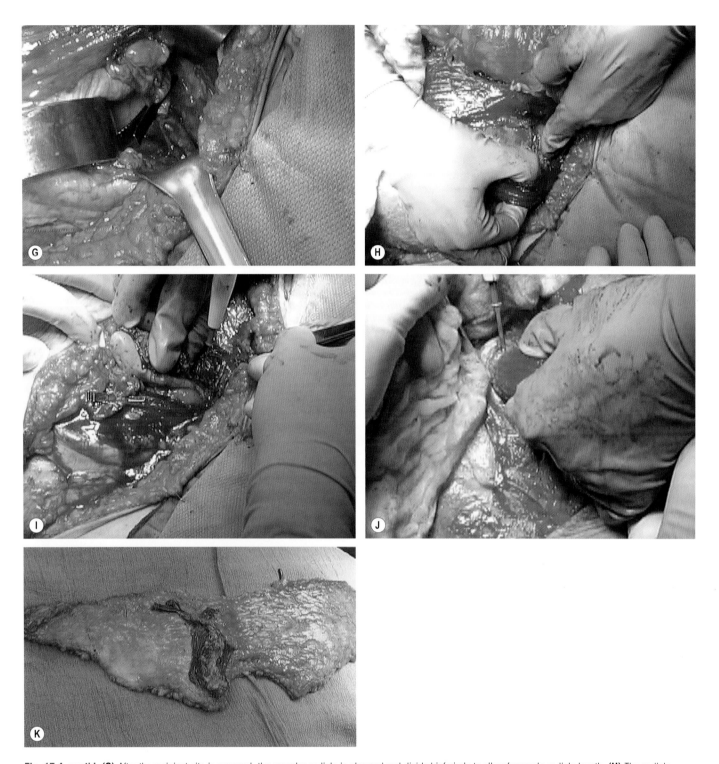

Fig. 17.4, cont'd **(G)** After the recipient site is prepared, the vascular pedicle is clamped and divided inferiorly to allow for ample pedicle length. **(H)** The pedicle is passed through the middle of the rectus muscle in the plane of the perforators. **(I)** The inferior muscle is divided. **(J)** The superior muscle is divided. **(K)** The flap is ready for anastomosis.

closure. This upper skin flap can be draped over the TRAM skin island to ensure an acceptable abdominal closure after complete removal of the flap. Following this, the incision of the lower border of the TRAM flap is performed. The superficial inferior epigastric vessels are encountered bilaterally in the mid-inguinal region and at this point, one should consider the possibility of performing an SIEA (discussed elsewhere). If insufficient for use, they may be ligated and divided, although preserving a large vein for additional or alternate drainage should be considered even if performing a TRAM. The dissection is carried down to the fascia using electrocautery and the lateral apices of the flap may be dissected off of the fascia as well. The dissection is carried from lateral to medial up to the point of the identification of the lateral row of perforators projecting through the rectus fascia into the subcutaneous tissue of the flap. If performing a unilateral reconstruction, the side of the flap opposite the vascular pedicle (zones II and IV) may be completely dissected off the abdominal wall and carried up to the point of the medial row of perforators on the pedicle side (across the midline). If a bilateral flap is being performed, division of the flap in the midline will aid in the medial row dissection on either side. A decision is made at this point to use the medial perforators, lateral perforators, or both. The fascia is incised vertically and circumferentially to incorporate the chosen perforators, thus creating an island of excised fascia as part of the flap. The size of this excised fascia depends on the number of perforators chosen, and may be as little as a linear fasciotomy if a single row, or single perforator is chosen. Next, the surgeon identifies the vascular pedicle posterior to, and at the lateral edge of the rectus muscle. It should be followed as far down to the external iliac vessels as possible, but should not be divided until the recipient site is ready for anastomosis and insetting. After division of the pedicle, the rectus muscle is divided inferiorly to the perforators, allowing for tension free release of the pedicle. Lastly, the superior muscle is divided; however, care must be taken to identify and oversew the superior pedicle to prevent bleeding. The degree of muscle sacrificed is dependent on the anatomic variability of the perforators and can range from no muscle sacrifice (DIEP or MS-III), central excision only (MS-II), medial or lateral excision (MS-I), or to complete transection of the lower rectus (MS-0) *(Fig. 17.5)*.

Recipient vessel

The two most common recipient vessel sites in free tissue reconstruction of the breast are the thoracodorsal vessels and the internal mammary vessels *(Fig. 17.6)*. In immediate breast reconstruction following a modified radical mastectomy, the thoracodorsal vessels are either fully or partially exposed. Only a short amount of surgical time is usually required for full preparation of these vessels in this setting. The thoracodorsal vessels are usually chosen as long as the autologous flap for reconstruction has a sufficiently long donor pedicle. This combination provides enough vessel length to allow for satisfactory medial placement of the reconstructed breast mound. The thoracodorsal artery and vein are dissected free from the takeoff of the scapular circumflex vessels and from the nerve, all other surrounding attachments, and each other for half of their length. A moistened sponge is placed in the depth of the axilla, filling this deep space and providing a horizontal platform for microsurgery. The free flap is not inset at this point but rather is temporarily secured so as to allow unencumbered positioning and viewing of both recipient and donor vessels during the anastomoses. The surgeon then performs end-to-end anastomoses either using interrupted 8-0 or 9-0 nylon sutures for both the artery and vein or using sutures for the artery and a coupler for the vein.

In the setting of delayed breast reconstruction, some surgeons choose the thoracodorsal recipient vessels because of their familiarity with flap insetting in immediate reconstruction and because of the proven efficacy of these vessels in delayed reconstruction.[51] After the mastectomy defect is recreated, the lateral chest wall skin is elevated until the anterior border of the latissimus muscle is identified. The border of this muscle is followed superiorly to just below its tendinous junction at the level of the axillary vein. Once the vein is identified, the soft tissue from the border of the latissimus toward the chest wall is dissected, within which should be the thoracodorsal artery and vein.

For many surgeons, the internal mammary vessels are the recipient vessels of choice in delayed free-flap breast reconstruction.[52,53] Choosing this recipient site has the advantage of avoiding surgery in the axilla previously subjected to an operation. Some surgeons use this recipient site primarily in immediate reconstruction

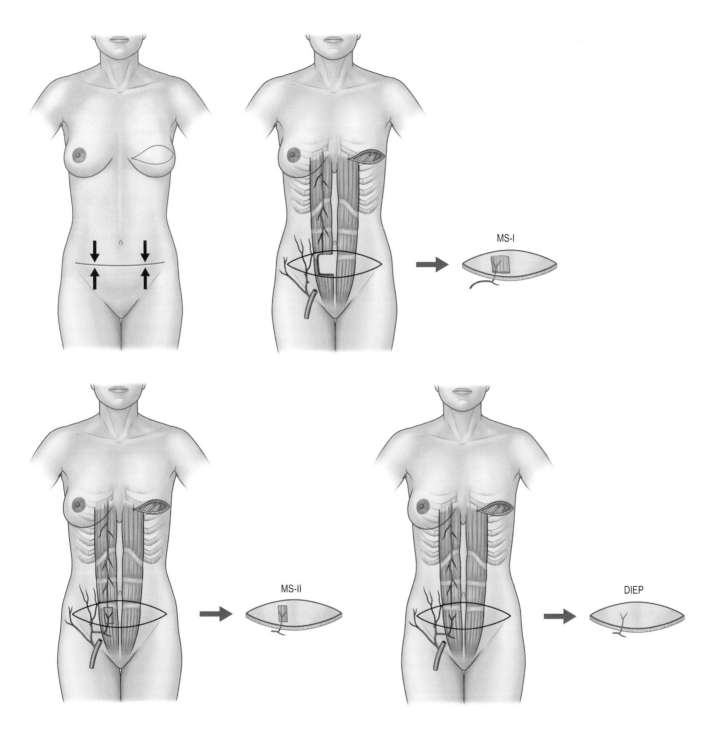

Fig. 17.5 The variations of a free TRAM. **(A)** The MS-0 flap in which the rectus muscle is completely transected. **(B)** The MS-I spares the lateral band preferably (as opposed to the medial band) of muscle with the goal of preserving the innervation of the muscle. **(C)** In an MS-II flap, only a small central portion of the rectus muscle around the perforators is transected. **(D)** The MS-III, otherwise known as a DIEP preserves the entire rectus muscle.

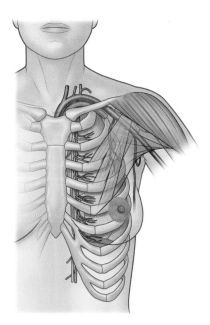

Fig. 17.6 The vascular anatomy of the chest wall. The two most common sites for recipient vessel harvest and subsequent vascular anastomoses are the internal mammary vessels and the thoracodorsal vessels.

as well because it allows a more medial positioning of the flap for improved symmetry and aesthetics. The internal mammary vessels have also been used preferentially when mastectomy combined with sentinel node biopsy is performed. There is limited axillary dissection with sentinel node biopsy, such that considerable further dissection is required for use of the thoracodorsal vessels. Although the results of a frozen-section biopsy of the sentinel node may be negative for malignancy, the final pathology result is occasionally positive, and secondary axillary dissection may be required. If the free flap is anastomosed to the thoracodorsal system, early secondary axillary node dissection can be challenging and runs the risk of pedicle damage. In addition, the internal mammary vessel site is usually selected in both immediate and delayed reconstruction when the flap chosen for breast reconstruction has a limited pedicle length, thus allowing medial placement of this tissue.[54,55]

The internal mammary vessels are first approached by separating the fibers of the pectoralis muscle overlying the third costal cartilage *(Fig. 17.7)*. Self-retaining retractors are placed perpendicularly, exposing the cartilage and intercostal musculature. The perichondrium is incised along the midanterior surface from the junction of the sternum to 1–2 cm medial to the costochondral junction. The perichondrium is separated off of the cartilage, first on the anterior surface and then extending to its posterior surface. Complete separation of the posterior perichondrium can be difficult and is unnecessary. Once the perichondrium is partially separated on the upper and lower edges of the costal cartilage, a rongeur is used to remove the cartilage. As this is being done, the cartilage usually separates from its attachments to the deep perichondrium, without perforation into the hemithorax. The deep perichondrium is then incised lateral to the internal mammary vessels and reflected lateral to medial. Care must be taken to avoid transection of the small intercostal vessel branches coming off of the internal mammary system. Once the vessels are identified and separated from the internal mammary lymphatics, the length of dissection is extended by dividing the intercostal musculature from the top of the fourth rib to the bottom of the second rib; this is done by staying lateral to the internal mammary vessels. As compared with most other recipient vessels throughout the body, the internal mammary artery is more susceptible to injury and thrombosis during its dissection. Minimal use of vascular forceps is recommended. The internal mammary vein tends to be larger on the right side than on the left side. Previous ways for approaching this site used the fifth costal cartilage; however, the size of the internal mammary vein was not routinely reliable for free tissue transfer at this location. Although the third cartilage is currently recommended, the second cartilage can be similarly removed for access to a recipient vein of greater diameter. Once fully dissected, the internal mammary artery and vein are divided at the level of the fourth rib and supported on their deep surfaces by a neurosurgical sponge. The free flap is temporarily positioned to allow easy performance of the anastomoses. Sutures of 9-0 nylon may be used for both anastomoses; however, the internal mammary artery is at times quite large, requiring 8-0 nylon. The vein is usually amenable to use of the coupler device.

Other potential recipient vessels include the scapular circumflex vessels, the thoracoacromial vessels, and the axillary artery and vein. These are rarely used as the planned primary recipient vessel site; rather, they are used when problems have occurred during surgery at one of the two routine recipient vessel sites. The scapular circumflex vessels are identified where they join the

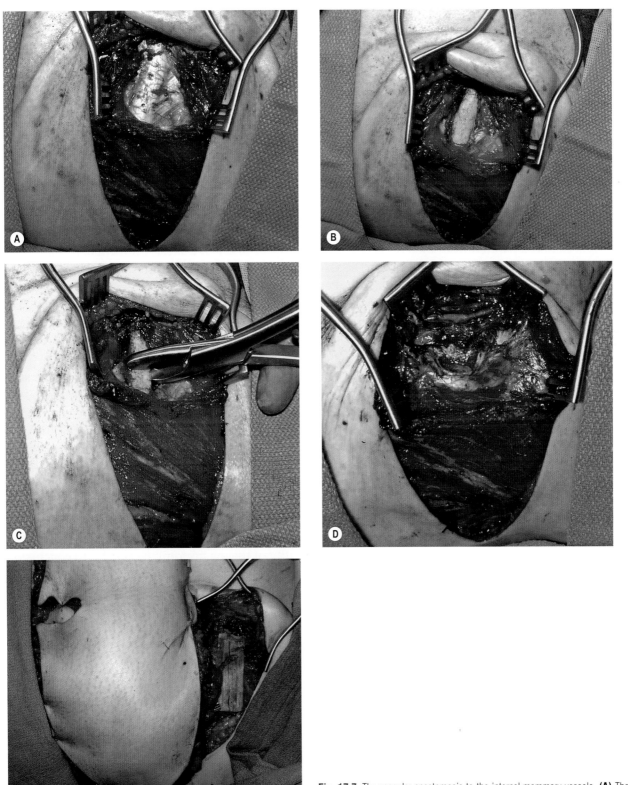

Fig. 17.7 The vascular anastomosis to the internal mammary vessels. **(A)** The third rib is cleaned off, followed by **(B)** incision of the anterior perichondrium. **(C)** The costochondral junction is removed with a rongeur. **(D)** Further dissection allows for exposure of the internal mammary vessels. **(E)** The anastomoses are performed.

thoracodorsal vessels to become the subscapular system. These are not usually injured during a previous axillary dissection, are of equal size to the thoracodorsal or internal mammary vessels and as a result should be considered the 3rd line recipient vessel site. In addition, the scapular circumflex vessels can be dissected from their origin to where they exit superficially onto the back, through the triangular space. When rotated down, they fall nicely into the axilla for anastomosis.

The thoracoacromial vessels are a primary blood supply to the pectoralis major and can be identified by Doppler in the midclavicular region, just inferior to the bone. The muscle fibers can be separated on top of the vessels. The vessels can be separated from their attachments to the pectoralis major and rotated superficially, providing for end-to-end anastomoses. The axillary vessels can be exposed with additional retraction. Care must be taken so as not to place undue traction on the brachial plexus, particularly when dissecting and preparing the axillary artery. Any free flap to the axillary vessels is performed end to side, usually with 9-0 nylon for the vein and 8-0 nylon for the artery. In addition, the external jugular vein and the cephalic vein can be transposed to the chest site to provide venous outflow for a free flap.[56,57] This usually is done when the typical recipient veins are inadequate, or for early postoperative correction of venous thrombosis.

Flap insetting

A decision as to whether to use an ipsilateral or contralateral free flap has usually been made preoperatively, based on the shape of the contralateral breast, the timing of reconstruction and the planned recipient vessels (*Fig. 17.8*). In general, when the thoracodorsals are used, a narrow ptotic breast is reconstructed with an ipsilateral flap which has been rotated 90° with the umbilicus positioned in an inferomedial orientation. As a result, the height of the TRAM flap design thus corresponds to the width of the base of the breast mound. To increase projection, the base may be folded over upon itself. A less ptotic, but wide breast is reconstructed with a contralateral free flap with the flap rotated approximately 140° such that the lateral aspect of the initial flap design becomes the tail of the neo-breast mound. This may be rotated up to 180° for increased width. If the internal mammary vessels are used, the concept is the same

except that the exact opposite is performed – a contralateral flap is used for a narrow, pendulous breast whereas an ipsilateral flap is used to construct a wider breast mound.

Once the anastomosis is complete and orientation established, the buried portions of the flap are de-epithelialized (*Fig. 17.9*). The goal is to remove the epidermis and a portion of the dermis; however, care should be exercised not to injury the subdermal vascular plexus which likely helps with more uniform perfusion of the edges of the flap. Various methods can be employed for deepithelialization including the use of a 10 blade, electrocautery, specifically designed curved blades, Ultrapulse CO_2 laser (Lumenis, Santa Clara, CA) and Versajet device (Smith and Nephew Inc., St Petersburg, FL). Regardless of the device, it is important to plan which portions of the flap are de-epithelialized. One must always be cognizant of the amount of TRAM skin needed to ensure proper closure of the recipient skin defect created by the mastectomy. In most cases of skin sparing mastectomy, the only exposed TRAM skin upon completion of insetting is the new site of the NAC. In delayed reconstruction, often times, there is a need to resect additional native skin during chest wall flap elevation. In addition, the skin may be inadequate for use as an envelope due to prior radiation therapy; thus, this defect must be replaced by the skin of the TRAM. Regardless, the flap is subsequently secured in place in multiple layers and the skin closed with running 4-0 absorbable monofilament. If there is a question about the viability of the mastectomy flaps prior to conclusion of the case, the TRAM may be "banked" under the mastectomy flaps without deepithelialization. The patient returns to the operating room 72 h later, after the skin flaps have fully demarcated, at which time the TRAM flap can be formally inset.[58]

Abdominal closure

After the TRAM flap is harvested, a fascial defect remains in the lower abdominal wall. Depending on the amount of fascia sacrificed, various techniques may be employed for closure. For instance, a MS-3 or MS-2 flap typically has a very small resultant fascial defect which may be closed primarily without tension. An MS-1 or MS-0 defect on the other hand, may preclude apposition of the free fascial edges. In this case, mesh in routinely

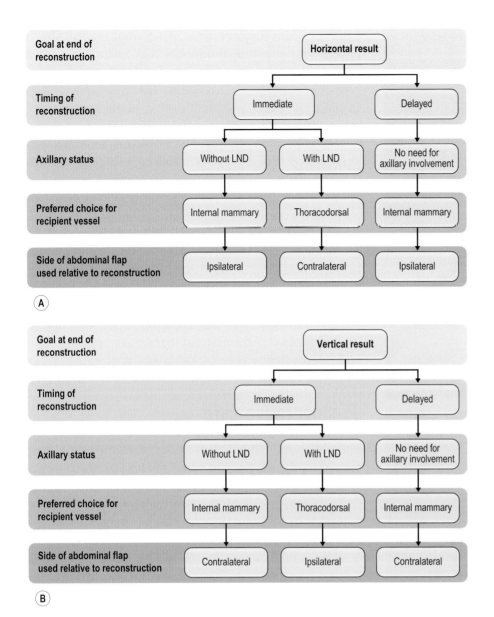

Fig. 17.8 Whether unilateral or bilateral, the standard approach to insetting is shown in this algorithm and takes in to consideration the overall goal, the timing of reconstruction, the axillary node status, choice of recipient vessels, and the laterality of the flap. The goal of a wider, more horizontal breast mound is shown in **(A)**; whereas, **(B)** depicts a more vertical, pendulous breast.

employed. Polypropylene mesh remains the most common subtype employed for fascial closure in a clean wound. It is permanent with incredible tensile strength. Unfortunately, the same qualities that give it durability also make it stiff and unnatural. Acellular dermal matrix (human, porcine or bovine), is one of many "biosynthetic" meshes which proponents argue are less prone to infection and result in a more natural contour. Alloderm (Lifecell Corporation, Branchburg, NJ) has been used successfully in free TRAM reconstruction;[59]

however, the long term results of abdominal wall integrity following biosynthetic mesh implantation remain to be seen. To date, there have been no prospective studies comparing results of abdominal wall closure techniques to guide an evidence based closure algorithm. Generally, small defects can be closed primarily with Prolene, whereas gaps are usually spanned with inlay mesh *(Fig. 17.10)*.

In unilateral reconstruction, after closure of the fascia, the abdominal wall and midline may no longer be

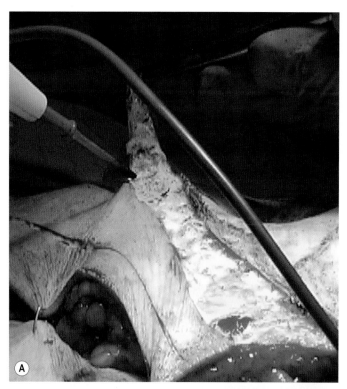

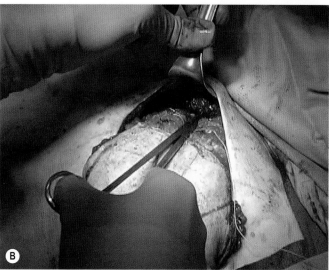

Fig. 17.9 Insetting of the flap. **(A)** The flap is de-epithelialized in all areas, except for the area where donor skin is needed to replace the mastectomy defect. **(B)** The flap is inset in multiple layers.

symmetrical. As a result, some surgeons recommend plication of the fascia on the contralateral side. Care must be taken however to not add to the tension of the fascial repair.

Prior to complete closure, the abdominal wound is temporarily closed and the patient raised to a near sitting position. This will allow for proper selection of

a site to resite the umbilicus. After marking the site, a hole in the superior abdominal flap is created, and a core of subcutaneous tissue is removed to allow for reimplantation of the umbilicus. The umbilicus is fixed in place by interrupted half-buried mattress monofilament sutures.

The abdominal donor site is closed in a manner similar to that of an aesthetic abdominoplasty. Scarpa's layer and the deep dermis are closed with interrupted absorbable polyglactin suture with the skin closed with a running 4-0 subcuticular closure. Alternatively, a Quill suture (Angiotech, Vancouver, BC) may be employed for faster closure. Multiple closed suction drains should be left in place and brought out inferiorly prior to closure to prevent seroma formation. Following complete closure, the wounds are dressed with sterile dressings; however, a window should be left over the free flap to be able to observe the skin color, measure capillary refill and intermittently check a Doppler signal.

Postoperative care

The patient is extubated, transferred to the PACU and subsequently admitted to either the ICU or a step-down type unit that has the capability for frequent nursing flap checks and Doppler evaluations. Our practice pattern is to continue Doppler checks every hour for the first 48 h, then every 4 h until discharge which typically is POD 3 or 4. Pain control is best managed with a patient controlled analgesic pump for the first 48 h at which point patients can usually be transferred over to an oral regimen. The patient remains NPO until the morning of POD 1 at which point they start clear liquids. A regular diet is instituted on POD 2 assuming they are not having any difficulties with clears. As for activity, patients are encouraged to get out of bed to a chair on POD 1 and to fully ambulate on POD 2 at which point the Foley catheter is removed. Sequential compression devices are placed preoperatively and are continued postoperatively while in bed until discharge.

Anticoagulation remains a controversial subject following free flap breast reconstruction. At our institution, all surgeons utilize subcutaneous heparin immediately after surgery both for DVT prophylaxis and to maintain a mildly hypocoagulable state following microanastomosis. The use of aspirin varies, with the goal of

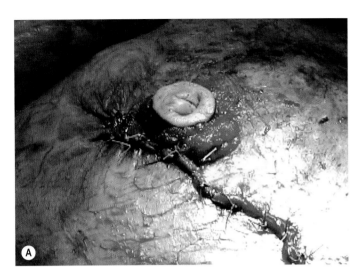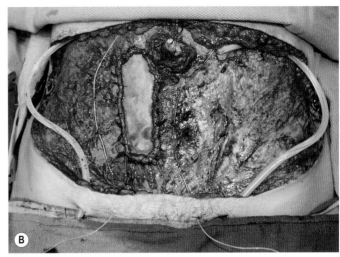

Fig. 17.10 Abdominal wall closure. **(A)** Standard primary closure without mesh. **(B)** In this case, the abdominal wall fascial defect was insufficient to allow primary closure. Polypropylene mesh was used to span the gap and provide added strength. On-Q infusion catheters (I-Flow Corporation, Lake Forest, CA) are placed for pain control and JP drains are left for drainage. The umbilical stalk is reset in an appropriate position as the superior flap is draped over the donor site.

decreasing the thrombosis rate without adding additional risk of hematoma postoperatively. The significance of aspirin's effect on either outcome remains unclear.

The use of prophylactic antibiotics for the prevention of surgical site infection (SSI) is another area of controversy, especially as governing oversight and public scrutiny have targeted SSIs as an area in need of improved outcomes. In breast surgery alone, several studies including two randomized controlled trials have failed to demonstrate a significant effect of preoperative antibiotics on the prevention of SSIs.[60–62] In addition, no difference in SSI rate have been shown between those patients receiving preoperative prophylactic antibiotics and postoperative prophylactic antibiotics in cases with drains.[63] In opposition, two separate meta-analyses and a large randomized control trial concluded that prophylactic antibiotics in breast cancer surgery did lead to a significant decrease in the rate of SSIs following an operation for cancer.[64–66] Breast reconstruction was not included in this analysis. Reconstruction has been identified as an independent risk factor for SSIs and as a result is considered higher risk and in this subgroup, preoperative antibiotics have been shown to significantly decrease the rate of SSI.[67,68] We recommend at the very least, preoperative dosing of Cefazolin within 30 min of incision, with redosing as needed intraoperatively in prolonged reconstruction. The data on postoperative prophylaxis while drains are

in remains limited and at this time should be at the discretion of the operating surgeon.

The patient is discharged home usually with a visiting nurse to help with drain management. The drains are removed in the office over the next several weeks, usually when the output of each is less than 30 cc/day. Over the next several weeks, the patient is instructed to slowly increase activity, but generally should avoid lifting for 6 weeks postoperatively.

Patients should be instructed to follow-up regularly with their medical and surgical oncologists. In unilateral reconstruction, patients will need to continue routine mammography of the contralateral breast as well as continue bilateral self examination. Unfortunately, both systemic metastatic disease and local recurrence do occur following mastectomy and reconstruction. Patients should be instructed to continue self examination of the reconstructed breast. Although fat necrosis can be mistaken for a neoplastic lesion, biopsy should be considered if a new mass is present. Mammography of the reconstructed mound has been shown to be less sensitive for picking up malignant lesions when compared to the native breast;[69] however, cases have been reported where calcifications have been identified which are not otherwise palpable on examination.[70,71] Currently, routine mammography of the reconstructed breast mound is not considered standard of care.

Complications

As with all surgery, the topic of autologous breast reconstruction would not be complete without a discussion of the potential complications. Wound infection occurs 3.5–9.5% of the time but is usually limited to simple cellulitis easily treated with antibiotics. Aside from infection, a broad category of noninfectious wound complications may arise including seroma, delayed wound healing, hematoma, autologous flap necrosis, mastectomy skin flap necrosis and fat necrosis. As a whole, the noninfectious wound complications may be as high as 28–43%; however, the vast majority of time, these heal without intervention or long-term sequelae.[44,72] Fat necrosis rates are highly variable between published reports as some have reported as little as 3.3%, where others have reported rates as high as 22.4%.[40,72–74] Total flap loss is thankfully rare, occurring 0.2–4.7% of the time.[40,41,72]

Due to the microvascular anastomosis and operative manipulation, the artery and vein are both subject to thrombosis *(Fig. 17.11)*. In a review of the last 700 free TRAM flaps performed at our institution, 2.7% experienced an intraoperative arterial thrombosis; 0.3% an intraoperative venous thrombosis; 0.9% a postoperative arterial thrombosis and 0.9% a postoperative venous thrombosis. Of the intraoperative thromboses, none resulted in eventual flap loss. Of the delayed arterial thromboses, 66.7% of the flaps were salvaged by returning to the operating room; whereas, only 50% of the delayed venous thromboses were salvaged. Clearly, delayed thromboses confer a more clinically detrimental outcome. In addition, unrecognized or delayed recognition of a thrombosis likely contributes to flap loss; therefore, close observation of these flaps is paramount in the immediate postoperative period. Venous congestion postoperatively can be treated with leach therapy; however, sudden changes in flap character or Doppler signal warrant exploration. Once in the operating room, the flap is explored through the same incision and the pedicle should be fully re-explored and managed according with standard microvascular techniques for reestablishing flow. The pedicle usually requires a completely new anastomosis.

The fascia, by the nature of its violation, is at risk for the development of either a hernia or a bulge. Hernias may require reoperation for repair. In addition, following manipulation of the abdominal wall, many patients may experience a permanent decrease in abdominal wall strength. A hot topic in autologous reconstruction remains the relative risks and benefits of free TRAM and muscle sparing free TRAM in comparison to more technically challenging muscle preserving procedures such as the SIEA or DIEP flaps. The proponents of the DIEP/SIEA group believe that sparing the rectus muscle leads to less donor site morbidity such as weakness or hernia formation with little downside.[75,76] The competing argument is that the blood supply to a perforator flap or SIEA may be less robust leading to increased flap complications. In addition, it remains unclear as to the significance of the donor site morbidity on patient functionality and satisfaction.[77,78] Although debate will likely continue, our interpretation of the existing data is that sparing muscle and fascia will lead to decreased abdominal wall morbidity over time; however, this must be weighed against a higher flap complication rate in procedures such as the DIEP and SIEA.

Aesthetic complications should be discussed with the patient preoperatively. These include breast mound asymmetry, contour irregularities, contracture and volume loss related to radiation or fat necrosis, poor wound healing and scaring. With proper planning, these setbacks can be ameliorated with revision surgery, reduction, implant augmentation and newer techniques such as fat grafting for contour irregularities. Proper counseling of patients preoperatively once again is imperative, as accurate expectations will most often yield the greatest patient satisfaction.

Revision

Following recreation of the breast mound with a TRAM, many women opt to recreate the nipple areolar complex (NAC) as a final step in restoring body image. The history of NAC reconstruction follows a similar timeline as autologous reconstruction, having been around for years and having undergone many permutations. Techniques employed in the past have included grafting from skin, buccal mucosa, labia minora or majora, thigh, buttocks, groin, upper eyelids or earlobes. Although the

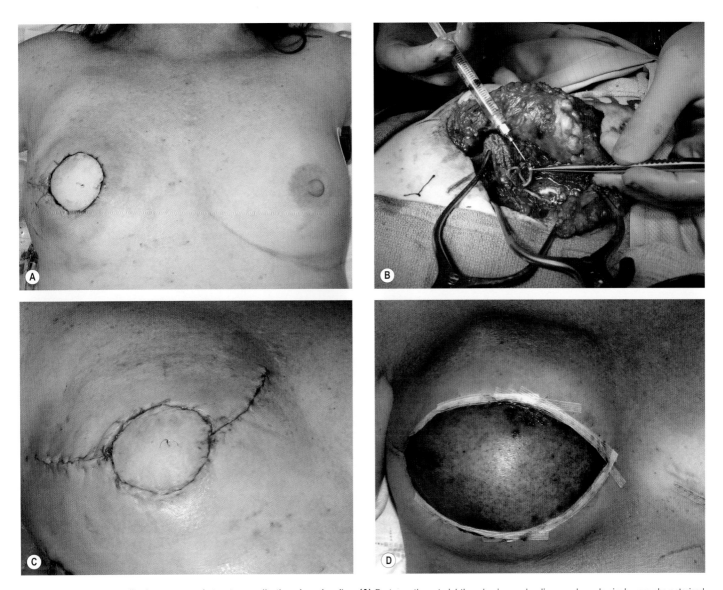

Fig. 17.11 Vascular complications are an unfortunate complication of any free flap. **(A)** Postoperative arterial thrombosis may be diagnosed on physical exam characterized by a pale flap with poor capillary refill, but use of a Doppler adds sensitivity. **(B)** Upon return to the operating room, the arterial anastomosis was taken down, the pedicle flushed with heparin and redone. **(C)** This flap was salvaged with good long-term results. **(D)** Venous thrombosis is often more dramatic, with significant engorgement and a blue hue – this flap was ultimately lost.

technique varies, the principles remain the same: to provide color, texture, size and projection which are all in line with the patients aesthetic wishes. The most common method used today consists of local skin flap rearrangement to create texture and projection followed by tattooing for color. NAC reconstruction in most cases is performed more than 3–4 months following mound reconstruction. This allows for complete healing of the flap and ensures stable mound symmetry which is a key

prerequisite prior to recreating a NAC. Immediate NAC recreation at the time of flap has been reported but by far is less common.[79]

Little literature exists on the frequency of revisional surgery following TRAM flap reconstruction. Aside from NAR, contour abnormalities, volume discrepancies, aesthetically displeasing scars and fat necrosis all contribute to the need for revisional surgery. We reviewed our most recent 100 unilateral free TRAM

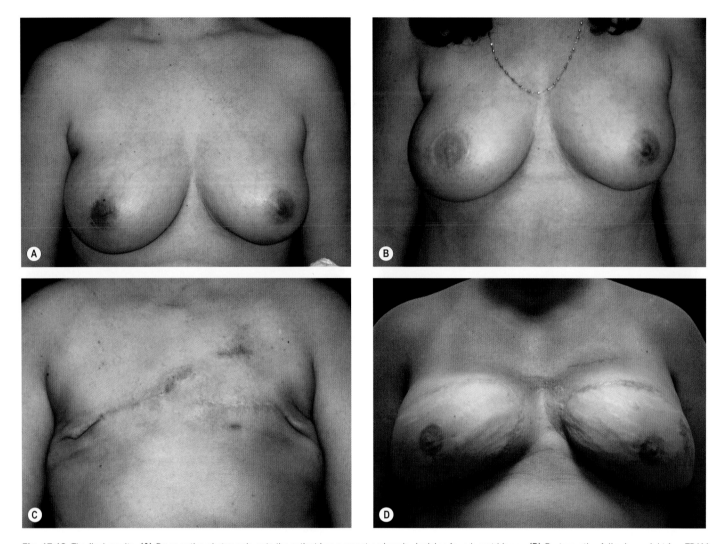

Fig. 17.12 The final results. **(A)** Preoperative photograph, note the patient has a recent periareolar incision for a breast biopsy. **(B)** Postoperative following a right free TRAM flap and subsequent NAR reconstruction with tattooing for color. **(C)** Preoperative photograph of a patient with previous bilateral mastectomies. **(D)** Postoperative following a bilateral muscle sparing free TRAM with subsequent NAR and reconstruction with tattooing for color. Note there is a significantly higher utilization of the skin from the flap for creation of an envelope.

reconstructions at our institution for this chapter. Overall, we found (excluding NAR) a nearly 50% revision rate overall, of which 15% went on to a repeat revision. Reasons for asymmetry included contour deformity in 45.2% and volume loss in 12.6%. Overall, 7.7% underwent implant augmentation; 18.3% local tissue rearrangement; 24.3% liposuction, but none required a second flap. To aid in creating symmetry, 21.2% of these patients underwent an operation on the contralateral healthy breast as well. The overriding theme of this data is that surgeons and patients alike should be prepared for the further, albeit usually minor, procedures in the future to eventually achieve a satisfactory result *(Fig. 17.12)*.

Conclusion

Autologous breast reconstruction using the free TRAM allows the creation of a generally soft, pliable, and ptotic breast mound with unmatched ability to mimic an intact native breast. Autologous reconstruction can be achieved in most patients despite advanced age or significant medical comorbidities. Flap selection and other issues related to the technical considerations of TRAM flap reconstruction should be based on the patient's needs and the surgeon's experience. With this in mind, autologous reconstruction can be successfully achieved in a broad spectrum of patients, with high patient satisfaction and a low incidence of complications.

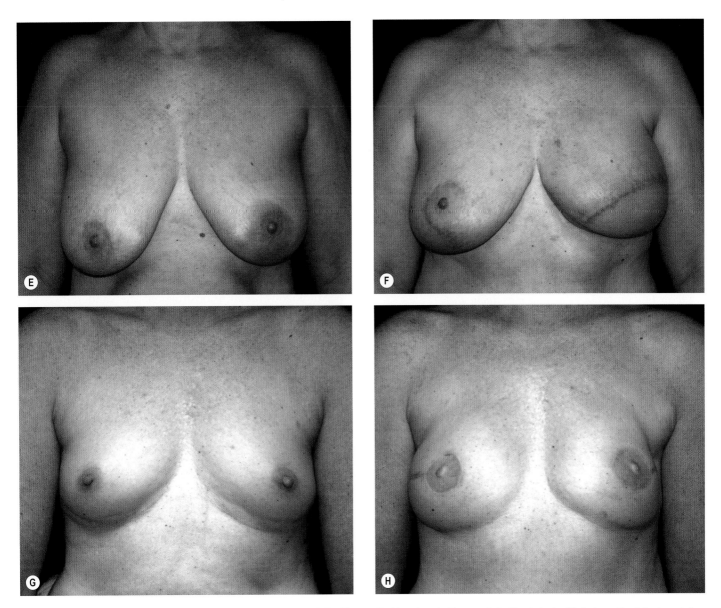

Fig. 17.12, cont'd **(E)** Preoperative photograph in a patient with a recent left axillary sentinel lymph node biopsy and significant ptosis. **(F)** Postoperative following a left free TRAM via a Wise pattern with concomitant balancing right mastopexy. She has yet to undergo NAR. **(G)** Preoperative photograph of a patient with bilateral malignancies. **(H)** Postoperative following bilateral skin sparing mastectomy with free TRAM reconstruction, NAR and tattooing.

Access the complete reference list online at **http://www.expertconsult.com**

15. Alderman AK, Kuhn LE, Lowery JC, et al. Does patient satisfaction with breast reconstruction change over time? Two-year results of the Michigan Breast Reconstruction Outcomes Study. *J Am Coll Surg.* 2007;204(1):7–12.

The Michigan Breast Reconstruction Outcomes Study was a well designed prospective analysis of patients undergoing breast reconstruction. This project resulted in several papers which contributed a plethora of prospective data comparing tissue expander, pedicled TRAM and free TRAM reconstruction. In this article, long-term patient satisfaction data is presented. Overall, patients undergoing free or pedicle TRAM have higher satisfaction rates than tissue expander/ implant reconstruction at 1 year as measured by survey quantifying overall satisfaction and aesthetic satisfaction. At 2 years, although the difference in overall satisfaction between treatment groups diminished, women who underwent autologous reconstruction had higher aesthetic satisfaction when compared with tissue expander/

implant reconstruction. This entire series of papers is worth reading for anyone interested in breast reconstruction.

21. Grotting JC, Urist MM, Maddox WA, et al. Conventional TRAM flap versus free microsurgical TRAM flap for immediate breast reconstruction. *Plast Reconstr Surg.* 1989;83(5):828–844.

22. Edsander-Nord A, Brandberg Y, Wickman M. Quality of life, patients' satisfaction, and aesthetic outcome after pedicled or free TRAM flap breast surgery. *Plast Reconstr Surg.* 2001;107(5):1142–1155.

23. Andrades P, Fix RJ, Danilla S, et al. Ischemic complications in pedicle, free, and muscle sparing transverse rectus abdominis myocutaneous flaps for breast reconstruction. *Ann Plast Surg.* 2008;60(5): 562–567.

   This was a retrospective review at one institution comparing ischemic complications between pedicled TRAM and MS-0 through MS-3 free TRAM reconstructions. Their data follows theoretical predictions based upon anatomy: there is a higher rate of fat necrosis in pedicled TRAMs when compared with free TRAM. There is a trend toward higher complication rates as the degree of muscle preservation increases. The bulge and hernia rates were however, no different between groups. Although limited by a retrospective design, this is one of many articles which give credence to improved outcomes with free versus pedicled TRAM.

27. Edsander-Nord A, Jurell G, Wickman M. Donor-site morbidity after pedicled or free TRAM flap surgery: a prospective and objective study. *Plast Reconstr Surg.* 1998;102(5):1508–1516.

37. Kronowitz SJ, Robb GL. Radiation therapy and breast reconstruction: a critical review of the literature. *Plast Reconstr Surg.* 2009;124(2):395–408.

   Radiation therapy can have dramatic effects on both the surgical field and overall outcomes in breast reconstruction. In particular, post reconstruction radiation therapy has been shown to lead to aesthetic and wound related complications. This excellent review article summarizes the current indications for radiation therapy and the existing literature on its effects on reconstruction. Although no cancer outcomes are presented showing a clinical impact, this article summarizes existing literature showing that reconstruction can compromise radiation delivery. In addition, the article discusses the "delayed-immediate" reconstructive algorithm.

40. Selber JC, Kurichi JE, Vega SJ, et al. Risk factors and complications in free TRAM flap breast reconstruction. *Ann Plast Surg.* 2006;56(5):492–497.

   In this retrospective review of 500 Free TRAM flap reconstructions performed by a single surgeon, the authors summarized the most common complications of TRAM reconstruction and work backward to find risk factors for poor outcomes. Overall, smoking was the most influential factor, leading to increased rates of wound infection, skin flap necrosis and fat necrosis. Obesity was an independent risk factor for mastectomy flap necrosis. Although limited by a retrospective design, this article offers nice data to help predict poor outcomes.

41. Greco III JA, Castaldo ET, Nanney LB, et al. Autologous breast reconstruction: The Vanderbilt Experience (1998 to 2005) of independent predictors of displeasing outcomes. *J Am Coll Surg.* 2008;207(1):49–56.

44. Mehrara BJ, Santoro TD, Arcilla E, et al. Complications after microvascular breast reconstruction: experience with 1195 flaps. *Plast Reconstr Surg.* 2006;118(5):1100–1111.

76. Wu LC, Bajaj A, Chang DW, et al. Comparison of donor-site morbidity of SIEA, DIEP, and muscle-sparing TRAM flaps for breast reconstruction. *Plast Reconstr Surg.* 2008;122(3):702–709.

   In this study, the authors combined a patient survey with a retrospective review to assess overall outcomes with donor-site morbidity following SIEA, DIEP and free TRAM flap reconstruction. This article suggests decreased abdominal wall morbidity of the SIEA flap in comparison to the free TRAM. Although more studies are needed, this article highlights one of the limitations of the free TRAM compared with more contemporary options – the donor site. Although sparing muscle likely limits the effect, by sacrificing muscle fibers of the rectus, patients are likely to experience some degree in overall decline of abdominal wall function which may never return to baseline.

18

The deep inferior epigastric artery perforator (DIEAP) flap

Philip N. Blondeel, Colin M. Morrison, and Robert J. Allen

SYNOPSIS

- The deep inferior epigastric artery perforator (DIEAP) flap provides a large volume of soft, malleable tissue that resembles the natural consistency of the breast.
- DIEAP flap dissection is comparable to conventional myocutaneous free flap surgery, once the initial learning curve is overcome.
- The main advantage of the DIEAP flap is the preservation of full rectus abdominis muscle function translating into less donor site morbidity
- In experienced hands, the DIEAP flap loss rate is less than 1%.
- The DIEAP flap is the perforator flap of choice for autologous breast reconstruction.

 Access the Historical Perspective section online at
http://www.expertconsult.com

Introduction

Perforator flaps have become increasingly popular over recent years. For this reason, they are positioned near the top of the reconstructive ladder and are considered a step advancement of musculocutaneous and fasciocutaneous flaps. Passive muscle and fascial carriers are no longer required to ensure flap vascularity and by virtue of their composition, perforator flaps permit excellent "like for like" tissue replacement with minimal aesthetic or functional donor morbidity. Perforator flaps

are usually thin, pliable, easily moldable flaps that are well suited to resurfacing work. They are also ideal for reconstructing pliable organs such as the tongue or for molding to complex contours as in head and neck surgery. Perforator flaps with large quantities of subcutaneous fat have proved ideal for reconstructing the breast.

A perforator flap is defined as a flap of skin and subcutaneous tissue, which is supplied by an isolated perforator vessel. Perforators pass from their source vessel to the skin surface either through or between the deep tissues (mostly muscle). Any vessel that traverses through muscle before perforating the outer layer of the deep fascia to supply the overlying skin is termed a myocutaneous perforator. A vessel that traverses through septum, i.e., between the muscle bellies, is designated a septocutaneous perforator.

Evolution of perforator flaps has been intimately related to growing knowledge of the blood supply to the skin and the history of musculocutaneous and fasciocutaneous flap development.

The deep inferior epigastric artery perforator (DIEAP) flap arose as a refinement of the conventional myocutaneous lower abdominal flap. The myocutaneous perforators of the inferior epigastric vessels were described[1] soon after the first transverse rectus abdominis myocutaneous (TRAM) flap was performed for breast reconstruction by Holmström and Robbins.[2,3] In the mid-1980s, following Taylor's landmark work on the vascular territory of the deep inferior epigastric artery, it became apparent that the lower abdominal flap could be perfused solely by a large periumbilical perforating vessel. That assumption was confirmed in 1989 when Koshima and Soeda[4] published two cases of "inferior epigastric skin flaps without rectus abdominis muscle".

Initially the DIEAP flap met with animosity from many in the surgical community, as it challenged conventional teaching and was thought to be unsafe. However, we are now in an era where DIEAP flaps are routinely performed in plastic surgery units throughout the world.

With an increased emphasis on optimizing the aesthetic result and minimizing donor site morbidity, in our opinion, the DIEAP flap is the current "gold standard" in breast reconstruction.

Basic science: anatomy

The deep inferior epigastric artery perforator (DIEAP) flap

The deep inferior epigastric artery arises from the external iliac, immediately above the inguinal ligament. It curves forwards in the sub-peritoneal tissue, and then ascends obliquely along the medial margin of the abdominal inguinal ring. Continuing its course upwards, it pierces the transversalis fascia, passing in front of the linea semicircularis, ascending between the rectus abdominis and the posterior lamella of its sheath.

The deep inferior epigastric artery finally divides into numerous branches, which anastomose, above the umbilicus, with the superior epigastric branch of the internal thoracic artery and with the lower intercostal arteries (*Figs 18.1, 18.2*).

The anatomy of the deep inferior epigastric artery system is very variable.[14,15] The average pedicle length is 10.3 cm and the average vessel diameter is 3.6 mm. Normally, the deep inferior epigastric artery divides into two branches, with a dominant lateral branch (54%). However, if the deep inferior epigastric artery does not divide, the vessel has a central course (28%) with multiple small branches to the muscle and centrally located perforators. If the medial branch is dominant (18%), flow appears to be significantly lower than in a central system or in patients with a dominant lateral branch.[16]

Blondeel et al.[16] found between two and eight large (>0.5 mm) perforators on each side of the midline. The majority of these perforators emerged from the anterior rectus fascia in a paramedian rectangular area 2 cm cranial and 6 cm caudal to the umbilicus and between 1 and 6 cm lateral to the umbilicus. Anatomical symmetry was hardly ever encountered. The closer a perforator is to the midline, the better the blood supply to the least vascularized part of the flap across the midline, as one choke vessel less has to be transgressed. However, the lateral perforators are often dominant and easier to dissect because they run more perpendicularly through the muscle. The sensory nerve that runs with these perforating vessels is also often much larger (*Fig. 18.3*). The medial perforators provide better perfusion of the flap but they have a longer intramuscular course, requiring more elaborate dissection with extensive longitudinal splitting of the muscle. An alternative is to extend the design of the flap to include more tissue from the flank. If one is uncertain as to whether or not enough volume can be transferred, the perforators can be dissected on both sides (Siamese flap).[5]

Preference is also given to perforators that pass through the rectus abdominis muscle at the level of the tendinous intersections. At this point, the perforators are frequently large and have few muscular side branches. The distance from the subcutaneous fat to the deep inferior epigastric vessels is also shorter, simplifying this most delicate part of the dissection.[17]

As a result, the design of a DIEAP flap is made over the most centrally located, dominant perforator, lateral or medial, as long as sufficient abdominal subcutaneous fat tissue is available and the least vascularized part of the flap across the midline can be discarded (*Fig. 18.4*). At the origin of the perforator, several nerves are encountered (*Fig. 18.3*). Although there is no constant anatomy, mixed segmental nerves run underneath or through the muscle from laterally and split into a sensate nerve running with the perforator into the flap and a motor nerve crossing on top of the deep inferior epigastric vessels distal to the bifurcation of the perforator, into the medial part of the rectus abdominis muscle.[18] One should always expect and anticipate a variety of anatomical differences.

The superficial inferior epigastric artery (SIEA) originates 2–3 cm below the inguinal ligament directly from the common femoral artery (17%) or from a common

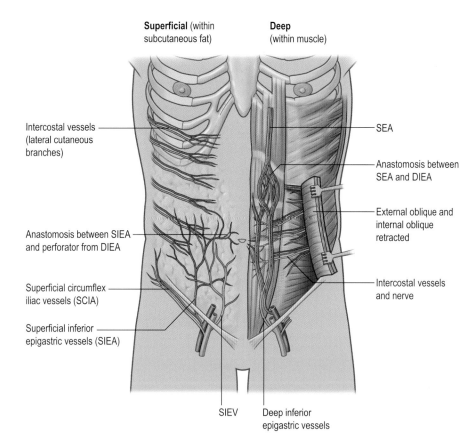

Superficial (within subcutaneous fat)   Deep (within muscle)

Intercostal vessels (lateral cutaneous branches)

SEA

Anastomosis between SEA and DIEA

External oblique and internal oblique retracted

Anastomosis between SIEA and perforator from DIEA

Superficial circumflex iliac vessels (SCIA)

Superficial inferior epigastric vessels (SIEA)

Intercostal vessels and nerve

SIEV   Deep inferior epigastric vessels

Fig. 18.1 The vascular anatomy of the lower abdomen. In the right hemi-abdomen the skin is removed down to the superficial inferior epigastric vessels. The artery with its common veins and the superficial inferior epigastric vein can be found medial to the superficial circumflex iliac vessels. Around the umbilicus the perforators of the deep inferior epigastric system connect with arteries and veins of the superficial system. The anterior branches of the intercostal arteries and veins move anterior and distally from their origin at the midaxillary line. Variable anastomoses between these different vessels make up for a complex and intense random network between the skin and the deep fascia. On the left side of the abdomen, the deep fascia of the rectus abdominis muscle is removed and the fascia of the external and internal oblique have been retracted. The deep inferior epigastric artery and vein pass deep to the lateral board of rectus abdominis as they move more cranially and enter into the rectus abdominis a few centimeters higher. Segmental branches of the deep inferior epigastric system connect with the anterior branch of the intercostal artery and veins (specially the lateral branch of the deep inferior epigastric artery). The anterior intercostal nerves run together with the segmental branches and branch into sensitive branches that run with the perforators into the subcutaneous tissues and motor branches that run medial and distally in the rectus abdominis muscle. More cranially, the deep inferior epigastric vessels anastomose in the diffuse network throughout the muscle with the superior epigastric artery.

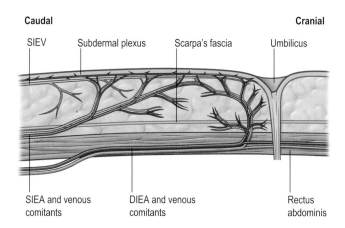

Caudal   Cranial

SIEV   Subdermal plexus   Scarpa's fascia   Umbilicus

SIEA and venous comitants   DIEA and venous comitants   Rectus abdominis

Fig. 18.2 The same anatomical structures as explained in **Figure 18.1** but seen in a paramedian sagittal view.

origin with the superficial circumflex iliac artery (48%). It then passes superiorly and laterally in the femoral triangle lying deep to Scarpa's fascia and crosses the inguinal ligament at the midpoint between the anterior superior iliac spine and the pubic tubercle. Above the inguinal ligament, the SIEA pierces Scarpa's fascia and

lies in the superficial subcutaneous tissue. During its course the SIEA lies deep to and parallel to the superficial inferior epigastric vein. The vein drains directly into the saphenous bulb.[19]

The superficial inferior epigastric artery is seen as a direct perforator to the skin while the perforators of the deep system are considered indirect perforators *(Fig. 18.5)*. Of all vessels, it is important to choose the largest, most dominant perforator destined to vascularize the fat and skin, that has few or no side branches to the muscle.

The superficial inferior epigastric vein is the largest vein draining the skin paddle of the DIEAP flap. It is located below the dermal plexus but above Scarpa's fascia, midway between the anterior superior iliac spine and the pubic symphysis. Harvesting an elliptical skin island transects this vein, redirecting the venous drainage through the smaller perforating veins. Connections between the superficial epigastric vein and the deep inferior epigastric system exist in every patient, but substantial medial branches crossing the

Video 1

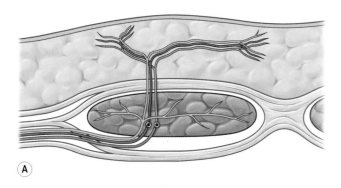

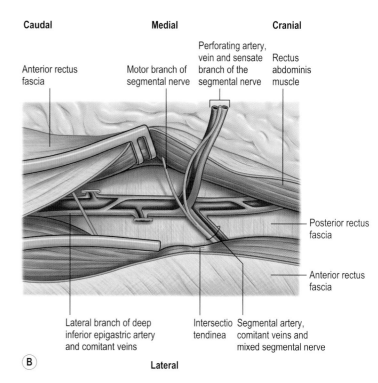

Fig. 18.3 (A,B) The anatomy of the intercostal nerves. The mixed intercostal nerves run below the fascia of the internal oblique and mostly enter the rectus abdominis muscle at its posterior surface at the level of the lateral branch of the deep inferior epigastric artery. They follow the intercostal and segmental vessels and mostly pass over the submuscular or intramuscular part of the lateral branch of the deep inferior epigastric artery. At that point it splits into two motor branches, one lateral and one medial, and additionally into a pure sensory nerve that accompanies the perforating artery and vein.

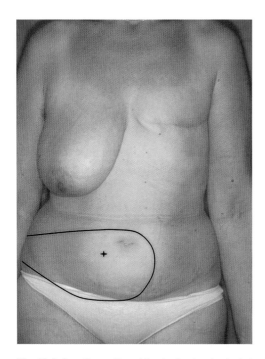

Fig. 18.4 Once the position of the dominant perforator is located on the abdomen, the flap is centered over this perforator. Finally, the incision on the abdomen will be symmetric over the midline but the least vascularized part of the flap will be discarded.

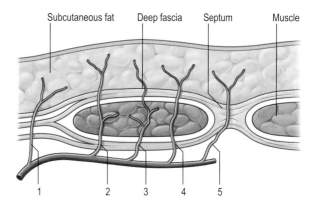

Fig. 18.5 The different types of perforators that can be found at the lower abdominal wall. (1) The branches of the superficial inferior epigastric artery are direct perforators that vascularize the subcutaneous fat and skin after perforating the deep and superficial fascia. All other perforators are indirect perforators; (2) perforators that have a predominant vascularization of the subcutaneous fat tissue and skin with few muscular branches; (3) perforators that branch off of side branches that have a predominant goal of nourishing the muscle; (4) perforators that pass through the rectus abdominis muscle without branching; (5) perforators that pass through the septum or around the rectus abdominis muscle with the sole goal of vascularizing the subcutaneous tissues.

midline have been found to be absent in 36% of cases.[20,21] In these flaps, venous connections are only present through the subdermal capillary network. This explains why the portion of a flap farthest from the midline may suffer from venous congestion and why the presence of this problem is so variable and unpredictable.

The lymphatic drainage of the DIEAP flap can be divided into a superficial and a deep system. The superficial collectors are located directly underneath the reticular dermis. Deep cuts performed during de-epithelialization may injure this system. The superficial collectors drain to the superficial lymph nodes in the groin. The deep system drains the deep structures of the abdominal wall, i.e., the muscles and fascia and is located in close proximity to the arteries and veins. Careful dissection of the vascular pedicle avoids iatrogenic damage to this lymphatic vasculature. The deep system drains to the inferior epigastric artery and then to the deep iliac nodes.[22]

Recipient vessels

The internal mammary artery and its accompanying veins are the first choice for DIEAP flap breast reconstruction.[9,11,23] Its central position on the chest wall facilitates microsurgery and offers the most flexibility during breast shaping. The vessels are easy to dissect and are usually protected from radiotherapy damage. In a number of irradiated vessels perivascular fibrosis can be encountered. Chest wall inflammation, following infected implant removal or extreme capsular fibrosis can sometimes cause severe peri-vascular scarring.

Although the artery is usually of sufficient caliber, the size of the veins is very variable. In general the veins on the left side of the chest wall are smaller than those on the right side. For this reason, we prefer to dissect the vessels at the level of the left third or fourth rib, but at the level of the fourth rib on the right side. A small segment of cartilage can be removed together with some intercostal muscles, both cranially and caudally *(Fig. 18.6)*. This provides sufficient exposure of the vessels and adequate recipient vessel length. One can also limit the dissection and exposure to the removal of only the intercostal muscles. Wider exposure can be obtained by nibbling away the lower border of the superior rib and the upper border of the inferior rib.

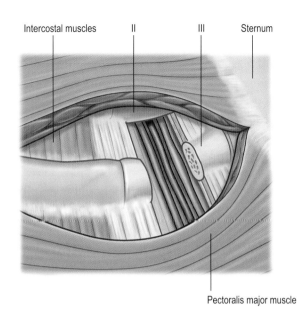

Fig. 18.6 The internal mammary artery and two common veins on the right side after removing a small part of the costal cartilage of the third rib.

At the level of the second and third intercostal space, large perforators sometimes emerge from between the intercostal muscles to perforate the medial part of the pectoralis major muscle. The size of these vessels is variable and it is estimated that they can only be used as recipient vessels for free flaps in about 5–10% of cases. These vessels can be identified and evaluated above and below the pectoralis during preparation of the recipient site. If no adequate perforators are found, the internal mammary artery and the accompanying veins are then prepared.

Diagnosis/patient presentation

When designing a DIEAP flap, the main factor is the amount of viable tissue that can be harvested on a particular perforator. The most accurate indicator of this is preoperative localization of the dominant source of blood inflow by duplex Doppler or CT imaging. In addition to defining the "safe" flap territory, these techniques provide a degree of reassurance by avoiding intraoperative surprises and considerably reduce operative time. A reduction of operative costs significantly decreases the over-all expense of the reconstructive procedure.

More recently, magnetic resonance angiography has shown promise in the imaging of perforators. In addition to producing accurate and detailed images, there is no radiation exposure,[24] unlike CT imaging.

Besides imaging with the purpose of identifying the main perforator, the conventional preoperative work-up includes blood work, oncologic screening and additional tests for concomitant diseases if necessary.

Ultrasound evaluation of perforator vessels

This is performed with a color Doppler, which employs a combination of grayscale and color Doppler imaging. This modality has 100% positive predictive value and few false negatives.[25]

Grayscale imaging shows the anatomical detail of fixed points, axial vessels and perforating branches. The addition of color Doppler allows identification of blood flow, direction (towards or away from probe), pattern of flow (i.e., venous or arterial) and finally a measure of blood flow velocity.[26–29]

The disadvantages of color duplex lie in its lack of anatomical detail and operator dependence. It requires a detailed knowledge of three dimensional vascular anatomy, as well as expertise in the handling of the devise. Whilst it provides dynamic information about blood flow this may lead to a false sense of security. It is essential to look for vessels with a minimum size and select the largest perforator in the region of interest. This is necessary because of the constant humeral and nervous stimuli that affect the microcirculation and cause fluctuations in vessel flow. Hence, flow rates do not always correlate with the size of the perforator.

In addition to preoperative imaging, it is possible to use a unidirectional hand-held pencil probe for identification of superficial vessels in the operating theatre. The perforators identified can be marked on the patient's skin to allow accurate flap design and aid intraoperative dissection. This is a simple and inexpensive technique, which provides a useful intraoperative adjunct.[30] There can, however, be false negative and positive signals as a result of interference from axial vessels or perforators that run parallel to the fascia, before entering their suprafascial course.

CT imaging

Multidetector-row helical CT is a recent innovation that permits rapid delineation of an anatomic area of interest, giving excellent resolution and low artifact rating. It takes less than 10 min to perform and is well tolerated by patients. This has become the modality of choice for the identification of abdominal wall perforators.[31–33] The use of magnetic resonance imaging to avoid the high X-ray dose is promising but still needs further sophistication.[34]

The scanning is performed in conjunction with intravenous contrast medium and allows evaluation of the donor and recipient vessels. Information collected includes the exact location and intramuscular course of vessels from their origin, the caliber of the perforators and also identifies the dominant vessel. Delineation of the relative dominance of the deep and superficial systems allows the surgeon to consider different options preoperatively. Not only can this modality be used to select suitable patients preoperatively but also operative times are reduced by a mean of 21%, with the obvious associated cost benefits.[35]

The disadvantages of multidetector-row helical CT lie in the X-ray dosage and use of intravenous contrast media, with the resultant risk of anaphylaxis. The X-ray dose, albeit significant, is less than a conventional liver CT scan and can be combined with staging investigations to reduce the overall exposure. Interpretation of the images can be done before and during surgery by the surgeon him/herself and correlated to intraoperative findings (*Figs 18.7, 18.8*).

Patient selection

Patients eligible for an autologous breast reconstruction with a DIEAP or SIEA flap are mainly those with sufficient lower abdominal subcutaneous fat tissue at the lower abdominal wall. Fortunately in our modern Western Society, many women are good candidates. Cultural differences may apply however. For example, Asian women are generally slimmer and might prefer other donor areas like the anterolateral thigh area. At the top of our preference list, the lower abdomen is our number one choice for autologous breast reconstruction. In microsurgical centers, the DIEAP flap is a preferred choice over implants. Only in very slender women or in cases where multiple scarring of the abdominal wall endangers the normal blood circulation of the free flap or the abdominoplasty flap, secondary options like

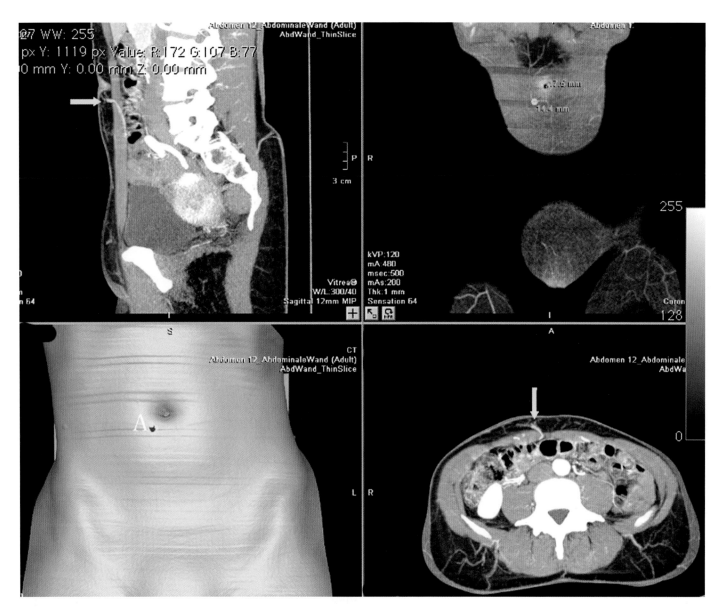

Fig. 18.7 Different views and 3-dimensional reproduction of a pararectal perforator on the right side. The sagittal view shows the course of the vessel through the rectus abdominis muscle. The location of the perforator is referenced to the umbilicus.

gluteal perforator flaps or internal thigh flaps are considered. Pedicled latissimus dorsi or thoracodorsal artery perforator flaps combined with an implant is at the bottom of the preference list. Contraindications concerning general health can also influence the decision. Morbid and severe obesity, uncontrolled diabetes, debilitating cardiovascular diseases and uncontrollable coagulopathies are the most frequent examples of absolute contraindications. Smokers and nonmotivated patients will be asked to postpone their surgery if oncologically possible. Implant reconstruction is recommended in patients with a limited oncological prognosis or with a limited life span because of age or concurrent diseases. Also, patients refusing additional scars at the donor site, refusing complex surgery or accepting the possible microsurgical complications, are seen as candidates for implant surgery. All other patients are good candidates for lower abdominal wall breast reconstruction.

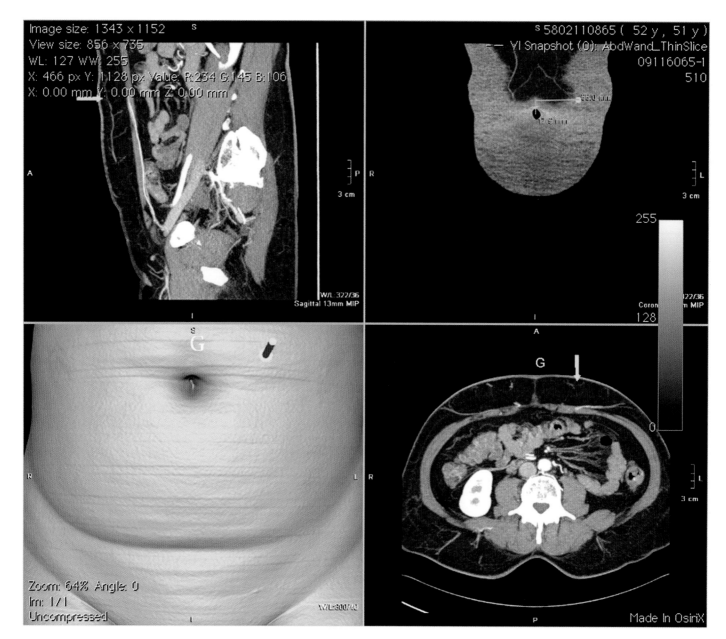

Fig. 18.8 CT-angio of a supraumbilical lateral perforator on the left side, symmetrical to a similar perforator on the right side, vascularizing only the most lateral parts of the lower abdomen. The sagittal view shows a relatively easy dissection as the vessel penetrates through the muscle relatively easy but choosing this perforator implies that tissues over the midline will certainly not be vascularized.

Surgical technique[36]

Preoperative marking

The patient is marked in a standing position. A fusiform skin island is drawn on the abdomen, similar to the one used for breast reconstruction with a free TRAM flap but the bulk of the flap is centered over the selected perforator. Although the size and shape may vary slightly, the borders of a DIEAP flap are generally located at the level of the suprapubic crease, the umbilicus and both anterior superior iliac spines, but the flap may be extended laterally to the mid-axillary lines.

A DIEAP flap generally measures 12–15 cm in height and 30–45 cm in width. However, the tension of the donor site following closure should be estimated, as this ultimately limits the size of the flap that can be harvested. A horizontal line is drawn just above the umbilicus and another one marked 12–15 cm below this. At a level 2 cm below the umbilicus the lateral limits of the flap are marked 15–23 cm on either side of the midline. The amount of subcutaneous fat present in the flanks is assessed, as this can be included in the flap if required *(Fig. 18.9A)*. All the outer markings are connected by a continuous line placed in natural skin creases.

Operative procedure

The patient is placed in a supine position with the arms positioned beside the trunk. If available, imaging data is drawn on the patient's abdomen using a 1 cm grid system based on the umbilicus. Two intravenous lines, an indwelling urinary catheter and antithrombotic stockings are applied. A warming blanket is used to keep the patients core body temperature at 37°C. The proposed incision lines are infiltrated with a dilute solution of local anesthetic and adrenaline (40 mL 1% Xylocaine with 1/100000 adrenaline in 40 mL sterile water), except in the region of the superficial epigastric veins. Three separate stab incisions are then placed around the umbilicus and connected with the aid of skin hooks. The umbilicus is incised circumferentially down to the fascia. While making the inferior incision, care is taken to preserve the superficial epigastric veins. If the venous drainage of the flap is insufficient or thrombosis of the perforating vein(s) occurs after the anastomosis, the superficial epigastric veins can be used as an additional venous conduit. Two or three veins may be present but they commonly unite further down the abdominal wall. The veins are dissected over a length of 2–3 cm and ligated with clips to make them easily retrievable later, if needed. If the caliber of the superficial epigastric artery is noted to be large enough, a similar skin island to the DIEAP flap can be harvested on these two vessels. The incisions are continued down to the fascia. Beveling is avoided unless extra volume is required as this may later lead to a depressed scar in the lower abdomen. Laterally however, the flap may be beveled to include more fat and reduce residual "dog-ears".

Dissection of the vascular pedicle of a DIEAP flap can be divided into three different technical stages; suprafascial, intramuscular and submuscular. The most demanding stage is the intramuscular dissection of the vascular pedicle.

Suprafascial dissection

Dissection begins laterally in the flanks and progresses medially with the aid of cutting and coagulating diathermy. The skin and subcutaneous fat are lifted off the external oblique fascia up to the lateral border of the rectus abdominis muscle. At this point dissection proceeds more cautiously as the perforators are identified. Gentle traction on the flap helps provide good exposure of the vessels. Again, if imaging data is available, the dissection can progress rapidly to the preselected perforator, with ligation of the more laterally placed perforators *(Fig. 18.9B)*. If only a unidirectional Doppler probe was used, one can try to visualize as many perforators as possible before selecting the largest one. This method needs some expertise, can be time-consuming and does not allow evaluation of all the medial perforators.

If the caliber of one vessel is estimated to be insufficient, an adjacent perforator located on the same vertical line can also be dissected. The abdominal wall muscles must be relaxed at all times and the perforating vessels kept moist with normal saline. No antispasmodic agents are routinely used. When dissecting a perforator from the lateral side, it is important to realize that a side branch may be located more medially. Extra care must be taken when dissecting the full circumference of a vessel, but complete dissection helps prevent vessel damage when raising the flap from the contralateral side *(Fig. 18.9C,D)*.

The anterior rectus fascia is then incised with a pair of scissors following the direction of the rectus abdominis muscle fibers at the rim of the tiny gap in the fascia through which the perforating vessel passes *(Fig. 18.9E)*. If more than one perforator is dissected, the different gaps can be connected with each other. A small cuff of fascia may be left around the perforator if the vessel is small or if the surgeon feels more comfortable doing so.

Lifting the fascia helps mobilize the perforator, which can be freed by blunt dissection, gently pushing away the loose connective tissue. The perforator can be adherent to the deep surface of the anterior rectus fascia for a variable distance before it plunges into the muscle. The division of the fascia is continued superiorly for a

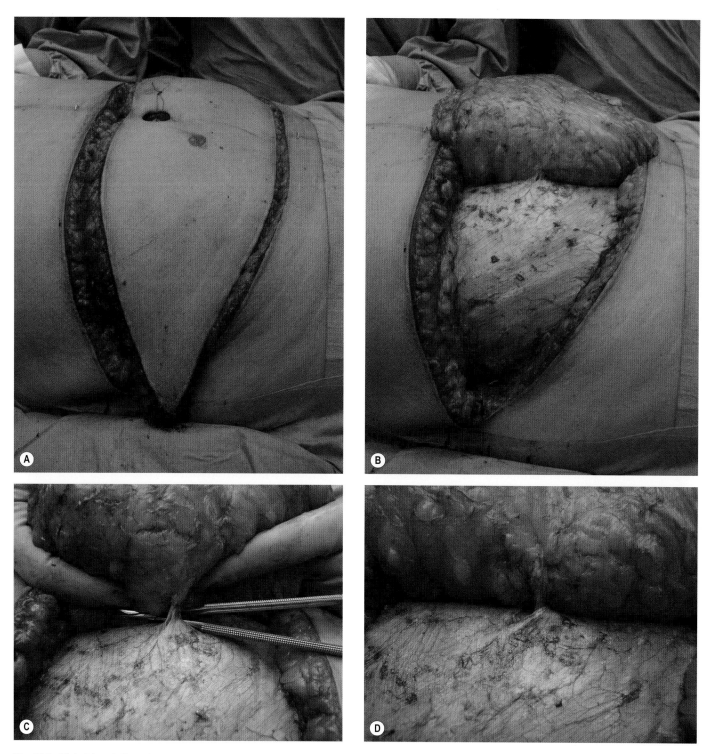

Fig. 18.9 (A) Incision of skin and subcutaneous tissue is extended towards the flanks if additional tissue is needed. The dominant perforator on the right side is marked with an "x" on the flap. **(B)** The flap is laterally undermined towards medial until the area around the preoperatively marked perforator is reached. Undermining of the fat is continued proximal and distal of the perforator. **(C)** Undermining continues around the perforator for a distance of about 2 cm. Lifting up the subcutaneous tissue is easier at this point when the deep fascia is still closed **(D)** Access to the perivascular loose connective tissue is sought by incising the gap in the deep fascia and the tissues surrounding the vessels.

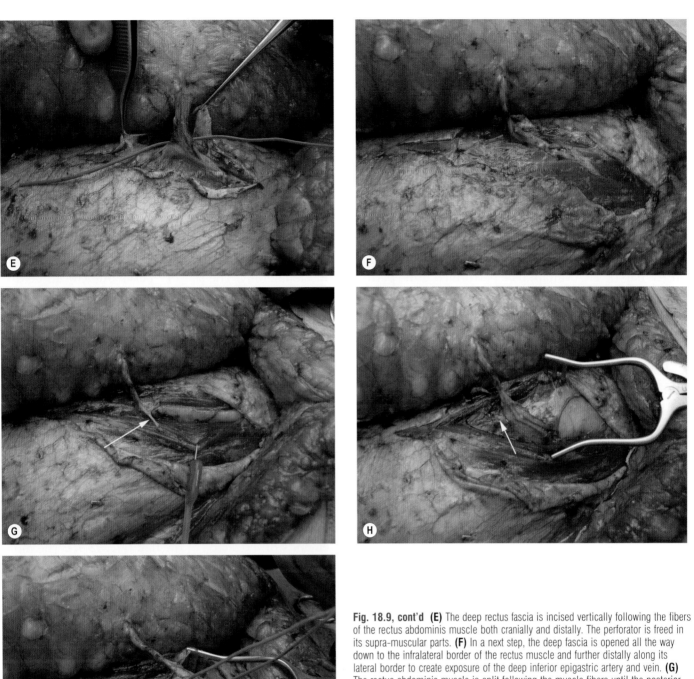

Fig. 18.9, cont'd (E) The deep rectus fascia is incised vertically following the fibers of the rectus abdominis muscle both cranially and distally. The perforator is freed in its supra-muscular parts. **(F)** In a next step, the deep fascia is opened all the way down to the infralateral border of the rectus muscle and further distally along its lateral border to create exposure of the deep inferior epigastric artery and vein. **(G)** The rectus abdominis muscle is split following the muscle fibers until the posterior fascia or the peritoneum can be seen. Sensory nerves come here from lateral and following the perforator can be transected. Motor nerves are left intact (white arrow). **(H)** Wide exposure is achieved with a self retaining retractor. A bloodless field allows perfect control of the dissection. The main axis of the deep inferior epigastric artery and its veins is clipped proximal to the perforators (white arrow). **(I)** Once the entire course of the perforator and the main vessels is clear, the posterior part of the perforator and the main vessels is dissected off the surrounding tissues. The distal part of the deep inferior epigastric vessels can be dissected either through the same incision through the rectus muscle or continued from lateral by pulling the rectus muscle medially.

distance of 3–4 cm and inferiorly to the lateral border of the rectus abdominis muscle in an oblique line towards the inguinal ligament *(Fig. 18.9F)*. At this point the direction of the division of the fascia is changed into the direction of the fibers of the external oblique muscle. This avoids a continuous area of weakness of the lower abdominal wall, as closure of the fascia is performed on top of the rectus abdominis muscle. Two separate incisions, one around the perforator and one over the deep inferior epigastric vessels at the lower lateral border of the rectus muscle can also be performed.

It is advisable to fully complete the dissection of the DIEAP flap on one side before progressing to the other. This allows a "life boat" in the form of a contralateral DIEAP flap or TRAM flap to be performed if the perforator is inadvertently damaged. It is important to emphasize that the vessels must be protected at all stages and complete muscle relaxation is necessary until donor site closure is obtained. As dissection progresses, the DIEAP flap should be secured to the abdominal wall with the aid of staples.

Intramuscular dissection

The rectus abdominis muscle should be split in a longitudinal direction in the perimysial plane through which the perforating vessel traverses. Splitting the muscle fibers makes dissection easier as the vessel becomes larger *(Fig. 18.9G)*. The perforator is again liberated by blunt dissection, staying close to the vessel at all times, as it remains covered by a thin layer of loose connective tissue. As a general rule, if resistance to dissection is encountered, a side branch or a nerve will be identified. Different muscular branches must be ligated with care and hemoclips are placed 1–2 mm away from the main vessel so that if one inadvertently comes off, it can easily be replaced. This technique avoids damage and spasm of the main perforating vessel. Placing a vessel loop around the vascular pedicle allows additional retraction without any unnecessary tension being placed on the vessel. Using bipolar coagulating diathermy and small hemoclips, one continues to ligate all the side branches until the origin of the perforator on the major branch of the deep inferior epigastric vessel is reached at the posterior surface of the rectus abdominis muscle *(Fig. 18.9H)*.

If two perforators have been selected, the rectus abdominis muscle must be widely separated. If the perforators run in two adjacent perimysial planes, the fibers may have to be cut. However, trans-section of large parts of the rectus abdominis muscle or division at the level where a motor nerve crosses from the lateral to the medial side should be avoided.

Submuscular dissection

The lateral border of the rectus abdominis is raised using noncrushing tissue forceps. Special care is taken not to injure the mixed segmental nerves entering the muscle laterally. The sensory nerve branch can be dissected by epineural splitting.[18] In this way, an additional 5–9 cm can be obtained, facilitating neural suturing at the recipient site. If possible, all the motor branches are left intact. However, in cases where a motor branch runs between two perforators, then this nerve has to be cut. Once the flap is harvested, it can be resutured.

Between the mixed segmental nerves, the plane posterior to the rectus abdominis muscle is opened, exposing the main deep inferior epigastric vessel. Side branches of the main stem are ligated and the dissection is continued by retracting the rectus abdominis muscle medially until the proximal part of the pedicle is completely liberated. The length of the pedicle can be tailored to meet the needs of different recipient sites or the demands of the shape of the flap *(Fig. 18.9I)*. The more distal the perforator is located in the flap, the further the deep inferior epigastric vessels need to be dissected into the groin. Frequently however, the pedicle can be transected at the lateral border of the rectus abdominis muscle. At this level, there is sufficient pedicle diameter and length to enable a safe microsurgical anastomosis.

If one is certain that the blood flow through the deep inferior epigastric vessel is sufficient (an ultrasonic flow meter can be used) the remainder of the flap can be raised. In cases of midline scars, or when a large flap is needed, the same vascular dissection can be performed on the contralateral side. Otherwise, all the remaining perforators are ligated, the umbilicus is released and the entire skin flap is raised. The pedicle is finally transected when the recipient vessels have been prepared. A hemoclip can be placed on the lateral comitant vein to help orientate the pedicle.

After division of the pedicle, the flap is turned over and the vessels placed carefully onto its undersurface. One has to be meticulous about the position of the pedicle, as it tends to rotate very easily, especially if only one perforator has been harvested. The flap is then weighed, photographed and transferred. The ischemia time is noted. The flap is placed on moist gauze at the recipient site to prevent desiccation and again stapled to the surrounding skin for security. The flap may be rotated to facilitate microsurgery, provided a note of this is made and the rotation reversed at the end of the procedure.

Hints and tips

10 golden rules in perforator flap surgery

1. Map the perforators preoperatively: identify the most dominant vessels on each side.
2. Start dissection on one side of the flap: leave the contralateral side intact until you finished the entire dissection of the pedicle.
3. Preserve every perforator until you encounter a larger one: discard only the smaller ones that you are sure you will not use. Select one or two perforators with the largest diameter that correspond with your preoperative mapping.
4. Consider the best location of the perforator within the flap: the more centrally located, the better blood flow to the outer parts of the flap.
5. Consider the easiest dissection through the muscle: long intramuscular dissections are more tedious, contain more risk for damaging the vessels and are more time-consuming.
6. Dissect close to the vessels, remaining within the perivascular loose connective tissue, thereby guaranteeing an absolute bloodless field.
7. Ensure sufficient and wide exposure by splitting the muscle along its fibers (avoid digging into a small hole).
8. Carefully ligate every side-branch at a distance of about 2 mm away from the main pedicle.
9. Avoid any traction on the perforator: intima rupture is a frequent cause of unexplained clotting of the perforator.
10. Trans-sect the other perforators after the entire pedicle is dissected.

Closure of the donor site and fashioning of the umbilicus

As no fascia has been resected, primary tension-free closure of the fascia with a running, nonabsorbable 1-0 suture is always possible. The upper skin flap is undermined using cutting diathermy to the level of the xiphoid and costal margin. Two suction drains are placed at the upper and lower margins of the skin flaps and brought out suprapubically on each side of the midline. The lower border of the umbilicus is marked on the anterior abdominal wall at the level of the anterior superior iliac spines and a 2 cm vertical line is drawn above this point. Only a vertical incision is performed. The anterior abdominal wall is extensively thinned at the site of the new umbilicus by trimming of the subcutaneous fat. The umbilicus is then passed through the defect and inset with a separate 4-0 absorbable suture.

The operating table is put in a flexed position to facilitate closure of the anterior abdominal wall. Scarpa's fascia is approximated with interrupted 1-0 absorbable sutures with particular attention being paid to medial advancement of the wound edges to reduce the "dog-ears" in the flanks. Finally, interrupted 3-0 sutures are placed intradermally to evert the skin edges and a skin adhesive is applied. No further abdominal dressing is used.

Shaping of the DIEAP flap in secondary autologous breast reconstruction

A systematic approach is applied to be able to create easy and reproducible results in shaping of autologous tissue by using the "3-step principle".[10,11] Recreating a 3-dimensional organ from a flat piece of abdominal fat and skin is broken down into three essential steps: (1) Redefining and recreating the basis and borders of the footprint of the breast (the interface of the posterior surface of the breast gland and the thorax) at the right location on the chest wall (*Fig. 18.10*); (2) molding the flap into a drop-shape like conus on top of the footprint by means of specific suturing (*Fig. 18.11*); and (3) redraping the skin envelope (*Fig. 18.12*) and the nipple areolar complex (*Fig. 18.13*) over the conus with the right tension.

The breast footprint

Any previous scars or severely damaged tissue that lies over the footprint of the new breast are excised. In modified radical mastectomy cases, the new inframammary fold is incised to a depth of approximately 1 cm

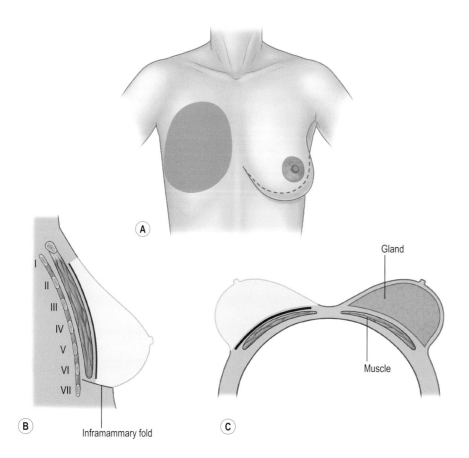

Fig. 18.10 (A) Coronal, **(B)** sagittal and **(C)** transverse view of the footprint of the breast.

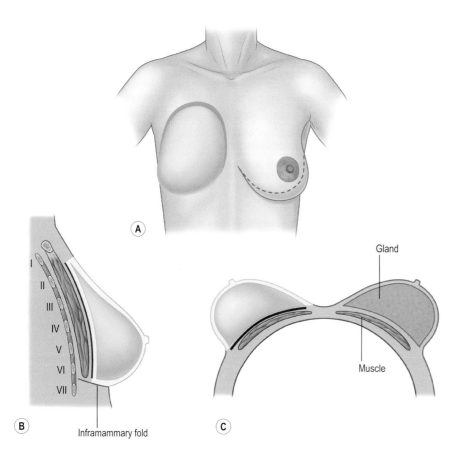

Fig. 18.11 (A) Coronal, **(B)** sagittal and **(C)** transverse view of the conus of the breast.

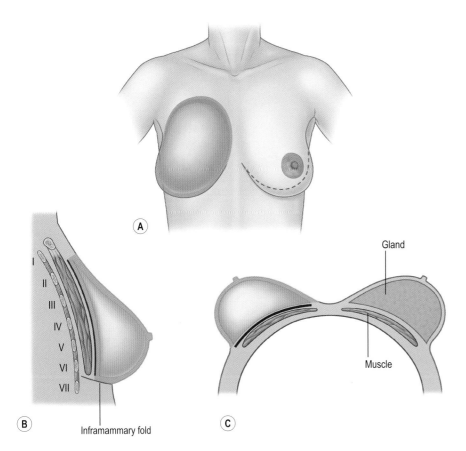

Fig. 18.12 **(A)** Coronal, **(B)** sagittal and **(C)** transverse view of the envelope of the breast.

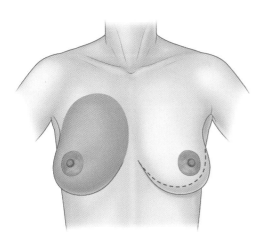

Fig. 18.13 The nipple areola complex is an integral part of the envelope of the breast.

to allow easy suturing of the DIEAP flap. While the position of the borders of the new footprint are at a mirror position of the contralateral footprint, the new inframammary fold position needs to be placed 2–3 cm higher than the contralateral inframammary fold depending on the laxity of the mastectomy flap skin

and tension exerted on the abdominoplasty flap later in the procedure. The skin in between the mastectomy scar and the inframammary fold is de-epithelialized. In this way, a layer of 1–2 cm of fat in the lower part of the breast is preserved, improving projection. The skin edges of the upper mastectomy flap are thinned down to the dermis for the first 5 mm and then progressively trimmed to obtain a seamless transition into the upper skin edge of the DIEAP flap. The upper mastectomy flap is then undermined on the lateral, cranial, and medial borders of the breast footprint to subsequently accommodate the flap.

In cases of primary breast reconstruction, the edges of the footprint are assumed to be intact. If for oncological reasons the edges of the footprint need to be undermined or resected, these borders will need to be repairs before transferring the flap.

The breast conus

We prefer to use the contralateral DIEAP flap in cases of delayed breast reconstruction. The flap is rotated

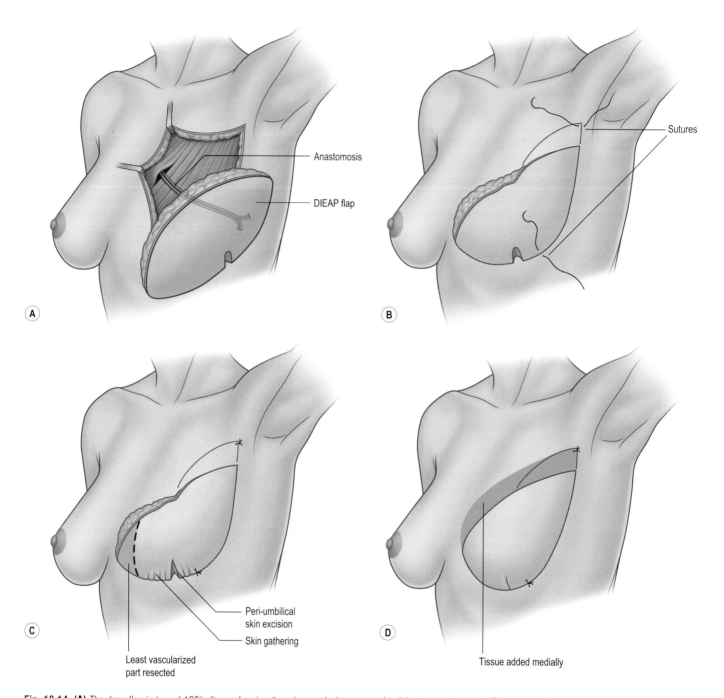

Fig. 18.14 **(A)** The deep flap is turned 180° after performing the microsurgical anastomosis of the vessels and then **(B)** sutured with two key sutures to the pectoral fascia at the anterior axillary fold and the lateral part of the new inframammary fold making sure to avoid any fullness of the inferolateral quadrant of the new breast. **(C)** A triangular excision of skin around the umbilical area and gathering of the skin at the inframammary fold around the midclavicular line will create projection of the flap and a sharp angle between the lower part of the breast and the abdominal wall. **(D)** The least vascularized part of the flap is then resected making sure to preserve enough tissue to fill the upper medial quadrant of the breast.

through 180° prior to transfer and shaping begins after the anastomosis has been completed *(Fig. 18.14A)*.

A wedge of skin is removed around the site of the umbilicus and closed in two layers. This simple maneuver gathers more volume in the lower half of the flap. The more skin that is removed, the more projection that can be achieved but it does result in compression of the subdermal plexus in this area.

The tendon of the pectoralis major muscle is then identified. The tip of the DIEAP flap is fixed just below the pectoralis tendon by suturing Scarpa's fascia to the pectoralis fascia 2–3 cm medial to the lateral pectoral muscle border. This first key suture recreates the anterior axillary fold *(Fig. 18.14B)*.

The lateral edge of the flap is then stapled to the most lateral part of the inframammary fold under slight tension to avoid excessive lateral fullness *(Fig. 18.14B)*. The transition from the lateral pectoral border into the lateral portion of the flap also recreates a natural lazy-S shape along the lateral border of the breast. The exact position of the second key suture is determined by moving the flap along the inframammary fold while assessing the lazy-S contour. It is always better to have minimal fullness in this location at the time of reconstruction, as the flap will shift laterally and distally in the postoperative period.

Medial to the second key suture, in the midclavicular line, the skin of the flap is then bunched up *(Fig. 18.14C)*. This, together with the triangular skin resection around the umbilicus dramatically increases flap projection. It also helps create a sharp angle between the skin of the flap and the abdominal skin below the inframammary fold.

The third key suture is placed at the medial end of the inframammary fold. The flap is not bunched in this location to avoid overfilling of the inferomedial quadrant of the new breast. However, one should be cautious, as if the flap is not placed medially enough, it can be difficult to achieve sufficient cleavage.

Two important components are then assessed; a volume estimation of the DIEAP flap compared to the contralateral breast and the poorly vascularized tissue in the flap that needs to be resected (previously called zone IV, *Fig. 18.14C*). The latter can be accomplished either by visual inspection of the skin, or by carving into the dermal plexus with a Bistouri in the most distal corner. Tissues that show mixed arterial and venous bleeding can be kept. When a DIEAP flap with an ipsilateral pedicle is used, poorly vascularized tissue is removed before placing the first key suture. We recommend making the reconstructed breast 5–10% larger than the contralateral side, anticipating a postoperative reduction in swelling.

The medial part of the flap is then rounded off, providing a smooth transition into the presternal region.

Overfilling of the superomedial regions of the breast is also recommended *(Fig. 18.14D)*, as gravity will be pulling the flap caudally over the ensuing 6 months. Excessive fat can easily be removed later, whereas a depression in this area can be very disturbing for the patient.

The breast envelope

Once the final volume of the flap is determined, one can make a rough estimate of how much skin overlying the DIEAP flap will be required. The flap can be pushed up into the pocket or pulled down, leaving more or less vertical skin height, respectively, on the skin paddle of the flap. The more skin that is left, the more ptosis that can be achieved. Also, the more skin resected in the lateral part of the flap, the more the flap will be pushed medially. Once again, the clinical and aesthetic assessment of the contralateral breast is key in fine-tuning the shape of the DIEAP flap. Finally, the upper part of the skin paddle covered by the mastectomy flap is de-epithelialized.

Postoperative care

The postoperative care is strongly simplified as the function of the rectus muscle is preserved. Preserving the integrity of the muscle also significantly decreases postoperative abdominal wall pain, facilitates rehabilitation and therefore reduces hospitalization time.

Flap monitoring is mainly clinical. Frequency of evaluation is hourly during the first 24 h, 2-hourly in the second 24 h and every 4 h during the following 2 days. Adhesive thermometer-strips are stuck to the skin island of the flap and the high sternal region. Differences of more than 2°C are reported to the physician on call. Besides temperature, color, consistency of the flap and capillary refill are registered on a specific microsurgical follow-up sheet. Unidirectional Doppler flowmetry and other more sophisticated devices are not used, as they can produce false positive signals.

Patients are mobilized within 24 h after removing the urinary catheter. Systemic antibiotics are given for 24 h. Except for daily subcutaneous prophylactic doses of low-molecular heparin no other anticoagulants are given. Besides paracetamol as pain relief and anti-inflammatory, no other drugs are given unless a specific medical condition would require it. Drinking starts 12 h postoperatively. Drains are left for 3–7 days depending on their daily output. Dressing changes are not necessary with the use of skin adhesives. A sterile towel covers the breast(s) and the abdomen to keep the flap warm for the first 5 days. After that a soft and elastic bra is adjusted. No compressive garments are applied.

Outcomes, prognosis, and complications

The dissection of a DIEAP flap has a certain learning curve, involving a very specific dissection technique of the perforating vessels. As long as dissection is performed close to the vessels in a plane of loose connective tissue surrounding the pedicle, side branches and crossing nerves can be easily identified and preserved. Dissection through other planes will cause excessive bleeding and slow the surgeon down. Two golden rules must be applied in any type of perforator flap surgery: bloodless field and wide exposure. A common mistake made is to be misled by the eagerness to follow the perforator vessels into the deep tissues in a small hole. Muscle, septum or other tissues through which the perforators travel should be opened widely to get a clear overview and to be able to deal with eventual bleeding.

A number of technical considerations are important in the planning and execution of the dissection. Evidently the wrong choice of perforator can lead to disastrous complications. With the help of imaging and direct intra-operative visualization, the most important perforator can be identified. Unusual courses of perforator as those rounding the medial or lateral edge of the rectus abdominis muscle must be taken into account. Dominance of the superficial system should be recognized at the beginning of the flap harvesting, at the time of incision of the lower edge of the flap.

During dissection of the pedicle overstretching of the vessels should be avoided. The use of vessel loops is limited to the actual dissection and should not be left in place as they accidentally can come under traction in a later phase of the operation.

Ligation of side branches should be performed at a distance of 2–3 mm away from the pedicle. When a vascular clip or a ligating suture is placed too close to the main pedicle, it can interrupt the arterial or venous flow. Care should be taken during the motor nerve dissection. Excessive traction or crushing of the nerve can permanently affect its function.

In case of a free flap, torsion of the pedicle can easily occur during transfer of the flap. Exact orientation with the help of vascular clips can avoid this problem. Following anastomosis, kinking of the pedicle can be avoided by placing the pedicle in smooth curves once the shaping has finished. During the shaping of the flap, excessive defatting can lead to areas of partial flap necrosis or fat necrosis. Delayed defatting using liposuction is a safer procedure. Poorly vascularized areas should be resected during the initial procedure to reduce the total amount of postoperative complications.

In inexperienced hands, the DIEAP flap dissection will require a longer operating time than a conventional myocutaneous flap. After a number of cases, operating time will fall back and be comparable to myocutaneous flap harvesting or even shorter if a limited pedicle length is needed.

Abdominal scarring is probably the most important risk factor for raising a DIEAP flap. It can cause major problems during the dissection of the perforators and the epigastric vessels. Intramuscular scarring is not always diagnosed on preoperative ultrasound and can spread out farther than suspected from the place and length of a previous incision.

Smoking is considered a relative contraindication to a raising a DIEAP flap. Our impression is that the area most distant from the vascular pedicle of smokers is not well perfused, with prolonged vascular spasm. Additionally, wound healing problems and wound infections have been observed more frequently in smokers. Smokers who request elective, delayed reconstructions are asked to stop smoking at least 3 months before becoming a candidate for surgery. This is an additional way to test the motivation of the patient. A nonmotivated patient or poor general medical health are the only absolute contraindications to DIEAP flap breast reconstruction.[36–38]

Secondary procedures

The free flap transfer and initial shaping is just the first step in achieving a full and natural breast reconstruction. Following the principles of a sculptor, we try to create a breast in the first step that is slightly bigger than the desired volume and resembles the final result as close as possible. Obtaining a definite result in one procedure is impossible. As removing tissues is so much easier than adding, specific areas of the flap can be aspirated or resected during the second operation 6 months later to achieve symmetry which is the final goal of this procedure. If more tissue is needed, the flap can be augmented by lipofilling in specific spots to improve the shape or throughout the flap if a pure volume augmentation is necessary. Augmentation by implants is possible as well but performed less and less as results of lipofilling become more predictable and successful. Nipple reconstruction is performed by using the modified CV flap *(Fig. 18.15)*. Scar revisions and adjustments of the borders of the footprint can easily be performed. During the second operation, the contralateral breast can also be corrected in case of unilateral reconstruction. Any preferred technique of breast augmentation, reduction or mastopexy can be performed as long as symmetry of shape and volume can be achieved.

In a final procedure, not really an operation, bilateral tattoo of the nipple-areola complex is performed under local anesthesia. Even if the contralateral breast has not been operated on, the nipple-areola complex is tattooed to obtain perfect color match of both sides, hereby creating an optical effect of camouflaging the reconstruction.

Primary reconstructions will always yield better aesthetic results than secondary or tertiary reconstructions as the natural footprint and skin envelope mostly remain intact, specifically if postoperative radiotherapy can be avoided. If the conus is properly shaped during the first procedure, many secondary procedures can be less complex and less frequent. For that reason, prophylactic mastectomies are performed more routinely today as a risk reducing operation in hereditary breast cancer

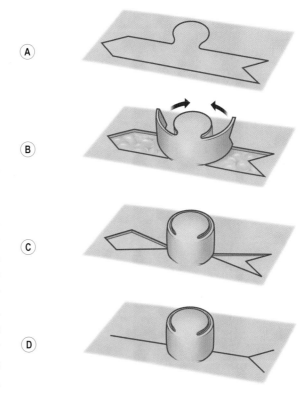

Fig. 18.15 The modified CV-flap technique for nipple reconstruction.

as in BRCA-1 and -2 mutations *(Fig. 18.16)* or for oncological reasons (i.e., invasive lobular carcinoma). Prophylactic mastectomy and immediate full breast reconstruction without adjuvant radiotherapy should also be weighed against a wide segmentectomy combined with aggressive radiotherapy leading to mutilation of the breast mound.

Secondary *(Fig. 18.17)* and specifically tertiary (implant crippled or failed previous autologous attempts) reconstructions are more complex as they involve corrections and adjustments at all 3 essential parts of the "3-step" principle. Applying this principle however lets the surgeon not only to analyze the problem but also to provide the opportunity to develop a clear preoperative strategy. In tertiary reconstructions, the surgeon is often left with no other choice than to remove all previous tissues, implants and scarring and to recommence the entire reconstructive process over again.

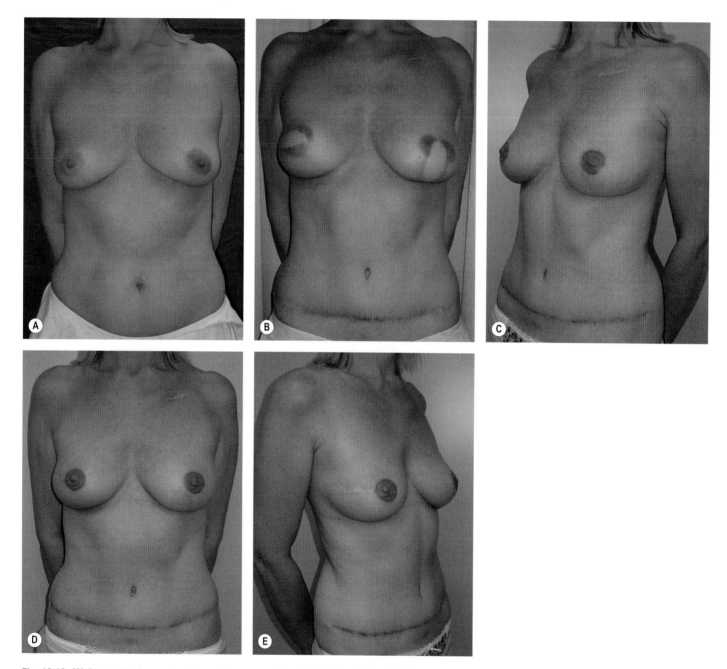

Fig. 18.16 **(A)** Preoperative image of a 46-year-old-woman, carrier of a BRCA-2 mutation, following tumorectomy through a horizontal racquet incision at the right breast. **(B)** intermediate phase after bilateral areola-sparing mastectomy, using the same scar on the right breast and a more conventional vertical scar on the left breast, and bilateral autologous reconstruction by means of a bilateral free DIEAP flap. **(C–E)** A 2-year-postoperative image after bilateral nipple reconstruction using the interposed skin island of the flap and bilateral tattoo.

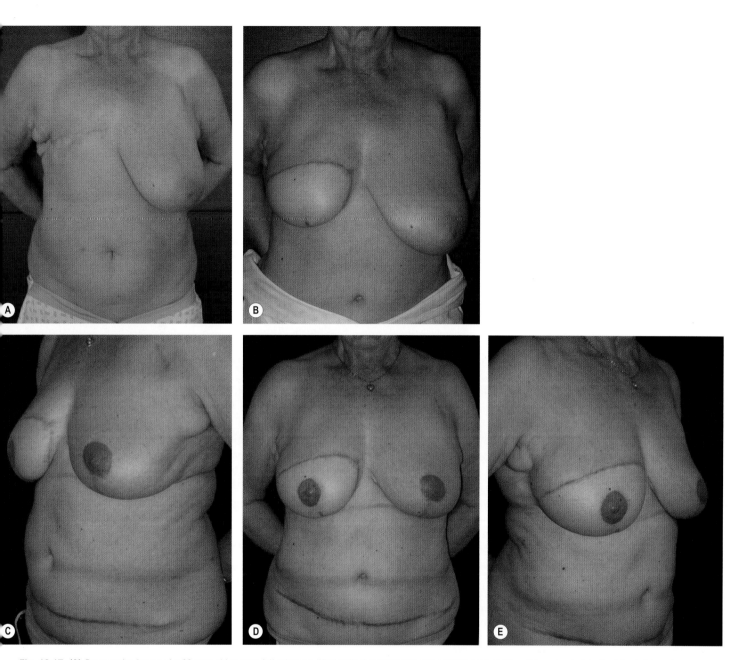

Fig. 18.17 **(A)** Preoperative image of a 62-year-old woman following modified radical mastectomy of the right breast and breast hypertrophy/ptosis of the left breast. **(B)** Intermediate phase after secondary autologous breast reconstruction by means of a unilateral free DIEAP flap. **(C–E)** Final result, 1 year postoperatively, after right nipple reconstruction (and later tattoo) and left breast reduction.

Access the complete reference list online at **http://www.expertconsult.com**

4. Koshima I, Soeda S. Inferior epigastric artery skin flaps without rectus abdominis muscle. *Br J Plast Surg.* 1989;42(6):645–648.

   The rectus abdominis musculocutaneous flap has many advantages, but its disadvantages are also well-known. These are the possibility of abdominal herniation and, in certain situations, its bulk. To overcome these problems, an inferior epigastric artery skin flap without rectus abdominis muscle, pedicled on the muscle perforators and the proximal inferior deep epigastric artery, have been used in two patients. A large flap without muscle can survive on a single muscle perforator.

5. Koshima I, Moriguchi T, Soeda S, et al. Free thin paraumbilical perforator-based flaps. *Ann Plast Surg.* 1992;29(1):12–17.

7. Allen RJ, Treece P. Deep inferior epigastric perforator flap for breast reconstruction. *Ann Plast Surg.* 1994;32(1):32–38.

8. Blondeel PN, Boeckx WD. Refinements in free flap breast reconstruction: the free bilateral deep inferior epigastric perforator flap anastomosed to the internal mammary artery. *Br J Plast Surg.* 1994;47(7):495–501.

    Besides the enormous advantages of reconstructing the amputated breast by means of a conventional TRAM flap, the main disadvantage remains the elevation of small (free TRAM) or larger (pedicled TRAM) parts of the rectus abdominis muscle. In order to overcome this disadvantage, the free deep inferior epigastric perforator (DIEP) skin flap has recently been used for breast mound reconstruction with excellent clinical results. After achieving favorable results with eight unilateral DIEP-flaps, we were challenged by an abdomen with a midline laparotomy scar. By dissecting a bilateral DIEP flap and making adjacent anastomoses to the internal mammary artery we were able to achieve sufficient flap mobility for easy free flap positioning and breast shaping. Intraoperative segmental nerve stimulation, postoperative functional abdominal wall tests and CT-scan examination showed normal abdominal muscle activity. On the basis of a case report, the technical considerations and advantages of anastomosing the bipedicled DIEP flap to the internal mammary artery are discussed.

9. Blondeel PN. One hundred free DIEP flap breast reconstructions: a personal experience. *Br J Plast Surg.* 1999;52(2):104–111.

    The transverse rectus abdominis myocutaneous (TRAM) flap has been the gold standard for breast reconstruction until recently. Not only autologous but also immediate reconstructions are now preferred to offer the patient a natural and cosmetically acceptable result. This study summarizes the prospectively gathered data of 100 free DIEP flaps used for breast reconstruction in 87 patients. Primary reconstructions were done in 35% of the patients. Well-known risk factors for free-flap breast reconstruction were present: smokers 23%, obesity 25%, abdominal scarring 28% and previous radiotherapy 45%. Mean operating time was 6 h 12 min for unilateral reconstruction and mean hospital stay was 7.9 days. These data indicate that the free DIEP flap is a new but reliable and safe technique for autologous breast reconstruction. This flap offers the patient the same advantages as the TRAM flap and discards the most important disadvantages of the myocutaneous flap by preserving the continuity of the rectus muscle.

10. Blondeel PN, Hijjawi J, Depypere H, et al. Shaping the breast in aesthetic and reconstructive breast surgery: an easy three-step principle. *Plast Reconstr Surg.* 2009;123(2):455–462.

11. Blondeel PN, Hijjawi J, Depypere H, et al. Shaping the breast in aesthetic and reconstructive breast surgery: an easy three-step principle. Part II. Breast reconstruction after total mastectomy. *Plast Reconstr Surg.* 2009;123(3):794–805.

    This is Part II of four parts describing the 3-step principle being applied in reconstructive and aesthetic breast surgery. Part I explains how to analyze a problematic breast by understanding the three main anatomical features of a breast and how they interact: the footprint, the conus of the breast and the skin envelope. This part describes how one can optimize his/her results with breast reconstructions after complete mastectomy. For both primary and secondary reconstructions, we explain how to analyze the mastectomized breast and the deformed chest wall before giving step-by-step guidelines how to rebuild the entire breast with either autologous tissue or implants. The differences in shaping unilateral or bilateral breast reconstructions with autologous tissue are clarified. Regardless of timing or method of reconstruction, it is shown that by breaking down the surgical strategy in three easy (anatomical) steps, the reconstructive surgeon will be able to provide more aesthetically pleasing and reproducible results.

19. Taylor GI, Daniel RK. The anatomy of several free flap donor sites. *Plast Reconstr Surg.* 1975;56(3):243–253.

35. Uppal RS, Casaer B, Van Landuyt K, et al. The efficacy of preoperative mapping of perforators in reducing operative times and complications in perforator flap breast reconstruction. *J Plast Reconstr Aesthet Surg.* 2009;62(7):859–864.

38. Massey MF, Spiegel AJ, Levine JL, et al. Perforator flaps: recent experience, current trends, and future directions based on 3974 microsurgical breast reconstructions. *Plast Reconstr Surg.* 2009;124:737–751.

    Perforator flap breast reconstruction is an accepted surgical option for breast cancer patients electing to restore their body image after mastectomy. Since the introduction of the deep inferior epigastric perforator flap, microsurgical techniques have evolved to support a 99% success rate for a variety of flaps with donor sites that include the abdomen, buttock, thigh, and trunk. Recent experience highlights the perforator flap as a proven solution for patients who have experienced failed breast implant-based reconstructions or those requiring irradiation. Current trends suggest an application of these techniques in patients previously felt to be unacceptable surgical candidates with a focus on safety, aesthetics, and increased sensitization. Future challenges include the propagation of these reconstructive techniques into the hands of future plastic surgeons with a focus on the development of septocutaneous flaps and vascularized lymph node transfers for the treatment of lymphedema.

19

Alternative flaps for breast reconstruction

Maria M. LoTempio, Robert J. Allen, and Phillip N. Blondeel

SYNOPSIS

- Many women today have undergone procedures on their abdomen, such as liposuction and abdominoplasty, that preclude the TRAM/DIEP breast reconstructive option.
- The skilled microsurgeon needs to be able to utilize other flaps for women in this category.
- Alternative flaps may include transverse upper gracilis free flap (TUG); superior gluteal artery free flap (SGAP); inferior gluteal myocutaneous flap (IGAP); deep femoral artery perforator (DFAP), and lumbar artery perforator flap (LAP).

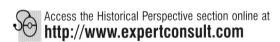

Access the Historical Perspective section online at
http://www.expertconsult.com

Introduction

The modern era of autogenous breast reconstruction began with the TRAM flap, popularized by Dr Carl Hartrampf in the early 1980s. This was the procedure of choice until the 1990s, when the goal of muscle preservation became more apparent. Perforator flap breast reconstruction in the early 1990s by the authors' group at Louisiana State University Medical Center was the next significant advance in breast reconstruction. By injecting fresh abdominoplasty specimens, it was determined that the skin and fat could be transferred without sacrifice of the rectus abdominus muscle. This led to the first DIEP flap for breast reconstruction by Allen in 1992.[1] The inception of free tissue transfer allowed an infinite range of possibilities to appropriately match donor and recipient sites.[2]

Not all women are candidates for autologous abdominal tissue transfer or simply, they prefer to use a different donor site. Since the increased popularity of plastic surgery and the widely accessible plastic surgeon, more women are choosing to have procedures, including liposuction and abdominoplasty. Many of these women are not aware that one in seven women may develop breast cancer in their lifetime. Having procedures on their abdomen diminishes their reconstructive options for autologous breast reconstruction. Many women who have had prior abdominal surgeries in the past are not candidates for abdominal free tissue transfer, depending on the placement of the scar and the extent of their prior surgery.

Patient preference and body habitus has played a role in determining where autologous tissue is taken. Some women do not like the long abdominal scar and prefer not to have surgery on their abdomen. Women's body shape plays a role in determining where to harvest tissue from. Many women can be categorized into two main body shapes: pear and apple. The apple shaped women predominantly have fat in their abdomen and pear shapes have more fat in their thighs and buttock.

The surgeon needs to take all this into consideration before determining the appropriate donor site that meets the needs of the patient. Now, with several options, the plastic surgeon has more to choose from in his/her armamentarium.

This chapter will review several alternative flaps for breast reconstruction with donor sites, including the medial thigh and the buttock region. The choices of medial thigh flaps discussed include the transverse upper gracilis, the medial circumflex femoral artery both the musculocutaneous and septocutaneous variations, and the superficial femoral artery perforator flap. In terms of the buttock donor site, the superior and inferior gluteal artery perforator flaps with the septocutaneous variations will be discussed. The lumbar artery perforator and the deep femoral artery perforator flap will also be considered.

Basic science/disease process

Patients with invasive ductal/lobular or DCIS/LCIS are most commonly seen in our practice. Detail about these diseases is outside the remit of this chapter and therefore the reader should review specific breast cancer texts to ascertain more information about these processes.

Diagnosis/patient presentation

Patients usually present to our practice with either active breast cancer or after they have completed treatment. The immediate reconstruction population is usually referred by their breast surgeon for surgical options for breast reconstruction at the same time as unilateral or bilateral mastectomy. The breast surgeons affiliated with our practice are performing more and more nipple sparing procedures, depending on the cancer diagnosis, location, size and lymph node involvement. These procedures allow us to bury the flap, and, ultimately, they have the best aesthetic appearance.

The delayed reconstruction population can either have an implant that has a capsular contracture, which can be painful or asymmetric, or the patient wishes to have them removed for personal reasons. In these patients, more skin is required to make up the original

tissue loss versus the buried flap in the immediate reconstruction group. The alternative breast flaps from the buttock/thigh will give most women the volume and skin they need, but one must consider adjunctive procedures if the volume match is not identical.

Transverse upper gracilis free flap (TUG)

Patient selection

As described previously, there are many factors the reconstructive surgeon must take into consideration when finding the ideal donor site for breast reconstruction. Certain questions need to be asked. Is this patient undergoing immediate or delayed reconstruction? Has the patient received radiation or are they going to receive postoperative radiation? Is a skin sparing or nipple sparing mastectomy going to be used? Do they want to be the same size, smaller or larger? The answers to these questions help the surgeon gauge if more skin is needed, the type of volume acquired, and types of incisions to be used.

A thorough history is obtained. It is important that there is a discussion with the breast surgeon to determine the oncological procedures needed as these may impact on the type or timing of breast reconstruction. Finally, consideration must be given to the patient's body habitus, as well as to their preference.

Anatomy

The gracilis muscle is a narrow muscle extending from the pubic tubercle to the medial upper surface of the tibia. Its actions include thigh adduction and flexion, as well as leg flexion and medial rotation. It is categorized as a type II muscle by Mathes and Nahai with one dominant and one minor pedicle.[13] The motor innervation is by the obturator nerve arising from the lumbar plexus L3–L4 with its anterior branch supplying the gracilis muscle. The blood supply is from the medial circumflex femoral artery from the profunda femoris artery in which the dominant pedicle enters the medial aspect of the gracilis 6–10 cm inferior to the pubic tubercle. This vasculature then divides into a musculocutaneous and sometimes a septocutaneous branch. This division usually takes place in the upper third of the muscle. The venae comitantes follow the perforators and enter into the femoral vein. The saphenous vein also augments drainage to this area.

Treatment/surgical technique

Many of our patients undergo a preoperative CTA or MRA of the medial thigh to determine the perforator location and size. This study also allows us to differentiate between musculocutaneous versus septocutaneous perforators. It can also help determine the presence of a superficial femoral artery perforator.

The patient is seen the day before surgery and the markings are placed at this time. Identifying the medial edge of the adductor longus and measuring 8–10 cm inferior from the pubic tubercle, a mark is placed on the skin. The hand held Doppler is used to isolate the arterial signal of the medial circumflex femoral artery and or perforator through the skin. The skin island measures roughly 7 cm in width and 20–26 cm in length. The markings start lateral to the adductor longus muscle and course to the midline of the posterior thigh, centered over the key perforator or medial circumflex femoral artery.

Using a 10-blade, the superior limits of the incision marking are incised first, starting laterally and extending medially to posterior. Identification and preservation of the saphenous vein is done, sparing superficial lymph nodes. The incision is continued to the inferior marking to identify the inferior extent of the saphenous vein. A suprafascial dissection begins lateral to medial, identifying the adductor muscle. The deep fascia of the adductor longus is incised vertically. A septocutaneous perforator will be first visualized here. If this is not present, then a musculocutaneous perforator identification commences, first dissecting from an anterior direction and then switching to a posterior direction over the gracilis muscle. In some instances, the perforators are too small and then the flap is converted to a TUG flap with a small section of muscle taken. If the perforator is observed, it is dissected through the muscle until it enters the medial circumflex femoral vessels. The pedicle is followed to its origin from the profunda femoris artery and vein. The pedicle is then clipped at its origin. The flap is weighed and brought to the recipient site. Anastomoses are to the internal mammary vessels or their perforators. The harvested flap is long, narrow,

Hints and tips

- Preoperative imaging will shorten your operative time by one-third.
- Always locate the adductor when the patient comes in for preoperative markings. It will make the dissection faster in the operating room due to the consistency of the anatomy in this flap.
- Once the vessels are identified, dissect under the adductor from its posterior border, then switch to the anterior border to finish the dissection to the superficial femoral artery/vein.
- Keep the saphenous vein intact to keep the percentage of lymphedema minimal.
- Use a knife when dissecting the superior portion of the flap so as not to stun the lymph nodes and again to minimize lymphedema.

and curved. Suturing the proximal and distal ends of the flap together results in a conical shape with a large base and pointed top. The flap coning creates an excellent breast shape. The donor site is closed in layers over a suction drain.

Complications

The complications of the TUG flap are similar to those of a medial thigh lift. We have seen the tendency for the drains to stay in for 2–7 weeks. With the prolonged drainage, the infection rate is around 20%. This is treated with adequate drainage and antibiotics. The patient may develop transient lower leg edema shortly after the procedure. We encourage a compressive garment over the donor site to be worn for 6 weeks, to compress the dead space and expedite healing.

Distortion of the external genitalia or inferior migration of the scar has not occurred in our 71 cases. Preoperative placement of the upper incision near the inguinal crease helps hide the scar. Aesthetically, the upper thigh can be scooped out compared with the lower part. There is a natural narrowing of the thigh superiorly, so this is usually not an issue. If this becomes an issue, liposuction at a second stage can improve contour *(Figs 19.1–19.5)*.

Superior/inferior gluteal artery perforator free flap (SGAP/IGAP)

Video 1,2

The superior and inferior (s/i) gluteal artery perforator flap for breast reconstruction was described by our group in 1993.[20] Advantages of the gluteal artery perforator flap versus the previous myocutaneous gluteal flaps include preservation of the gluteus maximus muscle and additional length of the pedicle. Bilateral simultaneous s/i gaps are often done by our group but require two microsurgeons in order to minimize operating time as well as minimizing ischemia time for the flaps.[21,22] Preoperative CT/MRI angiograms allow identification of the septocutaneous variants of the S/IGAPS for breast reconstruction.[23,24] The angiograms identify the key perforators being musculocutaneous or septocutaneous caliber, location and course, allowing

mapping to occur. As with other perforator flaps donor site morbidity is minimal and no sacrifice of muscle is required. Overall, the SGAP is slightly more popular than the IGAP, but the upper buttock donor site may have a scooped out appearance. When a patient has a saddlebag deformity, the IGAP is a good choice because of an improved donor site contour and a hidden scar, which lies in the crease.[20,25,26] These techniques can be difficult and complicated. The occasional microsurgeon needs to be aware of the learning curve. It has been estimated that it takes approximately 50–100 procedures to become an expert with GAP flaps.

Patient selection

Most women who have undergone or will undergo mastectomies and wish to be reconstructed with autologous tissue, are potential candidates for SGAP/IGAP flaps. If the abdomen cannot be used as a donor site due to previous abdominoplasty, liposuction, or the presence of multiple surgical scars, then the buttock should be considered. Also, patients with excess tissue in the buttock versus the abdomen are the ideal candidates. In general, the buttock has a high fat to skin ratio, whereas the abdomen has a high skin to fat ratio. Patients who require mostly fat and little skin may be candidates for SGAP/IGAPS flaps. A significant amount of tissue may be harvested and, in our series, the average final inset weights of our GAP flaps were slightly greater than weights of the mastectomy specimens removed.

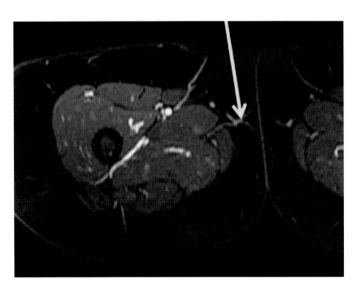

Fig. 19.1 MRA of transverse upper gracilis (TUG) free flap. The yellow arrow demonstrates the gracilis perforator from the gracilis branch of the medial circumflex femoral artery.

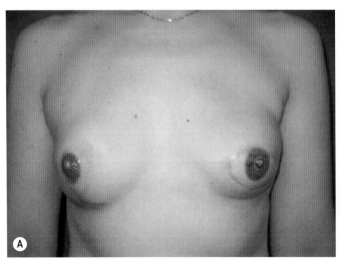
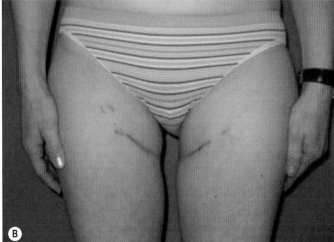

Fig. 19.2 (A,B) Postoperative bilateral TUG.

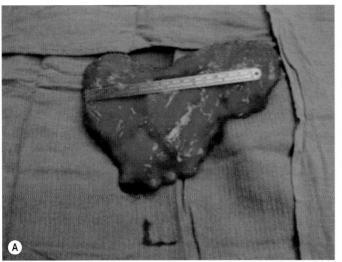
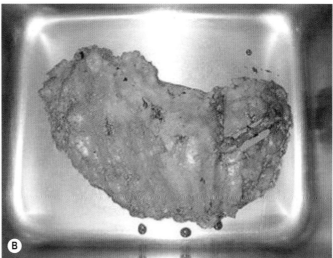

Fig. 19.3 Evolution of the TUG flap. **(A)** With and **(B)** without gracilis.

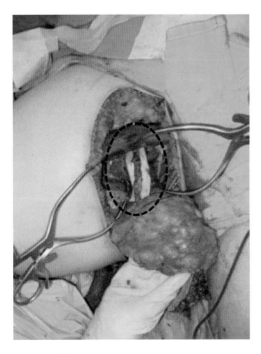

Fig. 19.4 TUG dissection.

Absolute contraindications specific to SGAP/IGAP flap breast reconstruction include previous liposuction at the donor site or active smoking within 1 month prior to surgery. Liposuction of the upper buttock is rare, so this typically does not often affect harvesting of the SGAP. Conversely, liposuction of the saddlebag area is more common, and this can affect the IGAP flap volume and circulation.

Anatomy

The superior gluteal artery is a continuation of the posterior division of the internal iliac artery. The artery has a limited length, which runs dorsally between the lumbosacral trunk and the first sacral nerve. It exits from the pelvis above the upper border of the piriformis muscle, where it quickly divides into both a superficial and deep branch. The deep branch travels between the iliac bone and gluteus medius muscle. The superficial branch continues to give off contributions to the upper portion of the gluteus muscle and overlying fat and skin. Anatomic location is planned when the femur is slightly flexed and rotated inward; a line is drawn from the posterior superior iliac spine to the posterior superior angle of the greater trochanter. The point of entrance of the superior gluteal artery from the upper part of the greater sciatic foramen corresponds to the junction of the upper and middle thirds of this line. Perforating vessels are found off the superficial branch of the superior gluteal artery.[27,28] Preoperatively CTA or MRA has greatly impacted planning of this procedure. Please provide either a drawing or a photograph of patient markings.

The inferior gluteal artery is a terminal branch of the anterior division of the internal iliac artery and exits the pelvis through the greater sciatic foramen.[29,30] A line is drawn from the posterior superior iliac spine to the outer part of the ischial tuberosity; the junction of its lower with its middle third marks the point of

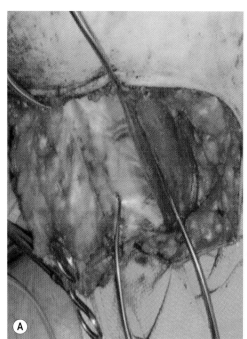

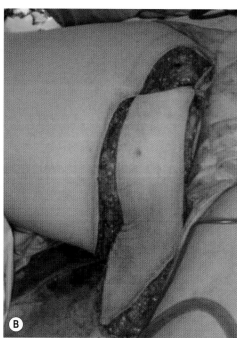

Fig. 19.5 (A,B) Intraoperative TUG.

emergence of the inferior gluteal and its surrounding vessels from the lower part of the greater sciatic foramen. The artery accompanies the greater sciatic nerve, internal pudendal vessels and the posterior femoral cutaneous nerve. In this sub-fascial recess, the inferior gluteal vein will receive tributaries from other pelvic veins. The inferior gluteal vasculature continues towards the surface by perforating the sacral fascia. It exits the pelvis caudal to the piriformis muscle. Once under the inferior portion of the gluteus maximus, perforating vessels are seen branching out through the substance of the muscle to feed the overlying skin and fat. The course of the inferior gluteal artery perforating vessels is more oblique through the substance of the gluteus maximus muscle than the course of the superior gluteal artery perforators, which tend to travel more directly to the superficial tissue up through the muscle. Thus, the length of the inferior gluteal artery perforator and the resultant pedicle length for the IGAP flap is 7–10 cm. The SGAP pedicle is 5–8 cm in length. Because the skin island is placed inferior to the origin of the inferior gluteal vessels, a longer pedicle is usually obtained.

The direction of the perforating vessels can be superior, lateral or inferior. Perforating vessels that nourish the medial and inferior portions of the buttock have relatively short intramuscular lengths; 5–7 cm, depending on the thickness of the muscle. Perforators,

which nourish the lateral portions of the overlying skin paddle, are observed traveling through the muscle substance in an oblique manner 4–6 cm before turning upwards towards the skin surface. By traveling through the muscle for relatively long distances, these vessels are longer than their medially based counterparts. The perforating vessels can be separated from the underlying gluteus maximus muscle and fascia and traced down to the parent vessel, forming the basis for the inferior gluteal artery perforator flap. Between 2 and 4 perforating vessels originating from the inferior gluteal artery will be located in the lower half of the gluteus maximus.[24]

After giving off perforators in the buttocks, the inferior gluteal artery then descends into the thigh accompanied by the posterior femoral cutaneous nerve and follows a long course, eventually surfacing to supply the skin of the posterior thigh.[26] The branches of the inferior gluteal nerve (L5, S1–2) supply the skin of the inferior buttock. A neurosensory flap can be elevated if these nerves are preserved in the dissection of the flap.[31,32]

The superior gluteal nerve arises from the dorsal divisions of the fourth and fifth lumbar and first sacral nerves. It exits the pelvis through the greater sciatic foramen above the piriformis muscle, accompanied by the superior gluteal vessels, and divides into both superior and inferior branches. The superior and inferior branches of the nerves travel with their corresponding arterial branches to end up in the gluteus medius, gluteus minimus, and tensor fasciae lata, respectively.

The inferior gluteal nerve arises from the dorsal divisions of the fifth lumbar and first and second sacral nerves. It exits the pelvis through the greater sciatic foramen below the piriformis muscle, and divides into branches that enter the deep surface of the gluteus maximus.

The posterior femoral cutaneous nerve innervates the skin of the perineum and posterior surface of the thigh and leg. It arises partly from the dorsal divisions of the first and second, and from the ventral divisions of the second and third sacral nerves, and issues from the pelvis through the greater sciatic foramen below the piriformis muscle, along with the inferior gluteal artery. It then descends beneath the gluteus maximus, the fascia lata, and travels over the long head of the biceps femoris to the posterior knee. Finally, it pierces the deep fascia and accompanies the lesser saphenous vein to the middle of the posterior leg. Some terminal branches communicate with the sural nerve. All its branches are cutaneous and distributed to the gluteal region, the perineum, and the posterior thigh and leg.

Surgical technique

The chest is marked in a sitting position. The midline and the inframammary crease on both sides are marked to be at the same level. If a patient is undergoing immediate breast reconstruction, skin markings are drawn on the breast, which include marks for the mastectomy as well as inframammary fold. In patients who are undergoing a nipple-sparring mastectomy vertical, lateral, or inframammary incision is marked.

For unilateral SGAP flap markings, the patient is placed in a lateral decubitus position. Preoperative CT or MR angiography along with the hand held Doppler probe are used to locate perforating vessels from the superior gluteal artery. These are usually located approximately one-third of the distance on a line from the posterior superior iliac crest to the greater trochanter. Additional perforators may be found slightly more lateral from above. It should be noted that perforators located laterally would produce longer pedicles thus allowing easier anastomosis.

Septocutaneous perforators are the most lateral and course between the gluteal maximus and medius. The skin paddle is marked in an oblique pattern from inferior medial to superior lateral to include these perforators. On average, the flap height and length is 7–10 cm and 18–24 cm. For bilateral SGAP planning, the patient is marked in the prone position.

For the IGAP flap, the gluteal fold is noted with the patient in a standing position. The inferior limit of the flap is marked 1 cm inferior and parallel to the gluteal fold. The patient is then placed in the lateral position for unilateral reconstruction and prone for bilateral reconstruction. CT or MRA, and the hand held Doppler probe is used to locate perforating vessels from the inferior gluteal artery. An ellipse is drawn for the skin paddle to include these perforators, which roughly parallels the gluteal fold with dimensions of approximately 7 × 18 cm. To include the "saddle bag" deformity, the skin pattern is shifted more laterally. This prevents harvesting the fat pad over the ischial tuberosity medial to the gluteus maximus muscle in order to prevent discomfort on sitting.

For unilateral procedures, the patient is placed in the lateral decubitus position and a two-team approach is used. The recipient vessels are prepared, while the SGAP/IGAP flap is harvested. For breast reconstruction, the internal mammary vessels or internal mammary perforators are preferred as anastomosis to these vessels allows easier medialization of the flap when it is inset. Often we need to remove some rib cartilage in order to gain length necessary to perform the anastomosis. The IGAP flap often has a long enough pedicle that will reach to the thoracodorsal vessels, however the SGAP may be challenging due to a shorter pedicle length. For bilateral simultaneous GAP flap reconstructions, the procedure is started supine. After mastectomy and recipient vessel preparation, the patient is positioned prone for flap harvest. Then the patient is repositioned supine for anastomosis and insetting.

The skin incisions are made and dissection circumferentially down to the gluteus maximus is performed. Beveling is performed as needed, particularly lateral to the muscle in the superior and inferior direction, to harvest enough tissue for width and volume to create a natural breast shape. The flap is elevated from the muscle in the subfascial plane, and the perforators are approached beginning from lateral to medial or medial to lateral. It is preferred to use a single large perforator, if present, but two perforators in the same plane and the direction of the gluteus maximus muscle fibers can be taken together as well. The muscle is then spread in the direction of the muscle fibers and the perforators are followed through the muscle. The dissection continues until both the artery and the vein are of sufficient size to be anastomosed to the recipient vessels in the chest. The artery usually is the limiting factor in this dissection. The arterial perforator is visualized and preserved as it enters the main ascending superior gluteal artery or the descending inferior gluteal artery. The preferable artery and vein diameter for anastomosis is 2.0–2.5 mm and 3.0–4.0 mm, respectively. When using the internal mammary vein (IMV) perforators as recipient, a shorter pedicle and smaller artery will suffice thereby simplifying flap harvest.

When the recipient vessels are ready, the gluteal artery and vein are divided and the flap is weighed. The skin and fat overlying the gluteus maximus muscle and posterior thigh with the IGAP are elevated superiorly and inferiorly to allow layered approximation of the fat of the donor site to prevent a contour deformity. The donor site is closed in several layers over a suction drain. Adding permanent removable skin suture increases the strength of the skin closure.

The anastomosis is performed to the recipient vessels under the operating microscope. The flap is inset over a suction drain into the breast pocket with care taken not to twist or kink the pedicle. To create a spherical flap, the ends of the ellipse are excised or approximated. The flap may be inset horizontally, vertically, or obliquely, depending on the situation.

Hints and tips

- Use preoperative imaging CTA/MRA to identify your perforators.
- Doppler out your perforator in the office once the CT/MR mapping is completed.
- Draw you skin paddle and take a photograph. Study this photograph the night before and morning of surgery; you may want to alter the pattern and make sure they are symmetrical.
- Use two skilled micro-surgeons so that simultaneous dissection can be accomplished.
- The first part of the dissection is predictable; the last 1 2-cm is where the most of the injuries occur because of the confluence of vessels.

Postoperative care

Our patients have a 1–2 hour stay in the recovery room and then are transferred to their private room with monitoring of the flap circulation every 2 hours for the night, then every 4 hours on postoperative day one. The ICU is not necessarily needed, though in institutions where experienced nursing staff is not available, it may be considered. Patients typically go home on the third or fourth postoperative day. The drain at the donor site usually will be left in place for at least 10 days and removed when draining <40 cc in a 24-hour period. Breast drains are usually removed on postoperative day three.

Complications

In a review of 492 GAP flaps performed by our unit for breast reconstruction, the incidence of complications was low. The overall take-back rate for vascular complications was 6%, mostly commonly venous being 4% with arterial 2%. The total flap failure rate was approximately 2%. Donor site seroma occurred in 15% of patients requiring aspiration. Approximately 20% of patients required revision of the donor site at the second stage of breast reconstruction.[19,21]

The most common reason for donor site revisions of the SGAP is contour deformity of the upper buttock. The most common revision for the donor site IGAP is liposuction of the lateral trochanter fat for contouring. 'Dog-ear' revisions are often done at the time of second stage breast reconstruction of both S/IGAP. Recipient site complications include fat necrosis rate of 8% with both S/IGAP flaps requiring revision. Breast flap contour asymmetry requires fat grafting or revision in approximately 10% of cases *(Figs 19.6–19.12)*.

The deep femoral artery perforator flap (DFAP)

The deep femoral artery perforator has one or two accompanying veins. At the site of the pedical harvest harvest the flap vein is 2–3 mm in diameter and a good match to the internal mammary recipient vein. Approximately 15% of patients have a large perforator from the profunda femoris artery. This perforator passes posterior to the proximal femur deep to the gluteus

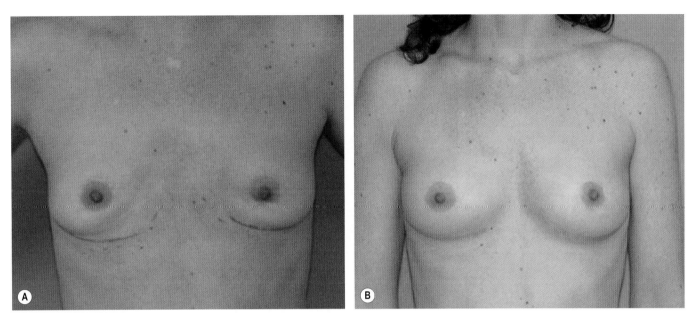

Fig. 19.6 (A,B) Superior gluteal artery free flap (SGAP) augmentation.

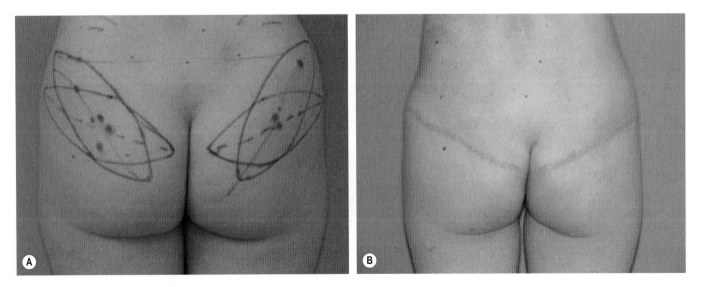

Fig. 19.7 (A,B) Pre- and postoperative photographs.

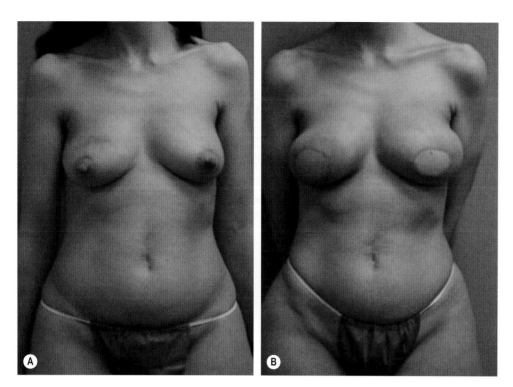

Fig. 19.8 (A,B) SGAP reconstruction.

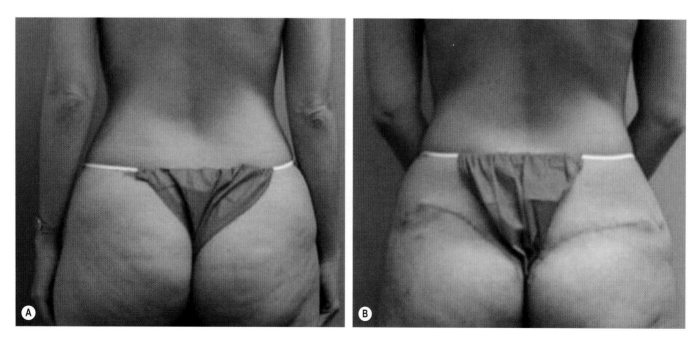

Fig. 19.9 (A,B) SGAP donor site.

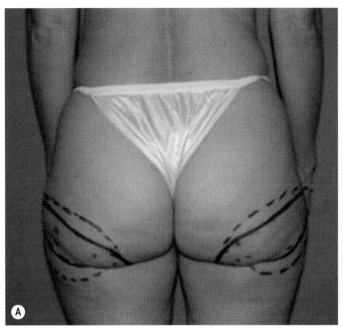

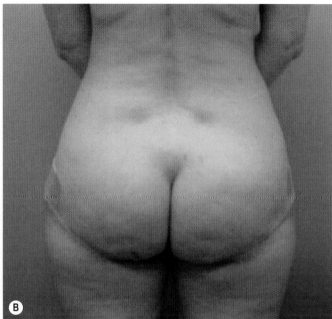

Fig. 19.10 **(A,B)** Improved buttock contour.

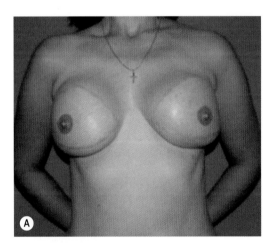

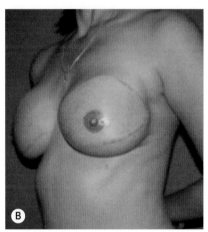

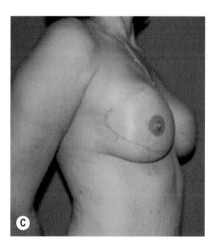

Fig. 19.11 **(A–C)** Bilateral inferior gluteal myocutaneous flap (IGAP) postoperative.

maximus and enters the trochanteric fat pad. MRA has been most important in identifying this perforator. The flap design has been the same as in the crease GAP flap described earlier. The advantage of this flap is a large septocutaneous perforator with excellent flap profusion. The disadvantage is a relatively short pedicle (6 cm) and an artery (2 mm) smaller than the internal mammary artery. We have used the DFAP flap for five cases of breast reconstruction, with excellent results. Recipient vessels are either the IMA/V or their perforators *(Figs 19.13–19.15)*.

Lumbar artery perforator flap (LAP)

The LAP flap for breast reconstruction was described by de Weerd et al. in 2003.[33] CTA or MRA demonstrates large perforators in the lower lumbar area. Either the 3rd or 4th lumbar perforator is selected based on the preoperative imaging with a MRA or CTA. The lumbar perforators arise from the aorta. Pedical length is short, approximately 5 cm. Arterial diameter is approximated 1.5 mm and venous diameter is approximately 2 mm. The LAP flap design captures the hip roll area above the

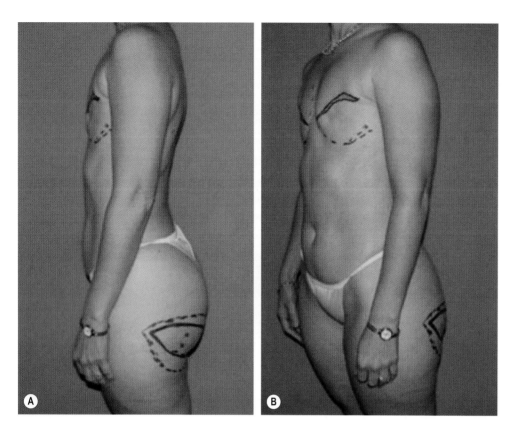

Fig. 19.12 (A,B) Bilateral IOGAP markings.

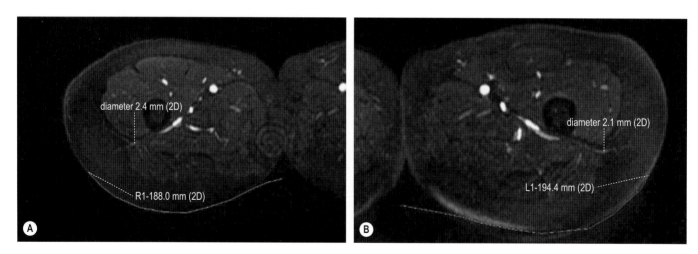

Fig. 19.13 Deep femoral artery perforator (DFAP) flap.

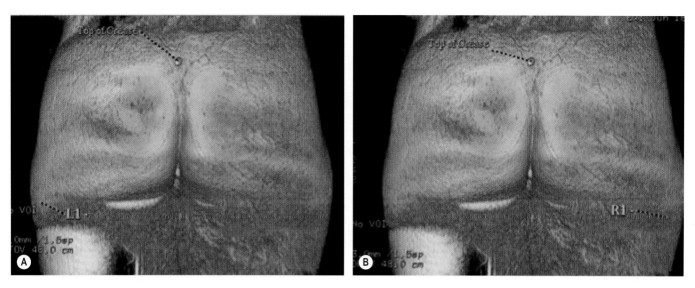

Fig. 19.14 3D MRA of DFAP flap.

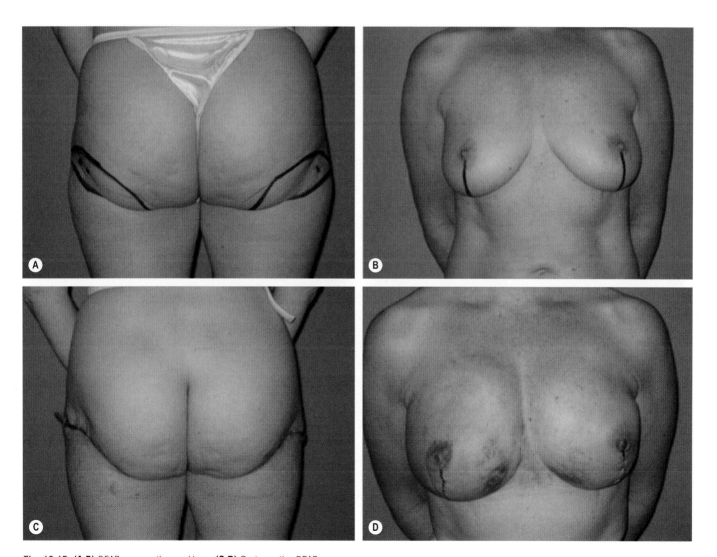

Fig. 19.15 (A,B) DFAP preoperative markings. **(C,D)** Postoperative DFAP.

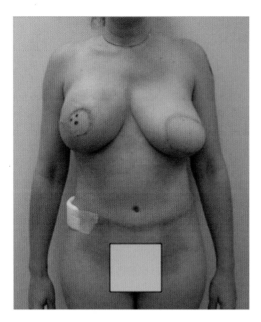

Fig. 19.16 Right lumbar artery perforator flap (LAP).

iliac crest. Advantage is good volume of fat in many patients without causing a contour deformity of the buttock. Disadvantages include a relatively short pedicle (5–6 cm) and a relatively small diameter artery (1.8–2 mm). We have used this in three breast reconstructions with good results *(Figs 19.16, 19.17)*.

Hints and tips

- Use preoperative imagining identifying the perforators.
- When dissecting the internal mammary vessels in the chest, leave the second perforator; it is often a good size match for the smaller vessels in these two flaps. It is also a good secondary blood supply if the internal mammary vein/artery becomes damaged.

Secondary procedures

We use several secondary procedures to enhance the volume or to refine the shape and symmetry. To add volume, we usually employ the ICAP (intercostal artery perforator) flap. This has a consistent blood supply at the anterior axillary line between the 7th and 8th rib. The flap measures 7 × 22 cm. It is harvested starting on the back in the bra-line; using sharp and blunt dissection it is dissected until at 2 cm of where the skin

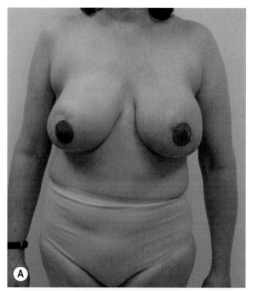

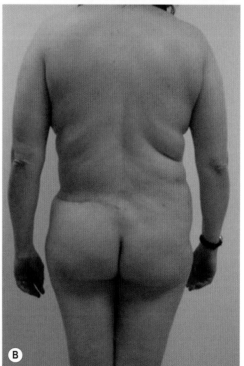

Fig. 19.17 (A,B) Right LAP postoperative photographs.

Doppler has a signal. Using a bipolar, the rest of the tissue is dissected until the perforator is met. The perforator is skeletonized 360° allowing the flap to be rotated superiorly or inferiorly to add the additional volume the breast requires. The coning of the flap gives the breast a natural shape.

Fat grafting has become one of our cornerstones of secondary procedures. The patient is under liposuction, the fat is filtered and centrifuged for 3 min and injected into the breast in several planes starting in the deep layer and moving more superficial with each 1 cc injection of fat. In one sitting, 350 cc of fat can be easily injected. Our fat survival is from 30–80%.

There are several ways one can design a nipple. We use an arrow-pattern flap with relatively good viability and projection. Each of these flaps has to be designed 30–50% larger because the flap will constrict with time. At the end of the process, the women will undergo tattooing to complete their journey.

Access the complete references list online at **http://www.expertconsult.com**

1. Allen RJ, Treece P. Deep inferior epigastric perforator flap for breast reconstruction. *Ann Plast Surg*. 1994;32:32.

5. Yousif NJ, Matloub HS, Kolachalam R, et al. The transverse gracilis musculocutaneous flap. *Ann Plast Surg*. 1992;29:482.

8. Hallock GG. The gracilis (medical circumflex femoral) perforator flap: a medial groin free flap. *Ann Plast Surg*. 2003;59(6):655–658.

14. Shaw WW. Breast reconstruction by superior gluteal microvascular free flaps without silicone implants. *Plast Reconstr Surg*. 1983;72(4):490–501.

15. Shaw WW. Microvascular free flap breast reconstruction. *Clin Plast Surg*. 1984;11:333.

20. Allen RJ, Tucker Jr C. Superior gluteal artery perforator free flap for breast reconstruction. *Plast Reconstr Surg*. 1995;95(7):1207–1212.

22. DellaCroce FJ, Sullivan SK. Application and refinement of the superior gluteal artery perforator free flap for bilateral simultaneous breast reconstruction. *Plast Reconstr Surg*. 2005;116(1):97–105.

25. Allen RJ, Levine, JL, Granzow JW. The in-the-crease inferior gluteal artery perforator flap for breast reconstruction. *Plast Reconstr Surg*. 2006;118(2):333–339.

26. Granzow JW, Levine JL, Chiu ES, et al. Breast reconstruction with gluteal artery perforator flaps. *J Plast Reconstr Aesthet Surg*. 2006;59(6):571–579.

31. Koshima I, Moriguchi T, Soeda S, et al. The gluteal perforator-based flap for repair of sacral pressure sores. *Plast Reconstr Surg*. 1993;91:678–683.

20

Omentum reconstruction of the breast

Joao Carlos Sampaio Góes and Antonio Luiz Vasconcellos Macedo

SYNOPSIS

- The use of the omentum flap is flexible, safe and provides several operative solutions.
- Videolaparoscopic approach is very safe, takes 60–90 min and provides fast postoperative recovery.
- This technique is mainly used in skin sparing mastectomy.
- The omentum flap can be used to create a central volume on the reconstructed breast or to cover a breast implant.
- It is a great surgery for repair of a failed reconstruction.

 Access the Historical Perspective sections online at
http://www.expertconsult.com

Introduction

Skin preservation in the treatment of breast cancer enables breast reconstruction with autologous tissue, differing from the traditional myocutaneous flaps. Implants are often an option for these cases, but when autogenous tissue is desired and skin not required, the omentum is an excellent choice. We have used video-laparoscopic total mobilization of the omentum since 1995. It has proven to be an excellent option to reconstruct total breast volume, in reoperations of inadequate reconstructions, reconstructing the soft tissues which cover silicone prostheses, and for bilateral use in pro-phylactic surgery to reduce the risk of breast cancer.

Basic science/disease process

Our technique was developed based on the experience of the senior author with skin-sparing mastectomy and the use of mesh support in breast surgery. This procedure follows the basic principles of breast recon-struction in an original way. First, the new breast's volume is obtained by insetting the laparoscopically harvested omental flap, based on the gastroepiploic vessels. Breast shape is defined and supported by an internal bra consisting of synthetic mixed mesh that wraps and fixates the flap to the thoracic wall. Finally, the skin-sparing mastectomy technique offers high-quality coverage with native skin and reduced and well-positioned scars.

Later, we started using the omentum to cover silicone implants, creating a protection tissue layer underneath the skin, partially conjugating it with the pectoralis major muscle and mixed mesh, whenever required. This composition of tissues covering the mesh and the silicone prosthesis creates a structure which simulates mammary tissue and does not enable skin adherence to the muscular plane, providing good aesthetic results in the reconstruction of skin sparing mastectomy similar to those obtained in augmentation mammoplasty. This tissue structure also creates an excellent protection for the mammary prosthesis, enabling good scarring adaptation and low complication rates.

Another advance of this technique was the use of mixed mesh to partially cover and support the lower hemisphere of the silicone prosthesis, which is then sutured to the lower edge of the pectoralis major muscle and to the inframammary fold (IMF). The pectoralis major is then released on the sternal region to decrease function, avoiding lateral projection without losing coverage of the upper hemisphere of the implants. The use of omentum flap is flexible, safe, and provides several solutions. Videolaparoscopic approach is very safe, takes 60–90 min, and provides good postoperative recovery.

Patient selection

The following points are important when selecting patients for this procedure. The patient needs to have enough good quality skin for the reconstruction; the omentum flap and the implant will provide the new breast volume. Abdominal cavity conditions for laparoscopic harvesting must be evaluated prior to surgery. Unfortunately, it is not possible to evaluate the volume of the omentum before surgery, but with the anatomical characteristics of the patient is possible to get an idea of the amount that may be used for the reconstruction. History of previous abdominal surgery near the omentum should be considered and any impact on the integrity of the pedicle.

Treatment/surgical technique

Laparoscopic harvesting of the omental flap

With the patient appropriately positioned, the abdominal cavity is inflated with CO_2 until intra-abdominal pressure is 10 mmHg. A Veress needle is then inserted through the umbilicus, followed by a 0-degree fiberoptic camera. Under direct visualization, two 12-mm trocars are symmetrically inserted 6 cm from the midline and 4 cm above the umbilicus. Two accesses for the surgeon's instruments and one for the assistant are established 4 cm caudal to the costal margin, at the level of the right midclavicular line.

The surgeon, positioned between the patient's legs, mobilizes the omentum using a forceps and an ultrasound-assisted dissector. Metallic clips are

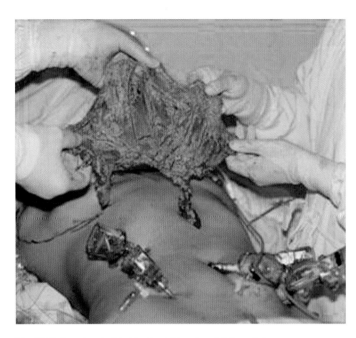

Fig. 20.1 Omentum isolated by the right gastroepiploic pedicle.

employed for hemostasis of vessels whose diameter exceeds 1 mm. Dissections between the omentum and colon progresses from left to right exposing the posterior portion of the stomach (from the duodenum to the gastric fundus), keeping the omentum connected to the stomach by its gastroepiploic pedicles *(Fig. 20.1)*. The left gastroepiploic pedicle is ligated using a 30-mm linear endoscopic stapler.

The omentum is exteriorized through a 5–6 cm midline incision in the upper epigastric region. The gastric branches of the gastroepiploic arcade are ligated from left to right until the right gastroepiploic pedicle is completely isolated. Extreme care must be taken when exteriorizing the flap to avoid torsion or kinking of the pedicle. The flap is then tunneled subcutaneously toward the mastectomy site *(Fig. 20.2)*. Aponeurosis is closed in the epigastric region using 0 Prolene sutures, leaving a 2 cm opening for the flap's pedicle. At this moment, the pedicle must be checked once more for kinking, compression, or torsion. The subcutaneous layers and skin are finally closed using Monocryl 4-0 sutures.

Omentum reconstruction

Immediate post-mastectomy reconstruction is performed by placing the omental flap anterior to the

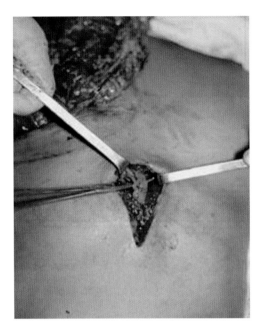

Fig. 20.2 Pedicle placed in the subcutaneous tunnel.

pectoralis major muscle and fixating it with Monocryl 4-0 sutures. Factors such as the breast's volume, limits, and projection are determined, and more volume is concentrated in the inferior hemisphere.

The synthetic mesh is then placed over the omentum to shape and support the new breast. Fixation of the mesh to the pectoralis major muscle is carried out using titanium clips or interrupted nylon 4-0 sutures *(Fig. 20.3)*. Skin closure is performed using a Mersilene 3-0 purse-string suture to completely cover the new breast cone, define its limits and complete the shaping process. Suction drains exteriorized at the level of the anterior axillary line are kept for 5 days or until drainage is <20 mL/day. *Figure 20.4* shows the preoperative condition for comparison purposes and *Figure 20.4B* demonstrates the immediate postoperative shape created.

Omentum reconstruction and implant

When patients have prior silicone prosthesis and the case enables the use of the previous prosthesis for reconstruction, the prostheses' capsule may be used to envelope a new prosthesis, and the omentum will cover it and replace only the volume of mammary tissue obtained at the skin-sparing mastectomy. This option provides good aesthetic results and does not

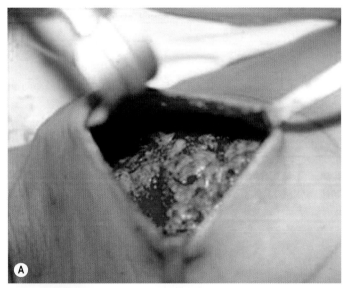

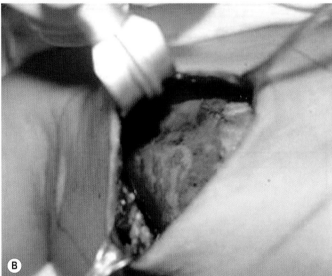

Fig. 20.3 (A,B) Omentum anterior to pectoralis major.

require surgical manipulation of thoracic muscles *(Figs 20.5–20.7)*.

Use of implants, pectoralis major muscle, mixed-mesh, and omental flap

This is a complex surgical option, however it provides excellent aesthetic results, with low complication rates, overcoming the disadvantages of mammary reconstruction using expanders.

The pectorals major muscle is used to cover the upper hemisphere of the implant and is inferiorly and

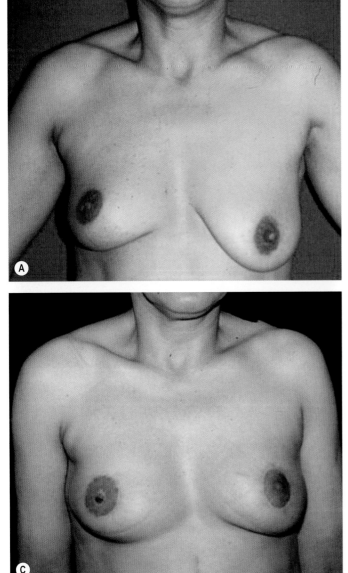

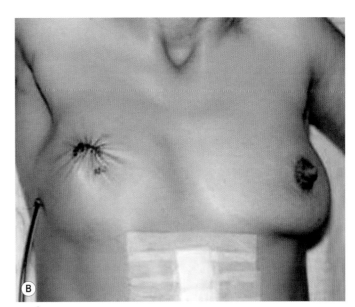

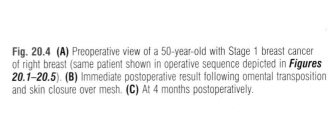

Fig. 20.4 **(A)** Preoperative view of a 50-year-old with Stage 1 breast cancer of right breast (same patient shown in operative sequence depicted in *Figures 20.1–20.5*). **(B)** Immediate postoperative result following omental transposition and skin closure over mesh. **(C)** At 4 months postoperatively.

medially released. The implant is laterally covered by the border of the serratus anterior muscle. We use anatomic implants with a thin cone-shaped upper pole which adapts well to submuscular space.

The lower hemisphere of the implant is covered by a mixed mesh or an acellular dermal matrix (ADM) layer, the inferior edge of the pectoralis major and to the IMF,

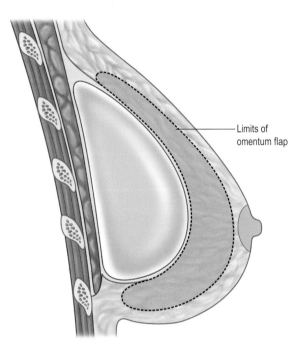

Limits of
omentum flap

Fig. 20.5 Reconstruction with implant covered by omental flap.

thus creating a deep coverage which will hold and position the implant.

The omentum is positioned and fixated with polyglactin 3-0 stitches covering the mixed mesh or AMD and the pectoralis major, creating a second intermediate coverage between the prosthesis and the superficial cutaneous coverage *(Fig. 20.8)*. Thus, the omentum provides a larger amount of tissue and volume similar to mammary tissue and does not allow skin adherent to deep planes, causing undesirable retractions due to contractions of the pectoralis major. Another advantage is the inferior release of the pectoralis major, avoiding lateral mobilization of the prosthesis caused by its dynamics when it fully covers the implant.

Complementing with lipofilling

Lipofilling is a frequently used alternative operation that increases the thickness of the skin flap in areas of interest, thus providing good fat coverage for the implants. Cannulas of 3 mm are used to harvest fat, and filling is performed in parallel tunnels in the subdermal space *(Figs 20.9, 20.10)*.

Bilateral reconstruction

The omentum may be used for bilateral reconstruction. The desired volume for each side should be defined

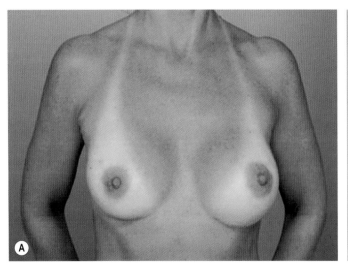

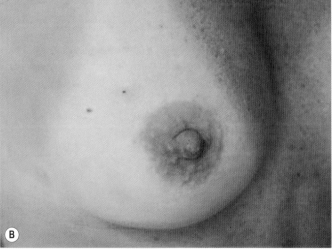

Fig. 20.6 (A) Mastectomy areolar approach. **(B)** reconstruction with implant covered by omental flap.

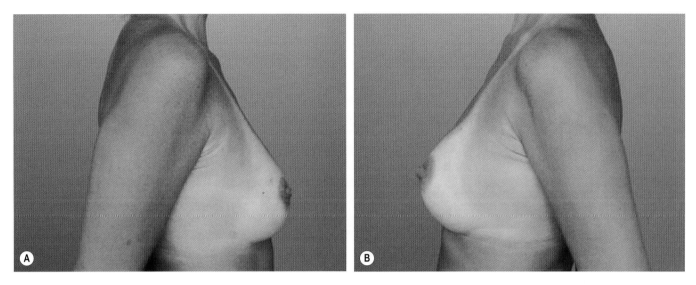

Fig. 20.7 (A) Mastectomy areolar approach and reconstruction with implant covered by omental flap. **(B)** Left breast shown with augmentation with an implant to show symmetry.

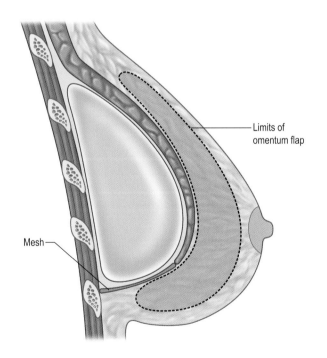

Limits of
omentum flap

Mesh

Fig. 20.8 Reconstruction with omental flap, anatomic implant and mixed mesh.

and the omentum should be divided among its branches, keeping the main pedicle of the gastroepiploic artery. A "Y" tunnel is created at the epigastric incision, through which each half of the omentum flap is passed to the breasts. This technique is often used in prophylactic bilateral mastectomy reconstructions *(Figs 20.11–20.13)*.

Closing the epigastric region

Since 1996, when we described the technique of omentum total approach with a pedicle in the right branch of the gastroepiploic artery and vein mobilized by videolaparoscopy, the procedure has been performed with subcutaneous tunnelization to the breast. The abdominal wall opening in the epigastric region should have a diameter of at least 3 cm to allow the passage of the omentum.

The epigastric skin incision mentioned by the author is optional. The authors personally favor it due to three important reasons:

1. The passage of the omentum through the tunnel is smoother and more controlled, avoiding injury to the vessels and enabling a better position of the omentum and its pedicle.

2. The opening in the abdominal wall must be closed to avoid epigastric herniation as a consequence. Presently, we use a small mixed mesh overlapping the pedicle fixed in the anterior fascia to create a local fibrosis controlling the development of omentum herniation in the area. A 4 cm skin

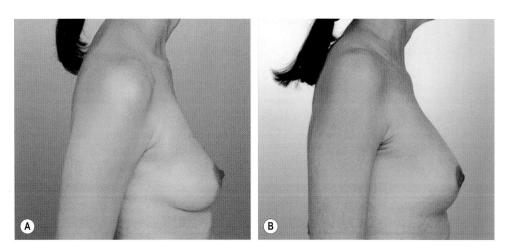

Fig. 20.9 Bilateral areolar mastectomy and reconstruction with implant covered by muscle, mixed mesh and omental flap. **(A)** Preoperative and **(B)** postoperative views.

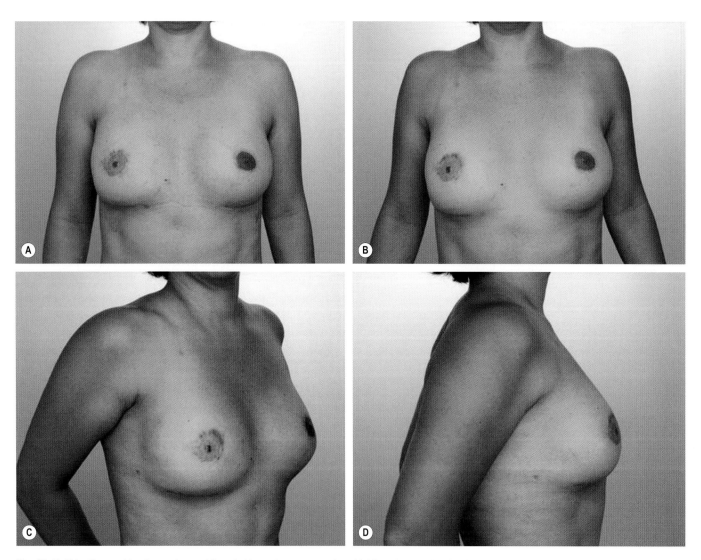

Fig. 20.10 This 42-year-old patient underwent bilateral skin-sparing mastectomies with bilateral anatomic cohesive gel implants partially covered by the pectoralis major muscle and mixed mesh. An omental flap was used on the right breast to increase soft tissue coverage and lipofilling in left breast. Two different techniques were used to improve coverage on each side with the same result achieved. The omentum is preferred when the mastectomy skin flap is thinner. **(A)** Postoperative result at 2 months. **(B–D)** Postoperative late result at 6 months.

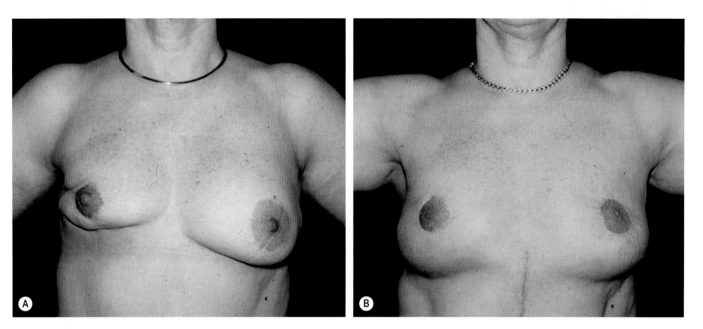

Fig. 20.11 (A) Preoperative view of a 63-year-old patient who is status post-quadrantectomy and radiotherapy with persistent deformity. **(B)** At 2 years postoperatively, after undergoing completion mastectomy on the right and implant removal on the left. Reconstruction was performed only with omentum without mesh. Some 80% of the omentum was used on the right and 20% to augment the volume on the left.

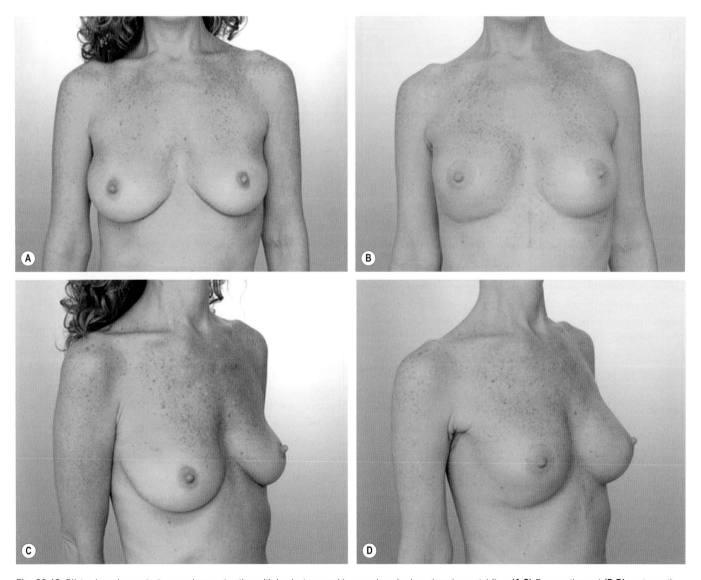

Fig. 20.12 Bilateral areolar mastectomy and reconstruction with implant covered by muscle, mixed mesh and omental flap. **(A,C)** Preoperative and **(B,D)** postoperative views.

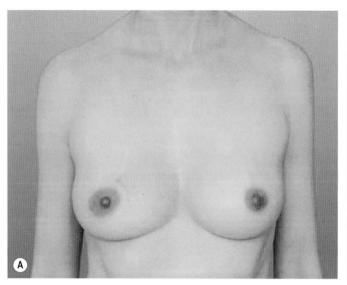
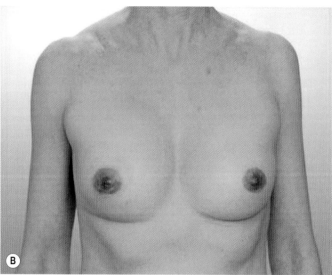

Fig. 20.13 Bilateral areolar mastectomy and reconstruction with implant covered by muscle, mixed mesh and omental flap. **(A)** Preoperative and **(B)** postoperative views.

incision in the area is fundamental to perform this procedure.

3. As in prophylactic surgery to reduce the risk of breast cancer, the epigastric skin incision is usually made to approach the omentum in bilateral reconstructions, splitting and manipulating it.

Symmetry and reconstruction of the nipple-areola complex

Symmetry

When symmetrization is performed as a second-stage procedure after 45–60 days, we prefer to reduce the opposite breast using the double-skin periareolar mammaplasty technique with or without mesh support. This provides a very similar breast in terms of shape and position of the nipple-areola complex.

Reconstruction of the nipple-areola complex

When necessary, reconstruction of the nipple-areola complex is also performed as a second-stage procedure. We prefer a full-thickness skin graft from the groin because it covers the mastectomy scar and results in an exclusive periareolar scar. The nipple is reconstructed using local flaps or a graft from the opposite nipple.

Postoperative care

Our patients stay in the hospital for 3 days postoperatively. There is no special care beside standard laparoscopic postoperative care. Vacuum drain is kept on the breast for 5 days and we use a bandage to mold the new breast in the ideal position and help to heal the skin to the inner structures. We do not use massage and patients are advised to avoid exercise for 2 months.

Outcomes, prognosis, and complications

Because it is a safe flap, with abundant vascularization, the complication rate with this technique is low. With 15 years' experience and 200 cases performed, we have not had any cases of omentum flap or mastectomy skin necrosis. We had one case of infection at the mixed mesh site, which was easily controlled by surgical cleansing and antibiotic therapy. There were no cases of seroma and four cases of small and easily absorbed hematomas were observed, which is probably due to the high scarring and absorption capacity of the omentum.

One case of intestinal adherence required laparotomy and enterolysis, and the patient subsequently had good resolution. No cases of thrombosis or pulmonary embolism were observed. Postoperative follow-up was uneventful with oral feeding on the first postoperative day and mean hospitalization time of 2.5 days.

We observed that, at the site of omentum exteriorization, the 5–7 mm passage left for the vascular pedicle did not result in hernia; however, the pedicle may have an unpleasant movement for the patient, increasing its subcutaneous volume. To correct this, a small mixed mesh was placed over the pedicle, at the time of surgery, fixating it on the fascia thus creating a coverage fibrosis at the outlet of the pedicle.

Secondary procedures

The omentum pedicle can be sectioned after 2 months without compromising blood supply. Any other surgical manipulation is very easily done as the omentum fat is soft and flexible. The mixed mesh can be incised surgically and sutured if necessary during the post operative time if needed without compromising the aesthetic result.

 Access the complete references list online at **http://www.expertconsult.com**

2. Góes JCS, Macedo ALV. Immediate reconstruction after mastectomy using a periareolar approach with an omental flap and mixed mesh support. *Perspect Plast Surg*. 1996;10(1):69–81.

   First publication using total laparoscopic harvesting omentum flap to breast reconstruction. Also the association with mixed mesh support was an innovation at that time. The authors present a series of five cases with a one and a half year follow-up with excellent results.

3. Góes JCS. Breast reconstruction after mastectomy by areolar approach. In: Figueira Fo ASS, Novais-Dias E, Salvador Silva HM, et al, eds. *Mastology: breast disease*. New York: Elsevier Science; 1995:375–378.

   First publication describing the skin sparing periareolar mastectomy. The author presents 34 patients with 4 years follow-up and immediate reconstruction with TRAM flap. The importance of this publication is that this kind of mastectomy opens up a great field to many modern breast reconstructive techniques, including the omentum flap use.

5. Góes JCS, Macedo ALV. Immediate reconstruction after skin-sparing mastectomy using the omental flap and synthetic mesh. In: Spear S, ed. *Surgery of the breast principles of the art*. 2nd ed. Philadelphia: Lippincott; 2006:786–793.

   Authors present an evolution of the technique with an update of the procedure. Also shown is a clinical radiological study of the omentum and the mixed mesh in the late follow-up.

9. Costa SS, Blotta RM, Mariano MB, et al. Laparoscopic treatment of Poland's syndrome using the omentum flap technique. *Clinics (Sao Paulo)*. 2010;65(4):401–406.

   For patients with Poland syndrome, a transverse skin fold in the anterior axillary pillar, infraclavicular depression and an anomalous breast contour are the most uncomfortable disfigurements. This study aims to demonstrate that superior aesthetic results can be achieved by using a laparoscopically harvested omentum flap to treat this condition. The outcomes of these patients revealed that the omentum flap technique provided superior amelioration of the deformities caused by Poland syndrome when compared with other reconstructive options.

11. Zaha H, Inamine S. Laparoscopically harvested omental flap: results for 96 patients. *Surg Endosc*. 2010;24(1):103–107.

    Recent advances in endoscopic surgery have allowed laparoscopic harvesting of the omental flap with minimal deformity of the donor site. This study aimed to assess the safety and long-term complication rate for laparoscopic harvest of the omental flap (LHOF). As a safe and minimally invasive procedure, LHOF has a low incidence of short- and long-term complications. This technique can expand the indications and usefulness of the omental flap.

14. Erol OO, Spira M. Reconstructing the breast mound employing a secondary island omental skin flap. *Plast Reconstr Surg*. 1990;86(3):510–518.

21

Local flaps in partial breast reconstruction

Moustapha Hamdi and Eugenia J. Kyriopoulos

SYNOPSIS

- Breast conserving therapy (BCT) is applied to most early stage of breast cancers.
- Oncoplastic surgery within multidisciplinary approach is "gold standard" in BCT.
- Using pedicled flaps is indicated in high tumor/breast size ratio.
- Partial breast reconstruction with pedicled flap is alternative to mastectomy in selected patients.
- Overcorrection is essential when pedicled flap is used in partial breast reconstruction.
- Perforator or muscle sparing latissimus dorsi flaps are the first choice of flap surgical techniques.
- Fat grafting and contralateral breast remodeling may be required to achieve breast symmetry at long-term follow-up.

Access the Historical Perspective section online at
http://www.expertconsult.com

Introduction

Breast-conserving therapy (BCT) with tumor resection and radiotherapy is a valuable component of breast cancer treatment, with an equivalent survival outcome to that of mastectomy. Quadrectomy or partial mastectomy offers wider, safe margins and reduces the rate of local recurrence. Partial breast reconstruction is required in most of the cases of quadrectomy to avoid post-BCT breast deformity. Every case requiring partial breast reconstruction should be addressed within a multidisciplinary approach. Local flaps are required in partial reconstruction of small-to-moderate size breasts. Pedicled perforator flaps provide adequate partial breast reconstruction with minimal donor site morbidity.

Basic science

Partial mastectomy combined with radiotherapy, often referred to as breast-conserving therapy (BCT) followed by breast irradiation, has replaced modified radical mastectomy as the preferred treatment for early stage invasive breast cancer. The 5-year survival rate of partial mastectomy with radiation is not statistically different when compared with mastectomy alone in patients with stage I or II breast cancer.[5,6] Women diagnosed at early stages of invasive breast cancer have equivalent outcomes when they are treated with lumpectomy and radiation therapy or modified radical mastectomy.[7]

It is interesting to point out that the surgical clearance of pathological margins has the most significant impact upon local recurrence in patients treated with BCT and RT. The presence of DCIS at the surgical margin is associated with the identification of residual DCIS in 40–82% of re-excised specimens and is correlated with margin widths of: 41% at 1 mm, 31% at 1–2 mm, and 0% with

2 mm of clearance.[5] A recent meta-analysis concluded that a margin width was significantly superior to lesser margins.[8]

The incidence of local recurrence depends upon certain factors, such as the tumor margin, nuclear grade-histology, radiation therapy and patient age. Most local recurrences occurred at the site of initial tumor excision (57–88%) or in the same breast quadrant (22–28%). In general, during the first 10 years after lumpectomy with radiation, the recurrence rate is 1.4% per year. The treatment of in-breast tumor recurrence in patients is completion mastectomy.[9] Therefore, more radical excision including the tumor with large surrounding tissue (quadrectomy or partial mastectomy) is recommended; however, it may result in an unacceptable aesthetic outcome.

Partial breast reconstruction has become a preferable option for an increasing number of patients. These techniques allow for local excision with oncologic benefits, while avoiding more extensive surgery with higher complications and increased morbidity rates associated with total mastectomy and immediate reconstruction. This chapter will discuss the use of the loco-regional flaps in partial breast reconstruction.

Diagnosis/patient presentation

The decision to undertake a partial mastectomy or alternatively, a total mastectomy to treat a patient with breast cancer, is ultimately an oncologic determination. In cases where the two treatment options are oncologically equivalent, the patient needs to participate in the decision-making in order to maximize their sense of satisfaction with their treatment.

Breast-conserving approaches may be preferable over a total mastectomy. This is especially true for patients with early stage disease, because the majority of the breast can be preserved and the operation is perceived as less invasive than a mastectomy. Most early-stage cancers (T1 and T2 cancers with or without nodal involvement) are indicated for BCT; however, there are some exceptions. Commonly known reasons for contraindications are: patients with a high probability for recurrence, especially those with multicentric disease; those who are pregnant; have collagen vascular disease; or those who have a history of prior radiation

therapy.[10] Relative contraindications include: patients with a high probability of subsequent cancers (BRCA mutations) and patients who are likely to have a poor cosmetic result, which includes patients with a high tumor/breast ratio, medially and inferiorly based tumors and tumors that require removal of the nipple-areola complex.

Approximately 10–30% of patients are dissatisfied with the aesthetic result after partial mastectomy with radiation.[11] Although the causes may vary, the factors that motivate patients to seek corrective surgery after partial mastectomy are: a volume discrepancy, contour deformity, and nipple malposition.[12] The resection of more than 15–20% of the breast parenchyma in a small-volume (A or B cup) and more than 30% in larger breasts will cause volumetric deformities and bilateral asymmetries. In addition, radiation therapy extenuates the image of the breast, initially causing breast edema and skin erythema and eventually causing parenchymal fibrosis, retraction, skin envelope atrophy, hyperpigmentation, hypopigmentation and telangiectasia. The long-term final effects of radiation are difficult to predict but seem to stabilize 1–3 years post-radiation.[13,14]

The intention of this chapter is not to extend on the indications of BCT, but to identify the complexity of partial breast reconstruction, to optimize reconstruction planning, and to indicate the importance of the use of local flaps in breast oncoplastic surgery.

Patient selection

The success of this procedure depends on the size of the cancer, the anatomical position, and the volume of resection needed to achieve clear margins in relation to the volume of the breast. Especially in cases of partial breast reconstruction after the excision of wide localized tumors, the value of oncoplastic surgery increases.

The choice of the technique used depends on many factors, including the extent of resection, the time of surgery, the breast size and tumor location and patient preferences.

Type of reconstruction

There are two basic types of surgery techniques in partial breast reconstruction. These are volume displacement and volume replacement.

1. Volume displacement techniques refer to advancement, rotation or transposition of large local breast flaps into the smaller created defect, redistributing the volume loss. The dissection involves the advancement of a full-thickness segment of breast fibroglandular tissue to fill the dead space. Volume displacement procedures and surgical scars are optimal when combined with mastopexy-reduction techniques. The tumor is excised within the planned markings of the reduction specimen in medium, large, or ptotic breasts, and the remaining parenchyma is sufficient enough to reshape the breast mound.[15]

2. Volume replacement techniques are technically more difficult and are used in small–moderate sized breasts or when the tumor/breast ratio is large and the remaining breast tissue is insufficient for the rearrangement and the replacement of the defect. Volume replacement with the use of non-breast local or distant flaps provides both tissue for the filling of the glandular defect and the skin deficiency of the reconstructed breast.[16]

Surgery for volume displacement avoids donor site morbidity, but is associated with ischemia of the dermo-glandular pedicle and may require contralateral breast surgery in order to achieve symmetry. The amount of tissue that is obtained for defect coverage and breast reconstruction is limited.

Volume replacement techniques maintain the original size and shape of the breast, without the need for any contralateral breast surgery, but are associated with longer operation times, require competent surgical skills, and possible complications in the flap and the donor site.

Timing of reconstruction

Reconstruction of partial mastectomies can either include delayed, immediate or immediate-delayed procedures. In delayed reconstruction, at least 6 months to 1 year is allowed to elapse after the last radiation therapy session, in order to evaluate the deformities of the breast and plan the appropriate reconstruction modality. In immediate reconstruction, the goal is to perform co-instantaneously tumor resection in oncologic appropriate margins and partial breast reconstruction. Immediate-delayed partial reconstruction is actually a two stage immediate surgical approach with delayed reconstruction (within a few days) until the results of the pathology report are known and the margins of the tumor excision are determined as sufficient or must be re-excised to clear margins before reconstruction. The final aesthetic outcomes are similar to those with immediate reconstruction.[17]

Immediate breast reconstruction offers many advantages over delayed breast reconstruction, such as a better aesthetic outcome due to the preservation of the three-dimensional breast skin envelope. The aim of immediate reconstruction after breast conserving therapy (BCT) is essentially to give better aesthetic results with the same oncological safety. Our target should be the reshaping of the treated breast with the alteration of the opposite breast for better symmetry, as part of the treatment, when indicated. Immediate reconstruction before radiation therapy is also preferred, because the breast can be better manipulated before radiation, with potentially decreased complication rates and improved aesthetic outcomes. In planning the approach on which method should be used to treat the partial mastectomy defect, the primary decision that must be made is whether reparative surgery will be needed after the tumor excision. If oncoplastic surgery is necessary, the next step is to choose the technique. If there is sufficient tissue, reshaping the breast, along with reduction of the opposite breast for symmetry is usually the best option. If there is not enough tissue left for breast reshaping, tissue must be added. If the defect is not too large, local tissue can be used, with simple techniques, such as rotation or transposition fasciocutaneous flaps from the axillary area or superiorly based composite flap of skin, subcutaneous fat and upper pole breast parenchyma. If the defect is too large to be filled by local tissue alone, a loco-regional pedicled or distal pedicled or free flap will be required (*Fig. 21.1*).

Breast and plastic surgeons must have a thorough understanding of breast anatomy, physiology, and the qualities of an aesthetically pleasing breast shape. Surgeons performing the oncoplastic approach should consider the aesthetic subunits when planning cosmetic quadrectomies, resections, and reconstructions.[18] Also, knowledge of the anatomical landmarks, breast proportions, and shape is essential in order to achieve a pleasing outcome.

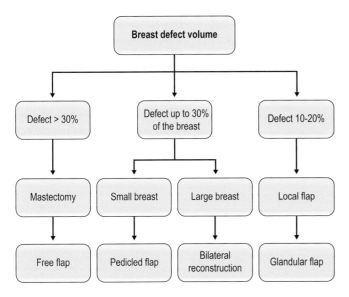

Fig. 21.1 Breast reconstruction: a decision-making process.

Preoperative evaluation of the patient and her breasts must be standard and detailed. The examination must include: evaluation of breast skin; elasticity; thickness; scars; and any defining marks such as tattoos, stretch marks, contour irregularities; and previous breast surgery. Palpation for masses or abnormalities in the breast parenchyma, nipple inspection and detailed documentation of breast sensation are integral. Breast shape, grade of ptosis, and size are determinants of success in surgical treatment.

The base and width of the breast, the width of the NAC, the height of the nipple and the distance from the sternal notch, midline and inframammary crease, must be recorded in detail.[18] Any natural breast asymmetry should be pointed out to the patient before surgery. Different body types, skin laxity and fat distribution are important factors in the decision-making process.

Treatment/surgical technique

Large defects in large breasts may be treated by converting a partial mastectomy into a reduction mammaplasty. Planning of skin incisions and parenchymal excisions follow templates using reduction mammaplasty and mastopexy techniques. The pattern can be rotated laterally or medially to fit the location of the defect. The choice of pedicle is related to the tumor location and the blood supply of the breast. It is important that skin incisions be planned, so that if mastectomy is

ultimately required for margin control, the incision site can be comfortably included within the mastectomy skin island.[6,15]

When volume replacement is necessary for BCT reconstruction, the decision of which technique will be used is determined mostly by the surgeon's experience and the size of the defect in relation to the size of the remaining breast. The use of nonbreast locoregional flaps offer the extra volume needed in large tumor excisions/quadrectomies for the replacement of the breast volume, however they can be more demanding procedures and associated with donor site and flap morbidity.

A small lateral defect can be easily covered with a skin rotation flap or a lateral thoracic axial flap. Especially in obese patients (with breast rolls), the lateral thoracic flap comes in handy. However, most of these fasciocutaneous flaps may be unavailable in the axillary lymph node dissection patients.

The latissimus dorsi muscle or musculocutaneous flaps have been very popular as a method of choice in partial breast reconstruction.[19]

On the other hand, pedicled perforator flaps have enabled surgeons to replace large defects with the minimum donor site morbidity. The advantage of perforator flaps, which are skin and subcutaneous flaps, is that they offer sufficient coverage without sacrificing the muscle and motor innervations and minimize seroma formation rate.

Classification and vascular anatomy of flaps

The latissimus dorsi (LD) flap has a constant anatomy.[20] The blood supply of the latissimus dorsi comes from a terminal branch of the subscapular artery (*Fig. 21.2*). The subscapular artery runs about 5 cm before dividing into the scapular circumflex and thoracodorsal arteries. The thoracodorsal artery is about 2–4 mm in diameter and it courses along the posterior portion of the axilla for about 8–14 cm, before it pierces the latissimus dorsi on its costal surface. The thoracodorsal artery gives off one or two branches to the serratus anterior muscle and one branch to the skin. The basic pattern of the thoracodorsal bundle (artery, nerve and 1–2 venae comitantes) branching is bifurcation into a lateral (vertical)

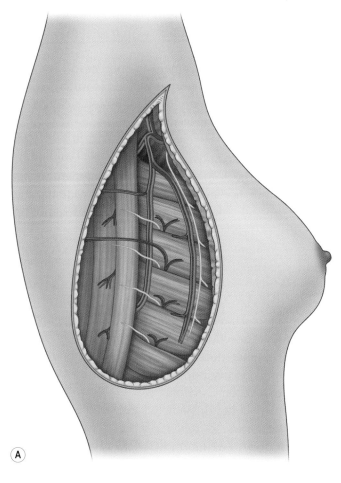

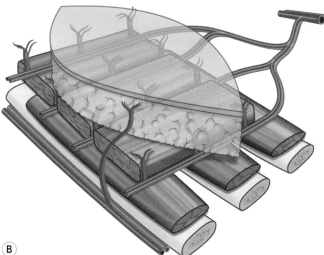

Fig. 21.2 (A) Vascular anatomy. TD, thoracodorsal; P, perforator; SA, serratus anterior; ICN, intercostal nerve. **(B)** The various nutrient artery sources and perforator branches are marked. TD, SA, and IC vessels are represented diagrammatically.

and a medial (horizontal) branch. The lateral branch follows a course parallel to the muscle fibers, 1–4 cm medial to the free-lateral border of the muscle and gives off perforating vessels that supply the skin. The smaller medial branch diverges at an angle of 45° and travels medially. A vigorous blood supply to the muscle is also available at its origin. Perforating vessels from the intercostal and lumbar arteries supply the muscle and overlying skin.[20,21]

The pedicled perforator flaps mostly used in our hands for partial breast reconstruction, classified according to the basic nutrient arteries and recommended by the "Gent" Consensus update in 2002[22] are *(Fig. 21.3)*:

- Thoracodorsal artery perforator (TDAP) flap
- Intercostal artery perforator (ICAP) flap
- Serratus anterior artery perforator (SAAP) flap
- Superior epigastric artery perforator (SEAP).

The TDAP flap

The TDAP flap is based on perforators originating from the descending (vertical) or horizontal branches of the thoracodorsal vessels. Anatomic studies on cadavers have reported the presence of 2–3 musculocutaneous perforators from the vertical branch.[23,24] The proximal perforator enters the subcutaneous plane obliquely 8–10 cm distal to the posterior axillary fold and 2–3 cm posterior to the anterior border of the muscle. The second perforator is found 2–4 cm distally to the first one. Occasionally, a direct cutaneous perforator arising from the thoracodorsal vessel passes around the anterior border of the muscle, making flap harvesting easier.

There may not always be a single reliable perforator for the TDAP flap, due to anatomical variations.[25] In this case, the surgeon must be aware and prepared to modify the flap dissection intraoperatively, as a muscle sparing TDAP flap.

The TDAP flaps are classified as followed[26]:

- TDAP flap, when no muscle component is included in the flap *(Fig. 21.3A)*.
- TDAP-MS-I, where a small segment of muscle (4×2 cm) kept attached to the back of the perforator vessels. The muscle segment protects the perforator from excessive tension and provides more freedom in flap positioning *(Fig. 21.3B)*.

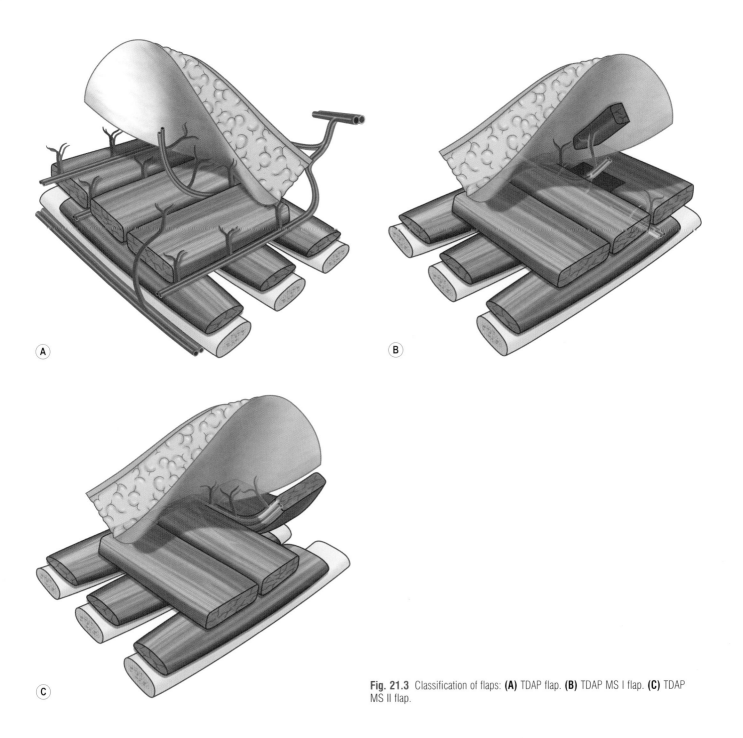

Fig. 21.3 Classification of flaps: **(A)** TDAP flap. **(B)** TDAP MS I flap. **(C)** TDAP MS II flap.

- TDAP-MS-II is indicated when multiple but small perforators are encountered. A larger segment, up to 5 cm wide along the anterior border of the latissimus dorsi muscle together with the descending branch of the thoracodorsal vessels is then included within the flap in order to insure a maximal blood supply to the skin paddle *(Fig. 21.3C)*.

The ICAP flap

The ICAP flap is based on perforators, arising from the intercostal vessels. The intercostal vessels form an arcade between the aorta and the internal mammary vessels and divide in four segments: vertebral, intercostal, intermuscular and rectus segments.[27]

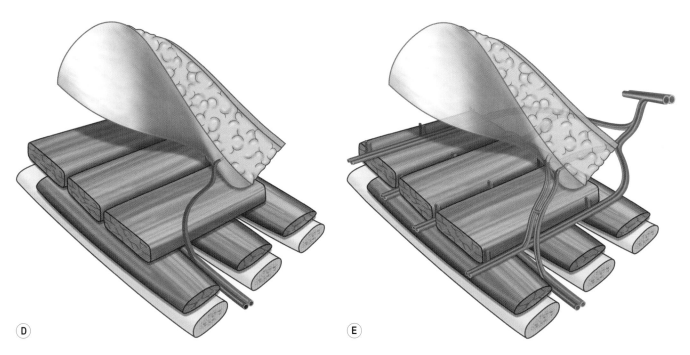

(D)   (E)

Fig. 21.3, cont'd (D) LICAP flap. **(E)** SAAP flap.

The ICAP flaps are classified as followed:

- The dorsal intercostal artery perforator (DICAP) flap. The flap is based on perforators originating from the vertebral segment of the intercostals vessels.
- The lateral intercostal artery perforator (LICAP) flap, based on perforators arising from the intercostal segment *(Fig. 21.3D)*.
- The anterior intercostal artery perforator (AICAP) flap. The nutrient perforators of this flap arise from the muscular or rectus segment.

The intercostal segment, which is the longest (12 cm), is very important because it gives 5–7 musculocutaneous perforators.[28]

The lateral intercostal artery perforator (LICAP), commonly used in breast surgery, originates from the costal segment of the intercostals vessels. The largest perforator is most frequently found in the 6th intercostal space, 0.8–3.5 cm from the anterior border of the Latissimus dorsi muscle.[29] The pedicle has adequate length, allowing the rotation of the flap up to 180° without tension and with no need to extend the dissection into the costal groove. An intercostal nerve may be included in the harvesting as an ICAP-sensate flap.

For small defects, the LICAP is designed on the lateral aspect of the thorax and for moderate-large defects the distal limit of the skin pad can reach the posterior thoracic region, planned in a fashion similar to the skin pad of a LD flap.[30]

The AICAP flap is outlined over the upper abdomen, so that the final scar will be hidden under the brassier strap. The donor site can be closed primarily if it is up to 6 cm wide (preoperative pinch test to be assured), or else in a reversed abdominoplasty fashion. The advantage of AICAP and SEAP flaps is that the patient is prepped in a supine position throughout the whole procedure. These flaps are mostly known for defects in the inferomedial quadrant of the breast.

The SAAP flap

The serratus anterior artery perforator flap is based on a connection between the thoracodorsal artery branch to the serratus anterior muscle and the intercostal perforators *(Fig. 21.3E)*. It is not a constant perforator (21%).[28] When an appropriately sized perforator is identified in front of the anterior border of the LD, it can be followed back to the nutrient artery, which in this case is the serratus anterior branch by dissecting the pedicle within the fascia and the fibers of the aforementioned muscle.

The SEAP flap

The SEAP flaps are based on perforators arising from either the superficial or the deep branch of the superior epigastric artery and the perforator flaps are named SSEAP and DSEAP respectively. As mentioned above, the superior epigastric artery perforator flap has similar indications as the anterior intercostals artery perforator flap;[31] however, it has a longer pedicle which allows it to reach the defect with less tension. Pedicled SEAP flaps should be used only in selected cases, since it may exclude the secondary use of abdominal tissue for autologous breast reconstruction (DIEAP, SIEAP, TRAM flaps) if completion mastectomy is later on indicated.

Indications for pedicled flaps

The main use for pedicled flaps is partial breast reconstruction (immediate or delayed) when volume replacement is necessary, however, other reasons include:

- Salvage procedure after partial/total free flap loss for breast reconstruction
- Post-mastectomy breast reconstruction in combination with implant
- Breast augmentation with autologous tissue
- Shoulder, back and chest wall defects.

Contraindications to pedicled flaps

The harvesting of a local perforator flap demands expertise of the technique and sufficient knowledge of the anatomy of the area. Less experienced surgeons may choose other reconstruction options to familiarize themselves with perforator flap harvesting, such as the deep inferior epigastric artery perforator or superior gluteal artery perforator flaps, with relatively larger and more perforator vessels.

The area of the defect may have limited access, especially when localized in the inferomedial quadrant and is difficult to be reached by a pedicled perforator flap based on the axillary vessels. However, the AICAP or SEAP flaps are ideal for such defects.

Previous axillary or thoracic surgery with damage to the thoracodorsal pedicle is a contraindication for LD or TDAP flap but might be not for harvesting a LICAP flap. Previous scars and radiation injury to the area may also result in the limitation of local pedicled perforator flaps.[26] When breast deformity after partial mastectomy with radiation is severe, the optimum choice is to perform a complete mastectomy and autologous reconstruction with a free flap transfer.

Flap design

Flap choice

Based on the thoracodorsal serratus, intercostal or superior epigastric vessels, several pedicle flaps can be raised on perforators in the axillary, back, anterior thoracic, and upper abdominal regions, depending on the location of the desired recipient site, the surgeon's preference and other anatomical and surgical indications.[32]

The pedicled TDAP flap is ideal for partial breast reconstructions, especially for defects located in the superior or inferolateral quadrants. The LICAP is a good alternative to TDAP flap for lateral and inferior breast defects (*Fig. 21.4*). However, the TDAP flap has a longer pedicle with a greater arc of rotation and reaches most of the breast, except for the inferomedial quadrants (*Fig. 21.5*).

Preoperative perforator mapping

Perforator mapping with correct flap design is the keystone in this technique. To localize the thoracodorsal perforators, a unidirectional Doppler (8 Hz) ultrasonography examination is performed for perforator mapping in the planned skin flap area. This device, although quite handy and less costly, has the disadvantage of generating false-negative and false-positive signals and provides less detailed anatomic vessel information. This is due to the misleading background signal from the thoracodorsal vessels, which can be confusing and difficult to distinguish from the perforator signal. To avoid this, the patient is positioned, as in surgery, at a lateral position with 90° of shoulder abduction and 90° of elbow flexion. Also, multidetector (MD) row CT scan can be used with accuracy to localize the perforator.[33]

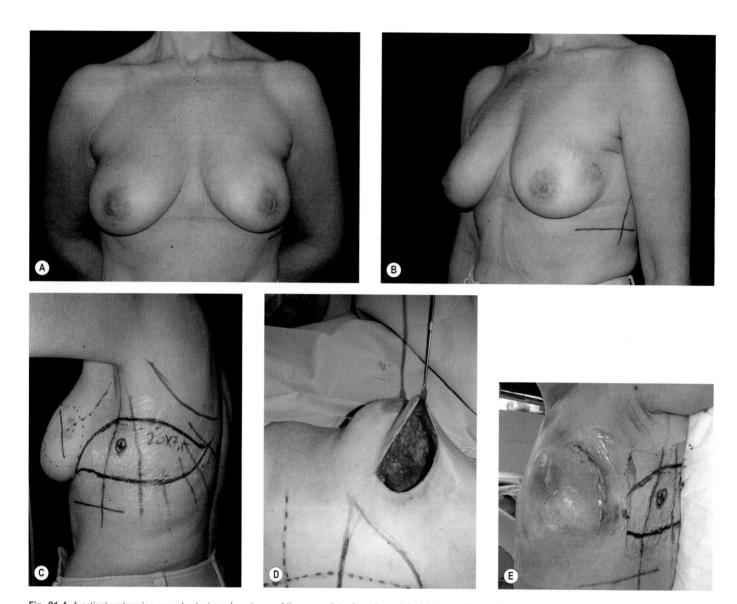

Fig. 21.4 A patient undergoing a quadrantectomy for a tumor of the supero-lateral quadrant of the left breast. The quadrantectomy specimen weighed 195 g. Reconstruction is with a completely de-epithelialized TDAP flap based on one perforator. **(A,B)** Preoperative views. **(C)** Flap design. The dominant Doppler was preoperatively located using MDCT. **(D,E)** The quadrantectomy was performed and the skin was closed in order to reposition the patient.

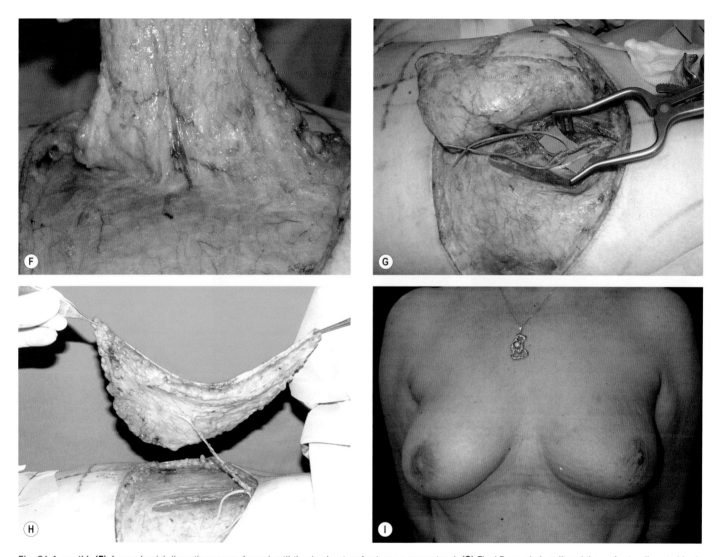

Fig. 21.4, cont'd (F) A suprafascial dissection was performed until the dominant perforator was encountered. **(G)** The LD muscle is split and the perforator dissected back to the main pedicle. **(H)** The TDAP flap was based on one perforator. **(I)** The flap is passed through the split LD muscle. The TD nerve is preserved.

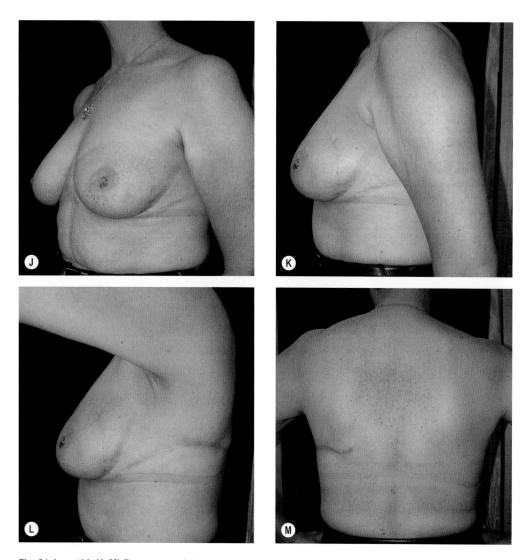

Fig. 21.4, cont'd (J–M) The outcome of the reconstruction and the donor site 18 months postoperatively.

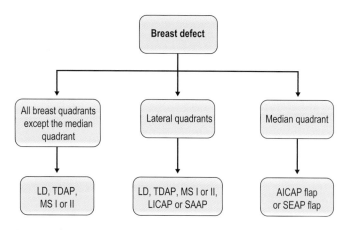

Fig. 21.5 Choosing pedicled perforator flaps for partial breast.

Using advanced image technology, such as color duplex flowmetry or MDCT when planning a perforator flap, is essential in order to make flap harvesting more reliable, shorten operative time and decrease complication rates due to poor perforator choice and surgical planning. The preoperative MDCT is performed a few days before surgery (*Fig. 21.4C*).

Markings

The patient is preferably marked the day before surgery. The breast size, tumor size and location, as well as the final defect size are estimated. The incisions for the tumor resection are chosen from an oncologic aspect but in the most aesthetically pleasing fashion. The TDAP flap planned for the partial breast reconstruction is designed to include the located perforators (one or more) at the proximal part if feasible, in the directions of relaxed skin lines, the bra-line, or even horizontally according to the patient's preference. Skin laxity and fat excess in the lateral thorax and back area are estimated by the pinch test. The size of the flap is determined by the need for defect coverage and is an average of 20×8 cm. The skin drawings are applied at first with the patient in an upright position and the anterior border of the LD muscle is palpated and marked also. Then the patient is placed in a lying position on her side, with the reconstruction side facing upwards, as in surgery, for the perforator mapping and the flap design in the lateral thorax. The skin island is always extended over the anterior border of the latissimus dorsi to include the pre-muscular perforators, if present. The proximal border of the flap approximates the inframammary fold *(Fig. 21.4C)*. If the defect is more medially, the flap is designed more distally, further in the back. The same design is applied for the LICAP, however, the flap is placed more anteriorly, towards the breast. The AICAP or SEAP flaps are usually designed under the IMF along the rib.

Surgical technique

The patient is prepped and positioned in the supine position for the tumor excision *(Fig. 21.4D,E)*. After the lumpectomy/quadrectomy at clear margins, clips are placed in the wound bed and left there, in order to indicate the area for future radiation therapy. If the plan is to proceed with TDAP, LICAP, or SAAP flap, the patient is positioned and prepped again in lateral position, as in the typical LD musculocutaneous flap dissection. Otherwise, for AICAP/SEAP flap the patient remains in the original position.

The flap harvesting starts with skin incisions. A posterior approach is usually used in TDAP flap. The surgeon continues dissection down to the LD suprafascial plane, while beveling in favor of the flap in order to gain as much of extra tissue as possible. Harvesting proceeds from the back towards the axillary region. Further harvesting under loop magnification continues meticulously, until the perforator vessel is visualized *(Fig. 21.4F)*. If the perforator is visibly pulsate and adequate in caliber (>0.5 mm), the dissection continues along the perforator course up to the nutrient thoraco-dorsal pedicle. If a large pedicle length is required, the TD vessels can be dissected up to their suprascapular vessel origin and included in the flap. If the perforators have an intramuscular course, dissection is performed in the direction of the muscle fibers and any nerves that come across are carefully preserved *(Fig. 21.4G)*. Within the muscle, all the perforator side branches are either ligated or coagulated. If two perforators are found along the same course, they can both be included within the flap, without sacrificing any muscle fibers *(Fig. 21.4H)*.

In case the perforators are inadequate in size, the flap harvesting is continued as muscle sparing LD, preserving a small piece of muscle attached to the posterior wall of the perforators, sacrificing only minimum fibers and most important, salvaging the muscle innervation. This modification is also useful when the flap is intended for the medial breast area, because it protects the perforators from presumed tension.

The flap harvesting carries on, with the skin incisions continued proximal to the axilla and lateral to the LD and the dissection proceeds anteriorly, until the flap is freed from the donor site tissues and left connected only to the vascular pedicle. The pedicle is carefully passed under a subcutaneous tunnel in the axilla-lateral thoracic area that has been previously prepared to the recipient breast area, avoiding any avulsion of the pedicle *(Fig. 21.4I)*. The donor site is sutured in three anatomical layers with a drain in place and the patient is returned again to the supine position.

Before final closure of the defect, the flap can be partially or totally de-epithelialized (depending on the native skin reservations of the recipient site) and folded accordingly, to give extra projection to the reconstructed breast mount but always in a tension free manner.

In LICAP flap dissection *(Fig. 21.6)*, an anterior approach is performed from the breast side towards the anterior-free border of LD muscle. Perforator dissection is done within the serratus muscle, until its origin from the costal groove. Further dissection is usually not needed.

Postoperative care

Postoperatively, protocol perforator flap monitoring is implemented and all patients receive piracetam for

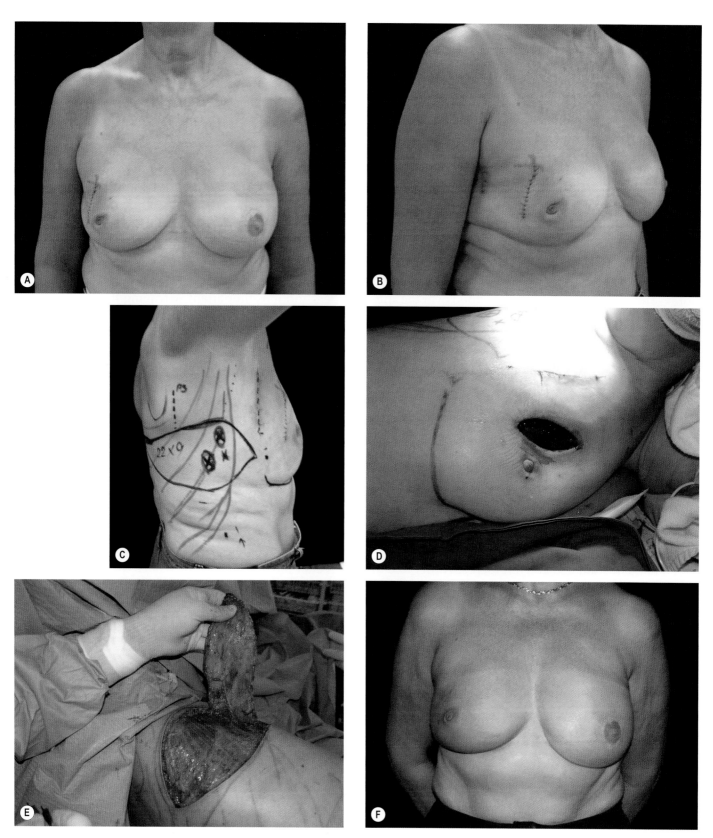

Fig. 21.6 A 59-year-old patient was admitted for quadrantectomy with partial breast reconstruction for right breast cancer located at supero-lateral quadrant. Two years previously, the patient had undergone a mastectomy at the left side with an immediate breast reconstruction using a DIEP flap. **(A,B)** Preoperative views. **(C)** A 22×9 cm flap was designed with the mapped perforators. **(D)** The defect after the quadrantectomy. **(E)** Preoperative view showing one intercostal perforator LICAP. The IC nerve was also included in the flap. The flap was completely de-epithelialized and folded to fill the defect. **(F–H)** Postoperative views.

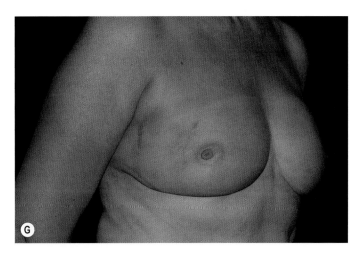

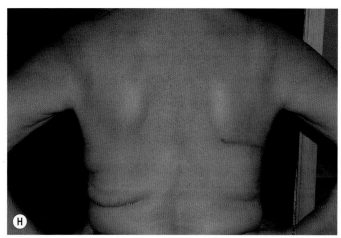

Fig. 21.6, cont'd

5 days IV (12 g/24 h) and for another 5 days per os (solution 20%, 25 cc ×4/24 h). The drug acts to increase the viability of the distal parts of the flap by increasing capillary blood flow. Patients leave the hospital when the drains are removed, which averages 3–5 days. The arm is held in 45° abduction. Arm stretching is restricted for a week. Physiotherapy can be started afterwards. Most patients require between 9 and 14 sessions of shoulder physiotherapy. Patients treated for BCT with pedicled perforator flaps have a short rehabilitation course.[6]

Adjuvant irradiation of the breast, if indicated, can be started at 6 weeks post-reconstruction. However, most of our patients received first adjuvant chemotherapy, which lasts usually 6 months. The chemotherapy, when applicable, can be started after 3 weeks postoperatively.

Outcomes, prognosis, and complications

Donor site morbidity after harvesting loco-regional pedicle perforator flaps for partial breast reconstruction is reduced to a minimum. Only a very limited rate of seroma formation has been observed and treated mainly conservatively. Wound dehiscence of the donor site usually, when closed under tension, is another infrequent event, managed with local treatment.

Partial or total flap losses are very rare incidents and one must exclude coagulopathies or other medical diseases and conditions. Unpleasing scars, flap contractures and volume loss are less rare sequelae and may need secondary surgical treatment. Also, flap reconstruction of breast defect may give a "plugged in" appearance, which seems to slightly improve after radiation therapy. It is hard to predict the long-term outcomes of partial breast reconstruction with pedicled perforator flaps due to the indefinite impact of irradiation to the final result.

Finally, some patients who undergo partial breast reconstruction with a TDAP flap document an initial decrease in forward arm elevation and passive abduction, which recovers over time.[34]

Secondary procedures

Our experience showed a stable result at long term (*Fig. 21.7*). However, one may expect breast asymmetry due to the different aging process between the two breasts. The nonirradiated side may become more ptotic compared with the irradiated one. On the other hand, the irradiated side may show signs of total breast atrophy. When the breast asymmetry becomes obvious, fat grafting alone, or with contralateral breast remodeling, is indicated.

The use of the lipofilling technique, alone or most commonly in combination with other reconstruction options for the treatment of breast defects after tumor resection, is gaining great popularity. In contrast to what was believed in the past, lipofilling of the breast is proven to be a safe, reliable method for the transposition of autologous fatty tissue in contour deformed areas of the breast.[35]

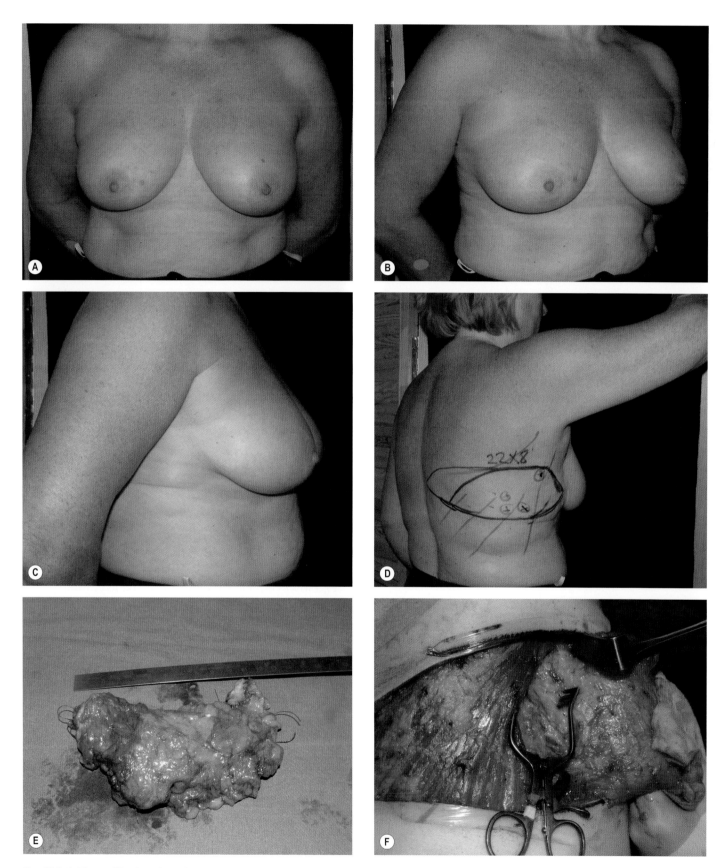

Fig. 21.7 A 65-year-old patient who underwent a partial right breast reconstruction with a pedicled SAAP flap. **(A–C)** preoperative views. **(D)** A 22×8 cm flap was designed with marked perforators. **(E)** The quadrantectomy specimen (120 g). **(F)** The flap was based on the communication between SA and the IC perforator.

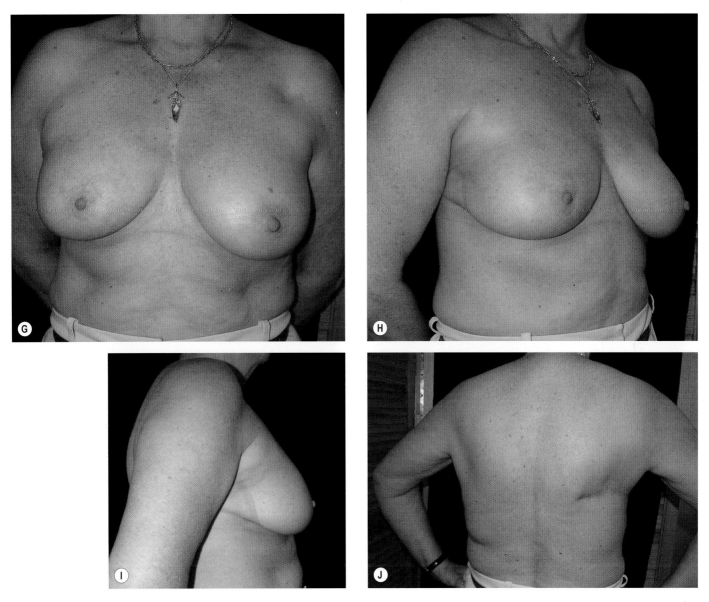

Fig. 21.7, cont'd (G–J) postoperative views with the donor site at 3 years postoperatively.

Fat injections into the breast can significantly improve small breast defects after limited lumpectomies. In larger excisions, partial breast reconstruction is preferably performed with other tissue replacement techniques described above, but when followed by fat grafting, it definitely improves the final outcome. Fat injections may be used primarily at the time of the breast conserving therapy to limit volume discrepancies between the two breasts, to add superomedial fullness for an aesthetically pleasing breast cleavage, or to correct the breast mound and shape. In second stage procedures, the fat grafting can be done in order to make refinements in volume, projection or contour irregularities due to fat necrosis or flap contractures. Fat grafting is also used for the treatment of skin atrophy of the breast after irradiation, which is explained by the stem cell mediated process of fat grafts in the intradermal plane. The major limitation of this technique is that it is time consuming and prolongs operation time significantly, especially in inexperienced hands and the requirement of staged applications. Also, it still raises some concerns about monitoring the breast and follow-up in breast conserving therapy patients.

6. Hamdi M, Wolfli J, Van Landuyt K. Partial mastectomy reconstruction. *Clin Plast Surg.* 2007;34(1):51–62.

Currently, the two main options for the management of primary breast cancer are total mastectomy and partial mastectomy with radiation. Although partial mastectomies (lumpectomy or quadrantectomy) conserve the nipple, areola complex and native breast tissue, asymmetry and distortion of the breast can still occur. Many methods of reconstruction have been described. The early and long-term effects of radiation also contribute to the complexity of these cases. This article reviews breast-conserving therapy, reconstruction options, and outcomes.

16. Kronowitz SJ, Kuerer HM, Buchholz TA, et al. A management algorithm and practical oncoplastic surgical techniques for repairing partial mastectomy defects. *Plast Reconstr Surg.* 2008;122(6):1631–1647.

Most patients with medium or large breasts will likely benefit from immediate repair, whereas some with small breasts may not. Immediate repair of partial mastectomy defects is preferred with the use of local breast tissue (local tissue rearrangement or breast reduction techniques) because of the simplicity of these approaches and because techniques using local tissue maintain the color and texture of the breast. Waiting to repair a large deformity until after whole-breast radiation therapy usually necessitates a complex transfer of a large volume of autologous tissue, which many patients who undergo breast conservation therapy are not willing to pursue. Use of lower abdominal flaps to repair partial breast defects is generally discouraged.

25. Hamdi M, Van Landuyt K, Hijjawi JB, et al. Surgical technique in pedicled thoracodorsal artery perforator flaps: a clinical experience with 99 patients. *Plast Reconstr Surg.* 2008;121(5):1632–1641.

Careful preoperative perforator mapping and a standardized approach to flap planning and harvest can significantly reduce the difficulty of executing pedicled thoracodorsal artery perforator flaps.

26. Hamdi M, Van Landuyt K. Pedicled perforator flaps in breast reconstruction. In: Spear SI, Willey SC, Robb GL, et al, eds. *Surgery of the breast: principles and art.* Philadelphia, PA: Lippincott-Raven; 2006:833–844.

27. Hamdi M, Van Landuyt K, de Frene B, et al. The versatility of the inter-costal artery perforator (ICAP) flaps. *J Plast Reconstr Aesthet Surg.* 2006;59(6):644–652.

The ICAP flaps provide valuable options in breast surgery; and for challenging defects on the trunk without sacrifice of the underlying muscle.

28. Hamdi M, Spano A, Van Landuyt K, et al. The lateral intercostal artery perforators: anatomical study and clinical application in breast surgery. *Plast Reconstr Surg.* 2008;121(2):389–396.

Lateral intercostal artery perforator flaps can be used to address challenging defects over the breast without sacrificing the pedicle of the latissimus dorsi muscle.

31. Hamdi M, Van Landuyt K, Ulens S, et al. Clinical applications of the superior epigastric artery perforator (SEAP) flap: anatomical studies and preoperative perforator mapping with multidetector CT. *J Plast Reconstr Aesthet Surg.* 2009;62(9):1127–1134.

The authors' clinical experience indicates that the SEAP flap provides a novel and useful approach for reconstruction of anterior chest wall defects. CT-based imaging allows for anatomical assessment of the perforators of the superior epigastric artery (SEA).

33. Hamdi M, Van Landuyt K, Van Hedent E, et al. Advances in autogenous breast reconstruction: the role of preoperative perforator mapping. *Ann Plast Surg.* 2007;58(1):18–26.

34. Hamdi M, Decorte T, Demuynck M, et al. Shoulder function after harvesting a thoracodorsal artery perforator flap. *Plast Reconstr Surg.* 2008;122(4):1111–1117.

Donor-site morbidity after harvesting a thoracodorsal artery perforator flap was reduced to a minimum. Therefore, perforator flaps should be considered in reconstruction whenever adequate perforators can be identified and safely dissected.

22

Reconstruction of the nipple-areola complex

Ketan M. Patel and Maurice Y. Nahabedian

SYNOPSIS

- Creation of the nipple-areola complex allows the reconstructed breast mound to truly resemble the natural breast.
- The overall plan for the resection and reconstruction is a collaborative effort between the medical oncologist, general surgeon, and plastic surgeon.
- Many of the currently used flaps are derivatives of the basic design of the skate flap and star flap.
- The most common complications with local flap techniques are projection loss, flap/nipple necrosis, dehiscence, malposition, and infection. When other graft types are used, complications related to graft loss, extrusion, and exposure are possible.

 Access the Historical Perspective sections online at **http://www.expertconsult.com**

Introduction

For many women, nipple-areola reconstruction provides closure to the long journey associated with mastectomy and breast reconstruction. Much of this journey has been associated with complicated decisions and operations that required hospitalization and prolonged recovery time. Of all the procedures associated with the reconstructive process, nipple reconstruction represents the simplest from a technical perspective but is among the most important from an aesthetic perspective. Creation of the nipple-areola complex will allow the reconstructed breast mound to truly resemble the natural breast. Fortunately, nipple reconstruction can be performed with all types of breast reconstructive procedures and at any time following completion. This chapter will review the indications, patient selection criteria, and many of the techniques associated with reconstruction of the nipple-areola complex.

Diagnosis and patient presentation

Most patients will have the nipple and areola resected during skin-sparing mastectomies and included in the specimen as the nipple contains ductal breast tissue. Only a select few patients will be eligible for a nipple-sparing mastectomy, which is usually determined by the size and proximity of the cancer to the nipple.[15] Although preservation of the nipple leads to improved patient satisfaction,[16] most patients are not candidates for keeping the native nipple. The overall plan for the resection and reconstruction is a collaborative effort between the medical oncologist, general surgeon, and plastic surgeon. Most times, patients will have the entire nipple-areolar complex (NAC) removed. Regardless of the disease process, recreation of the NAC represents a challenging issue with multiple possible reconstructive options.

The NAC is ideally located on the point of most projection on the breast mound. There are a wide variety of

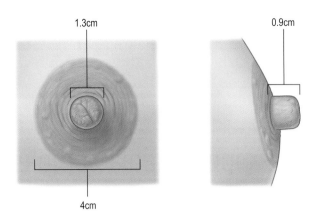

1.3cm   0.9cm

4cm

Fig. 22.1 The average proportions of the nipple-areola complex. The average areolar diameter is 4 cm. The average nipple diameter is 1.3 cm and the nipple height is 0.9 cm.

NAC characteristics regarding nipple size, diameter, shape, areola size, and color among women. Measurements from the contralateral breast, if available, should include the sternal notch-nipple distance and the inframammary fold to areola distance. These measurements will guide the surgeon to uncover any asymmetries or subtle abnormalities that may affect nipple reconstruction.

In bilateral reconstruction, the surgeon must make use of standard values to create a nipple position, size, and areola size. A review of 600 breasts showed that the mean diameter of the areola is approximately 4 cm, with average nipple diameter being 1.3 cm and the average nipple projection being 0.9 cm *(Fig. 22.1)*.[17] The average nipple-areola and areola-breast proportion is approximately 1.3.[18] These numbers can be useful guiding principles, in particular, in bilateral cases where symmetry and ideal NAC creation is desired.

Timing of NAC reconstruction is crucial to the final aesthetic result. Surgical decisions made too early may result in asymmetric placement of the nipple. Key factors in the decision-making mainly focus on adjuvant breast cancer therapies and revisional reconstructive procedures. Adjuvant therapies need to be taken into consideration as the tissue healing effects of radiation and chemotherapy may compromise final outcomes. Also, revisional procedures can change breast dimensions and may lead to asymmetry of a previously symmetrically reconstructed nipple. Taking these points into consideration, the ideal timing for reconstruction is approximately 3–5 months after the last revisional reconstructive surgery. This allows for swelling and inflammation to subside, while allowing for settling of the reconstructed breast mound into its final position.[19]

Patient selection

The type of previous breast reconstruction is another important factor to consider in patient selection. Patients who undergo prosthetic-based breast reconstruction will have a thin, expanded skin-subcutaneous tissue base, usually with a centrally placed mastectomy scar. On the other hand, in autologous reconstruction, patients will typically have a variable sized donor tissue skin paddle with an elliptical or circular shaped scar with a thick base. As discussed later, these factors are important in eventual NAC reconstruction as thin flaps can potentially decrease nipple projection and poorly located scars can prohibit the use of certain flap techniques due to interference with blood supply *(Table 22.1)*.

Surgical techniques

There are many innovative ways to create a NAC. Although many claim some methods are superior to others, each method has unique characteristics that apply to certain breast types. In this section, multiple categories of reconstructive techniques will be explored, focusing on the desirable and undesirable aspects of each.

Composite nipple graft

Many of the initial methods for nipple reconstruction were by way of various types of skin and composite grafts. The initial descriptions of using grafts involved ipsilateral nipple-areola grafts.[2] Eventually, the concept of contralateral nipple grafting and distant site composite grafting were attempted and proven successful.[3,4,24,25] Labial tissue and toe pulp were initially used and advocated, but donor site morbidity has led to reluctant use of these grafts.[3,6,24] Nipple-banking was also used, but uncertainty of the oncologic safety of this method has led surgeons to abandon this technique. Nipple-sharing

Table 22.1 Studies comparing projection of various flaps constructed on either an implant-based or an autologous-based breast mound

Author(s)	Flap type	Residual projection (%)		Significance (p)
		Implant base	Autologous base	
Rubino et al. (2003)[20]	Arrow	49.10	49	>0.05
	Modified star	30.1	38.5	<0.01
Banducci et al. (1999)[21]	Modified star	23.3	36.7	<0.005
Few et al. (1999)[22]	Modified star	41	41	>0.1
Shestak et al. (2002)[23]	Skate	61.6	59.8	NA
	Modified star	60.6	59.5	NA
	Bell	28.0	32.1	NA

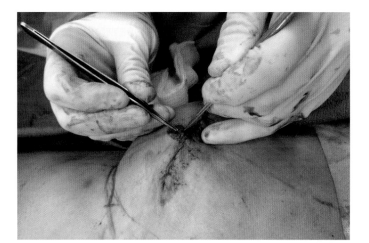

Fig. 22.2 De-epithelialization of the proposed nipple site.

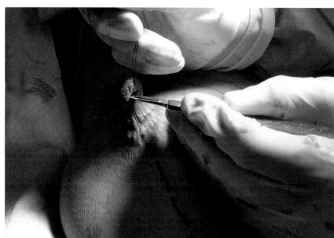

Fig. 22.3 Traction is placed to elongate the nipple and scalpel is used to transect 40–50% of the distal nipple.

technique continues to be a popular method for nipple reconstruction with the presence of a prominent contralateral nipple.

Initiated by Adams in 1944[2] and described by Millard in 1972,[4] contralateral nipple grafts have remained as a popular method for nipple reconstruction in patients with excess contralateral nipple projection. Patients with projection in excess of 5–6 mm are ideal candidates for composite nipple grafts. Many patients have reservations about this method of nipple reconstruction due to: (1) fear of contralateral surgery; (2) donor site morbidity, and (3) decreased contralateral nipple sensation.

When excess projection is present, the technique for composite nipple grafting is straightforward. The basic technique first entails de-epithelialization of the future nipple site of reconstructed breast *(Fig. 22.2)*. Then, a scalpel is used to transversely remove the distal 40–50% of the contralateral nipple *(Fig. 22.3)*. The harvested nipple is then placed in the proposed site and sutured into place *(Fig. 22.4)*. The donor nipple is then closed with either a purse-string suture or interrupted sutures. Close attention is paid to avoid fluid accumulation beneath the grafted site. Skin grafting of the areola can be performed at this time if excess tissue is available or from donor sites such as the inner thigh.[26,27] After the procedure, a bolster dressing or gel-filled silicone nipple protector is used to avoid shearing.

As previously mentioned, one of the feared aspects of composite nipple grafts is the donor site morbidity. One study showed that patients subjectively felt that the donor nipple had the same sensation as prior to surgery and that erectile function was similar. Statistically, the study found that punctate touch

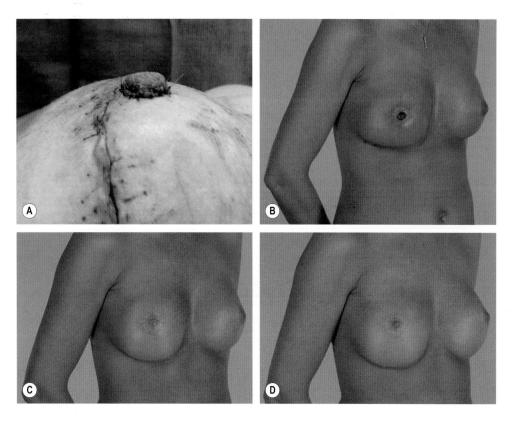

Fig. 22.4 (A) Placement of the composite nipple graft and secured with interrupted chromic suture. **(B)** At 2 weeks postoperatively from composite nipple grafting. The nipple commonly will have a discolored and ischemic appearance. **(C)** At 9 weeks postoperatively from composite nipple grafting. Notice that the nipple color becomes more pink and natural looking. **(D)** At 6 months postoperatively from composite nipple grafting. The nipple appears uniform in color and closely matches the contralateral nipple.

stimulus to monofilament was normal 6 months postoperatively.[28]

Zenn *et al.* reviewed 57 patients who underwent composite nipple grafting. They found that only 47% of patients considered donor site sensation as "normal," but found that 96% of patients were happy with the overall appearance, with 87% retaining erectile function in the donor nipple. In contrast, in the grafted nipple, the study found that 35% of patients had sensation in the reconstructed nipple within an average of 6 months. Interestingly, 42% of patients reported to having erectile function in the reconstructed nipple within an average of 3 months. In addition, they found complete graft take in both patients that had previous irradiation.[29]

Hints and tips

- Excellent option for patients with contralateral nipple >1 cm projection
- Countertraction suture and No. 11 blade help to harvest nipple accurately
- Early postoperative discoloration is normal and expected
- Irrigate blood and clot beneath the nipple with an 18-gauge catheter after securing to prevent fluid accumulation.

Traditional flaps

Many of the currently used flaps are derivatives of the basic design of the skate flap and star flap. This section describes the basic concepts, designs, and uses of these two flaps and many of the newer modifications and derived flap designs *(Table 22.2)*.

Skate flap

Since Little's initial description on how to design the skate flap in the 1987,[11] there has been many attempts at modifying the technique. The original design of the skate flap as described by Little, is shown in *Figure 22.5*. This flap has reliably produced long-term projection and is used when a projected appearance is required. Traditionally, this type of flap is used in conjunction with a skin graft for immediate areola reconstruction. The design is based on a central axis. After the appropriate site is selected, the diameter of the areola is determined; either from the opposite side or averaging 4 cm. A line bisecting the intended areola is marked and used to determine the base of the flap. The base should be directed away from the mastectomy scar in order to

Table 22.2 Studies reporting projection and projection loss with commonly used flaps

Flap design	Author(s)	Projection (mm)	Follow-up (months)	Projection loss (%)
Skate	Shestak et al. (2002)[23]	NA	12	40.94
	Richter et al. (2004)[30]	9.24	6	45
	Zhong et al. (2009)[31]	2.5	44	NA
Star	Shestak et al. (2002)[23]	NA	12	43.36
	Banducci et al. (1999)[21]	NA	38	71.3
	Few et al. (1999)[22]	4–8.3	12	59
	Kroll et al. (1997)[32]	1.97	24	NA
	Rubino et al. (2003)[20]	3.25	12	66.7
C-V flap	Losken et al. (2001)[33]	3.77	60	NA
	Valdatta et al. (2009)[34]	3.52	12	32
	El-Ali et al. (2009)[35]	2.17	15	45
Arrow flap	Li et al. (2008)[36]	NA	3	50
	Rubino et al. (2003)[20]	4.75	12	50.9

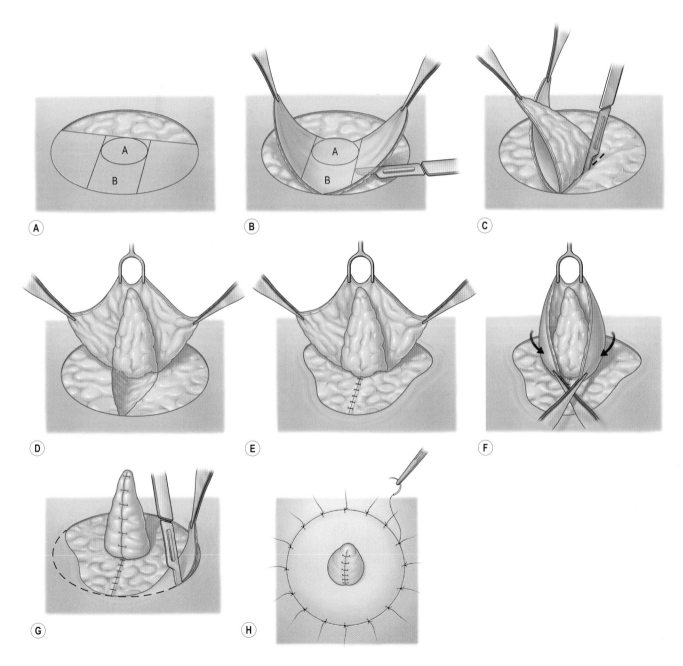

Fig. 22.5 The traditional skate flap is elevated with only a thin layer of subdermal fat on the outer wings and approximately 7–8 mm of fat on the underside of the central axis. This fat is the main contributor to the core of the nipple.

maximize blood flow. The line is then split into thirds. The inner and outer thirds will be used as the wings that fold to form the sidewalls of the nipple. After this line is established, a semicircular line is drawn from the two edges of the bisected line. The midpoint of this arc will represent the most projected portion of the future nipple. Varying this distance will add/lessen projection to the nipple and thoughtful placement of this arc is recommended.

Dissection begins at the outer wings and proceeds toward the inner third central segment, paying close attention to elevate in the subdermal level and to include a thin layer of subdermal fat. After the two wings have been elevated, the central segment dissection begins. The central segment typically includes 7–8 mm of subdermal fat. As dissection proceeds proximally to the flap base, care must be taken to avoid dissecting past the flap base. The wings are then rotated into place opposite the base and sutured. The subdermal fat of the central pedicle adds bulk to the nipple.

The traditional design of the skate flap de-epithelializes the remainder of the areola. A doughnut shaped skin graft is then prepared and secured on the donor site and de-epithelialized area. This approach allows for a texture and color difference to the areola more closely resembling a native areola.[11]

Modifications to the skate flap have been developed to improve long-term outcomes and decrease donor site morbidities. Many of these techniques attempt to limit distant skin graft harvests. Bogue *et al*. describes a modification that closes the skate flap donor site primarily *(Fig. 22.6)*. His modification, similar to Nahabedian's

elongated C-flap *(Figs 22.7)*,[19] decrease the tension required to close the donor site left from a traditional skate flap. They evaluated 31 nipple-areolar reconstructions using a skate flap design with tapered distal ends in order to facilitate primary closure. After elevation and nipple creation, the donor site is primarily closed. Then, a round template is used to outline an areola. The areola is then elevated as a full-thickness graft up to the base of the flap and then laid back down and a bolster dressing applied. Although all patients had satisfactory results, immediate and long-term projection is compromised by the tapered flap design.[37]

Richter *et al*. found that the skate flap was the best local flap to give projection. They followed 29 patients who had skate flap nipple reconstruction for an average of 10.9 months. Although they found an average decrease in projection of 45%, the skate flap group produced a mean nipple projection of 9.24 mm at least 6 months after reconstruction.[30]

Shestak *et al*. found that the skate flap gave a predictable long term projection after 12 months. They followed a subset of 23 patients who underwent skate flap nipple reconstruction at 3-month intervals in order to assess projection loss. They found that the skate flap was an appropriate choice when the projection goal is >5 mm. The greatest amount of projection loss occurred within the 6 months of surgery and seemed to stabilize after that time period. After 12 months, they found an average projection loss of 40%.[23]

Hints and tips

- Including more subdermal fat in central base gives more reliable projection
- Longer flaps increase tension if primary closure desired leading to flattening of breast
- Skin graft from scar revision areas can be used to minimize donor sites
- Will give the most projected appearance of flap techniques.

Star flap

The star flap was first described by Anton *et al*. using a three-wing flap to create moderate projection.[12] The star flap utilizes similar principles in flap design as the skate flap. As originally described, this flap has the advantage of eliminating skin graft donor site morbidity by allowing for primary closure and possibly an

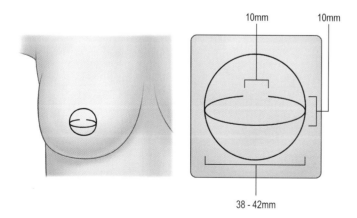

10mm   10mm

38 - 42mm

Fig. 22.6 Modified skate flap proportions are shown. Flap length is decreased in order to primarily close the donor site.

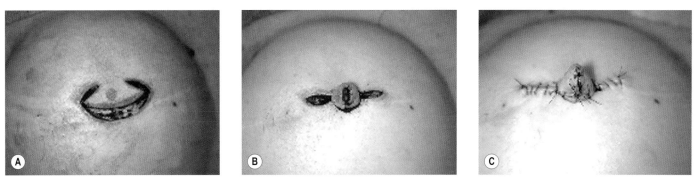

Fig. 22.7 **(A)** Modified skate flap, or elongated C flap, shown with the proposed nipple site marked. **(B)** The donor site is primarily closed and the outer wings are rotated to the midline and secured. **(C)** Interrupted sutures are used to close the nipple and donor site.

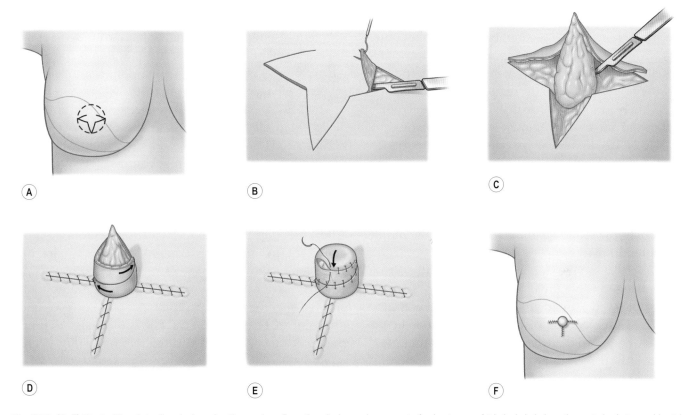

Fig. 22.8 (A–F) The traditional star flap design, elevation, and configuration. An increasing amount of subcutaneous fat is included along the central axis to provide stability to the base of the nipple.

improved cosmetic result. On the other hand, the main disadvantages of the star flap are the lack of projection when compared with the skate flap, and loss of long-term projection.[38] Kroll *et al.* followed 47 patients who underwent star flap nipple reconstruction. He found that mean projection achieved was 1.97 mm after a 2-year follow-up.[32] Few *et al.* used a modified star-dermal fat flap technique on 93 nipple reconstructions. They designed a flap with a blunted central wing and

two opposing lateral triangles, or wings. The flap lengths directly correlated to the gain in projection. They found that 1 cm in flap length gave 0.16 cm in projection. In addition, long-term projection loss was 59% using their modification.[22]

The basic design of the star flap is based on a three-wing pattern *(Fig. 22.8)*. Similar to the skate flap, the central wing base width determines the width of the nipple. The outer star wing lengths vary depending on

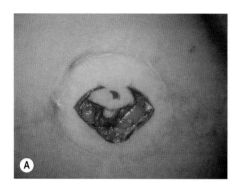 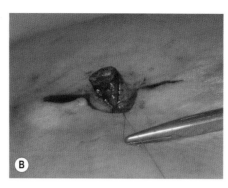 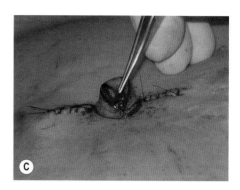

Fig. 22.9 (A) The basic design of the C–V flap. The outer V-segments can have variable degrees of angulation from sharp to blunted edges. **(B)** Sutures are first placed to approximate the donor site. The outer wings are then approximated at the midline and sutured together. **(C)** The central C-segment is then rotated down to form the rounded dome of the nipple.

the size of the contralateral NAC. After drawing the appropriate pattern, dissection begins on the outer wings. In contrast to skate flap elevation, the outer wings are elevated in the subdermal fat plane paying close attention to include subcutaneous fat. The central wing is then elevated from distal to proximal while including an increasing amount of subcutaneous fat. After flap elevation, one of the outer wings are rotated along the nipple base and sutured into position. The second outer wing is then rotated around the nipple and the distal end is sutured anterior to the base of the first outer wing. After secured in place, central wing is brought over the top to form the distal tip of the nipple and secured in place.

Shestak *et al.* used the star flap in patients with <5 mm of contralateral nipple projection and no areola projection. He followed 28 patients for 12 months and analyzed the degree of loss of projection. Similar to the skate flap, he found that the greatest loss of projection occurred in the first 3 months and stabilized at 6 months. They found an average of 43% loss of projection at 12 months postoperatively.[23]

Hints and tips

- Provides low-moderate projection
- Limited breast flattening on closure
- May use de-epithelialization on redundant wing tips to add bulk.

C–V flap

The C–V flap is so named for the shape of the flap segments used for nipple creation. Taking elements of both the star and skate flaps, the C–V flap is composed

of two lateral wings, or V-shaped segments. The central segment resembles a C shape, or has a rounded appearance. The main advantage of the C–V flap is the ease of elevation and ability to close the donor site primarily without the use of a skin graft.

The basic design of the flap is represented in *Figure 22.9A*. Flap elevation begins at the outer V-segments and proceeds toward the central, C-segment. Dissection will typically include a thin subdermal fat layer. After elevation, the donor site is closed directly. The central segment will then be elevated with a deeper layer of subdermal fat in order to provide bulk to the nipple. After the flap has been elevated, the donor site is approximated and the two outer V-flaps are rotated into place similar to that of the skate flap *(Fig. 22.9B)*. The two flaps are rotated along the base of the nipple and sutured together to provide the support for projection opposite the base. The central flap is then used to round the tip of the nipple and sutured into place *(Fig. 22.9C)*.

Valdatta *et al.* found good overall satisfaction when using the C–V flap in 29 patients. He also found that average nipple projection was 3.52 mm compared with 4.96 mm on the native nipple at 1 year postoperatively. Projection loss after 1 year was 32%, but found an increase in diameter of the reconstructed nipple of 17%. In fact, the volume calculated of the reconstructed nipple was maintained after 1 year.[34]

Losken *et al.* found maintained projection using the C–V flap after 5-year follow-up. In comparison with the native nipple, projection was not statistically different with the reconstructed nipple measuring 3.87 mm compared with 4.71 mm on the native side. Overall patient satisfaction was 81%, with satisfaction with nipple projection being only 42% after the 5-year follow-up.[33]

Modifications to the C-V flap have been developed in attempts to improve long-term outcomes and stability.[35,39,40] In attempts to add volume to the nipple, Mori and Hata[39] and Brackley and Iqbal,[40] report de-epithelialization of the lateral V-segments, providing increased bulk and possibly increasing long-term projection. Importantly, in nipple reconstruction to expander/implant patients, providing increased vascular tissue to the nipple core can compensate for dermal thinning commonly seen in implant-based reconstruction.

Hints and tips

- Versatile flap
- Shape of outer distal segments can vary with little change in outcome
- Can de-epithelialize outer segments to provide bulk.

Arrow flap

Originally described and designed by Thomas in 1996 as a method for geometrically analyzing nipple proportions, the nipple design later used to construct the arrow flap was introduced.[41] Rubino *et al.* introduced his "arrow flap" modification to prevent nipple flattening and retraction.[20] The basic design is similar to the C–V flap design except the outer wings are designed to resemble the two sides of an arrow. Rubino added a modification to include an area of de-epithelialization to the flap design, which adds bulk to the nipple construct *(Fig. 22.10)*. Dissection of this flap employs the same techniques used for the previous flaps described. As shown in the figure, the two arrow ends are designed to oppose one another along the base of the flap and the closure resembles a Z-plasty in that the vertical scar becomes re-oriented *(Fig. 22.11)*.

Rubino *et al.* compared the long-term results of using the arrow flap compared with the modified star flap. Each group contained 16 nipple reconstructions and he found that the arrow flap maintained 49.1% projection after 12 months, with an average projection of 4.75 mm.[20]

Hints and tips

- Z-plasty configuration may decrease contraction and nipple distortion
- Pay close attention to avoid de-vascularization of outer segment tips.

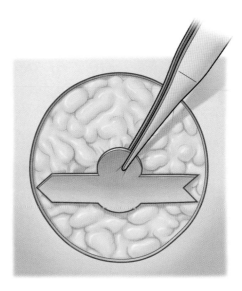

Fig. 22.10 The outer lines represent the entire flap. The shaded areas represent the de-epithelialized areas that can be used to add bulk to the nipple construct.

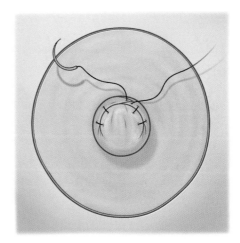

Fig. 22.11 The outer segments are rotated to form the base of the nipple and the two sides of the "arrow shape" (see *Fig. 22.10*) as closed in a V-configuration.

Pull-out/purse-string flap techniques

The designs described in the following section represent unique methods to create nipple and/or areolar projection using surrounding tissue mobilization and purse-string techniques. These flaps are best used when the breast mound tissue is supple and able to be mobilized to enhance projection *(Table 22.3)*.

Table 22.3 Studies reporting projection and projection loss with pull-out flaps

Flap design	Author(s)	Projection (mm)	Follow-up (months)	Projection loss (%)
Bell	Shestak *et al.* (2002)[23]	NA	12	73.95
Peri-areolar/purse-string	Dolmans *et al.* (2008)[42]	5	12	50

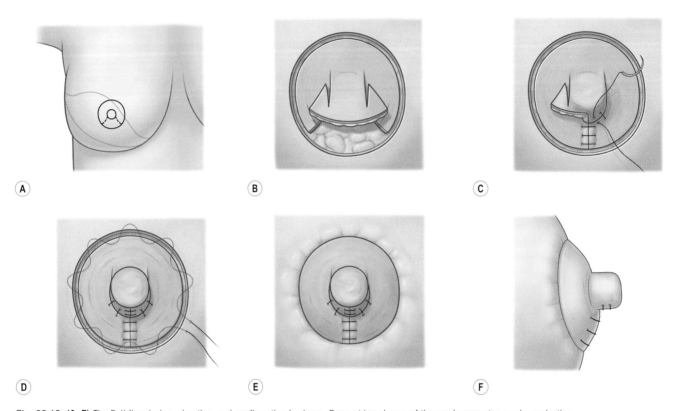

Fig. 22.12 **(A–F)** The Bell flap design, elevation, and configuration is shown. Purse string closure of the areola promotes areolar projection.

Bell flap

Described by Eng in 1996, the bell flap is so termed to describe its design. The unique design also incorporates a purse-string areola closure that provides slight areolar projection.[13] The basic design of the flap is shown *(Fig. 22.12)*. Slight overestimation of the areola needs to be considered as the purse-string effect will decrease the final diameter. The intended nipple is then drawn and the bell-shaped flap is raised in the subdermal plane. The flap is then wrapped upon itself in an inverted box configuration and sutured into place.[13]

In a long-term comparison study, Shestak *et al.* found the Bell flap was the least reliable at providing long-term projection compared with the skate and star flap.

After 12 months of follow-up, 73% projection loss was found using the Bell flap technique.[23] The unreliable projection maintenance has led to reluctant use of this flap.

Hints and tips

- May be used if contralateral nipple projection of 2–3 mm
- Lacks long-term projection maintenance.

Double opposing peri-areolar/purse-string flap

Described by Shestak *et al.* and Hammond *et al.* in 2007, the nipple portion of the double opposing peri-areolar

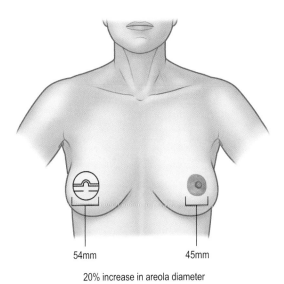

54mm 45mm

20% increase in areola diameter

Fig. 22.13 The basic design of the peri-areola/purse-string flap is shown. Overcorrection of the areola will account for purse-string effect.

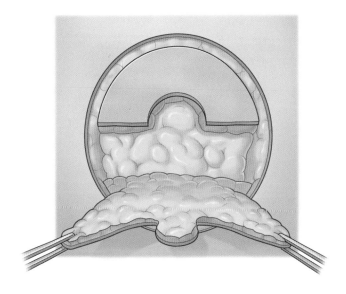

Fig. 22.14 Flap elevation begins with the outer wings and moves central. As dissection begins under the central segment, increasing amounts of subdermal fat is included.

flap/skate flap purse-string design is a derivative of the original skate flap. They sought to design a projecting nipple with donor site scarring conspicuously contained within the areola. The "pull-out" flap design attempts to project at a level above the breast mound, adding another degree of projection.[43,44]

Flap design begins with critical assessment of the contralateral nipple in the case of unilateral reconstruction or following some basic measurements for bilateral reconstruction. The nipple base width is first measured, which is approximately 12 mm. The width of the outer limbs are roughly between 10–12 mm with the length being roughly between 20–22 mm. The intended diameter of the areola is overestimated by 20–25% in order to account for the final purse-string closure *(Fig. 22.13)*.

Dissection begins by elevating the outer wings including a thin layer of subdermal fat *(Fig. 22.14)*. As the base is approached, subcutaneous fat is included in order to provide substance and projection. In contrast, Hammond describes elevating the base and wings with an even layer of subdermal fat.[43] Next, the outlined areolar border is incised into the subcutaneous tissue in order to allow these areolar flaps to slide along subcutaneous pedicles *(Fig. 22.15)*. The nipple is then assembled and sutured together similar to previous flaps *(Fig. 22.16)*. The areolar flaps are then sutured

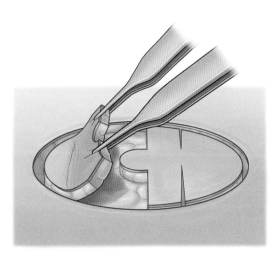

Fig. 22.15 Slight undermining of the areolar flap is performed in order to allow for mobility of this segment.

together and sutured to the nipple base *(Fig. 22.17)*. Lastly, the areola is closed via purse-string suture using 2-0 or 3-0 nonabsorbable suture *(Fig. 22.18)*.[44]

In Shestak's series of 47 nipples reconstructed using this technique, he found no flap loss, dehiscence, or separation. One patient required revision for a downward inclined nipple and one patient, who was a smoker, developed distal tip ischemia.[44] Dolman *et al.* evaluated 14 nipple-areola reconstructions using the skate flap purse-string technique. After 12 months,

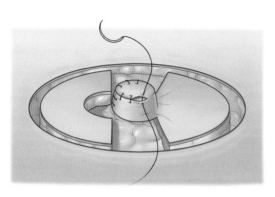

Fig. 22.16 Nipple assembly with rotation of the outer segments toward the midline and approximation of the central segment to form the dome of the nipple.

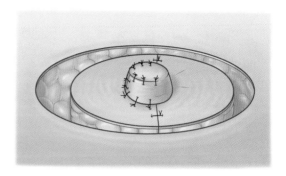

Fig. 22.17 Areolar flaps are approximated and sutured into place.

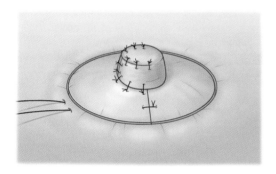

Fig. 22.18 Areola closed with a purse-string suture to create areolar projection.

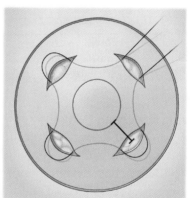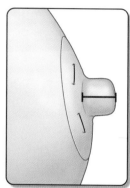

Fig. 22.19 The traditional top-hat flap is shown. Four incisions are made to allow for purse-string suture placement. The incisions are then closed in a radially oriented fashion.

average nipple projection was 5 mm representing a 50% loss in projection.[42]

Hints and tips

- Nipple distortion can occur if tension present on base sutures
- Good option in autologous reconstruction with large skin paddles
- Wide or excessive undermining will lead to ischemia and nonhealing issues.

Top-hat flap

The original description of the top-hat flap was based on creating nipple projection by a "purse-string" effect.[45] The design is unique compared with other techniques, as no true flaps are created, thus eliminating much of the undesirable donor site issues when local tissue is used.

The first four incisions are placed at the base of the intended nipple, making sure to leave 2–4 mm of space between each incision and the intended nipple diameter **(Fig. 22.19)**. Dissection is carried down into the subcutaneous tissue at each site. A nonabsorbable purse string suture is placed from each incision to the next. The tension is then adjusted to create projection. The horizontal incisions will typically be closed in a radially oriented fashion.[46]

Gamboa-Bobadilla *et al.* found success when using this method of nipple reconstruction. The evaluated 23 patients with an average follow-up of 18 months and found 6 mm of maintained projection with a nipple diameter of 10 mm. In addition, two patients were found to have projection loss at follow-up, but found that 90% of their patients were satisfied with the reconstruction.[46]

Table 22.4 Studies reporting projection and projection loss with flap designs adjacent to scars

Flap design	Author(s)	Projection (mm)	Follow-up (months)	Projection loss (%)
Double-opposing tab	Kroll et al. (1997)[32]	2.43	24	NA
	Kroll and Hamilton (1989)[47]	3.8	≥10	66
S-Flap	Cheng et al. (2004)[48]	3.27	18	NA
	Lossing et al. (1998)[49]	3.9	36	80

Hints and tips

- Good option when flaps cannot be used
- Unlikely to maintain projection in scarred or radiated tissue
- Can add peri-areolar purse-string suture to give a small amount of areolar projection.

Flap designs adjacent to scars

Many of the previous flaps described as useful when a reliable, continuous blood supply is present within the entirety of the flap. In circumstances related to a centrally located mastectomy scar, such as those commonly found in immediate prosthetic-based reconstruction, the following section will provide options for creating a successful nipple without the compromised blood flow *(Table 22.4)*.

S-flap

The S-flap, described initially by Cronin *et al.* in 1988, provides a method of nipple reconstruction when the scar traverses the proposed nipple site. The S-flap uses opposing dermal pedicles opposite each other receiving transversely oriented blood supply. This allows for nipple creation with the presence of a scar.[14]

The original flap design is based on opposing dermal flaps oriented in a S-configuration. Each flap measures approximately 1.5 cm in width and 2.5 cm in length. The projection of the nipple is determined by the length created by the rotated, interfacing flaps *(Fig. 22.20)*. As originally described, entire nipple-areola site is de-epithelialized first. Each flap is then elevated in the sub-dermal fat plane to provide bulk and a robust vascular supply. After rotating the segments, the flaps are sutured together loosely to allow for swelling *(Fig. 22.21)*. This was followed by a full-thickness skin graft secured with a bolster dressing.[14] Modifications in the S-flap have

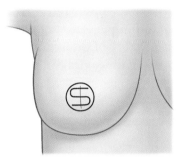

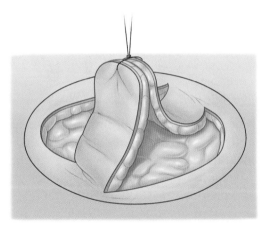

Fig. 22.20 The modified S-flap is shown with the native breast skin. The traditional flap as described starts with a de-epithelialized area.

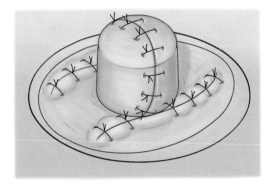

Fig. 22.21 The S-configuration is sutured into place and the donor site is closed primarily.

allowed for minimal donor site morbidity by eliminating skin grafting, thus providing a simpler method of S-flap creation.[47,49–51]

Lossing *et al.* used a modified S-flap technique that eliminated the need for skin grafting by maintaining the native skin on each flap. The design is similar to the classic S-flap with the addition of a 1 cm back-cut made on each flap allowing for proper rotation at the expense of blood supply. They found that the nipple maintained 3.9 mm of projection in a series of 25 nipple reconstructions using a modified S-flap technique. After a follow-up of 36 months, approximately 80% of projection was lost. In addition, five nipples had complications of nipple necrosis.[49]

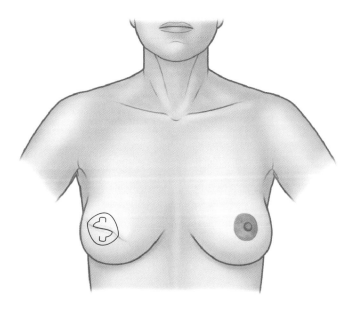

Fig. 22.22 The double-opposing tab flap is shown centered around a mastectomy scar.

Hints and tips

- Unreliable long-term projection
- May cause distortion if flaps too wide
- Modified S-flap back-cuts can lead to distal tip necrosis.

Double-opposing tab flap

Similar to the S-flap, the double-opposing tab flap was described by Kroll in 1989 as a method for nipple reconstruction that includes native skin on each flap can be placed directly over a previous scar. This nipple design is ideal when the previous mastectomy scar traverses the ideal nipple position.

The flap design is shown *(Fig. 22.22)*. If a scar is present, the two flaps should be positioned on either side of the scar. First, the two tabs are initially elevated at the level of the deep dermis. As dissection is carried more proximally on each flap, the dissection is deepened to the level of the subdermal fat. This thickness will provide the bulk to the nipple and should be half the diameter of the desired nipple *(Fig. 22.23)*. The donor sites are then closed like Burrow's triangles, allowing the two flaps to lie in opposition to each other. The tabs are then wrapped around and sutured to the opposing flap, creating the base of the nipple. The flap tips are then moved into position at the tip of the nipple and sutured to the opposing flap to create a rounded appearance *(Fig. 22.24)*. An areola design is then made and de-epithelialized. A skin graft is placed with a bolster dressing.[47]

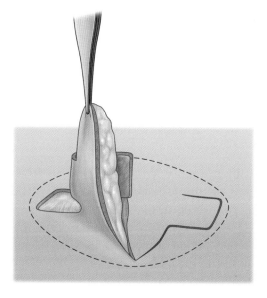

Fig. 22.23 The flap thickness represents half the nipple diameter.

Using this method, Kroll found satisfactory long-term projection. After having 11.1 mm of initial projection, 3.8 mm of projection was maintained longer than 10 months, resulting in 34% of maintained projection.[47] In addition, Kroll *et al.* compared the double-opposing tab flap to the star flap and found improved long-term results with the tab flap. Their group found, after 2 years, that the tab flaps had an average of 2.43 mm of

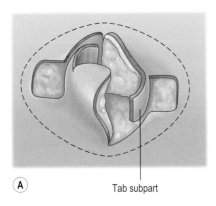

Tab subpart

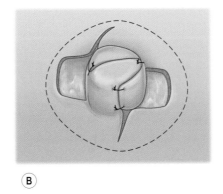

A

B

Fig. 22.24 **(A)** The tab portion of the flap is sutured into place first followed by **(B)** creation of the nipple dome.

projection compared with 1.97 mm of projection with the star flap group.[32]

Hints and tips

- Better option than S-flap
- Produces average long-term projection.

Spiral flap

Similar to the previous two flaps mentioned, the spiral flap is a practical and simple method for nipple creation when the mastectomy scar traverses the intended nipple site. The benefit of the spiral is in the ease of elevation and limited use of breast skin. Described by Di Benedetto *et al.*, the spiral flap is composed of residual scar tissue. As seen in *Figure 22.25*, 5–6 cm of scar medial to the projected nipple site is marked with the flap width being approximately 1 cm. Rotating the elevated flap and progressively suturing the flap into place in a circular spiral configuration then creates the nipple.[52]

Long-term data lacks in the use of this flap for nipple reconstruction, but the simplicity and lack of a donor site make this alternative a valuable tool when tissue is scarce and the mastectomy scar lies in the plane of the nipple site.

Hints and tips

- Unreliable long-term survival and projection
- Easy and simple technique
- Minimal distortion due to small donor site.

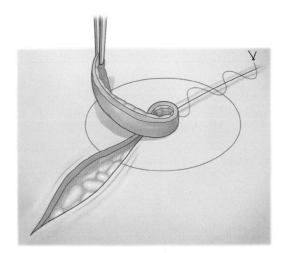

A

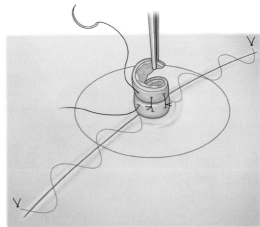

B

Fig. 22.25 The spiral flap is composed of 5–6 cm of scar rolled upon itself and sutured together to create nipple height.

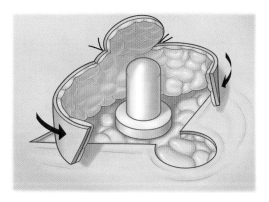

Fig. 22.26 Cartilage graft is shown and is placed at nipple base prior to flap closure.

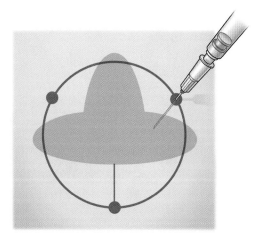

Fig. 22.27 The proposed areola is marked prior to fat grafting. Fat injection entry points are made at the periphery as to camouflage scarring. The shaded area represents the intended fat graft sites.

Flaps with autologous graft augmentation

Cartilage grafts

Auricular cartilage was first advocated by Brent and Bostwick in 1977 as method to augment nipple reconstruction.[5] This method was then modified by Tanabe et al. to be included within a dermal-fat flap to maintain projection.[53] Long-term results are lacking with using auricular cartilages but some authors believe that the cartilaginous structure provides long lasting results with minimal loss of projection *(Fig. 22.26)*.[25,54]

Costal cartilage grafts have been advocated by Guerra and colleagues in autologous breast reconstruction.[55] They report successful use of the arrow flap in a large series of 454 patients in conjunction with a costal cartilage graft harvested and banked during the initial free flap reconstruction. Their group found a 4% cartilage graft loss attributed to local flap ischemia and infection. Despite these complications, long-term projection was maintained.[55] Cheng et al. also described maintaining nipple projection in Asian females with the use of a modified top-hat flap in combination with costal cartilage banked at the initial flap inset.[56] After long-term follow-up of 58 patients, they found an average of 26.1% projection loss after 45 months. In addition, they had a 12% complication rate, mostly related to partial flap loss, nipple malposition, and cartilage exposure.[57]

Fat grafts

Fat grafting has become an increasingly popular method as a surgical adjunct for soft tissue augmentation in all

Hints and tips

- Warping of graft due to residual perichondrium presence can lead to nipple malposition
- Neo-nipple with rigid appearance and feel
- High rate of cartilage extrusion/exposure.

aspects of plastic surgery. Therefore, the use in nipple reconstruction seems to be a logical step in fat grafting utility. Bernard outlines steps for the use of fat grafting in primary and secondary nipple reconstruction.[58] In primary reconstruction, the proposed neo-nipple location is marked but not incised. Donor fat is harvesting from the abdominal or other donor region using Coleman aspiration cannulas. After concentrating the fat, 1 cc syringes are prepared and instilled into the proposed nipple site. Only 1–2 cc are needed and this process may be repeated in interval settings. After sufficient time passes to allow for partial fat resorption, the original flap is elevated and sutured into place. This technique may be useful in patients who have had tissue expansion leading to thinned dermis and subdermal fat. *Figure 22.27* shows the proposed area of fat grafting. Bernard and Beran used this technique in combination with a C-V flap and found satisfactory results at 1-year follow-up.[58]

Dermal fat grafts can also be used and harvested from discarded breast tissue. Eo et al. used a small dermofat graft taken from the excised portion of breast tissue and prepared a $1 \times 1 \times 2$ cm piece. This was then placed at the center of a C–V flap. They found successful results with long-term projection by using this method.[59]

> **Hints and tips**
>
> - Can be done simultaneously to other revisional breast fat grafting
> - High resorption rate and projection loss in radiated tissue.

Flaps with alloplastic augmentation

Alloplastic grafts have been used for nipple reconstruction to provide stable projection. The main disadvantage to using nonautologous tissue is the risk of infection and extrusion. Some of the currently used materials include hyaluronic acid and calcium hydroxylapatite.[60–62]

Hallock advocated the use of a polyurethane-coated silicone gel implant for nipple creation as a salvage-type procedure. He reported the use of silicone implants for two nipple reconstructions with no reported capsule contracture at 1 year.[63] This type of implant is only reserved for special cases and is rarely used today.

Evans et al. used Radiesse, injectable calcium hydroxylapatite embedded in a cellulose gel, to augment the reconstructed nipple. The gel scaffold allows for tissue ingrowth to aid in stability. The initial study included evaluation of six patients over an average of 6 months of follow-up. The average time from the original nipple reconstruction to the injection was 237 days. A majority of the group indicated major improvements to the appearance of the nipple and one patient reported a little decrease in projection. Overall, they found that all patients were satisfied with the use of Radiesse.[60]

Hyaluronic acid is an attractive option for nipple projection augmentation. Panettiere et al. used this to augment nipple reconstruction and performed injections at 2, 4, and 7 months after nipple creation. Reliable projection was maintained at 12 months, but they found that one patient had a false-positive result on PET scan.[61]

Yanaga et al. evaluated 100 patients who underwent nipple reconstruction with bilobed dermal flaps an skin graft with an artificial bone substance, Ceratite at the center to provide projection. He found maintained long-term projection with an average of 80.5% nipple height

symmetry to the contralateral side. In addition, there was a 5% exposure rate, which was related to dermal flap tension.[64]

Wong et al. used polytetrafluoroethylene (PTFE) as a method to create nipple projection. This method was utilized in selected patients: either is secondary reconstruction or when there was a lack of donor tissue for a local flap. A total of 17 patients underwent placement of PTFE into a subcutaneous pocket at the desired nipple location. An amount of 3.5 mm PTFE are used to create the initial desired projection with 3.0 mm pieces used for added contour. In the series, all patients were reported to be satisfied or very satisfied with their results. One patient had implant extrusion secondary to infection, but was later replaced after the infection subsided. Overall, they found projection of 4–5 mm.[65]

> **Hints and tips**
>
> - Limited use due to foreign body reaction and extrusion
> - Fillers can bleed into surrounding tissues
> - May interfere with oncologic surveillance.

Flaps with allograft augmentation

Acellular dermal allografts represent a new and revolutionary product in the field of breast reconstruction. After gaining wide acceptance for the use in implant-based reconstruction, the use of acellular dermis has expanded to all aspects of revisional and secondary breast reconstruction, including nipple reconstruction. Allografts have many of the ideal properties of an implantable material, as they have a high rate of incorporation with limited resorption. Because of the ability to incorporate into surrounding tissues, infection is limited.

Nahabedian first used AlloDerm, human-derived acellular dermis, for revisional nipple reconstruction in 2005. A small piece (1×2 cm) of AlloDerm is cut and folded upon itself and sutured in place with absorbable suture. The dimensions of the AlloDerm piece were 2×6 mm. This piece is then oriented vertically to serve as a strut within the pocket made by the wings of the flap. Among the five secondary nipple reconstructions using Alloderm, four of the nipple exhibited 4–5 mm of maintained projection at follow-up, ranging 6 months to 1 year. In addition, tertiary nipple reconstruction with AlloDerm occurred in three patients. A total of 4–5 mm of projection was maintained in these patients as well at follow-up ranging from 6–8 months. AlloDerm was incorporated into the base of the reconstructed nipple using the C–V flap or elongated C-flap.[66]

Garramone and Lam evaluated the long-term nipple projection after using AlloDerm in primary reconstruction. A total of 30 nipple reconstructions (16 implant-based breast mounds and 14 TRAM breast mounds) using a star dermal flap, were evaluated. In contrast to Nahabedian, the AlloDerm piece was cut into a strip measuring 1.5 × 4.5 cm. This piece was then rolled upon itself and sutured together. This then was secured into the pocket formed by the flaps. Among the 16 patients who had TRAM flaps, the average initial projection was 1.2 cm, with the average 12-month projection being 0.7 cm. In the implant-based group, the average initial projection was 1.15 cm and the 12-month average projection was 0.5 cm. Maintained projection after 12 months was 56% for the TRAM group and 47% for the implant group. Overall, the average maintained projection was 51.2% after 12 months follow-up.[67]

Recently developed, the Cook medical nipple reconstruction cylinder is another good option for acellular dermal augmentation *(Fig. 22.28A)*. This cylindrically shaped product is shaped perfectly to fit into a subcutaneous pocket *(Fig. 22.28B)*. This product eliminates the need to shape or roll acellular dermal products and eliminates any size discrepancies that would cause asymmetries *(Fig. 22.28C)*.

Areola reconstruction

The major challenges of areola reconstruction are to recreate the pigmentation and texture typically associated with a native areola. The most commonly employed techniques involve using skin grafts, tattooing, and/or a combination of these two techniques. Also, the surgeon must choose an appropriate timing for the reconstruction. Skin grafting is preferentially performed in the immediate setting or at the time of nipple reconstruction. Tattooing usually occurs at 6–8 weeks after nipple reconstruction, but some have good results and advocate for simultaneous nipple creation and tattooing.[69]

Skin grafting of the areola has the advantages of providing a textured, wrinkled surface and distinct pigment differences, both of which resemble a normal areola with Montgomery tubercles *(Fig. 22.29)*. Common donor sites for areola skin grafting include contralateral areola, inner thigh/groin region, revised/excess breast skin, or other body areas, where revisional surgery is needed *(Fig. 22.30 and Box 22.1)*. In addition, to avoid a donor

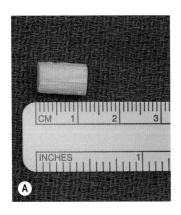 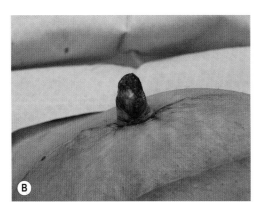 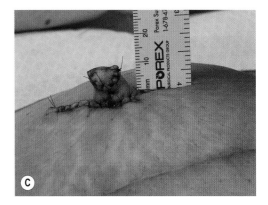

Fig. 22.28 (A) The nipple reconstruction cylinder is shown used for incorporation in a local flap for projection augmentation. **(B)** The nipple reconstruction cylinder is placed in the subcutaneous pocket made from rotation of the V segments of a C–V flap. **(C)** The C segment is rotated over the top of the reconstruction cylinder to finish the nipple reconstruction.

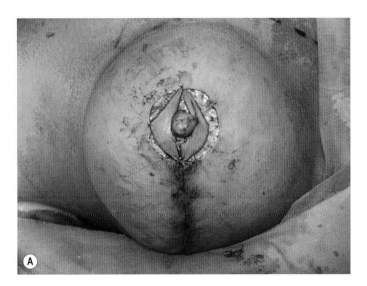

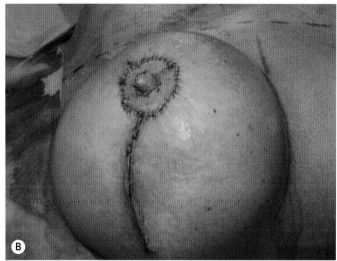

Fig. 22.29 (A) Two skin grafts being placed at the areola site is shown. **(B)** The completed skin graft on the areolar site is shown.

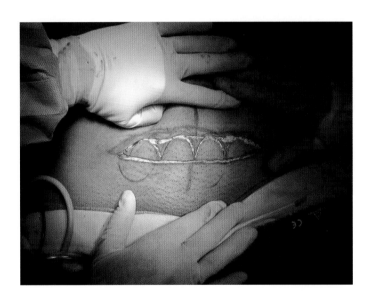

Fig. 22.30 A previous C-section scar is used to obtain skin grafts for areolar grafting. Half-circle configurations are made and elevated.

Box 22.1 **Common areola donor sites**

- Contralateral areola
- Inner thigh
- Excess/discarded skin
- Scar revision skin
- Labial tissue (rarely used).

site, the planned areola can be elevated and raised as a skin graft and re-placed into its original position.[70]

Tattooing is the other major adjunct to areola reconstruction. Either used by itself or in conjunction with skin grafting, tattooing can provide excellent areolar color match with limited morbidity. Initially introduced by Rees in 1975[71] and popularized by Spear et al.,[72] tattooing uses intradermal pigments, typically mixtures of iron and titanium oxide chosen from a color plate *(Fig. 22.31A)*. These pigments are then electrically deposited into the upper and mid-papillary dermis *(Fig. 22.31B)*. Sterile technique is mandatory as disease and viral transmission is possible. Pigment placement too superficially will result in pigment extrusion and sloughing, while deeper placement leads to macrophage processing and removal, both resulting in early pigment fading *(Fig. 22.31C)*.[73]

In unilateral cases, colors should be chosen that are slightly more pigmented than the contralateral areola. Spear and Arias found that 9.5% of areolas needed touch ups for pigment fading and that 60% of all areolas were described as being too light during the study interval.[74] Thus, many patients will likely need touch-up tattooing after several months or years to achieve an aesthetically symmetric color match.

After tattooing is performed, the area will usually undergo sloughing and crusting for 3–5 days. The area should be kept moist with bacitracin or other type of petroleum jelly and dressings should be changed daily. After this period, slight de-pigmentation may occur

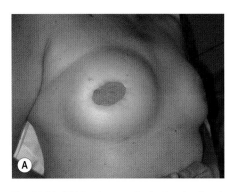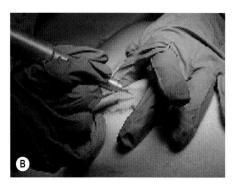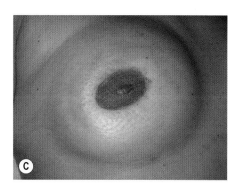

Fig. 22.31 **(A)** The chosen color is placed uniformly on the proposed tattoo site. **(B)** The tattoo pigment is electrically deposited with the use of a tattoo gun. **(C)** After the tattooing is finished, a nice uniform deposition of pigment should be observed.

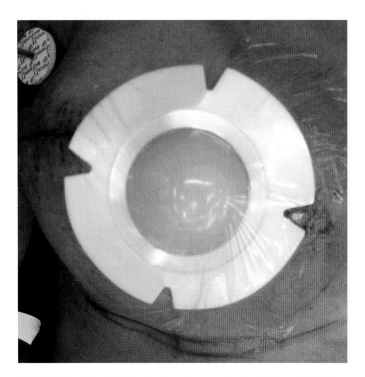

Fig. 22.32 A nipple shield is placed over the reconstructed nipple and is filled with hydrating jelly to promoting healing.

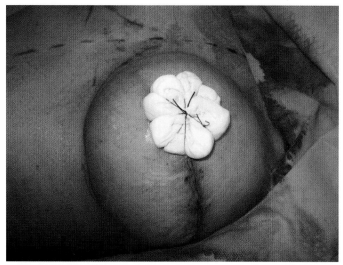

Fig. 22.33 A standard bolster dressing with Vaseline gauze is applied over an areola graft. Silk sutures are placed at the periphery of the areola to avoid later scarring.

and many patients will require touch-ups in the next few months.

Postoperative care

Currently, for local tissue flaps for nipple reconstruction, many nipple shields are available for use to protect the neo-nipple for the first few weeks after reconstruction. As seen in *Figure 22.32*, the silicone-based nipple shield protects the newly formed nipple from shearing stresses and mechanical forces that increase the likelihood of infection and flap loss.[19] This shield is kept in place for 1 week postoperatively and usually contains bacitracin or another hydrating gel to keep the healing nipple moist.

For composite nipple grafts and skin grafts, a standard bolster dressing is fashioned using silk sutures placed at the periphery and secured over the top of a cushioned pad of Vaseline gauze *(Fig. 22.33)*. Some degree of sloughing is to be expected. Standard bolster dressing may be removed between 3–5 days and gentle routine care afterwards with a nipple shield is encouraged as not to damage the new grafts.

Outcomes and satisfaction

Representing the final hurdle in breast reconstruction, nipple reconstruction has a large variety of different outcomes. Many studies have reported success with seemingly every type of flap. Flap choice, however, is best tailored to the individual person and previous oncologist surgery, as outcomes will vary from person to person using the same methods. The key factors in outcomes related to nipple reconstruction continue to be the preservation of long-term projection and contralateral symmetry. As seen throughout the chapter, multiple studies have reported the use of many of flaps described. Authors have reported varying amounts of projection maintained and absolute nipple height achieved.

Most studies report patient satisfaction after NAC reconstruction from 60–90%.[29,33,75] Although overall patient satisfaction is high in NAC reconstruction, Jabor *et al.* reports that approximately one-third of patients rate their NAC reconstruction as fair to poor. They found that the most common reasons for lack of satisfaction were the lack of projection, color mismatch, and shape/size discrepancies. They found no significance in the type of method used for reconstruction. Interestingly, they found that longer time intervals between breast mound and NAC reconstruction negatively impacted patient satisfaction.[75]

Complications

The most common complications with local flap techniques are projection loss, flap/nipple necrosis, dehiscence, malposition, and infection. When other graft types are used, complications related to graft loss, extrusion, and exposure are possible *(Box 22.2)*.

Most of the treatment options for these complications can be accomplished with antibiotics, minor office procedures, and/or operating room visits. Local wound care options promoting secondary healing

Box 22.2 **Common complications associated with nipple reconstruction**

- Loss of projection
- Partial flap loss
- Dehiscence
- Infection
- Malposition.

may, in fact, provide additional texture and color variations that add to the NAC reconstruction goals. Projection loss and malposition represent common and difficult complications following NAC reconstruction. Mainstay treatment options rely on revisional procedures to correct any asymmetrical projection loss or malposition.

Secondary and revisional reconstruction

Revisional and secondary procedures for nipple reconstruction are done mainly for the occurrence of common complications, and usually can be expected in 4–10% of patients.[31,57,76] In the setting of projection loss, some of the indwelling adjuncts, such as fat grafting, AlloDerm placement, and injectable fillers, are helpful at increasing projection. These techniques, though, may require additional procedures as projection loss will likely recur in the long term. Luckily, these adjuncts have no/minimal donor site morbidity, which makes them desirable alternative and repeatable procedures.

Caution must be taken if flap elevation is attempted as a secondary procedure. Scar and previous nipple position may lead to unsuccessful placement and survivability of any revisional flap.

When dealing with graft-related complications, many times removal and antibiotics are necessary to resolve any superficial infection that may be present. Revisional procedures should be delayed to allow for resolution of infection and tissue swelling.

Access the complete references list online at **http://www.expertconsult.com**

12. Anton MA, Eskenazi LB, Hartrampf CR Jr. Nipple reconstruction with local flaps: star and wrap flaps. *Perspect Plast Surg.* 1991;5:67–78.

22. Few JW, Marcus JR, Casas LA, et al. Long-term predictable nipple projection following reconstruction. *Plast Reconstr Surg.* 1999;104(5):1321–1324.

    Prospective evaluation of 93 nipple reconstructions using a modified star dermal fat flap technique. They found that flap length was a strong predictor of intra-operative and long-term projection. A linear relationship existed such that every 1-cm increase in flap length lead to an increase in 0.16 cm of nipple projection. At 2-years follow-up, 41% projection maintenance was achieved in both implant-based and TRAM-based reconstruction.

23. Shestak KC, Gabriel A, Landecker A, et al. Assessment of long-term nipple projection: a comparison of three techniques. *Plast Reconstr Surg.* 2002;110(3):780–786.

    Long-term assessment of patients who underwent NAC reconstruction with either a bell flap, a modified star flap, or a skate flap. If patients had areolar projection and <5 mm of nipple projection, a Bell flap (n=19) was used. If there was no areolar projection and <5 mm of projection, a modified star flap (n=30) was used. A subset of patients with >5 mm of projection had a skate flap and skin graft (n=25) placed. Projection was assessed at 3-month intervals for 12-month follow-up period. The study found that the Bell flap lost 70% projection, while the star and skate flap both lost 40% projection at 12-months follow-up. They found that projection loss stabilizes at 6 month postoperatively.

33. Losken A, Mackay GJ, Bostwick J 3rd. Nipple reconstruction using the C-V flap technique: a long-term evaluation. *Plast Reconstr Surg.* 2001;108(2):361–369.

43. Hammond DC, Khuthaila D, Kim J. The skate flap purse-string technique for nipple-areola complex reconstruction. *Plast Reconstr Surg.* 2007;120(2):399–406.

44. Shestak KC, Nguyen TD. The double opposing periareola flap: a novel concept for nipple-areola reconstruction. *Plast Reconstr Surg.* 2007;119(2):473–480.

66. Nahabedian MY. Secondary nipple reconstruction using local flaps and AlloDerm. *Plast Reconstr Surg.* 2005;115(7):2056–2061.

    Described the use of AlloDerm in revisional nipple reconstruction. He used AlloDerm in eight nipples to increase projection. A C–V flap or elongated C flap were for nipple reconstruction. Five of these were done in a secondary stage, while the remaining three were performed as tertiary reconstruction. One of five nipples reconstructed secondarily resulted in flattening and led to one of three tertiary reconstructions. Some 80% of patients had acceptable projection.

74. Spear SL, Arias J. Long-term experience with nipple-areola tattooing. *Ann Plast Surg.* 1995;35(3):232–236.

    Performed a long-term evaluation of 151 patients who underwent nipple-areola tattooing. A total of 57% of patients indicated that tattooed areola was similar to normal areola; 68% of patients graded the color as a close match or only 'slightly off in color'. Also, they found that there was a re-tattoo rate of 9.5% to correct for fading. There was a reported 3% infection rate and rare occurrences of rash and sloughing. In terms of satisfaction, 84% of patients reported somewhat-definitely satisfaction with tattooing. Some 86% of patients reported that they would undergo tattooing again.

75. Jabor MA, Shayani P, Collins DR Jr, et al. Nipple-areola reconstruction: satisfaction and clinical determinants. *Plast Reconstr Surg.* 2002;110(2):457–465.

    Performed a retrospective analysis of 120 patients who underwent breast mound and nipple reconstruction in order to assess patient satisfaction and long-term outcomes. The number of procedures needed to complete NAC reconstruction was one in 66% of patients, two in 32% of patients, and three or more in 2% of patients. Satisfaction for breast mound reconstruction was rated as excellent/good in 81% and fair in 14% of patients.

76. Eskenazi L. A one-stage nipple reconstruction with the "modified star" flap and immediate tattoo: a review of 100 cases. *Plast Reconstr Surg.* 1993;92(4):671–680.

23.1

Congenital anomalies of the breast

Egle Muti

SYNOPSIS

- The term "tuberous breast" is used to indicate a great variety of breast deformities that may present very different anatomical-morphologic characteristics, with differing degrees of severity.
- Hypoplastic tuberous breasts can be classified into three main types: type I, type II, and type III.
- Glandular flap tissue is transferred from the area of surplus to the area of deficiency. There are four main types of flaps used to correct these deformities: Flap type I (variously shaped) is used to correct type I breast deformity. Flap type II is used for type II breast deformity, in order to correct the typical deformity of the mammary profile due to retroareolar glandular protrusion. Flap type III and flap type IV are used in different ways to correct other breast type II deformities, according to the particular characteristics present in each single case.

Introduction

The term "tuberous breast" was described for the first time by Rees and Aston in 1976,[1] and is used to indicate a great variety of breast deformities, which may present very different anatomical-morphologic characteristics with differing degrees of severity. Various names are used to describe the deformity such as: tuberous breast; tubular breast; Snoopy breast; nipple breast; domed breast; herniated areolar complex; narrowed-based breast; constricted breast; lower pole hypoplasia. This creates great confusion, especially when describing the

different types of surgical technique utilized for its correction. An author often describes a precise surgical technique for the treatment of such malformations, without making a precise distinction between the different types of anatomical deformity or degree of severity of such malformations.

There is no single surgical technique suitable to correct all types of different malformations, however we can trace a common denominator such as: transferring the dislocated, retained, or constricted tissue through glandular flaps, which will correct the existing deformity and at the same time allow the opening and the extension of the retained and constricted fibrotic mammary base. In other words, through the use of glandular flaps, glandular tissue is transferred from the area of surplus to the area of deficiency.

This chapter considers the different forms of highly hypoplastic tuberous breast and some nontuberous congenital mammary asymmetry, without taking into consideration complex malformations of the chest wall such as pectus excavatum. (However, malformation of the muscular apparatus found in Poland syndrome is discussed Chapter 23.2).

The different types of tuberous breast deformities carry a psychological weight on the young patient and it highly influences young girls' relationships because of the unusual shape and appearance of their breasts.

The right time to intervene surgically is usually considered when the development of the breasts is clearly complete. But sometimes the decision to intervene more precociously may be taken due to the impact and emotional distress such deformity has on the patient. Of course, such decision should be taken together with the help of a psychologist and with the parent's approval.

Basic science/disease process

From the embryological development point of view, we can summarize by saying that the mammary bud is differentiated and formed during intrauterine life until birth[2] but its full development as the mammary organ occurs at the time of puberty. Such a period may vary from 7–9 to 15–16 years of age depending on different racial and constitutional characteristics.[3]

From an anatomical point of view, the mammary organ is formed by the split of two superficial layers of the superficial fascia, which continues into the superficial abdominal fascia ("fascia of Scarpa"). The superficial layer and the deeper layer of the superficial fascia lie anterior to the fascia pectoralis. These layers are penetrated by fibrous attachments that originate deeply behind the thoracic muscle, penetrating the parenchyma and the superficial layer of the superficial fascia, anchoring them in front of the derma that covers the breast in a more or less consistent manner.[4] These fibrous attachments are called Cooper's ligaments and represent the so-called suspension system of the breast, which determines the degree of effectiveness of the cutaneous glandular adhesion.

The etiology of the tuberous deformities is neither clear nor well-defined; some authors consider the absence of the superficial layer of the superficial fascia at the level of the areola an important element. Others stress the importance of objective clinical data in which we can observe, in different types of tuberous breast, the presence of a fibrous constricting ring around the areola.[5,6] Such a constricting ring can be more or less dense and more or less complete; sometimes, this ring is present only around the inferior half of the areola and extends itself to the inferior pole of the breast, like a fibrotic fascia, preventing or holding back the growth of the mammary gland. According to Mandrekas *et al.*, this fibrotic ring represents a thickening with fibrosis of the superficial fascia or hypertrophy of the Cooper's

ligaments.[2] The result, in any case, is that the mammary gland cannot expand in its inferior quadrants.

Almost all publications that discuss the subject of the tuberous breast describe a gland more or less herniated into the areola, with consequent areolar widening. Almost all classifications of the tuberous breast take into consideration this concept and distinguish the various types of deformities according to their location, degree of severity and lack of mammary development in the various quadrants.[1–36] However, in my opinion we should accept this definition and classification only for one type of tuberous breast, defined here as type I *(Figs 23.1.1, 23.1.2)*, and which is characterized by severe hypotrophy of Cooper's ligaments. The definition is not suitable to describe, e.g., the breast deformity in Case III right breast (see below), which is classified here as tuberous breast type II *(Fig. 23.1.3)*. This type of tuberous breast presents a very small and compacted areola with the gland protruding behind it and pushing the areola forward, without widening it. The areola also presents a strong cutaneous glandular adherence due to hypertrophy of Cooper's ligaments *(Fig. 23.1.6A,B)*. These morphological clinical features are indeed completely different from those we observe in a type I tuberous breast. ⊛ FIGS 23.1.1C–F; I–O, 23.1.2C; E–G, O, Q, 23.1.3E, F, H, J APPEAR ONLINE ONLY

In the pathogenesis of these malformations we could assume the existence of a common initial pathogenic element, which differentiating in a precocious manner, produces the formation of different morphological entities which require, in the author's opinion, a different corrective surgical approach. (See, e.g., the difference between Case II, *Figure 23.1.2* and the right breast in Case III, *Figure 23.1.3*.)

Diagnosis/patient presentation

An accurate diagnosis is a fundamental first step to obtain a successful good result in any medical surgical field, but it is particularly important in aesthetic or dysmorphia surgery which, as for tuberous breast, is more closely related to reconstructive surgery than the purely aesthetic surgery. Such a diagnosis should include not only the patient's objective examination, localized to the mammary organ, but should also take into consideration a complete examination of the general clinical

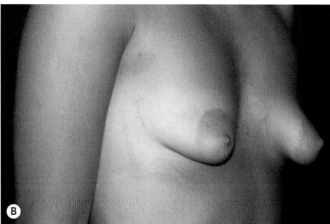

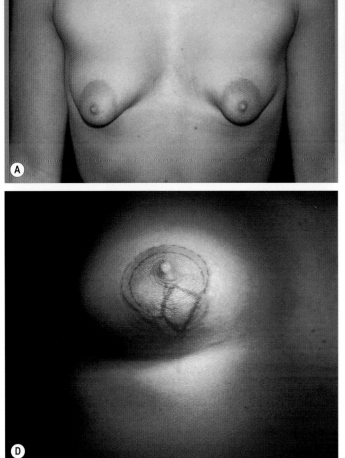

Fig. 23.1.1 (A,B) Typical example of bilateral symmetric tuberous breast type I in a 23-year-old female patient, showing a degree of glandular prolapse into the inferior half of the expanded areola. **(D)** Intraoperative sequence: the preoperative evaluation marks a peripheral ring of deepithelialization to lift the areola in order to reduce its diameter thus enhancing its conicity of the areolae, a rhombus of skin is marked in the central inferior portion of the areola which will be excised. This rhombus will correspond to the projection of the glandular herniation. (A,B,D, reproduced with permission from Muti E. Personal approach to surgical correction of the extre mely hypoplastic tuberous breast. *Aesthetic Plastic Surgery Review*, New York: Springer-Verlag. 1996;20:385–390.)

status and psychological attitude of the patient. Correct assessment of the patient's general health status and thorough questioning with regard to detailed clinical family and personal history, with specific instrumental examination will greatly reduce or even avoid general postoperative complications. A correct preoperative diagnosis of any morphological malformations enables the most proper surgical correction technique to be chosen.

It is essential that careful attention should be paid to assess the patient's psychological attitude and her real expectations before any operative planning is made. Such attention will greatly reduce, or even avoid dissatisfaction of the result, and avoid or reduce any potential legal issues. This aspect is often underestimated and represents an elevated risk for the surgeon because it may lead him/her to a "wrong" evaluation. In fact, a young patient is often unable to express clearly her own aesthetic ideas, fears and expectations, and the surgeon may not always possess the necessary skill and preparation to understand this aspect of their patient. The author recommends a private interview with the young patient without the presence of her parents, as they may influence her attitude.

Hints and tips

- A disturbed patient is a good candidate to be an unsatisfied patient
- An "unsuitable" psychological attitude should be sufficient reason to refuse surgical procedure to a patient seeking this type of surgery

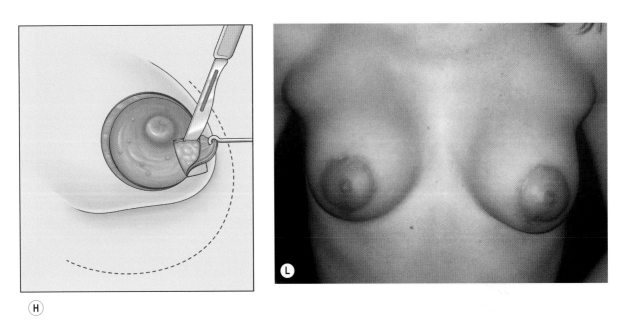

Fig. 23.1.1, cont'd (H) The flap type I is sculpted down to the deep plane and lifted. **(L)** The prosthesis is implanted in a pre-pectoral plane, the areola is lifted and reduced, and the skin is sutured with a periareolar and a very short vertical scar.

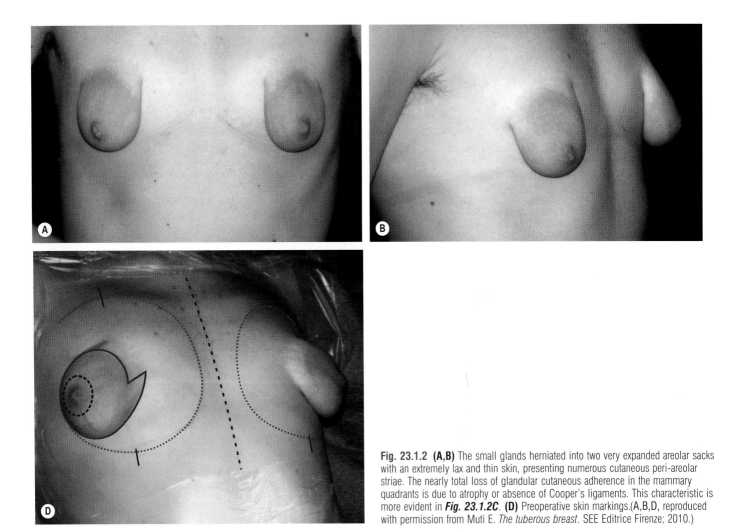

Fig. 23.1.2 (A,B) The small glands herniated into two very expanded areolar sacks with an extremely lax and thin skin, presenting numerous cutaneous peri-areolar striae. The nearly total loss of glandular cutaneous adherence in the mammary quadrants is due to atrophy or absence of Cooper's ligaments. This characteristic is more evident in **Fig. 23.1.2C. (D)** Preoperative skin markings.(A,B,D, reproduced with permission from Muti E. *The tuberous breast*. SEE Editrice Firenze; 2010.)

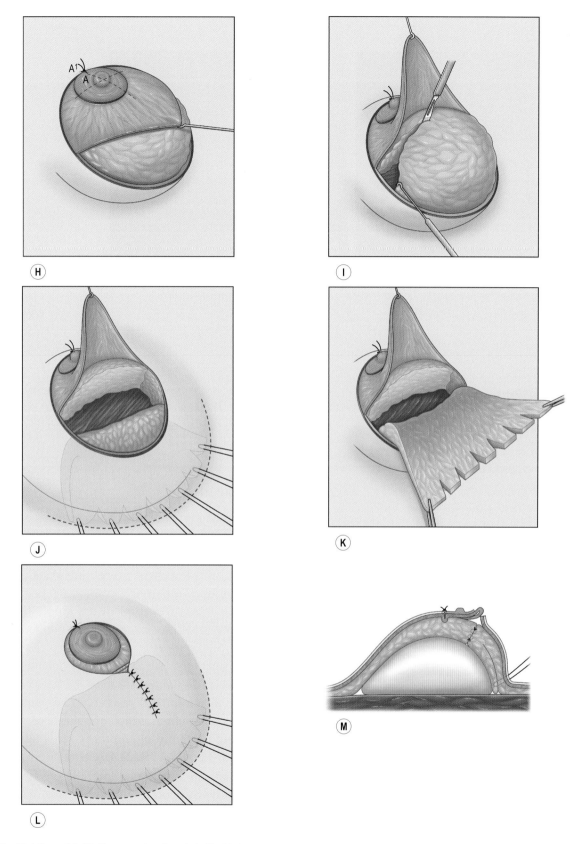

Fig. 23.1.2, cont'd (H) The new reduced areola is lifted in its new position. The dermis of the inferior pole is undermined up to the inferior border of the areola. **(I)** The dermal flap is lifted. The herniated gland is transversally incised at full thickness from the inferior border of the new areola, down to the muscle-thoracic plane. **(J)** A square-shaped glandular flap is exposed, multiple small incisions on its free margins are performed in order to spread it in fan like shape, allowing a wider distribution along the new inframammary fold. **(K)** Few transcutaneous stitches are performed fixing into the desired position the free margins of the flap. **(L)** The flap is fixed into position, the prosthesis is implanted in the pre-pectoral plane, the skin is sutured with a periareolar and a short vertical scar in the inferior pole. **(M)** Lateral vision at the end of surgery. The prosthesis is placed in a pre-pectoral plane. The glandular flap is folded under the skin of the inferior pole, with the margins fixed at the new IMF with few transcutaneous stitches. The dermal flap from the inferior pole, in this unusual solution, is folded under the areola between the ducts, through blunt dissection, to increase areolar projection.

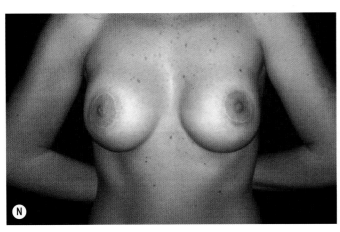
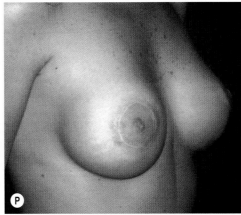

Fig. 23.1.2, cont'd **(N)** This 10-year postoperative result still shows the good shape, volume and symmetry achieved. **(P)** This oblique 10-year postoperative result shows the good anatomical shape of the breast with a smooth superior pole and a full inferior pole, although round prosthesis were utilized.

Examination of the patient

Carefully evaluate details such as:

- The shape of the breast and its essential anatomical features, which allows classification of the breast into the proper typology
- Possible breast asymmetry, even if minimal, and also any asymmetry of the thoracic wall
- Cutaneous quality, degree of skin laxity, presence of any cutaneous striae
- Presence of scars due to previous surgery.

The objective and detailed exam enables placement of the patient into the correct morphological type, corresponding to the author's own classification (see below), in order to choose the proper preoperative planning.

Classification of the different types of tuberous breast deformity

For long time I (the author) reflected over the necessity for a classification for the numerous and diverse types of tuberous breast, but could not find agreement with the various current proposed classifications.[2] However, I can now identify the most important elements that combine into a broad family of similar groups of the numerous diverse forms of tuberous-tubular deformity. After careful consideration, I have distinguished three

different types of hypoplastic tuberous breasts: type I, type II, and type III. This chapter presents some significant clinical examples which I have encountered in my practice.

Type I: tuberous breast

The most significant morphologic characteristics are as follows:

- Mammary tissue herniating into an expanded areola with lax and thin skin presenting poor cutaneous glandular adherence, sometimes occurs only in the half inferior portion of the areola *(Fig. 23.1.1A–C)*, but sometimes in the whole areola, which is generally very expanded *(Fig. 23.1.2A–C)*. The Cooper's ligaments seem to be hypoplastic or absent.
- The inframammary fold (IMF) is very cranialized with a fibrotic constriction, which appears like a constricting ring surrounding, almost completely, the small gland *(Figs 23.1.1B, 23.1.2C)*
- Often, the breasts are positioned laterally on the chest wall with a wide intermammary space.

Type II: tuberous breast

The most significant morphologic characteristics are as follows:

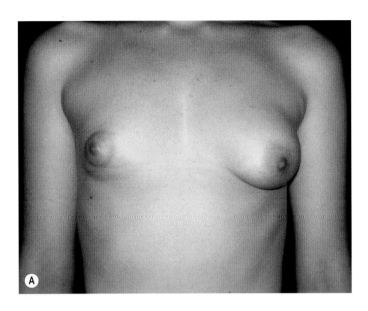

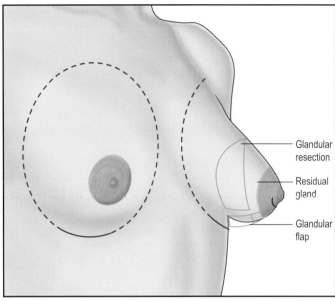

Fig. 23.1.3 (A) This preoperative frontal view shows, besides the deformity and the asymmetry, the extreme lateralization of the breasts on the thorax, which makes this case much more difficult to correct. **(B)** In this case of asymmetry, the author follows his preferred choice: to reduce the bigger breast to the same size and shape of the smaller one by using two equal prosthetic implants on both breasts. This figure shows the drawing of a yellow area with a red dotted line indicating the expected subcutaneous glandular resection to be performed on the left breast in order to match the volume of the right breast. On the right side, it is marked with a red line the new inframammary-fold and the access to the prosthetic pocket. **(C)** Preoperative view. This view shows the right breast deformity in profile (marked with a red line). The fundamental characteristics of type II tuberous deformity are clearly evident. (A–C, reproduced with permission from Muti E. Local flaps for tuberous and asymmetric breasts. In: Hall-Findlay EJ, ed. *Breast surgery*. Philadelphia: Saunders Elsevier; 2010.)

- Severely hypoplastic breast with solid skin, small or very small areola, and strong cutaneous glandular adherence
- The mammary base is constricted, although the constricting ring is not so evident
- The inferior pole is absent, flat, or concave
- The inframammary fold is absent

- Typical glandular protrusion behind the areola with deformity of the inferior border of the areola; such deformity is enhanced after the introduction of the prosthesis, even when releasing incisions of the inferior pole are performed.[19,26]
- The areolas are mostly positioned on the most lateral aspect of thorax quadrants (see the right breast in *Fig. 23.1.3A,C*).

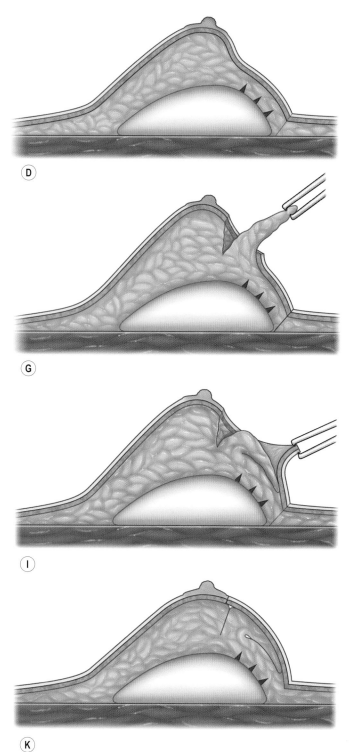

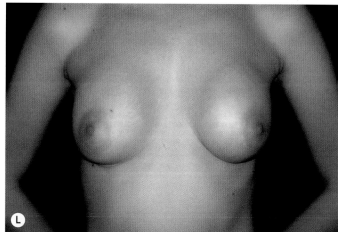

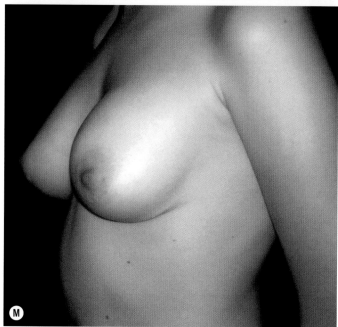

Fig. 23.1.3, cont'd **(D)** After BAM, and even though some releasing incisions of the glandular and subcutaneous tissue of the inferior pole have been performed, the breast still appears flat and a certain infra-retro areolar protrusion is still evident. **(G)** Creation of the glandular pedicled small flap is seen. **(I)** The flap is inserted under the undermined skin from the central region of the inferior pole. **(K)** The apex of the flap is positioned and fixed in the desired place, sometimes with few transcutaneous stitches. The inferior pole profile appears completely changed with a round convex shape. **(L)** This 4-year postoperative result shows the good shape and symmetrization of both breasts is retained. **(M)** The shape, symmetry, and the natural aspects of the breasts with complete correction of the single lateral deformity are seen. (D,G, reproduced with permission from Muti E. Local flaps for tuberous and asymmetric breasts. In: Hall-Findlay EJ, ed. *Breast surgery*. Philadelphia: Saunders Elsevier; 2010.)

Type III: tuberous breast

The most significant morphologic characteristics are as follows:

- The breasts are normoplastic
- Breasts appear basically tubular
- A "dive" ptosis and a nipple-areola-complex turning downward
- A circular "mammary footprint" positioned generally high, although not excessively lateralized, on the thorax
- Reduced distance of the nipple-areola-complex.

Hints and tips

Type III tuberous breast on the left side is often associated with type II tuberous breast on the right side *(Fig. 23.1.3A–C)*. Is this pure coincidence or is there a genetic link?

Treatment/surgical technique

General considerations

A number of techniques have been described to correct these breast malformations[1–36] but because of their great polymorphism, it is impossible to adopt a single ideal surgical technique suitable to each single morphological feature or for every type of tuberous deformity. Therefore, in trying to resolve this difficulty, I came to the conclusion that there could be a solution to this problem by adopting a common basic concept which could be modified, adapted and tailored to each single case.

The concept includes the creation of glandular flaps of different shapes designed in such a way to mobilize the mammary tissue and redistributing it according to the need of each single case. Furthermore, with the creation of these flaps, we are able to obtain the opening of the constricted and fibrotic mammary base. The glandular flap sculpted at full thickness down to the pectoralis fascia allows the opening of the mammary base, interrupting the fibrotic constriction present at the base of the breast. To complete the above described manoeuvres, the author performs gland and subcutaneous deep releasing radial incisions according to Rees and Aston[1] and Maxwell.[6]

In less hypoplastic breasts, the desired result is obtained through the so-called deep glandular unfurling flap manoeuvre, also defined as unfurling of the deep surface of the mammary base.[4,9,16] Moreover, according to each specific morphologic characteristic, possible correction is performed, such as lifting and reduction of the areola or areolas, tailored reduction of the mammary gland, in cases of asymmetry and reduction of the cutaneous sack. Once the deformity has been completely corrected, we can implant the mammary prosthesis.

Hints and tips

The mammary deformity should be completely corrected before the insertion of the prosthesis. I totally disagree with those aesthetic surgeons who recommend the use of larger prosthesis in order to attain a better control of the deformity.

The selection of the type of prosthesis (round or anatomical, etc.), the choice of prosthetic pocket, and access for the implant will vary from case to case and is explained during the description of the surgical technique adopted for each single case. In the author's opinion, it is very important to avoid the use of heavy and large size prosthesis. It is important to remember the young age of many of patients and that the bigger and heavier the prosthesis, the more frequent and more important will be the inconvenience caused by its size and weight: relaxation and thinning of the skin, lowering of the prosthesis with pseudoptosis, and visibility and wrinkling of the prosthetic borders. Smaller and lighter prostheses result in less or inexistent future potential problems. Furthermore, it is now possible to supplement prosthesis where the size is considered insufficient, or to soften the mammary contour through the use of lipostructure according to the Coleman technique.[13] With this technique, we may even be able to substitute the use of prosthesis completely. This is a future ideal goal.

Surgical technique

Glandular correction flaps

As discussed above, tuberous deformity of the breast may be classified into three different types, each of them presenting some fundamental common characteristics that can be corrected with its relative type of glandular flap.

The types of glandular flaps are:

- *Flap type I* (see Cases I and II)
- *Flap type II* (see Case III – right breast)
- *Flap type III* (see Case VI)
- *Flap type IV* (see Case IV)

Flap type I (variously shaped) is used to correct type I breast deformity. *Flap type II* is used for type II breast deformity in order to correct the typical deformity of the mammary profile due to retroareolar glandular protrusion. *Flap type III* and *flap type IV* are used in different ways to correct other breast type II deformities, according to the particular characteristics present in each single case.

Glandular flap type I

Video 1

Glandular flap type I is created with a central inferior glandular flap with an inferior superficial pedicle, which will be sculpted at full thickness down to the thoracic plane, presenting its apex toward the base of the nipple and its pedicle based on the subcutaneous vascular blood net, at the level of the inferior constrictive border or pseudo infra mammary fold. The size and shape of the flap will vary from case to case, but it usually includes the gland that appears herniated into the areola. The flap is horizontally incised at the level of the inferior border of the areola down to the muscle-thoracic plane, then it is deeply and caudally folded over, bringing its apex toward the new inframammary fold *(Fig. 23.1.1D–M)*. This surgical procedure will be then completed according to each particular case with other details such as lifting/reduction of the areola, remodeling of the retroareolar glandular tissue, conization of the mammary cone, placement of the prosthesis and closure of the skin incisions.

The aims of this flap are as follows:

- The transference of the herniated gland into the insufficient or inexistent inferior pole in order to thicken it
- The interruption of the fibrotic mammary base allowing its opening
- The reduction of the enlarged areola.

Glandular flap type II

Glandular flap type II is correlated with tuberous breast deformity type II (see right breast of Case III, *Fig. 23.1.3A,C*).

This is a glandular flap, glandular pedicled and superficially, subcutaneously rotated. It is used to transfer a certain amount of gland protruding behind the small areola to the center of the inferior pole under the tense skin. This flap can be defined as a small retroareolar glandular flap. The aims of this flap are as follows:

- To eliminate the retroareolar glandular protrusion that determines the deformity of the breast profile
- To undermine the tense skin below the areola on the central part of the inferior pole. This allows the detachment of the Cooper's ligaments, eliminating the strong adherence between the skin and the gland
- To interpose the small flap between the skin and the gland thus avoiding the recurrence of the defect
- The transfer of a flap on the inferior pole. Even if it is a small one, will entirely change the shape of the breast profile giving the inferior pole a nice round shape *(Fig. 23.1.3F–J)*.

Glandular flap type III

Glandular flap type III is created from the deep retroareolar surface used to mobilize a certain amount of tissue from the upper side to the inferior side of the areola both superiorly and inferiorly to it. This flap is used to modify certain type II deformity, where the very small gland is protruding completely behind the small areola *(Fig. 23.1.6A)*. The aims of this flap are as follows:

- To smooth the superior border of the areola, transferring the protruding gland to the inferior pole below the inferior border of the areola, thus obtaining continuity between them with a nice breast profile
- To open the central, deep fibrotic surface of the gland.

Glandular flap type IV

Glandular flap type IV is a deep flap created using some part of the deep surface of the breast from the upper retroareolar region to the inferior border of the gland

and creating a flap "a", which is freed and caudally stretched under the inferior pole, with a movement mimicking the opening of a clenched fist. This flap is used to correct tuberous breast deformity type II, when sufficient thickness of the breast and soft tissue covering the thoracic wall are present, and the base is not too narrow. The aims of this flap are as follows:

- To open the fibrotic glandular base
- To thicken the inferior pole.

Clinical examples

Case I

A 23-year-old female patient presented with a typical example of bilateral symmetric tuberous breast type I *(Fig. 23.1.1C)*. A certain degree of glandular prolapse into the inferior half of the expanded areola was evident. The IMF was cranialized and tense, with a very short distance between the inferior border of the areola and the inframammary fold. The inferior mammary pole was practically absent. The mammary base was quite well positioned on the thoracic wall. The skin was of good quality, with a relatively acceptable intermammary space. The preoperative evaluation marked a peripheral ring of de-epithelialization to lift the areola in order to reduce its diameter thus enhancing conicity of the areola. A rhombus of skin was marked in the central inferior portion of the areola, which will be excised. This rhombus will correspond to the projection of the glandular herniation *(Fig. 23.1.1D)*. The glandular herniation, which will be used to create the glandular flap type I was clearly evident *(Fig. 23.1.1E)*. The glandular flap sculpted at full thickness down to the deep plane was stretched outward *(Fig. 23.1.1F)*.

Intraoperative result

The flap has been deeply and caudally rotated with its apex toward the new lowered inframammary fold. It is pedicled on the inferior subcutaneous vascular net. The areola has been lifted and flattened in half inferiorly. The mammary prosthesis has been inserted through the existing incisions in a pre-pectoral plane. In this case, a Dow Corning round micro-structured Prosthesis of 210 cc has been utilized *(Fig. 23.1.1G)*. The flap type I is

sculpted down to the deep plane and lifted. The flap is rotated deeply and caudally under the skin of the inferior pole with its apex reaching the new inframammary fold. The prosthesis is implanted in a pre-pectoral plane, the areola is lifted and reduced, and the skin is sutured with a periareolar and a very short vertical scar *(Fig. 23.1.1H–M)*. Postoperative results are shown in *Figure 23.1.1N,O* and demonstrate the optimal stability of the result with a natural and pleasant appearance of the upper and lower pole and good symmetry of the breasts without residual deformity.

Case II

A young 17-year-old patient presents with severe tuberous breast deformity *(Fig. 23.1.2A–C)*. Because of the severity of this malformation we can consider this case as a variation of tuberous breast type I. This is a more difficult case because of the wide areolar expansion conditioning the preoperative markings necessary for the cutaneous resection.

Intraoperative result

The difficulty is shown by the wide extension of the areolar skin which covers and comprises practically the whole mammary gland. This influences the preoperative skin markings *(Fig. 23.1.2D)*, forcing us to perform a cutaneous resection that will comprise the residual areolar skin around the new areola. This is in contrast with what could have been our ideal resection whether we want to choose the periareolar technique or to perform a cutaneous resection with periareolar and vertical redistribution on the inferior pole. This last choice is by far the most appropriate one. In this case, once the periareolar deepithelialization is performed, the dermis of the inferior pole is incised on its lateral and medial borders, up to the equatorial line of the areola, then the dermis is undermined and lifted up to the inferior border of the new areola *(Fig. 23.1.2E,F)*. The small gland which becomes still more prolapsed and evident, is incised at the level of the inferior border of the new areola, transversally at full thickness down to the thoracic-muscle plane thus creating a square shaped flap, which can be seen in *Figure 23.1.2F,I*. The retro-glandular plane is then appropriately undermined in order to create the prosthetic pocket, in this case, pre-pectoral. The glandular flap remains as subcutaneous inferior pedicle based on the superficial cutaneous vascular net. The flap is than folded over on itself (with finger flexion-like movement), bringing its apex toward the new inframammary fold *(Fig. 23.1.2G,M)*.

Furthermore in this case, the free margins of the flap are stretched in a fan like shape through numerous, small peripheral incisions, in order to fully redistribute the flap in the inferior pole, above the prosthesis *(Fig. 23.1.2L)*. The newly widened free margin of the flap is fixed into the desired position with few transcutaneous stitches, we then proceed to the placement of the prosthesis; to the reconstruction of the glandular continuity between the upper pole and inferior pole, and at the end suturing of cutaneous incisions *(Fig. 23.1.2D–G)*.

Intraoperative sequence

The new reduced areola is lifted in its new position. The dermis of the inferior pole is undermined up to the inferior border of the areola *(Fig. 23.1.2H)*. The dermal flap is lifted. The herniated gland is transversally incised at full thickness from the inferior border of the new areola, down to the muscle-thoracic plane *(Fig. 23.1.2I)*.

A square-shaped glandular flap is exposed and multiple small incisions on its free margins are performed in order to spread it in fan-like shape allowing a wider distribution along the new IMF *(Fig. 23.1.2L)*. Few transcutaneous stitches are performed fixing into the desired position the free margins of the flap *(Fig. 23.1.2M)*.

The flap is fixed into position, the prosthesis is implanted in the pre-pectoral plane, the skin is sutured with a periareolar and a short vertical scar in the inferior pole *(Fig. 23.1.2N)*. Lateral vision at the end of surgery. The prosthesis is placed in a pre-pectoral plane *(Fig. 23.1.2O)*. The glandular flap is folded under the skin of the inferior pole, with the margins fixed at the new IMF with few transcutaneous stitches. In this unusual solution, the dermal flap from the inferior pole is folded under the areola between the ducts, through blunt dissection, to increase areolar projection.

Postoperative result

The 10-year postoperative result still shows the good shape, volume and symmetry achieved *(Fig. 23.1.2P)*.

The scars are slightly evident due to bad skin quality and initial cutaneous suturing tension 18 years postoperatively *(Fig. 23.1.2Q)*. The oblique 10-year postoperative result showed they achieved good anatomical shape of the breast with a smooth superior pole and a full inferior pole although round prosthesis were utilized. In this case, two round Dow Corning, micro-structured, high profile prosthesis of 270 cc were used. The implant was inserted in a pre-pectoral pocket through periareolar incisions.

Asymmetric tuberous breast deformity

General considerations

Asymmetric tuberous breast deformity always present a real challenge even to the most skilled and experienced surgeon, especially when he/she wants to attain the goal of one surgical stage procedure. This type of malformation often presents a greater surgical difficulty because it includes not only the general difficulty associated with asymmetry, but also includes difficulty associated with tuberous breast deformity. Asymmetry of shape associated with asymmetry of volume is challenging, and because we are treating mostly young patients, the long-term result should be carefully evaluated taking into consideration all the possible changes, such as those associated with weight variations, pregnancy or body aging. On the basis of these criteria, it is very important to use a very similar strategy on both breasts, e.g., if the case requires the use of prosthesis on one side of the breast, I might use the same size prosthesis on the other side. This will avoid the inconvenience of having one prosthetic breast and one nonprosthetic breast. For this reason I strongly recommend, whenever possible, to reduce the size of the bigger breast to the size and shape of the smaller one in order to place, if the case permits it, two equal prosthesis. This objective achieved through the use of an Aimed subcutaneous segmentary glandular resection (ASSGR), preoperatively calculated through careful observation and palpation of the breast, with the patient in a standing position. This represents the author's preferred choice whenever possible.

Case III

This is an example of bilateral tuberous breast with asymmetry in a young patient, presenting *type II right* tuberous deformity and *type III left* tuberous deformity. The preoperative frontal view *(Fig. 23.1.3A)* shows the deformity and the asymmetry, as well as the extreme lateralization of the breasts on the thorax, which makes this case much more difficult to correct.

Preoperative planning

In this case of asymmetry, I follow my preferred choice: to reduce the bigger breast to the same size and shape as that of the smaller breast in order to use two equal prosthetic implants on both breasts. *Figure 23.1.3B* shows the drawing of a yellow area with a red dotted line, indicating the expected subcutaneous glandular resection to be performed on the left breast in order to match the volume of the right breast. On the right side, it is marked with a red line the new inframammary-fold and the access to the prosthetic pocket. *Figure 23.1.3C* shows, with a white line, the right breast profile deformity. The fundamental characteristics of *type II* tuberous deformity are clearly evident:

- severe mammary hypoplasia
- firm skin with strong cutaneous glandular adherence
- small or very small areola
- constricted mammary base
- flat or often concave inferior pole
- absent inframammary fold
- typical glandular protrusion behind the areola with subsequent deformity of the mammary profile which, if not properly corrected, will be enhanced by the insertion of the prosthesis even if releasing incisions of the inferior pole are performed
- the areolas are mostly positioned on most lateral aspect of the quadrants.

Surgical procedure right breast type II tuberous deformity with type II glandular flap

The type II tuberous breast deformity is frequently underestimated. Many surgeons consider that relaxing the tension of the inferior pole through radial glandular and/or subcutaneous incisions, according to Rees and Aston[1] and Maxwell,[6] and introducing an adequate prosthesis, the deformity will be corrected. The author's opinion is on the contrary, this small but clearly evident irregularity of the inferior pole profile will be enhanced after the introduction of the prosthesis. For this reason, an appropriate and careful evaluation of this detail and its correction using the correct flap is essential. According to my experience, a simple but effective and precise correction can be obtained utilizing flap type II, shown in *Figures 23.1.3D–J*. It is important to stress that even a small flap inserted under the undermined skin of the inferior pole will definitely change the shape and profile of the breast *(Fig. 23.1.3L)*. In this patient, the anatomical shaped prosthesis were inserted in a retro-pectoral plane.

Case IV

A 25-year-old patient presenting with *type II* tuberous breasts, more evident on the right side. The typical features of this type of deformity can be observed:

- The inferior pole is concave and tense
- The gland is protruding under the areola
- The inframammary fold is very cranialized
- Small areolas
- The skin is tonic with strong adherence between the skin and the gland.

In this particular case, the breast and the thoracic skin envelope present good thickness and quite a large glandular base *(Fig. 23.1.4A)*.

Preoperative planning

Because of the particular large thorax, thick soft tissue and relatively large glandular foot print in this case, we chose a different correction flap: flap *type IV* formed by tackling the gland from its deep surface *(Fig. 23.1.4B)*.

Operative sequence of flap type IV

Starting from the deep retroareolar region, we incised the deep surface of the gland continuing toward the sulcus, creating a horizontal flap caudally pedicled on the gland (Flap A) *(Fig. 23.1.4C–E)*. This flap is stretched toward the new sulcus, thus obtaining the following effects:

- The opening of the constricted fibrotic mammary base
- The flattening of the abnormal retroareolar glandular protrusion
- The thickening of the insufficient inferior pole.

This technique has been also described by Benelli,[7,8] Botti[4] and Persichetti et al.,[29] with few differing details.

Postoperative result

The two inframammary folds are in good and symmetric position at 2 years postoperatively. The two nipple areola complexes are also well positioned. The volume appears sufficient and in harmony with the whole thoracic feature. The final appearance of the breast is very natural and soft. Shape, symmetry, natural appearance, and beauty of the breasts are shown in the frontal and two oblique views *(Fig. 23.1.4F–H)*.

Case V

A 23-year-old patient presented with severe bilateral mammary hypoplasia and monolateral tuberous

deformity *type II* on the left breast corrected with flap type II *(Fig. 23.1.5A–D)*.

Result after lipostructure

To improve the general natural appearance of the breasts, the patient underwent a lipostructure treatment, with Coleman technique 6-months after surgery *(Fig. 23.1.5E,F)*.

Case VI

Figure 23.1.6A–D shows an example of the use of flap *type III* for a different case of tuberous breast deformity *type II*. The protrusion of the gland is evident behind the areola with a fibrotic ring around its periphery. This postoperative view shows the corrected shape of the areola *(Fig. 23.1.6B)*. A rectangular shaped flap is

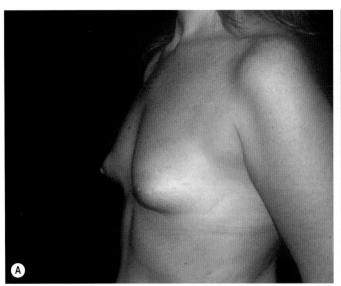

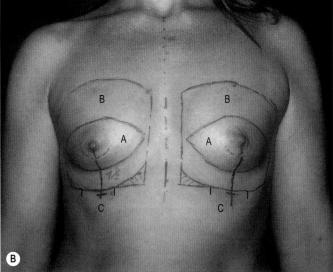

Fig. 23.1.4 (A) The deformity of the contour of the right breast, the retroareolar protrusion, the tense inferior pole and the cranialized IMF are visible. The contour of the base of the gland is outlined. **(B)** Preoperative skin markings are marked. The contour of the prosthetic pocket is outlined. (A,B reproduced with permission from Muti E. The tuberous breast. SEE Editrice Firenze; 2010.)

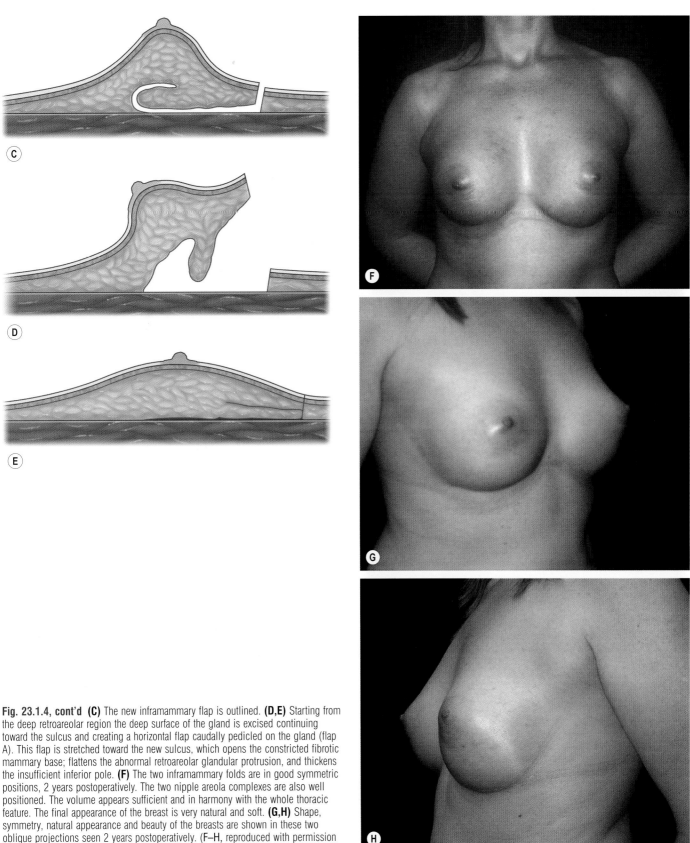

Fig. 23.1.4, cont'd (C) The new inframammary flap is outlined. **(D,E)** Starting from the deep retroareolar region the deep surface of the gland is excised continuing toward the sulcus and creating a horizontal flap caudally pedicled on the gland (flap A). This flap is stretched toward the new sulcus, which opens the constricted fibrotic mammary base; flattens the abnormal retroareolar glandular protrusion, and thickens the insufficient inferior pole. **(F)** The two inframammary folds are in good symmetric positions, 2 years postoperatively. The two nipple areola complexes are also well positioned. The volume appears sufficient and in harmony with the whole thoracic feature. The final appearance of the breast is very natural and soft. **(G,H)** Shape, symmetry, natural appearance and beauty of the breasts are shown in these two oblique projections seen 2 years postoperatively. (F–H, reproduced with permission from Muti E. *The tuberous breast*. SEE Editrice Firenze; 2010.)

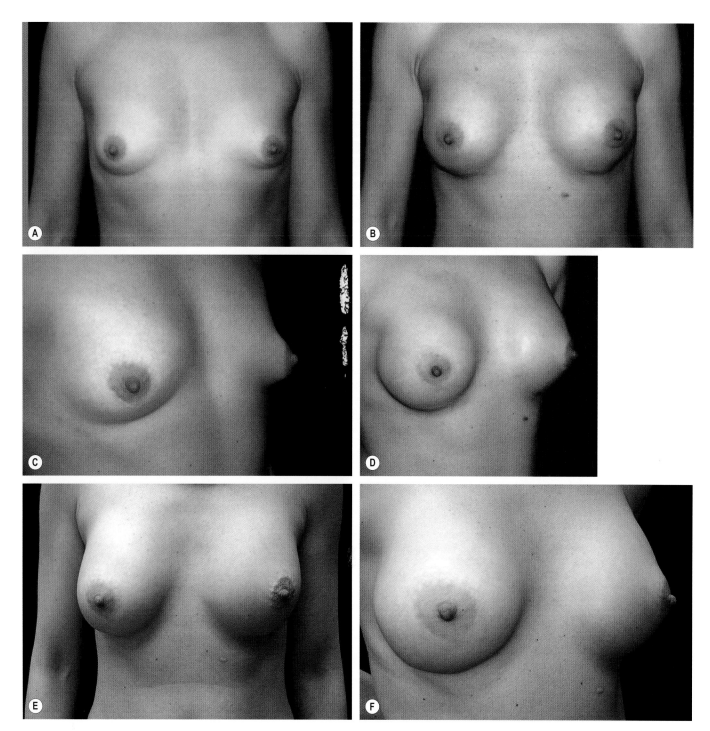

Fig. 23.1.5 (A) Severe bilateral hypoplasia with tuberous deformity type II on left breast and mild volume asymmetry for prevalence of right breast is shown. **(B)** Good symmetrization has been obtained at 6 months postoperatively, although the intermammary space is still too wide and the breasts appear solid and fixed. **(C)** The typical retro-glandular protrusion of the small gland projects as a cylinder like shape. **(D)** Seen here at 6 months postoperatively, the left breast has been corrected with flap type II (also used for the right breast of Case III). A certain capsular contracture and fixity of the prosthesis with an unnatural appearance of the breast is evident. **(E,F)** At 1 year after one lipostructure, the appearance of the breasts have completely changed; the capsular contracture is almost gone and the breasts have a more natural look with a smooth contour. (A–F, reproduced with permission from Muti E. *The tuberous breast*. SEE Editrice Firenze; 2010.)

transferred from the superior half of the deep surface of the areola to the inferior half of it *(Fig. 23.1.6C)*. This flap is created to obtain a smooth superior breast profile and a better continuity between the areola and the inferior pole. At the same time, the base of the gland has been open and relaxed, allowing its redistribution over the prosthesis *(Fig. 23.1.6D)*. ⊛ FIG **23.1.6** APPEARS ONLINE ONLY

Nontuberous congenital breast asymmetry

General considerations

A certain degree of breast asymmetry is very often present in women and if it is within certain limits, this is accepted as normal, especially if we have asymmetry of volume, but becomes a problem when there is asymmetry of shape or asymmetry of the areolas. Correcting mammary asymmetries, although less difficult than correcting asymmetric tuberous breast deformity represent the same surgical challenge.

Hints and tips

The surgeon who undertakes the correction of this kind of pathology should possess great competence and skills in the different surgical techniques and should exercise observation and scrupulous perseverance to achieve the result without overlooking even the smallest detail.

Congenital mammary asymmetries present a wide variety of situations and as many variable degrees of surgical difficulties. Asymmetries can be distinguished according to three different levels of difficulty and each level is based on the specific surgical procedure needed to correct the asymmetry.

First level: bilateral similar surgical procedure on both breasts

- Bilateral ptosis
- Bilateral hypertrophy more or less asymmetric
- Bilateral hypoplasia.

It is quite obvious that by intervening simultaneously on both breasts presenting the same pathology, it is possible to adapt the correction to each breast in order to obtain symmetry. In these cases, we can consider the result to be easy, predictable and stable (see Case VII, below).

Second level: monolateral operation

There could be two different situations:
- Monolateral hypertrophy with > < ptosis
- Monolateral hypotrophy needing augmentation mammaplasty

In these cases, we can consider the result to be more difficult, less predictable and more or less stable *(Fig. 23.1.8)*. If we need to intervene only on one breast, the challenge is obtaining, as much as possible, volume and shape equal to the contralateral breast, without intervening on the latter. In the case of mastopexy or breast reduction mammaplasty, we should be able to plan and foresee the necessary adjustment of movement and stabilization that the operated breast will require during the first 6 months post-surgery. We should keep in mind that these modifications will be greater for predominantly adipose breasts and lesser for mostly glandular breast. Furthermore, we should not forget that the bigger and heavier the breast, the more will be its caudal sliding. The mammary remodelling should entirely depend on the glandular tissue and not on the skin resection, whose quality has certain importance: a young, tonic, elastic skin without striae with good skin glandular adherence will give support in holding the breast, just like any common brassiere. Therefore it is very important to pay particular attention, through a careful and precise evaluation with the patient in the upright position, to the correct quantity and site of the gland being resected and to the type of remodelling flap used because this flap will determine the shape and volume of the breast we will be operating on.

Although my tenaciously pursued goal is to obtain the desired result with a one stage only procedure, it is absolutely advisable to inform the patient on the likelihood of a possible second surgical procedure, in order to attain a more satisfactory result. The difficulty of any surgical procedure should be fully explained and discussed with the patient. Obtaining a better result than promised can definitely be considered a success.

Third level: bilateral but different operation (see Case IX, below)

- Monolateral hypoplastic breast with contralateral ptosis with or without hypertrophy. In these cases, we consider the result to be very difficult, unpredictable and less stable.

This represents a more challenging situation because we are dealing with a ptotic, more or less hypertrophic breast, which we have to match in volume and shape with the contralateral prosthetic breast.

This is certainly not easy to accomplish, but the surgeon should try to reach this goal with passion and skilful precision. We should not forget that any body changes such as those associated with weight loss, weight gain, pregnancy, or body aging will greatly modify the result, compromising the surgeon's work and the good result obtained because the non prosthetic breast will undergo modification that the prosthetic breast will not experience. For this reason, I prefer and advise whenever possible to reduce the bigger breast to match the size of the smaller one, and to match not only the shape but also the volume of the small breast in order to implant an equal prosthesis. Equalizing shape and volume of the breasts and using two identical prosthesis allows a more secure and stable result.

Case VII

A young girl presented with clearly evident volume asymmetry and different degree of ptosis. She considers the volume of her left breast quite satisfactory, but she does not like its shape and does not want a bigger breast by introducing prosthesis. Her skin is of good quality, with the gland consisting mostly of glandular tissue. These qualities will help to obtain a good long-term and stable result. Both breasts underwent the same surgical procedure, helping to maintain the symmetry postoperatively to be maintained long term. In these cases, we can consider the result to be easy, predictable, and stable.

Clinical example

The volume asymmetry and degree of ptosis is evident in the preoperative view *(Fig. 23.1.7A)*. Good symmetry of volume and shape has been achieved 1 year postoperatively *(Fig. 23.1.7B)*. I (the author) criticized the size of the areola, which is too large in my opinion. Bilateral ptosis with evident asymmetry in volume and different degree of ptosis is seen in *Figure 23.1.7C*. Volume and shape are fairly symmetric at 1 year postoperatively *(Fig. 23.1.7D)*. Good scar quality is seen at 1 year postoperatively *(Fig. 23.1.7E)*. On the left side, there is only one vertical scar, while on the right side there is a vertical and a very short horizontal scar.

Case VIII

A young girl presents with a monolateral tubular like deformity and volume asymmetry on the left breast. The right breast has a nice shape, well positioned on the thorax, and its volume is considered to be sufficient by the patient and the surgeon. The skin is of very good quality, with tenacious cutaneous glandular adherence, and Cooper's ligaments are optimal. The structure of the breast is fundamentally of glandular type, this fact facilitates the hold of the mammary reshaping, which is performed through an aimed subcutaneous segmentary glandular excision (ASSGR) of the mammary base and of the lateral quadrants with the central reapproximation of the medial and lateral pillars. In such a case, we can consider the result to be difficult, less predictable, and more or less stable.

Clinical example

The volume and shape asymmetry is evident *(Fig. 23.1.8A)* and its result is stable at 3 years postoperatively *(Fig. 23.1.8B)*. We can expect this result to hold in the long term. The tubular shape of the left breast is evident preoperatively *(Fig. 23.1.8C)*. The left breast volume and shape continues to match the contralateral breast at 3 years postoperatively, thanks to a careful and precise glandular resection and breast reshaping *(Fig. 23.1.8D)*. The quality of the vertical scar and the $2\frac{1}{2}$ cm horizontal scar can be seen in *Figure 23.1.8E*.

Case IX

A young patient presented with severe hypoplasia of the left breast requiring augmentation mammaplasty, and a right ptotic breast, considered sufficient in volume by the patient but requiring mastopexy without augmentation mammaplasty. This type of asymmetry is the most difficult to deal with because we cannot reduce the bigger breast to the size of the smaller one, as the difference in volume is too pronounced. Moreover the patient does not like this solution. Therefore the surgeon

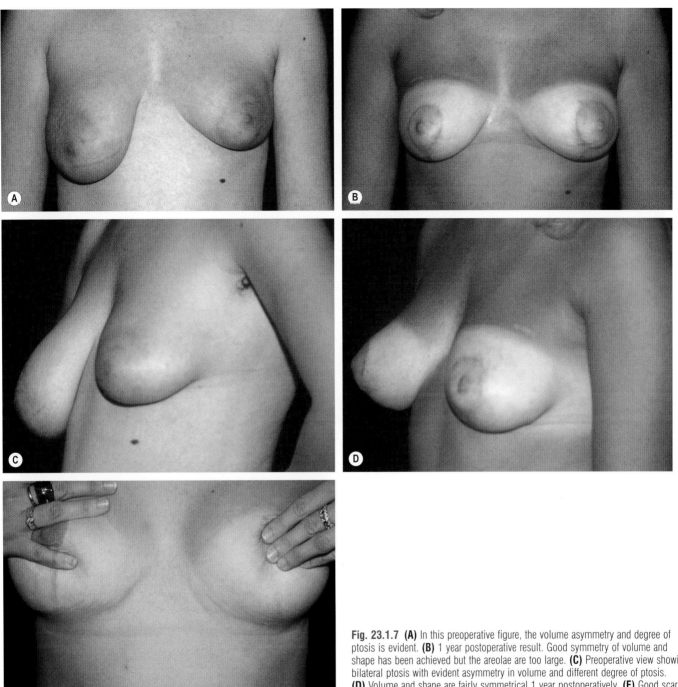

Fig. 23.1.7 (A) In this preoperative figure, the volume asymmetry and degree of ptosis is evident. **(B)** 1 year postoperative result. Good symmetry of volume and shape has been achieved but the areolae are too large. **(C)** Preoperative view showing bilateral ptosis with evident asymmetry in volume and different degree of ptosis. **(D)** Volume and shape are fairly symmetrical 1 year postoperatively. **(E)** Good scar quality 1 year postoperatively. On the left side, there is only one vertical scar, while on the right side there is a vertical scar and a very short horizontal one.

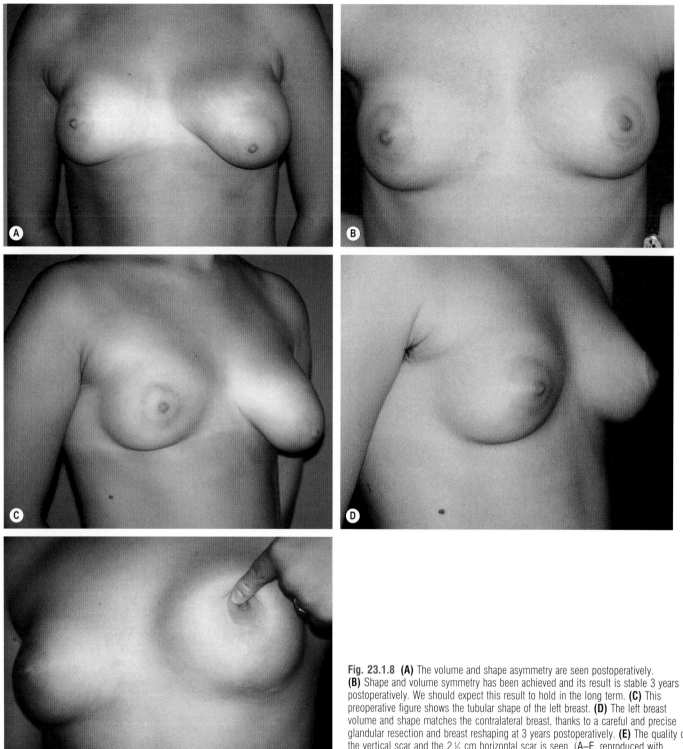

Fig. 23.1.8 (A) The volume and shape asymmetry are seen postoperatively.
(B) Shape and volume symmetry has been achieved and its result is stable 3 years postoperatively. We should expect this result to hold in the long term. **(C)** This preoperative figure shows the tubular shape of the left breast. **(D)** The left breast volume and shape matches the contralateral breast, thanks to a careful and precise glandular resection and breast reshaping at 3 years postoperatively. **(E)** The quality of the vertical scar and the $2\frac{1}{2}$ cm horizontal scar is seen. (A–E, reproduced with permission from: Muti E. Trattamento della mammella tuberosa ipoplastica. In: Lauro R, Dominici D, eds. *Chirurgia Plastica Della Mammella*. Padova: Piccin Nuova Libraria; 1996:192–206.)

must, after performing augmentation mammaplasty on the left side, perform a mastopexy on the right breast, in order to bring symmetry of volume and shape with the prosthetic breast; this is not always easy to attain. The big unknown factor in these cases is the uncertain long-term maintenance of the surgical result because the "natural" or nonprosthetic breast will change over the course of time following the natural modification of the body, due to weight change, pregnancy and aging, while the prosthetic breast will undergo a different modification. All these modifications with recurrent asymmetry will be much less evident if the "natural" breast is lighter or less heavy. In these cases, we should consider the result to be very difficult, less predictable, and unstable.

Clinical example

The volume and shape asymmetry is evident: we can see a sufficient in volume but ptotic breast on the right side, and on the left side, we can see a highly hypoplastic breast (see *Fig. 23.1.9A*). Despite the patient gaining 10 kg, the symmetry of volume but especially symmetry of shape are still very good *(Fig. 23.1.9B,D,F)*. In this particular case, symmetrization between the prosthetic breast and the nonprosthetic one is maintained in time for various reasons, which we can sum up as follows:

- The difference in volume between the two breasts is such that it is quite impossible to reduce the bigger right breast to the size of the small left breast, allowing the placement of two equal prostheses.
- The right ptotic breast is not excessively heavy, the skin is of good quality, and a mastopexy with a pedicled superior flap will fill the superior pole, allowing an adequate glandular reshaping. This will enable us to create a breast similar to the contralateral prosthetic breast with a good chance of a long-term stable result.

The stable, long-term result, despite weight changes and body aging, is my opinion due to the utilization of two procedures as "support/stabilization": the use of fascia pectoralis flap and the dermal flap of the inferior pole *(Fig. 23.1.9G,H)*. These two flaps will be explained below.

Hints and tips

All the results of the cases presented here have been obtained with a single stage surgical procedure, without the necessity to perform a secondary surgical stage or refinement. Only for *Figure 23.1.5* has a secondary lipostructure according to Coleman been performed. This technique may be more frequently employed in the future in cases requiring trimming or correction of breast asymmetry or for moderate breast volume augmentation.

Long-term stabilization in mammary asymmetry

As mentioned previously, the most secure long-term support is achieved when we can create two equal breasts of same weight/volume either with or without prosthesis. The factors which generally favor long-term stabilization of the result in a mastopexy or in a reductive mammaplasty are as follows:

- The type of reduction
- The type of the reshaped gland
- The breast residual weight
- To a lesser degree: the quality of the glandular tissue (a mostly glandular tissue will ensure a better support. In contrast a mostly adipose tissue will result in a poor support); the quality of the cutaneous tissue (obviously a lax skin with striae will tend to relax even more in time, while a solid skin will give, even if small, a better support to the breast.)

Additional procedures to improve long-term support include the pectoralis fascial flap and the dermal flap of the inferior pole (or dermal apron).

Pectoralis fascial flap

The pectoralis fascial flap (PFF) was conceived by Muti and Fontana[25] and was born from clinical and surgical observation of the tenacious glandular-muscular adherence available in nonptotic breasts, which were operated for other reasons. It was observed that ptotic breast presenting caudal sliding of the mammary gland with an empty and concave superior pole showed poor muscular glandular adherence. This observation has

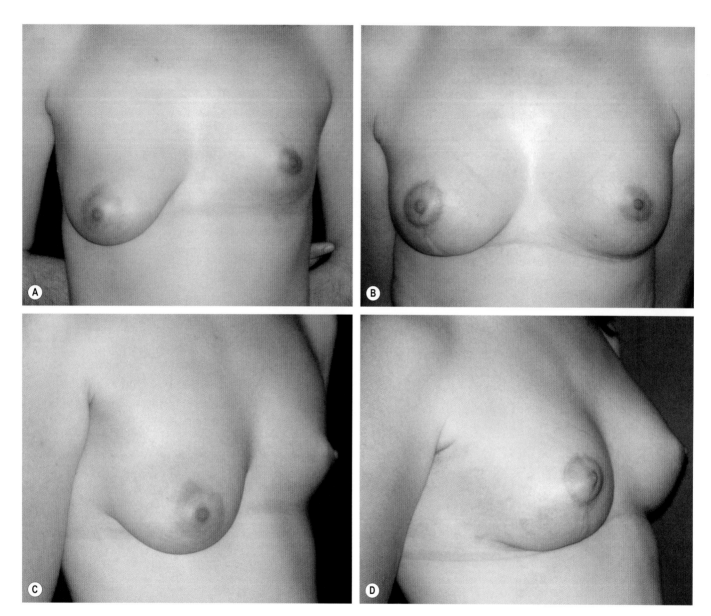

Fig. 23.1.9 (A) The volume and shape asymmetry are shown in this patient: on the right side a volume sufficiency but ptotic breast is seen, while on the left side we see a highly hypoplastic breast. **(B)** 1 year postoperative result. Good shape and volume symmetry as been attained. **(C)** This preoperative view shows the left hypoplastic breast with a tense, flat inferior pole. **(D)** 1-year postoperative result: the right breast has the same volume and shape as that of the left breast. (**A–D,** reproduced with permission from Muti E. Trattamento della mammella tuberosa ipoplastica. In: Lauro R, Dominici D, eds. *Chirurgia Plastica Della Mammella*. Padova: Piccin Nuova Libraria; 1996:192–206.)

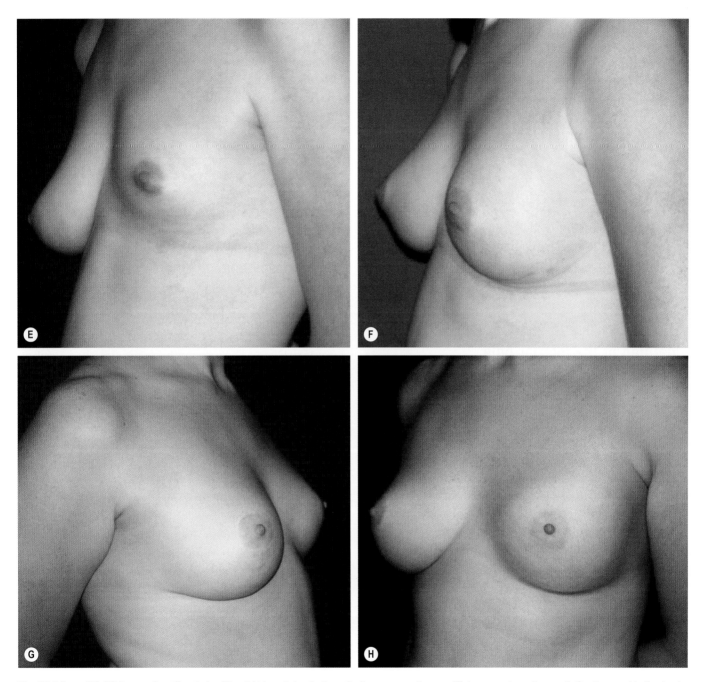

Fig. 23.1.9, cont'd (E) Preoperative. The ptosis of the right breast despite the patient's young age is seen. **(F)** 1-year postoperative result. Good symmetrization has been attained between the prosthetic left breast and the nonprosthetic right breast. **(G,H)** 10 years postoperatively. (E–F, reproduced with permission from Muti E. *Trattamento della mammella tuberosa ipoplastica.* In: Lauro R, Dominici D, eds. *Chirurgia Plastica Della Mammella*. Padova: Piccin Nuova Libraria; 1996:192–206.)

brought us the idea of incrementing the adherence between the reshaped mammary base and the surface of the pectoral muscle. The easiest way to obtain such adherence without utilizing foreign material is to de-fascialize the pectoral muscle in the seat of the mammary footprint, but instead of discarding the fascia, we utilize it as a flap folding it over caudally (like a book page), with its free margins reaching the inferior border of the new mammary base. This also helps us to maintain, to a certain degree, the reapproximation of the two pillars, lateral and medial, of the reshaped gland *(Fig. 23.1.10A–C)*. ⊛ FIG **21.1.10** APPEARS ONLINE ONLY

What have we achieved with this flap?

We obtain an increasing of the adherence between the deep surface of the reshaped gland and the muscular plane, reducing the usual caudal sliding of the gland, and with a better stabilization of the result obtained intraoperatively.

Dermal flap of the inferior pole or "dermal apron"

In mastopexy and reductive mammaplasty with a superior pedicle and cutaneous drawings/mark-up such as those performed by Pexioto,[28] once we have finished the periareolar and inferior pole de-epithelialization, the medial and lateral margins of the dermis of the inferior pole are incised and separated from the skin, up to the level of the areolar equatorial line. Then the dermis of the inferior pole is undermined from the mammary gland up to the level of the inferior border of the reduced areola, following a precise practically unbleeding plane *(Fig. 23.1.11A)*. The flap is then placed on one side during the other reshaping manoeuvres of the breast *(Fig. 23.1.11B)*. Before performing the vertical sutures on the inferior pole, the flap is placed back low in its previous position with a lateral–medial tension similar to its original one. At this point, the skin is laterally and medially undermined from the gland, enough to allow the flap to be sutured on the gland *(Fig. 23.1.11C)*. Once the dermal flap has been sutured on the gland, the two cutaneous flaps are approximated on the median line and then sutured together *(Fig. 23.1.11D)*.

What have we achieved with this flap?

The objectives of the dermal apron are the following:
- To improve the blood circulation of the areola
- To help to maintain the approximation of the lateral pillar to the medial pillar of the breast
- To support the inferior pole by doubling the dermal plane
- To improve the quality of the vertical scar
- To avoid tissue ectopy.

Case X

In this case *(Fig. 23.1.12)* of severe asymmetry with level 2 difficulty, we intervened only on the right breast, which is considerably hypertrophic and ptotic compared with the left breast, which the patient did not want to modify. According to Botti's classification,[8] this type of right breast should be classified as PAR 4–CAC 4, which means a higher grade of difficulty. In addition, a further element of difficulty for any long-term result is given by the fundamentally adipose characteristic of the mammary tissue. The two methods previously described (PFF and dermal apron) had not been performed in this early case. The postoperative 1-year result is mediocre and shows a caudal sliding of the gland and contextual hollowing of the areola, with its relative elevation and loss of retroareolar projection. A certain degree of weight gain does not justify this outcome. The vertical scar is of poor quality *(Fig. 23.1.12C,D)*. Can we say that if I had performed the PFF and the dermal apron, the long-term result could have been better? My honest answer is "Yes", although a certain importance for the outcome was due to the type of glandular reshaping flap utilized. In this early case, a lozenge resection of the inferior pole and the conization was performed with a simple plication of the gland of the inferior pole. Such a technique has been proven certainly insufficient to achieve a good outcome, especially in the long-term *(Fig. 23.1.12A–E)*. ⊛ FIG **23.1.12** APPEARS ONLINE ONLY

Suturing techniques/ postoperative care

The author's standard choice when performing skin suture is by applying single stitches, in two or

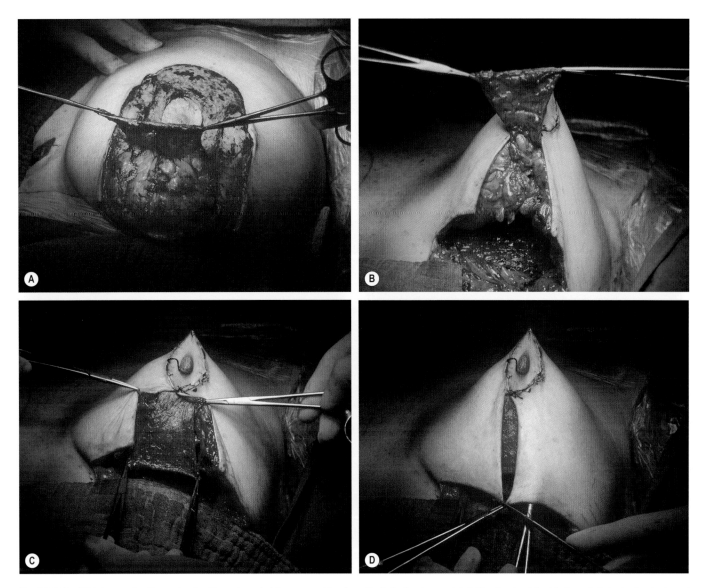

Fig. 23.1.11 **(A)** Intraoperative figure showing the early part of the surgery. The de-epithelialization is completed. The dermis of the inferior pole is incised and released from the skin borders up to the equatorial line of the areola, and undermined and elevated up to the inferior border of the reduced areola. **(B)** Intraoperative figure showing the end of the procedure. The breast has already been reshaped, and the two edges of the skin of the inferior pole are slightly undermined in order to make room for the repositioning of the dermal apron. **(C)** The dermal flap is repositioned on the lower pole with a transversal tension similar to the original. **(D)** The dermal flap is sutured on the glandular surface and the flaps are approximated to the central line over the dermal flap so they can be sutured together. (A–D, reproduced with permission from Muti E. *The tuberous breast.* Editrice Firenze; 2010.)

three layers, starting from the deep to the superficial plane, using reabsorbable materials such as 2-0, 3-0, 4-0, until I obtain a perfect approximation of the two incision margins. On the incision line, I use superficial glue and above it I place a paper taping or Steri-strips to be kept in place for at least 2 months, changing them approximately every 2 weeks. With these types of paper tapes, patients can lead a normal active life and take showers without changing the tapes too often. The use of paper tapes helps to reduce or even prevent the scars hypertrophic phase, with a more secure final result.

Bonus images for this chapter can be found online at http://www.expertconsult.com

Fig. 23.1.1 (C) Typical example of bilateral symmetric tuberous breast type I in a 23-year-old female patient, showing a degree of glandular prolapse into the inferior half of the expanded areola. **(E–G)** Intraoperative sequence: the preoperative evaluation marks a peripheral ring of deepithelialization to lift the areola in order to reduce its diameter thus enhancing its conicity of the areolae, a rhombus of skin is marked in the central inferior portion of the areola which will be excised. This rhombus will correspond to the projection of the glandular herniation. **(E)** The glandular herniation, which will be used to create the glandular flap type I is clearly evident. **(F)** The glandular flap sculpted at full thickness down to the deep plane is stretched outward. The flap has been deeply and caudally rotated with its apex toward the new lowered inframammary fold. It is pedicled on the inferior subcutaneous vascular net. The areola has been lifted and flattened in half inferiorly. The mammary prosthesis has been inserted through the existing incisions in a pre-pectoral plane. In this case, a Dow Corning round micro-structured prosthesis of 210 cc has been utilized. **(I)** The flap is rotated deeply and caudally under the skin of the inferior pole with its apex reaching the new intramammary fold **(J)**. **(K,M)** The prosthesis is implanted in a pre-pectoral plane, the areola is lifted and reduced, and the skin is sutured with a periareolar and a very short vertical scar. **(N)** The 1-year postoperative result. **(O)** The five-year postoperative result. (**C–G**, reproduced with permission from Muti E. Personal approach to surgical correction of the extremely hypoplastic tuberous breast. *Aesthetic Plastic Surgery Review*, New York: Springer-Verlag 1996; 20:385–390. **N,O** reproduced with permission from Muti E. *The tuberous breast*. SEE Editrice Firenze; 2010.)

Fig. 23.1.2 (C) The small breasts are positioned rather high on the chest wall and very lateralized on the thorax externally to the hemi-clavicular lines. The glandular base, herniated into the areolar sack, is surrounded by a well defined fibrotic constrictive ring which makes the breast appear like hanging on the chest wall. **(E)** After the de-epithelialization, the reduced areola is lifted and the gland is shown appearing totally herniated and leaning on the thorax. **(F)** We can observe the thin dermal flap which was covering the inferior pole being undermined and cranially lifted. The mammary gland, seen in Fig. 23.1.2E, exposed and leaning on the thorax, is transversally incised to the level of the inferior border of the new reduced areola. We then proceed to incise the gland at full thickness up to the muscle thoracic plane and to vertically open it in its deep surface, thus creating a wide square shaped flap with an inferior subcutaneous pedicle based on the superficial blood net. **(G)** The glandular flap has been deeply and caudally folded over toward the new inframammary fold, creating a sort of thin lower pole. **(O)** The 18-year postoperative result. The scars are slightly evident due to bad skin quality and initial cutaneous suturing tension. **(Q)** 18 years postoperatively. The result is unchanged over the years, and actually enhancing the natural look of the breast. (**E–G**, reproduced with permission from Muti E. *The Tuberous Breast – See Editrice Firenze*, 2010.)

Fig. 23.1.3 (E) The residual type II deformity is seen after BAM has been performed. **(F)** A small periareolar inferior incision with minimal undermining of the inferior areolar skin shows a certain amount of gland transversally incised toward the glandular surface, thus creating a small flap which is seen stretched externally. **(H)** The flap is inserted under the undermined skin from the central region of the inferior pole. **(J)** The apex of the flap is positioned and fixed in the desired place, sometimes with few transcutaneous stitches. The inferior pole profile appears completely changed with a round convex shape. (**E–H**, reproduced with permission from Muti E. Local flaps for tuberous and asymmetric breasts, in Hall-Findlay EJ, ed. Breast surgery. Philadelphia: Saunders Elsevier; 2010.)

Fig. 23.1.6 (A) The protrusion of the gland behind the areola with a fibrotic ring around its periphery is seen. **(B)** The corrected shape of the areola postoperatively is seen. **(C)** A rectangular shaped flap is transferred from the superior half of the deep surface of the areola to the inferior half. **(D)** The use of this flap results in a smooth superior breast profile and a better continuity between the areola and the inferior pole. At the same time, the base of the gland has been open and relaxed, allowing its redistribution over the prosthesis.

Fig. 23.1.10 (A) Intraoperative figure showing the drawing of the fascial flap on the pectoral muscle, with a horizontal line at the level corresponding to the superior border of the mammary footprint, and two vertical lines, more or less to the medial and lateral border of the pectoral muscle. **(B)** Intraoperative figure showing the undermined flap, in this case comprising a few muscular fibers, which is lifted and folded over like a book page, caudally toward the IMF. **(C)** Intraoperative figure showing the free margins of the flap which is sutured to the inferior border of the reshaped mammary base with a slight lateral-medial tension. (**A–C**, reproduced with permission from Muti E. *The tuberous breast*. SEE Editrice Firenze; 2010.)

Fig. 23.1.12 (A) The preoperative skin markings on the right breast. The left breast will not be modified. **(B)** This figure shows in blue the area to be de-epithelialized and the lozenge of glandular resection **(yellow)**. **(C)** The outcome is to be considered "mediocre" in this patient 2 years postoperatively. The inferior pole is slightly heavy and in its caudal sliding has drag deeply the retroareolar tissue with consequent hollowing of the nipple-areolar-complex. The vertical scar is of poor quality. **(D)** The asymmetry of volume and shape and the peculiar shape of the left breast with a concave superior pole is seen. However, the patient does not want to modify the left breast. **(E)** Patient 1 year postoperatively. The defects have already described in the frontal view. The patient's weight gain is more evident and is also noticeable on the left breast. (Reproduced with permission from Muti E. Trattamento della mammella tuberosa ipoplastica. In: Lauro R, Dominici D, eds. *Chirurgia Plastica Della Mammella*. Padova: Piccin Nuova Libraria; 1996:192–206.)

Access the complete references list online at http://www.expertconsult.com

2. Mandrekas AD, Zambacos GJ, Anastasopoulos A, et al. Aesthetic reconstruction of tuberous breast deformity. *Plast Reconstr Surg*. 2003;112(4):1099–1109.

4. Botti G, ed. Mammelle tubulari e tuberose. In: *Mastoplastiche estetiche*. SEE Editrice Firenze; 2004:280–295.

The authors describe, in a clear and precise manner, his technique regarding the unfurling of the breast for the correction of some types of tuberous breasts.

5. Bass U. Herniated areola complex. *Ann Plast Surg*. 1978;1:203.

9. Berrino P. *Operative strategies in breast plastic surgery*. SEE Editrice Firenze; 2007:380–382.

10. Bostwick J. *Plastic and reconstructive breast surgery: anatomy and physiology*. 2nd ed. St Louis: Quality Medical; 2000:76–123.

13. Coleman SR. Long-term survival of fat transplant controlled demonstration. *Aesthetic Plast Surg*. 1995;19:421–425.

   In this study the author demonstrates, through the work of 400 infiltrations of fatty tissue into the naso-labial folds, the potential of the long lasting nature of this type of grafting.

17. Góes CS. Periareolar mammaplasty: double-skin technique with application of mesh support. In: Spear SL, ed. Surgery of the breast: principles and art, Vol. 2. Philadelphia: Lippincott Williams & Wilkins; 2006:991–1007.

   The author's surgery techniques on aesthetic breast surgery are very interesting and internationally well known. His techniques have added new possibility for the surgical correction of the breast.

19. Hammond DC. Augmentation mammaplasty in the patient with tuberous breasts and other complex anomalies. In: Spear SL, ed. Surgery of the breast principles and art, Vol. 2. Philadelphia: Lippincott Williams & Wilkins; 2006:1367–1375.

   In this paper the author has provided an algorithm that could facilitate the planning and the extension of these procedure.

23. Mottura AA. Circumvertical reduction mastoplasty: new consideration. *Aesthetic Plast Surg Rev*. 2003;27:83–85.

   The author describes a technique for the reduction of mammaplasty that summarize most of my own procedure and details. I have utilized the same technique since 1980s, but I have never published my considerations and my work. The author describes very well this technique, this case demonstrates how the same procedure can be conceived in two different setting and how two different surgeons can come up with the same approach in dealing with this specific breast surgery.

28. Peixoto G. Reduction mammaplasty: a personal technique. *Plast Reconstr Surg*. 1980;65(2):217–225.

   The author has represented for me a revolution, a total new approach in the field of breast surgery. He has clinically demonstrated the actual possibility of the mammary gland to survive trough the superficial vascular net. Freeing me from the bondage of the deep vascular pedicles, allowing me, instead, to create and mobilize different "glandular flaps". This technique has been very useful to me as I mastered this method and applied to correct the different types of tuberous breast and for the mastopexy as well.

23.2

Poland syndrome

Pietro Berrino and Valeria Berrino

SYNOPSIS

- Poland syndrome is a unilateral congenital chest deformity characterized by the absence of the sternal portion of the pectoralis major muscle.
- The anterior axillary fold is absent.
- The incidence of this anomaly ranges from 1 in 10 000 to 1 in 100 000 births.
- Breast tissues are often fibrotic, since the missing pectoralis major muscle is replaced by fibrotic bands or by a compact fibrous layer.
- Associated features may include:
  - Absence of the pectoralis minor muscle
  - Absence of one or two ribs or costal cartilages
  - Ipsilateral latissimus dorsi muscle agenesia or hypoplasia
  - Atrophy of the ipsilateral chest skin and subcutaneous tissue
  - Sternal rotation
  - Ipsilateral anomalies of the hand, lower arm or entire upper limb
  - Multi-organ anomalies involving the gastrointestinal tract, liver and heart.

 Access the Historical Perspective sections online at
http://www.expertconsult.com

Introduction

Poland syndrome is a unilateral congenital chest deformity characterized by the absence of the sternal portion of the pectoralis major muscle. The morphological consequence of the missing muscle is that the anterior axillary fold is absent. The incidence of this anomaly ranges from 1 in 10 000 to 1 in 100 000 births. In females the diagnosis is often made only after breast development and patients are often referred to specialists because of breast asymmetry. Ipsilateral breast anomalies range from mild hypoplasia to total agenesia. Breast tissues are often fibrotic since the missing pectoralis major muscle is replaced by fibrotic bands or by a compact fibrous layer. In males, Poland syndrome is often misdiagnosed as a "chest asymmetry" and it is often recognized only after full development. The absence of the sternal component of the pectoralis major and breast anomalies can be associated with one or more of the following malformations:

- Absence of the pectoralis minor muscle
- Absence of one or two ribs or costal cartilages
- Ipsilateral latissimus dorsi muscle agenesia or hypoplasia
- Atrophy of the ipsilateral chest skin and subcutaneous tissue
- Sternal rotation
- Ipsilateral anomalies of the hand, lower arm or entire upper limb
- Multi-organ anomalies involving the gastrointestinal tract, the liver, the heart.

There is a known male predilection of 2:1 and a corresponding right-sided predilection in males of 2–3:1. A sidedness predilection does not however exist in females with Poland syndrome.

Basic science/disease process

Absence of the sternal component of the pectoralis major and the associated breast anomalies can be also associated with several other malformations, though presence of all of these phenomena is rarely seen and presence or absence of these associated lesions is not necessary to make the diagnosis of Poland syndrome. Absence of the pectoralis minor muscle is frequently seen in patients with this condition. Furthermore, aplasia or hypoplasia of ribs 3–5 have been reported. In fact, ipsilateral anomalies of the hand, lower arm or even the entire upper limb have been associated with Poland syndrome. These have ranged in severity from a simple partial syndactyly, to a complete mitten hand. Occasionally, digital anomalies are also associated, particularly in digits 2, 3 and 4. This has led to descriptions of shortened hands and even limbs in association. Several theories have been advanced to explain these anomalies. These include the temporary disruption of blood supply to the subclavian/vertebral systems during weeks 6–7 of embryological development. Another theory is that there is disruption of the mesodermal plate during weeks 3–4 of embryonal development. Though this syndrome appears sporadically, a small number of patients appear to have a heritable component to their condition.

Diagnosis/patient presentation

The most frequent presentation is that of chest wall asymmetry. In both male and female, this is often unnoticed in childhood. In boys it generally is noticed at full or near full skeletal maturity whereas in girls, it is generally noticed at the time of breast development. It should always be suspected in a young patient presenting with chest wall deformity. At presentation, a full history should be taken. Physical examination should include examination of the chest wall, and, particularly, palpation of the ribs, looking for hypoplasia. The status of the pectoralis major and minor, latissimus, serratus anterior muscles should be documented. Also, the ipsilateral upper limb should be carefully examined with particular attention being paid to the hand, looking for syndactyly and digital abnormalities. Imaging tests

(such as chest X-ray, ultrasound, CT scan, or MRI – and what the indications for these are), etc. should be used. There has been a diagnosis of Poland syndrome made by mammography in the past, with a rate of 1:19 000.

Treatment/surgical technique

Correction of the thoracic anomaly in males

Reconstruction of the missing muscle

In all groups of patients, the absent sternal head of the pectoralis muscle should be replaced by anterior transposition of the ipsilateral latissimus dorsi muscle. The following minimal incisions are used in these usually young patients:

1. The latissimus muscle flap is harvested through a dorsal incision positioned above the lateral border of the muscle: this 5–8 cm long incision can be either vertically or horizontally oriented. The S-shaped vertical incision proposed in 1985 provides easy visualization of the whole muscle.[2,3] However, a straight incision along the brassiere line is easier to hide and is the authors' current preferred option.[4] Through this approach, the entire surface of the anterior fascia of the latissimus dorsi is detached from the subcutaneous layer. The deep surface of the muscle is then freed from underlying structures. Care must be taken at the inferior angle of the scapula in order to avoid dissection under the Teres major muscle. The inferior border of the muscle flap is then severed as distally as possible using bipolar forceps.

2. An incision positioned in an axillary horizontal crease is used to gain access to the posterior axillary fold: the latissimus dorsi muscle is freed until the tendon is reached. The tendon is then transected at its insertion on the humerus. The whole muscle is isolated on the thoracodorsal neurovascular pedicle as in a microsurgical operation. The tendon is then sutured to the anterior bicipital sulcus of the humerus, in the position where the pectoralis major is inserted when anatomy is normal.

3. A periareolar incision is carried out anteriorly. Through this approach, the skin of the entire

hemi-chest is undermined. A subcutaneous tunnel is created to join the mammary and the axillary undermining. The muscle flap is then transferred anteriorly on the neurovascular pedicle, and sutured to the lateral border of the sternum, to the fascia along the new submammary fold and the lower border of the clavicular portion of the pectoralis major muscle. The muscle flap should be sutured with moderate tension in order to maintain function and to avoid atrophy. If the areola is small, the incision is carried out some millimeters below the areola border and the intervening skin is resected in order to obtain a sufficiently large approach. Alternatively, the periareolar incision can be lengthened horizontally at the two extremities and converted in a pure periareolar incision by minor skin resection at the end of the operation.

If the ipsilateral latissimus dorsi muscle is atrophic, the following options are available:

1. The contralateral latissimus dorsi muscle can be transferred microsurgically; in this case the flap is re-innervated by anastomosing the donor thoracodorsal nerve to an anterior serratus motor nerve at the recipient site.

2. A transverse abdominal flap can be transferred either as a pedicled or as a free flap to fill the subcutaneous defect. Although tissue obtained by this procedure can be sufficient both for axillary fold reconstruction and for creation of the new breast mound, the missing muscle is not replaced. Therefore, the axillary defect is filled but a real fold is not obtained and the dynamic defect is not corrected.

3. As a simpler and less demanding option, fat injections can be used to fill the anterior axillary fold area. An anatomically shaped fold, however, is not provided by this option and no dynamic effect is obtained.

Classification of the chest deformity in females

The surgical strategy for correction of the chest deformity in women depends on the severity of the condition. In order to devise a protocol for surgical treatment, we have classified patients into three different groups. In all three groups, the sternal head of the pectoralis major muscle is absent and the anterior axillary fold is missing.

- *Group I*: mild ipsilateral breast hypotrophy. Breast shape and elasticity of mammary tissues on the two sides are similar.
- *Group II*: severe hypotrophy of the ipsilateral breast, severe asymmetry. Breast parenchyma is fibrotic and adherent to the chest cage since the pectoralis muscular tissue is substituted by collagen bands.
- *Group III*: total breast agenesis. The skin is tight, subcutaneous tissues are thin or absent, the dermis can be adherent to the chest cage or to the thoracic fascia if one or more ribs are absent. The nipple areola complex is missing or severely hypoplastic.

Reconstruction of the breast mound is approached differently in the three groups of patients.

Group I

In these patients, breast tissue compliance makes the operation easier. The latissimus dorsi muscle is transposed and through the periareolar incision, an anatomical implant is positioned under the muscle flap. Contralaterally, if the breast is small or a more rounded shape is desirable, an implant is positioned, thus improving symmetry durability.

Correction in group I patient (Case I)

This 17-year-old patient *(Fig. 23.2.1)* presented with breast asymmetry. The missing axillary fold suggested the immediate diagnosis of Poland syndrome. Breast tissues on the affected side appeared to be elastic and expandable; the contralateral breast was small and the patient and her parents asked for augmentation. Anterior transposition of the latissimus dorsi muscle was carried out using a 7 cm long horizontal incision. Bilateral anatomical implants (275 g on the left side, 200 g on the right side) were positioned in the submuscular plane. After 5 months, the patient required improvement of the hypoplastic left nipple. This was accomplished by a keel-shaped graft harvested from the contralateral nipple. Long-term follow-ups showed good symmetry and satisfactory reconstruction of the left axillary deformity. Residual dorsal scarring was acceptable but the donor area showed subcutaneous

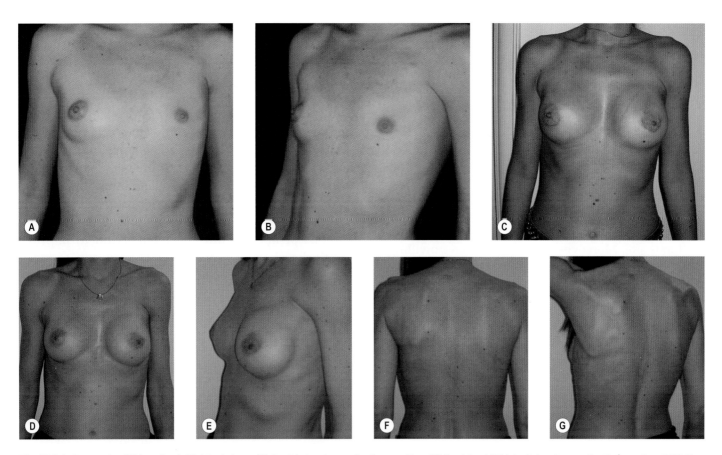

Fig. 23.2.1 Preoperative **(A)** frontal and **(B)** lateral views. **(C)** Frontal view 1 year after the operation. **(D)** Frontal and **(E)** lateral view 6 years after the operation. **(F,G)** The dorsal donor site at the 6-year follow-up: residual scarring is minimal, but thinning of the subcutaneous layer and mild "scapula alata" can be observed and are obvious stigmata of the operation. (Reproduced with permission from: Berrino P. Operative strategies in breast plastic surgery. SEE Editrice Firenze; 2007.)

thinning due to the absence of the latissimus dorsi muscle.

Group II patients

In these women, fibrosis of the breast base makes it difficult to obtain expansion of the breast mound. The gland must be scored in order to interrupt all fibrotic bands. The incisions on the deep surface of the gland are carried out after complete undermining and exposure of the breast base. Incisions must be performed perpendicularly to the desired direction of tissue expansion (i.e., if the inferior breast pole appears too short in the vertical direction, horizontal scoring of the fibrotic bands is performed). This procedure allows the breast base to expand in the desired direction and the final shape is maintained by suturing the glandular flaps in the new position. An anatomical expander

is then positioned. The location of the tissue expander can be pre-muscular or retro-muscular. This choice is conditioned by the type of reconstruction that is planned after removal of the expander: if autogenous tissue reconstruction is chosen, the expander should be positioned above the muscle. If an implant is to be used, the expander is positioned in the submuscular plane. Expansion is carried out to a volume which is larger by 20% than the expected final breast volume. Full expansion is achieved in 4–6 weeks.

The tissue expander can be replaced by three different options:

1. The expander is removed and an anatomical implant is positioned. The capsule of the expander is incised by multiple scoring in order to obtain tissue gain in the desired direction. This maneuver is crucial in order to obtain the appropriate final shape. Symmetry obtained

with this option is usually temporary since breast aging will be different. When a contralateral implant is positioned, symmetry will last longer.

2. The expander is removed and a vascularized abdominal flap is transferred either as a free flap or as a pedicled flap. The skin island is completely de-epithelialized and sutured in the proper position. This procedure provides a tissue-to-tissue reconstruction with a rewarding final outcome and permanent symmetry. However, the abdomen in these usually young patients is often an unsuitable donor site. Moreover patients are often unwilling to undergo two extensive surgical procedures.

3. The expander can be deflated by approximately one-third of its volume and fat injections can be simultaneously carried out in the subcutaneous pre-capsular plane to compensate for the reduced volume. In 3–5 operative stages the whole volume provided by the expander is thus replaced by the injected fat. This simple multi-stage outpatient procedure shows excellent patient compliance and appreciation in post-mastectomy patients and can be profitably used in Poland syndrome.

Correction in group II patient (Case II)

This 29-year-old woman presented with a diagnosed Poland syndrome and showed an evident axillary defect *(Fig. 23.2.2)*. The breast on the affected side was small and retracted, with a deep compact fibrotic layer anchoring the breast mound to the chest cage. The ipsilateral latissimus dorsi muscle was severely hypotrophic. She had a large ptotic contralateral breast and abdominal tissue redundancy and a retracted vertical appendicectomy scar. A two-stage procedure was planned: in the first operative stage an anatomical expander was positioned and the breast base was scored in order to facilitate expansion. The implant was inflated to 350 mL in 5 weeks. A rapid inflation of the expander was carried out in order to take advantage of the surgical expansion of the retracted breast base. At 2 months later, the second operative stage was planned: (1) expander removal; (2) transposition of a de-epithelialized pedicled abdominal flap; (3) contralateral vertical mammoplasty using a modified Lejour technique. The follow-ups at 3 years, 13 years, and 16-years show that satisfactory long-term symmetry is achieved when autogenous reconstruction is carried out.

Group III patients

This condition resembles postradical-mastectomy deformity and requires a completely different reconstructive approach. The areola is missing and therefore an incision positioned in the future submammary fold is used to suture the transposed latissimus dorsi muscle to the chest wall. The skin is often very tight and the subcutaneous fat layer is thin or absent: one or more sessions of lipostructure are often useful to improve the thickness of the subcutaneous layer and to make skin more elastic. After latissimus dorsi muscle transfer, the expander is always positioned submuscularly. The costal defect, when present, can be disregarded as it will be hidden by the implant and by transposed tissues, but care must be taken during dissection of the pocket, since the dermis is adherent to the thoracic fascia and a risk of pneumothorax exists. Expansion is carried out more slowly because overlaying tissue is tight. In group III patients, the expander is replaced by an anatomical implant. One or more sessions of lipostructure are often required to refine the result: a more natural cleavage is created at the upper pole, the thinness of subcutaneous defective tissue at the inner quadrants is corrected and the inferior pole is made more rounded. Moreover, costal irregularities can be at least partially camouflaged by fat injections. Reconstruction of the nipple and areola is carried out during the last stage of the procedure. A contralateral graft is used if the nipple-areola complex is totally missing: an external peripheral strip of the contralateral areola and a keel-shaped nipple fragment are harvested and grafted at the proper de-epithelialized recipient site on the reconstructed breast. When the nipple areola complex on the affected site is present but hypoplastic, enlargement of the areola is obtained by tattooing, while a more prominent nipple is obtained by eversion (as in a retracted nipple operation) or by a contralateral graft.

Correction in group III patient (Case III)

This 17-year-old patient showed severe Poland syndrome *(Fig. 23.2.3)*. The left breast is missing (Amazon syndrome), the subcutaneous layer at the affected site is

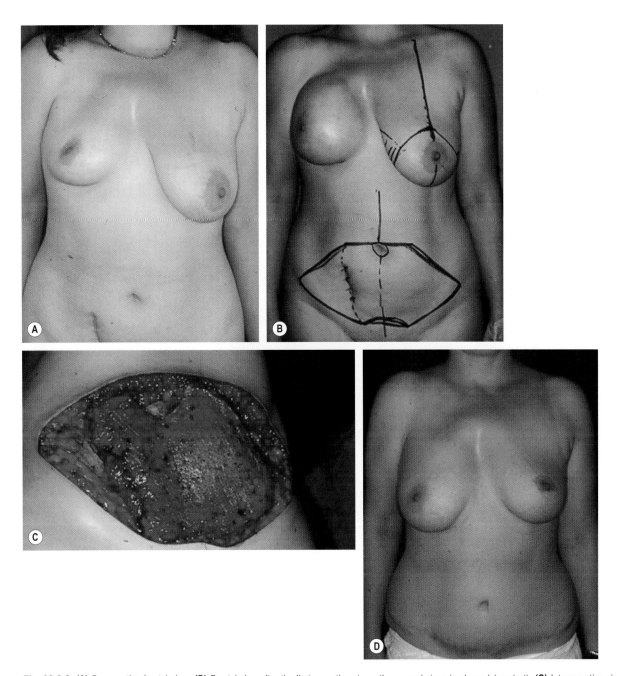

Fig. 23.2.2 **(A)** Preoperative frontal view. **(B)** Frontal view after the first operative stage: the second stage is planned (see text). **(C)** Intraoperative view of the deepithelialized abdominal flap. **(D)** Postoperative view at the 3-year follow-up. (Reproduced with permission from: P. Berrino: Operative strategies in breast plastic surgery, SEE Ed. Firenze 2007.)

absent and the dermis is in contact with the thoracic fascia. The fourth rib is missing. Total transposition of the latissimus dorsi was planned and an expander was positioned under the muscle flap. The expander was slowly inflated to 330 mL during 4 months. At 5 months after the first operation, the expander was removed and a 300 mL anatomical implant was positioned. As a final stage, the nipple-areola complex was reconstructed by contralateral grafts and lipostructure was carried out at the superior quadrants and at the inferior pole. At 2 years later, the patient required contralateral breast reduction, which was obtained by sectorial parenchyma removal through a 3 cm incision in the right submammary fold. At 1 year after the last operation, and 40

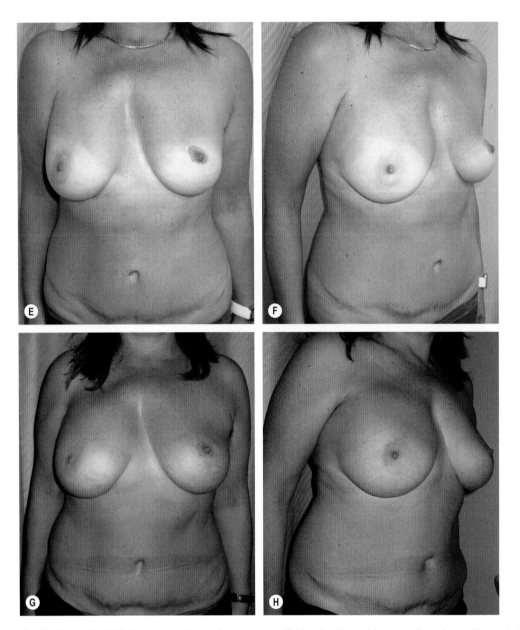

Fig. 23.2.2, cont'd **(E,F)** Postoperative views at the 13-year and **(G,H)** at the 15-year follow-ups. (Reproduced with permission from: Berrino P. Operative strategies in breast plastic surgery. SEE Editrice Firenze; 2007.)

months after the first operation, symmetry is satisfactory. At 5 years later, the patient requested a new lipofilling session to improve the upper cleavage and to camouflage chest asymmetry. At 9 years after the first operation, the patient showed stable symmetry.

Long-term results after correction in females

Symmetry after correction of the chest anomaly in Poland syndrome can be permanent in group I patients,

when bilateral implants are used. In group II patients, symmetry is long lasting only when autogenous tissue is used to replace the expander.

Secondary procedures

Group II and group III patients who undergo reconstruction using implants often require long-term symmetry adjustments. Procedures used to maintain

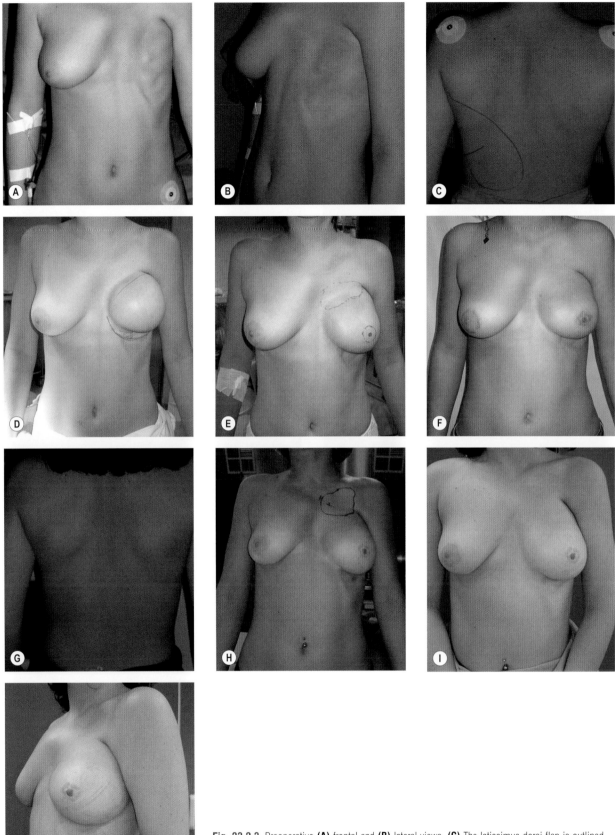

Fig. 23.2.3 Preoperative **(A)** frontal and **(B)** lateral views. **(C)** The latissimus dorsi flap is outlined. **(D)** The result after the first stage. **(E)** Frontal view after the second stage: reconstruction of the nipple-areola complex and lipostructure of the upper quadrants is planned. **(F)** The result 1 year after. **(G)** the dorsal defect is less conspicuous when a good subcutaneous layer is present. **(H)** Frontal view 5 years later when the patient required subclavicular lipofilling. **(I,J)** The result 7 years after the first operation. (Reproduced with permission from: Berrino P. Operative strategies in breast plastic surgery. SEE Editrice Firenze; 2007.)

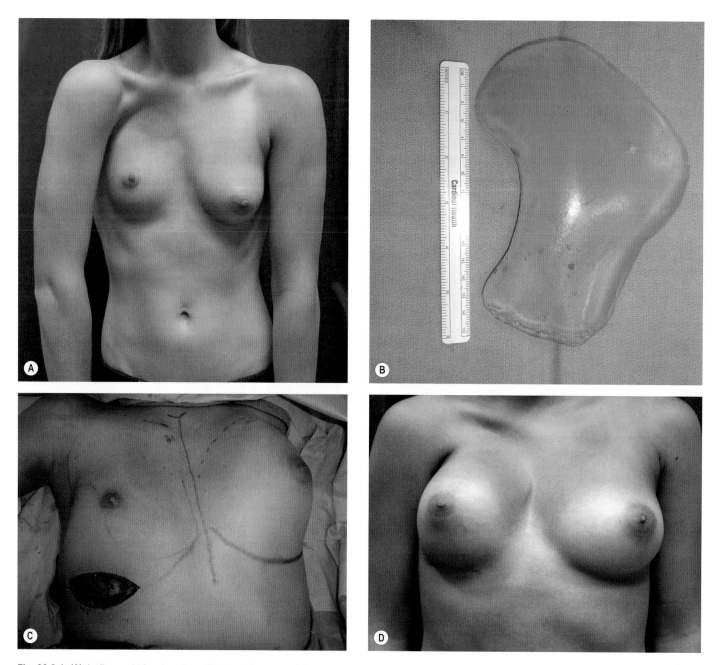

Fig. 23.2.4 (A) A 17-year-old female patient with Poland Syndrome. **(B)** Custom silicone chest wall implant made from moulage. **(C)** Chest wall implant placed through inframammary incision. **(D)** Breast implant placed in front of chest wall implant at separate stage.

symmetry include implant replacement, contralateral mammoplasty (to maintain symmetry of position) and, most often, lipostructure, which represents an extraordinarily effective procedure to allow the breast to maintain a symmetrical shape when differences in the thickness of local tissues appear.

Correction of the thoracic anomaly in males

Males with Poland syndrome usually complain of the flatness of the affected hemi-chest but rarely notice the missing fold. Correction is obtained by anterior transposition of the latissimus dorsi muscle. The procedure is performed as described in females, but a submammary approach is often used because the areola is usually very small. Since in most males the latissimus dorsi muscle is much smaller that the pectoralis major muscle, reconstruction of the axillary fold is less satisfactory than in females. Moreover, in the mammary region, there is no breast implant camouflaging the residual asymmetry. Lipostructure is therefore often used to improve the result.

Alternative method of reconstruction

While it can be argued that latissimus transfer, as described above, yields the best results, this deformity can also be corrected using customized chest wall implants. This can be applied in both males and females.[5,6] A moulage is made of the chest wall defect. A customized implant made of silicone is then manufactured. In the male, this is generally a one-stage procedure and, depending on the extent of the deformity, can give very satisfying results. In the female, the customized chest implant is usually combined with a breast implant so that the chest implant addresses the chest wall component of the deformity, while the breast implant addresses the breast deformity. Usually, the chest implant is placed first with subsequent placement of the breast implant. Once again, depending on the extent of the deformity, this can yield very satisfying results *(Fig. 23.2.4)*.

Postoperative care

Standard incisional postoperative care is required. If implants are used, postoperative implant protocols are used.

Outcomes, prognosis, and complications

Long term results tend to be lasting. However the long term complications of implants, especially capsular contracture, occur in this situation as in all cases involving implants.

References

1. Poland A. Deficiency of the pectoral muscles. *Guy's Hosp Rep.* 1841;6:191–193.
2. Santi P, Berrino P, Galli A, et al. Anterior transposition of the latissimus dorsi muscle through minimal incisions. *Scand J Plast Reconstr Surg.* 1986;20(1):89–92.
3. Santi P, Berrino P, Galli A. Poland's syndrome: correction of thoracic anomaly through minimal incision. *Plast Reconstr Surg.* 1985;76(4):639–641.
4. Berrino P. Poland's syndrome. In: *Operative strategies in breast plastic surgery.* SEE Editrice Firenze; 2007: 423–435.
5. Pereira LH, Sabatovich O, Santana KP, et al. Surgical correction of Poland's syndrome in males – a purposely designed implant. *J Plast Reconstr Aesthet Surg.* 2008;61(4):393–399.
6. Saour S, Shaaban H, McPhail J, et al. Customised silicone prostheses for the reconstruction of chest wall defects: technique of manufacture and final outcome. *J Plast Reconstr Aesthet Surg.* 2008;61(10):1205–1209.

24

Contouring of the arms, breast, upper trunk, and male chest in the massive weight loss patient

Jonathan W. Toy and J. Peter Rubin

SYNOPSIS

- Upper body contouring procedures in the massive weight loss (MWL) patient requires accurate assessment of the deformity and sound surgical planning.
- Patients must be willing to exchange improved body contour for lengthy scars in some cases.
- Multiple body contouring procedures may be performed in a single stage. Upper body and breast procedures may be done at the same time as lower body procedures in well selected cases with an understanding that significant opposing vectors of pull should be avoided.
- The breast deformity following MWL is complex. The technique of dermal suspension mastopexy with total parenchymal reshaping is a long-lasting and reproducible technique that utilizes the patient's own tissues to autoaugment breast volume.
- Pseudogynecomastia in males following MWL is common, with varying degrees of deformity. For more severe cases, extensive skin envelope excess and nipple descent may be treated with a transverse elliptical excision with repositioning of the nipple areolar complex on a thin dermoglandular pedicle.

 Access the Historical Perspective sections online at
http://www.expertconsult.com

Introduction to brachioplasty and axillary contouring

Upper extremity contouring procedures have exploded in popularity in the past decade. According to the American Society of Plastic Surgeons, arm contouring procedures increased by almost 4200% from 2000 to 2009.[1] Following massive weight loss (MWL), varying degrees of upper arm deformity are seen, from minor residual fat deposits to large aprons of skin. Patients commonly complain of a "bat wing" deformity that may include the upper brachium, axilla, and lateral chest wall.[2] Many techniques to contour the arm have been described. However, the severity of deformity following MWL requires new procedures and technical modifications to existing operations.

Basic science/disease process

Although individual variation occurs, changes in the arm following massive weight loss include: laxity and displacement of the posterior axillary fold, residual lipodystrophy of the arm, and loose, hanging skin. Sagging of the arm is most often seen in the posterior aspect from the axilla to the elbow. Although the greatest area of descent and excess usually occurs at the proximal arm, the lowest point of descent is the arm midpoint.

Commonly, the posterior axillary fold becomes deflated, causing significant descent, resulting in broadening of the attachment of the arm to the chest wall. This area originates from the lateral chest wall, and by definition, the skin excess merges with this area. The anterior axillary fold is enlarged and elongated. It is formed along the lateral border of the pectoralis major muscle, beginning at the pectoralis humeral insertion and ending at the superior-lateral breast.[12] Axillary enlargement may be seen.

Diagnosis/patient presentation

Examination should note position and amounts of residual lipodystrophy, skin excess, along with their relative amounts, and assessment of the lateral thoracic wall. There have been a number of proposed classifications for the arm deformity following MWL.[6] The Pittsburgh Rating Scale assesses adiposity, skin tone, and the extent of loose, hanging skin present.[13] As a part of a complete history, key points that need to be elicited include:

- Weight loss history, including type of weight loss surgery
- History of lymphedema, or risk factors for upper extremity lymphedema such as prior lymph node dissection, axillary radiation
- Prior surgeries on the upper extremities
- History of nerve compression syndromes
- Specific goals and expectations

Physical examination of the upper extremities should include:

- Determination of excess skin and fat (pinch test) and their relations – this is important to assess and record in the proximal, middle, and distal arm
- Degree of arm deflation
- Lateral chest wall deformity (include contiguous rolls with the breasts, back), presence/amount of axillary descent
- Asymmetries
- Presence of lymphedema
- Identification of prior upper extremity surgical scars.

Patient selection

Choice of procedure is dependent on patient expectations, surgeon preference, as well as physical properties of the arms. The patient's skin tone, amount of adiposity, and the extent of skin redundancy, all play a role. Patient selection is vital for a good outcome *(Table 24.1)*.[14]

Table 24.1 Pittsburgh Rating Scale for contour deformities after bariatric weight loss: arm deformities

	Clinical findings	Preferred procedure
0.	Normal	None
1.	Adiposity with good skin tone	UAL and/or SAL
2.	Loose, hanging skin without severe adiposity	Brachioplasty
3.	Loose, hanging skin with severe adiposity	Brachioplasty ± UAL and/or SAL

(Adapted from Song AY, Jean RD, Hurwitz DJ, et al. Classification of contour deformities after bariatric weight loss: the Pittsburgh Rating Scale. Plast Reconstr Surg 2005; 116:1535–1546.)

In patients with good skin tone and adiposity with minimal skin excess, liposuction alone may be adequate, thus improving contour while omitting lengthy scarring. Ultrasound assisted liposuction is an excellent technique for arm contouring and may lead to greater postoperative skin contraction than traditional liposuction.[15,16] Patients unwilling to have scars on the arms may be given the option of having conservative ultrasound assisted liposuction of the arms, followed by a dermolipectomy procedure to correct skin redundancy if retraction does not occur satisfactorily.

Patients with adiposity and moderate skin redundancy in the proximal arm may benefit from liposuction in conjunction with an excisional procedure (mini-brachioplasty) in the inner proximal arm.[17-19] This may be in the form of an ellipse, or a T-shape. Patients with isolated horizontal laxity may require an elliptical excision in the axilla that results in a well-concealed scar. The addition of vertical laxity requires a T-type excision.

Patients with significant adiposity with moderate to severe skin redundancy may have liposuction and an excisional procedure performed in two separate stages, or at the same time.

A mini-brachioplasty alone may be all that is necessary to treat mild to moderate skin redundancy in the proximal arm in the absence of significant adiposity, although this is a rare situation after massive weight loss.[17] Patients with loose hanging skin down the length of the arm, without severe adiposity and with poor skin tone, good contour results can be obtained using excisional brachioplasty from axilla to elbow. Extension of the excision to the level of and distal to the elbow is sometimes necessary to deal with significant proximal forearm laxity. Extension into the axilla and down to the lateral chest directly contours these areas. Alternatively, a technique described by Goddio involves correction of ptosis, without excision based on rolling a de-epithelialized flap around from posterior to anterior.[20]

The ideal patient for a full-scar traditional brachioplasty procedure is one with loose hanging skin that more than doubles the width of the upper arm. In patients with severe adiposity and hanging skin, liposuction in conjunction with brachioplasty is necessary. The aggressiveness of brachioplasty is dependent on the extent of skin excess. Brachioplasty is commonly done in conjunction with other body contouring procedures and rarely performed in isolation.[21]

Special precautions need to be taken to avoid undue complications. Pre-existing scars and prior surgeries need to be noted. Modifications may be needed to avoid violation of blood supply. Patients with prior axillary nodal dissections or otherwise at high risk of lymphedema postoperatively should be approached with caution and carefully counseled on risk of prolonged or permanent swelling. Importantly, if undergoing longitudinal excisional brachioplasty, patients need to be accepting of the trade-off between arm tightening and scars.

Numerous procedures have been described in the treatment of arm deformities following MWL.[2,7,8,10,11,20,22–27] Controversy exists among surgeons regarding the position of the arms scar in full brachioplasty. Some advocate placement posteriorly on the arm, while some prefer placement in the brachial groove.[9,22,27–29] While a posteriorly placed scar remains hidden to the patient looking in the mirror, others may see it from behind. The more anteriorly situated scar allows it to be hidden between the arm and chest wall with the arm at rest. Therefore, it is the preference of the authors to place the final scar in this position.

In the standing position and the patient's arm in the "victory position", the proposed scar position in the brachial groove is marked from apex of the axilla to the distal extent of skin excision. Scar length may be altered depending on the amount of skin laxity. For skin redundancy in the elbow region, the scar must continue distally for adequate tightening. Next, inferior traction on the medial arm skin simulates brachioplasty vector of pull. The superior resection line is determined using this maneuver and continues proximally into the axilla just posterior to the anterior axillary fold.

The posterior axillary fold is pinched up to meet the new superior resection apex and marked, simulating correction of axillary ptosis. This point is often 4–5 cm from the axillary dome. This will be the point that is defined to elevate the posterior axillary fold and lateral chest wall. Handling the axillary excess in this fashion obviates the need for Z-plasties in this region. Superior displacement with pinch test determines the inferior resection margin. The inferior margin is checked and remarked intraoperatively. If liposuction is necessary, the posterior arm area is marked, with small incision port placed just posterior to the elbow.

Treatment/surgical technique

With arms prepped and draped circumferentially to the lateral chest wall, the superior excision line is incised and carried into the axilla (*Figs 24.1, 24.2*). A posteriorly based flap is elevated superficial to brachial fascia. Care is taken to preserve any sensory nerves encountered. Medially, the flap is elevated just superficial to brachial fascia. Dissection in the axilla is more superficial.

Video 2

Distally, the dissection becomes more superficial to protect the medial antebrachial cutaneous (MAC) nerve, which is usually found in conjunction with the basilic vein at the distal upper arm. A cadaveric study by Knoetgen and Moran demonstrated that although variable, the MAC nerve pierced the deep fascia at approximately 14 cm proximal to the medial epicondyle. They also noted that the MAC nerve did not always run in conjunction with the basilic vein, with some instances where the nerve was >5 cm anterior to the vein in the midarm.[21] The medial brachial cutaneous (MBC) nerve is vulnerable during surgical flap elevation in the medial arm. It runs with the basilic vein and sends 2–4 branches to the skin 7 cm proximal to the medial epicondyle, and another few branches that pierce fascia to innervate skin 15 cm proximal to the medial epicondyle.[30]

An assistant elevates the arm off of the operating table to ensure no tethering of the posterior arm

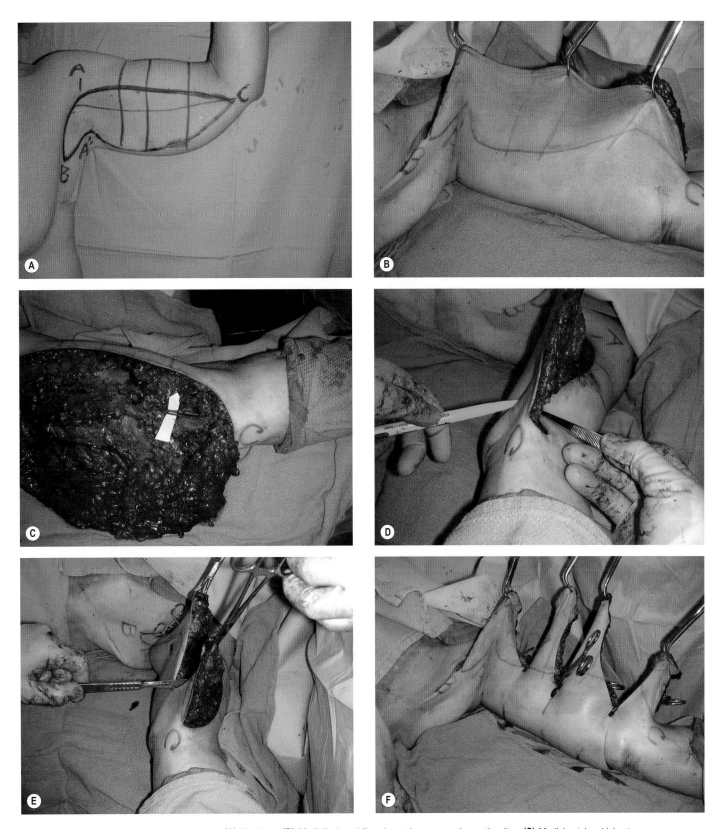

Fig. 24.1 Brachioplasty: intraoperative technique. **(A)** Markings. **(B)** Medially-based flap elevated to proposed resection line. **(C)** Medial antebrachial cutaneous nerve (MABC) in proximity to basilic vein. **(D)** Flap marking technique with heavy forceps to assess medial resection margin. Preoperative markings may require adjustment. **(E)** Flap splitting at 6 cm intervals to level of proposed line of resection. **(F)** Multiple flaps following division.

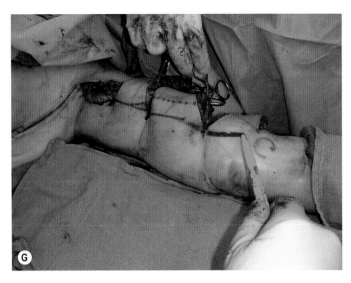
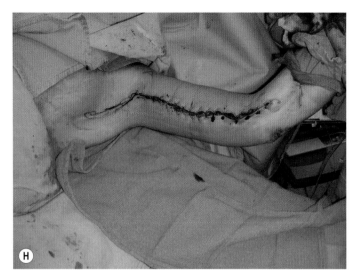

Fig. 24.1, cont'd (G) Proposed medial line of resection re-marked to be incised. **(H)** Closure in three layers. Note extension into axilla, similar to Bruner incision in the hand, with no requirement for axillary Z-plasty.

tissues. A flap marking technique is used to precisely define the inferior margin of resection. A heavy forceps is used to transpose the superior margin of resection beneath the dissected flap to estimate extent of resection at three points. Towel clips are used to temporarily secure the tissues. The flap is then segmentally cut and excised using these three points. The posterior apex point is secured to the clavipectoral fascia with braided nylon sutures at the dome of the axilla in order to prevent possible tissue descent.

Closure should progress quickly following resection to minimize edema that could prevent wound edge opposition. When liposuction is performed in conjunction with excisional brachioplasty, it is advised to infiltrate tumescent fluid followed by immediate liposuction and by segmental resection of arm skin in rapid succession to minimize the spread if edema in the operative field. Communication with the anesthesiologist is imperative to avoid fluid overload that may increase edema and make closure excessively tight, or not possible. It is the author's preference to give the least amount of intravenous fluid possible to maintain adequate perfusion and urine output, and to administer colloid if appropriate. Closure over drains, first of the superficial fascial system (SFS), followed by deep dermis and subcuticular, is performed.

Hints and tips

Arm contouring

- Communication with the anesthesiologist is imperative to avoid fluid overload that may increase edema and make closure excessively tight, or not possible.
- Various techniques may be performed to contour the arms. The surgeon must assess the amount of lipodystrophy, skin quality, and skin excess. The patient must be willing to trade possible extensive scars for improved contour.
- Prevent a tight or impossible closure of skin flaps during excisional brachioplasty by keeping IV fluid volume to the minimum necessary in order to reduce the soft tissue edema, double check excision markings of the flaps prior to incising flaps, performing excision immediately after liposuction of the arm (if liposuction is needed) and closing flaps as quickly as possible after excision.
- Leave a carpet of soft tissue over the brachial fascia in the distal third during flap elevation to protect sensory nerves.
- Brachioplasty procedures may safely be combined with other body contouring procedures in well-selected patients.

Postoperative care

Arms are wrapped in an ACE wrap compressive dressing. Elevation is encouraged. Compressive arm sleeves are substituted at the first postoperative visit. Drains are removed when output is <30 cc over a 24-h period,

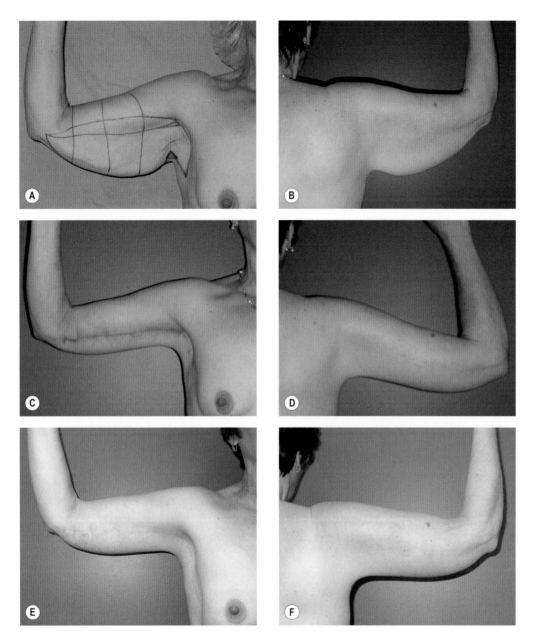

Fig. 24.2 Brachioplasty. A 43-year-old woman s/p 60 kg weight loss. Preoperative views including markings for brachioplasty. **(A,B)** Characteristic changes following MWL are seen including laxity and displacement of the posterior axillary fold with resultant broadening of the attachment of the arm to the chest wall, residual lipodystrophy of the arm, and skin laxity and excess. Postoperative views shown at 4 months **(C,D)**, and 2 years. **(E,F)** Note progression of scar maturation.

usually lasting from 2 to 5 days. Patients are instructed to avoid heavy lifting and elevation of arms over 90° for 2 weeks. Abduction exercises are begun at this time with gentle active range of motion.

Outcomes, prognosis, and complications

Complication rates following brachioplasty have been reported to range from 25% to 40%.[21,28] The majority of these complications were considered minor. A major disadvantage with a full-scar brachioplasty is a visible scar with variable scar quality and prolonged scar maturation.[8,28,31] The scar may be red and raised for up to a year postoperatively. Other adverse events include edema, seroma and lymphoceles, paresthesias, neurapraxia or transection of the MAC or MBC nerves (possible neuroma formation), wound infection, suture extrusion or abscess, under-resection, and wound dehiscence.[21,28] Possible over-resection of tissue with the inability to close is a complication that is generally avoidable with intraoperative confirmation of markings.

Hypertrophic scarring may be reduced by SFS approximation. Scar treatments may include silicone based products, scar massage, and other scar modalities. Injection of dilute steroid may be helpful.[32] The surgeon should have a lower threshold for scar revision in the arm areas. At times, significant and poorly formed scars may occur and are difficult for the patient to conceal. Scar revision rates following brachioplasty range from 3–12%.[21,24,28]

Seromas following brachioplasty are often found on a delayed basis (4–6 weeks postoperatively). These tend to be distal on the arm and discrete low volume localized collections (often 5–10 cc). Treatment of seromas typically involves aspiration in the office, with excision rarely necessary.

Injury to the MAC and MBC nerves also may occur during excisional brachioplasty.[30] A 5% rate of injury has been reported for the MAC nerve. On average, the MAC nerve became superficial in at a point approximately 14 cm proximal to the medial epicondyle.[21] Depth of resection, with dissection more superficial in the distal arm region will leave an important amount of soft tissue coverage over this nerve and prevent injury.

Mastopexy and breast reshaping in the MWL patient

The youthful breast has been a symbol of femininity and beauty throughout the ages. Nipple descent and loss of parenchymal volume is suggestive of aging and loss of attractiveness. Regnault described a widely utilized classification for breast ptosis relying on nipple position relative to the inframammary fold.[33] However, the breast deformity following MWL is more complex.

As increasing numbers of patients are presenting to plastic surgeons following MWL, traditional mastopexy techniques have been challenged and the surgeon forced to adopt newer techniques for this challenging deformity. These patients differ from candidates for typical breast reshaping.

Box 24.1 Characteristic features of the breast following massive weight loss

- Volume deflation
- Stretched skin envelope
- Significant ptosis
- Flattening of shape
- Medialized nipple areola complex
- Lateral chest roll

Box 24.2 Pitfalls in the treatment of breasts after massive weight loss

- Inadequate treatment of the lateral chest wall roll
- Failure to reposition and lateralize the usually medialized nipple areola complex
- Failure to restore aesthetic breast shape.

Basic science/disease process

Characteristic changes in the breast typically follow massive weight loss (**Box 24.1**). Volume deflation resulting in a stretched skin envelope, significant ptosis, and flattening of the overall breast shape occur. The nipple areola complex is medialized, and lateral chest rolls develop contiguous with the breast. The chest roll is a difficult area to treat and obscures the lateral curvature of the breast, blunting its shape. Breast asymmetry is the norm. A significant amount of skin excess occurs, while parenchymal volume may be deficient. The skin envelope may be thin and relatively inelastic. Internal supporting structures of the breast may be attenuated. Traditional techniques for breast ptosis are usually inadequate for these deformities.[34,35]

Traditional classification schemes to describe breast ptosis fall short in the MWL patient.[33] To better describe deformities following MWL, the Pittsburgh Rating Scale was developed to classify contour deformities in this group of patients.[13] Specific to breasts, the scale combines the Regnault grade of breast ptosis with volume loss, loose skin, and the presence or absence of lateral chest wall skin rolls (**Box 24.2**).

Diagnosis/patient presentation

Goals in mastopexy after massive weight loss are listed in **Box 24.3**.

Variations in technique have been described, many using local flaps to autoaugment breast volume.

Parenchymal suspension to chest wall structures, including pectoralis fascia, or rib periosteum have also been included.[36–39]

As in any breast procedure, a complete breast and medical history collected:

- Weight history (including history of weight loss surgery, lowest, highest, and current weight and BMI, recent weight fluctuations, length of time weight has been stable)
- Bra size: largest, current, ideal
- Personal, family history of breast cancer
- Prior breast abnormalities, masses
- Prior breast surgeries or biopsies
- Previous mammographic history
- Breast-feeding history, future plans for breast-feeding
- Genetic pre-disposition to breast cancer, history of ovarian, colon cancer.

Physical examination should include distances (suprasternal notch to nipple, breast meridian at clavicle to nipple, nipple to inframammary fold), asymmetries, position of the nipple areola complex, examination for masses or irregularities, presence of lateral chest wall roll, breast, scars, quality of skin envelope, parenchymal volume, and mobility of the inframammary fold.

Mammography should be performed according to American Cancer Society guidelines.[40]

Operative planning/patient selection

Many approaches to mastopexy have been described.[41–47] After weight loss, the breasts usually are lacking in upper pole fullness, and it is difficult in the MWL to produce and maintain upper pole fullness with some techniques. Traditional breast reduction (Wise pattern or vertical) using a variety of pedicles to carry the nipple areola complex (inferior, lateral, superior, medial), augmentation with implant, and augmentation mastopexy may fall short in the MWL patient. Some methods to reshape the breast include dermal suspension techniques, while others discuss techniques to use local tissues for autoaugmentation. Graf *et al.* describe using a lateral thoracic wall flap suspended with a loop of pectoralis muscle to reshape the breast and add upper pole fullness.[37]

In patients with Pittsburgh grade I breast changes, traditional augmentation, reduction, or mastopexy techniques may be performed based on patient desires. The Pittsburgh grade II breast may also be treated with mastopexy ± augmentation with implants. Breast implants may be used to supplement insufficient volume and provide upper pole fullness in Wise pattern and vertical mastopexy techniques.

Grade III changes are best treated with parenchymal reshaping techniques with dermal suspension and autoaugmentation if volume deficient. Ignoring deformities of structures adjacent to the breast in the MWL patient (axillary fold, lateral chest wall) tends to lead to aesthetic disharmony and unsatisfactory results.[36] Techniques dealing with grade III changes include the recruitment of laterally based thoracic flaps, the rotation-advancement of a supero-medial pedicle, as well as the simultaneous use of implants for additional parenchymal volume.[48]

The addition of a lateral thoracic flap based on intercostal perforators allows the recruitment of soft tissue to augment insufficient breast volume, along with simultaneous removal of commonly found lateral thoracic soft tissue excess. The intercostal perforators that require preservation are located along the anterior axillary line, parallel to the lateral border of the breast.[49] It is not possible to preserve perforators through the latissimus muscle however. Dissection is generally carried out in a plane deep to the fascia.

A Wise pattern technique with use of a variety of pedicles, including the supero-medial pedicle may be utilized in patients with adequate parenchymal volume in order to provide parenchymal reshaping. The addition of implants to supplement volume and improve upon upper pole fullness may be considered. In any patient with inelastic skin, the size of implant should remain conservative. Larger implants will not be adequately supported by the remaining breast structures

Table 24.2 Surgical options for the breast after massive weight loss

Pittsburgh scale rating		Preferred surgical technique
0.	Normal	None
1.	Ptosis grade I/II or severe macromastia	Traditional mastopexy (preference for vertical), reduction, or augmentation techniques with implants ± nipple elevation
2.	Ptosis grade III or moderate volume loss or constricted breast	Traditional mastopexy (traditional Wise pattern) ± augmentation
3.	Severe lateral roll and/ or severe volume loss with loose skin	Parenchymal reshaping techniques with dermal suspension, consider autoaugmentation. Avoid implants if at all possible if autoaugmentation produces sufficient volume

(Adapted from Song AY, Jean RD, Hurwitz DJ, et al. Classification of contour deformities after bariatric weight loss: the Pittsburgh Rating Scale. Plast Reconstr Surg 2005; 116:1535–1546.)

and lead to implant descent and recurrent ptosis. If mastopexy with augmentation is planned, the safest method to manage more severe cases of breast ptosis is to stage the procedure. If larger implants are considered, additional support with cadaveric dermal products may be used to minimize the risk of implant descent.[50,51]

A de-epithelialized inferior pedicle used in conjunction with a separate pedicle to carry the nipple areola complex may also reshape the breasts with addition of superior pole fullness.[47] Parenchymal tissues may be either suspended to stable chest wall structures (pectoralis fascia, rib periosteum) or by a loop of pectoralis muscle.[37,52] Plication of parenchymal or de-epithelialized dermis allows for increased projection and reshaping of the underlying glandular structure.[34,48]

Choice of technique is dependent on breast morphology, patient desires and expectations, and surgeon preference (Table 24.2). An important assessment is whether or not the patient is happy with the current volume of the breasts in a bra. This will guide the surgeon as to the need for only parenchymal reshaping, breast reduction, or addition of volume (autoaugmentation or implant placement).[53]

The senior author has developed a technique based on an extended Wise pattern that achieves all of the goals of mastopexy following MWL.[34,35,54] Goals of this procedure include: elevation of the nipple areola

complex, tightening of the breast skin envelope and reshaping the breast mound, recruiting a laterally-based dermoglandular flap for breast autoaugmentation and simultaneous ablation of the lateral chest wall roll, establishing a stable result (see *Figs 24.4, 24.5*).

Dermal suspension and total parenchymal reshaping mastopexy

Surgical markings

The patient is marked standing. The suprasternal notch is identified and the breast meridians are marked. In many MWL patients, the nipple areola complexes are medialized and will need to be lateralized. The new nipple position is referenced to the existing inframammary fold. A standard Wise pattern is then drawn with extension laterally to encompass the thoracic roll. The keyhole pattern, is placed with the superior extent 2 cm above the proposed new nipple position, with 5 cm vertical limbs and a 42 mm diameter areola.[55] Back rolls may be treated with horizontal upper bodylift excision that merges with the lateral extent of the mastopexy, extending to the posterior axillary line, and beyond if necessary.[35] If rolls are more vertically oriented, a vertical excision may be performed in the mid-axillary line, ultimately merging with the excision for a concomitant brachioplasty. The nipple areola complex is transposed on a 10 cm infero-central pedicle, resulting in a reliable vascular supply.

Treatment/surgical technique

The nipple areola complex (NAC) is reduced using a 42 mm marker. De-epithelialization is carried out over the entire Wise pattern marking. The lateral extent of de-epithelialization depends on the amount of lateral tissue needed for volume augmentation. The inferocentrally based pedicle is raised down to pectoralis fascia by completely degloving the breast parenchyma with 1–1.5 cm thick flaps overlying the breast capsule. The base of the pedicle is maintained at a width of 10 cm. Care is taken to avoid release of sternal attachments. The lateral and medial extensions of the Wise pattern are raised off the chest wall. The lateral wing is vascularized by intercostals perforators. Once the chest

Video
3

wall is reached, dissection continues cephalad to the level of the clavicles *(Fig. 24.3)*.

Suspension is performed utilizing the central keyhole dermoglandular extension. Nonabsorbable braided nylon sutures affix this to rib periosteum along the breast meridian in the position of the second or third rib, depending on the elevation required. This suspension should raise the nipple to its intended position and allow stable elevation with long-lasting fullness. Care is taken to palpate directly over rib, while the needle is passed through pectoralis. One should feel the needle pass against the rib.

The lateral breast flap is rotated medially to auto-augment breast volume. It is suspended to a position one rib lower than the initial suture. This re-establishes a natural lateral breast curvature. The medial flap is also suspended. It is helpful to perform bilateral suspensions concomitantly to improve symmetry.

Parenchymal reshaping with plication of dermal elements is performed with absorbable sutures to enhance projection. The lateral flap is sutured to the central extension. Medially, the flaps are approximated. Laterally, the breast flaps are sutured to serratus fascia to emphasize the lateral curve and further increase projection. If necessary, the inferior pole of the breast is plicated to shorten the distance from the nipple to the inframammary fold.

The remaining skin-parenchymal envelope is redraped over the new breast scaffold. Constant assessment for symmetry occurs during this procedure, with the patient sitting up. Closure to the SFS of the abdominal wall may be required if the abdominal wall tissues are mobile. Release of the dermis adjacent to a portion of the nipple areola complex may be necessary to allow better inset if tethered. Multi-layered closure over drains is performed.

Disadvantages to the dermal-suspension with parenchymal reshaping technique include the need to create lengthy scars, a longer operative time for extensive de-epithelialization, and a great deal of intraoperative tailoring.

The dermal suspension with parenchymal reshaping technique is a safe and reliable procedure that may be performed in conjunction with other body contouring procedures. However, when adding abdominal contouring procedures, the abdominal region should be treated prior to the breast, as the resultant pull may lower the inframammary fold and require remarking of the mastopexy pattern before starting the breast procedure.[54] If further volume is needed, implant placement in the subpectoral plane may be added.

Hints and tips

Mastopexy after MWL

- Changes in the breast following MWL may include volume deflation, excess skin envelope, ptosis and flattening of the overall breast shape. A lateral chest wall roll is common.
- Careful assessment of the breast deformity aids in technique selection. Addressing the skin envelope, deficiencies in parenchymal volume, and glandular reshaping in more severe cases is necessary.
- Various mastopexy techniques utilizing lateral chest wall-based flaps add volume to commonly deflated breasts.
- If implants are to be considered for augmentation of breast volume, larger sizes may further stretch a poorly elastic skin envelope and the implant is prone to descent. Smaller sized implants, or the use of additional support (such as an cadaveric dermis sling) may prevent this recurrent ptosis and worsening implant descent

---

Postoperative care

A lightly compressive dressing is applied postoperatively and maintained until the first postoperative visit *(Figs 24.4, 24.5)*. Drains are removed once drainage is <30 cc over a 24-h period. Patients are instructed to wear a supportive bra and avoid underwire bras for 4 weeks. Heavy lifting of items >10 lb for 4–6 weeks postoperatively is discouraged.

Outcomes, prognosis, and complications

The technique of dermal suspension with parenchymal reshaping mastopexy is a reliable and safe method of dealing with the difficult deformities in the breast after MWL. More common complications related to this procedure include minor wound dehiscences, primarily at "triple-point" (5%), seroma (3%), and hematoma (1%).[54] Other complications include: asymmetry, "dog-ears" at the ends of resection (requiring in-office revision in 5% of patients), scarring, as well as changes to nipple sensation. Small wound dehiscences are managed conservatively in the office with bedside debridements and dressings. All have healed without the need for formal surgical revision. Seromas are most common in the

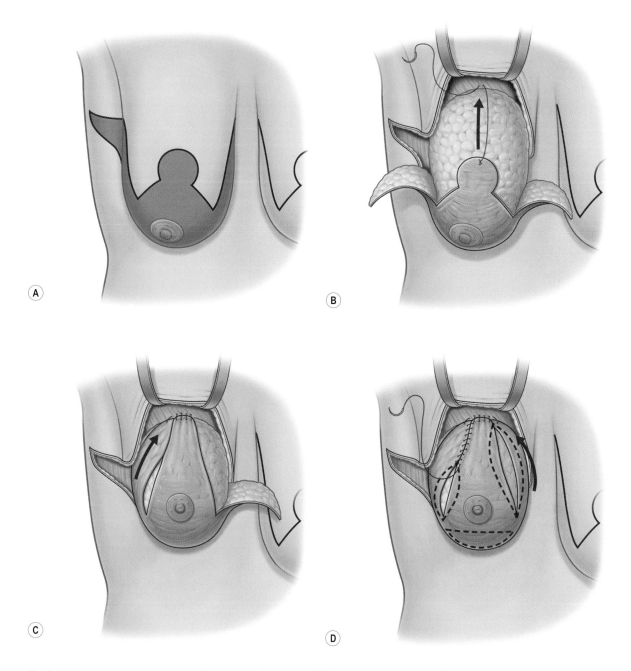

Fig. 24.3 Dermal suspension mastopexy with parenchymal reshaping. **(A)** The patient is marked with a Wise pattern that extends laterally to encompass the redundant axillary roll. The entire area of the Wise pattern is de-epithelialized, preserving an extensive dermal surface. **(B)** The breast parenchyma is degloved by raising a 1 cm-thick flap and then continuing the dissection superiorly just superficial to the pectoralis fascia. Medial and lateral flaps of dermis/breast tissue are mobilized from the chest wall. The central dermal extension is elevated and secured to the chest wall (usually rib periosteum) using braided nylon suture. **(C)** The lateral breast flap is elevated to create the lateral curvature of the breast mound, and the dermis secured to the chest wall near the previous fixation point. The lateral flap can be extended posteriorly on the chest wall to provide extra tissue for autologous volume augmentation. **(D)** The dermal edge of the medial breast flap is fixed to the chest wall. A running absorbable braided suture is used to approximate the dermal edges of the lateral flap and central dermal extension. Dashed lines show the pattern of plications used. The pattern of placation may be individualized to achieve the best breast shape in each patient. In general, there is a later component, a medial component, and an inferior component that corrects the "bottomed out" appearance and increases projection. (Reproduced with permission from Rubin JP, Gusenoff J. Bodylifts and post massive weight loss body contouring. In: Guyuron B, Eriksson A, Persing J, et al., eds. Plastic surgery: indications and practice. Philadelphia: Elsevier; 2008:1648–1649.)

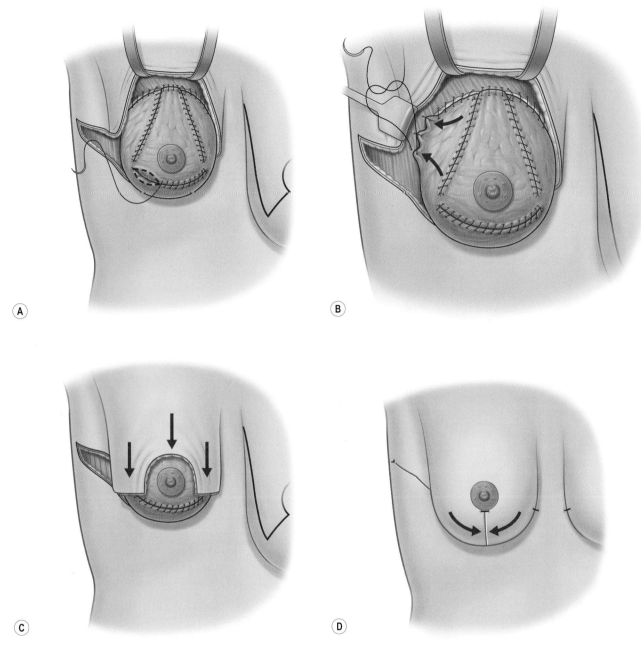

Fig. 24.4 (A) The dermis of the medial breast flap is approximated to the central dermal extension using a running suture. The dermis on the inferior pole of the breast is plicated with a running suture to shorten the distance between areola and inferior mammary fold to approximately 5 cm. **(B)** The dermis along the lateral breast is secured to the lateral chest fascia (not rib periosteum) with permanent sutures to increase projection and accentuate the lateral curve of the breast. The breast parenchyma is now firmly secured to the chest wall, and the shape has been adjusted using the placation sutures. **(C,D)** The breast skin flap is redraped and closed with absorbable intradermal sutures over the drain. If the nipple is tethered and pointing in an approximate direction, the dermis adjacent to the nipple is scored to release the tension. Because of the robust pedicle, scoring of the dermis can be safely performed along part of the circumference, if necessary. (Reproduced with permission from Rubin JP, Gusenoff J. Bodylifts and post massive weight loss body contouring. In: Guyuron B, Eriksson A, Persing J, *et al.*, eds. Plastic surgery: indications and practice. Philadelphia: Elsevier; 2008:1648–1649.

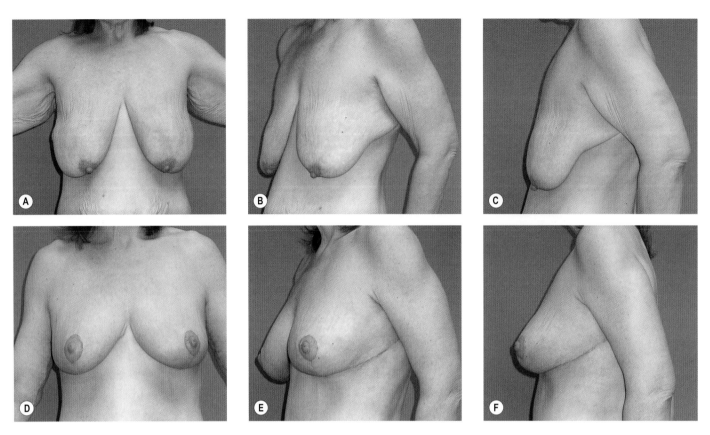

Fig. 24.5 A 46-year-old patient treated with this mastopexy technique following a 160 lb (73 kg) weight loss. **(A–C)** Preoperative and **(D–F)** 6-month postoperative views.

lateral aspect of the breast, and like most other seromas seen following body contouring, respond well to serial aspiration, requiring no re-operation.

The robust blood supply of the centrally and inferiorly based dermoglandular flap that supplies the nipple areola complex provides a safe method of nipple elevation. In our series, we have had no incidences of nipple necrosis with this technique. As with any procedure involving the elevation of flaps for autoaugmentation, one must be aware of the possibility of fat necrosis, especially of the distal flaps. Caution not to extend the lateral autoaugmentation flap past the posterior axillary line, as well as ensuring viability by healthy bleeding edges intraoperatively help to prevent fat necrosis. The authors also consider active smoking a contraindication for this procedure.

Upper bodylift

Good results in body contouring incorporate scars in the position of the borders of existing aesthetic units.

Increasing interest exists in the contouring of rolls of excess skin and lipodystrophy in the back area. In the past, back rolls were more commonly treated with suction lipectomy alone, but excisional procedures are quickly gaining in popularity. This upper bodylift may be combined with breast procedures or reverse abdominoplasty in females and with excisional gynecomastia procedures in males. One advantage of the upper bodylift in conjunction with breast reshaping procedures, is that the lateral skin and subcutaneous flap may be medially rotated to restore volume to a deflated breast based on the lateral intercostals perforators.

Basic science/disease process

Accompanying the residual deformities of the chest and abdomen in the MWL are varying degrees of back rolls, which may extend from the chest and cross the axilla. These rolls are composed of skin and subcutaneous tissue of varying degrees, the assessment of which determines the choice of surgical procedure. Patients may complain about lack of a smooth back silhouette or unaesthetic bulges at the bra-line. Rolls may range in number from one to four on either side of the midline.[56] It is essential that the surgeon understands these deformities.

The highest of the back rolls that may be present is the posterolateral extension of the breast roll.[56] Lateral descent of the breast mound itself is an associated finding. Other possible rolls in descending order, include the scapular, lower thoracic, and hip rolls. The fifth roll seen in the chest wall may be in the axilla. These rolls tend to be tethered at zones of adherence in the midlines of the chest and back, producing maximum tissue descent laterally (inverted-V deformity).[57] Other potential thoracic deformities include breast changes in females, and variable degrees of gynecomastia in males.

Patient evaluation

In the MWL patient, back rolls are uncommonly an isolated deformity. With today's fashion trends in women's clothing, lipodystrophy and excess rolls in the trunk may be accentuated. Excess skin and fat may be seen bulging above and below bra-lines, or be visible through tight fitting blouses.

Along with tempering patient expectations, the surgeon must preoperatively counsel the patient on the lengthy scars that are produced with large skin and soft tissue resections. In upper body lifting of the trunk, transverse excisions may be hidden within the bra-line, but vertical truncal excisions may be visible while wearing only a bra and not follow boundaries of aesthetic units. If breast or arm surgeries are planned, appropriate history, physical examination, and counseling are required.

As with any elective body contouring procedure, the patient is assessed for medical co-morbidities, which are preoperatively optimized. A complete weight history, including minimum, maximum, and current weights and BMIs are recorded. Any fluctuations in weight in the past 3 months are probed. If multiple procedures are to be performed, second stage is delayed at least 3 months or longer, depending on the patient's overall status. Patients are counseled about smoking cessation if they actively smoke. Agents that may increase the risk of surgical bleeding (e.g., aspirin) are stopped if possible at least 14 days prior to surgery.

Physical examination should include assessment of the back, but also other adjacent areas that may require contouring (e.g., arms, breasts, abdomen). The level of skin redundancy and elasticity, along with the thickness of fat overlying the muscle is noted. Documentation of the number of rolls, especially lateral breast or chest roll and its level of descent is important, along with the position of the inframammary crease.

Operative planning/patient selection

Back contouring procedures are selected based on the deformity present, surgeon preference, as well as the patient's expectations and acceptability of final scar placement. The predominance of excess skin versus fat is also an important consideration.

In patients with mild amounts of skin excess, good skin elasticity accompanying lipodystrophy, back rolls may be treated with liposuction alone (ultrasound-assisted liposuction is a good adjunct).[58] If following liposuction, the skin does not satisfactorily retract, a second stage skin excision may be performed.

If moderate to severe amounts of skin redundancy is present, excisional procedures are necessary. The key to decision-making in this area is descent of the lateral inframammary crease.[57] In these cases, three main options in the management of back rolls are possible.

The first is a transversely based excision that extends from the mid-axial line (or merged with anteriorly based breast or chest excisions) to the midline of the back. The extent of resection toward the midline may be shortened, based on deformity. Maximal resection occurs more laterally, with less amounts of excision on the midline. The advantage of this procedure is the ability to plan the final scar to lie within the patient's bra-line.

The second option is a vertically based excision in the midaxillary line that extends from the axilla to as far inferiorly as the iliac crest.[59] This excision may be modified and shortened if necessary to include only the upper chest tissues.[60] The advantage of this vertically based procedure is possible transverse tightening of the abdomen and back without creating scars anteriorly or posteriorly, thereby avoiding a fleur-de-lis type resection in the abdomen. The inferior descent of the breast mound may also be corrected with this procedure. This procedure should be performed as a second stage if combined with any abdominoplasty or circumferential body lift type procedure, as it may disrupt the blood supply of abdominal flaps.[59]

The third option is a valuable option in females presenting with minimal upper back laxity, clinically seen as tissue redundancy above a worn bra. Extension from an excisional brachioplasty is performed down through the lateral chest to the inframammary crease. The result is elevation of the inframammary crease, in conjunction with upward rotation of the upper back tissues.[61] Both the horizontally and vertically-based excision may be merged into brachioplasty, breast, or reverse abdominoplasty excisions.

It is possible that skin resection surgeries adjacent to the back may improve contour in select patients, thereby avoiding the morbidity of an excisional back procedure.[58] For example, the lower thoracic and hip rolls seen in the lower trunk are improved with circumferential bodylifting procedures. If breast surgery is concomitantly performed, the lateral breast roll may be excised to the posterior axillary line and used to autoaugment breast volume. Care must be taken to preserve the intercostal perforators supplying this flap, and caution in the patient who has previously had breast reduction surgery is important.

Surgical markings

Transverse excisional upper bodylift (Fig. 24.5)

The patient is marked standing. If chest procedures such as mastopexy, reduction mammaplasty, or excision of gynecomastia are to be performed, these anterior markings are made first. It is important to mark the inferior aspect of the descended inframammary fold, extending to the lateral chest. In female patients, the patient is asked to bring in a bra of their choice to enable final scar position to be hidden in the outline of her bra-line. The proposed final scar position is marked. The excision may be modified and need not reach the midline. The superior margin of the resection is made within the bra-line extending the midaxillary line, which will act as an anchor point. The inferior tissues are then pinched upward to simulate resection. Using this maneuver, the inferior resection is marked to the

midaxillary line, where it merges with anterior chest markings. Vertical reference lines are made every 6 cm. Symmetry is assessed and adjustments are made if necessary.

Treatment/surgical technique

The procedure is begun in the prone position. If concomitant chest or abdominal procedures are planned, they are performed after the upper bodylift procedure. The superior mark is incised and dissection carried to the deep fascia. A strong layer of SFS will be encountered. An inferiorly based flap is elevated superficial to the muscle fascia to the proposed inferior resection line, continued laterally to the midaxillary line. Towel clips are used to estimate the safety of resection. Laterally, the vertical mark in the midaxillary line that is the merge point with the chest procedure is incised and resection is completed. Towel clips temporarily close the wound, which is subsequently closed with 2-0 braided absorbable sutures to close the SFS deeply, followed by deep dermal and subcuticular layers with absorbable monofilament sutures. The resultant lateral 'dog-ears' are closed temporarily with staples, and will be resected with the anterior chest procedures in the supine position. Skin glue is applied topically. Gauze followed by strips of occlusive dressings is placed. Drains usually come anteriorly from the chest. The patient may now be flipped to the supine position for further anterior procedures. A representative case is shown (*Fig. 24.6*).

Hints and tips

Upper bodylift

- Choice of procedure for back contouring depends on the relative excesses of skin and fat, along with the patient's skin elasticity. Many excisional procedures result in extensive scars that patients must be willing to accept.
- Upper bodylift excisions may be merged with brachioplasty, gynecomastia, and breast procedures in the same stage.
- Upper bodylifts should be performed in a second stage to most abdominal or circumferential dermolipectomy procedures.
- Full transverse upper bodylifts should not be performed concurrently with a lower body lift in most cases because there may be significant concurrent opposing vectors of pull.

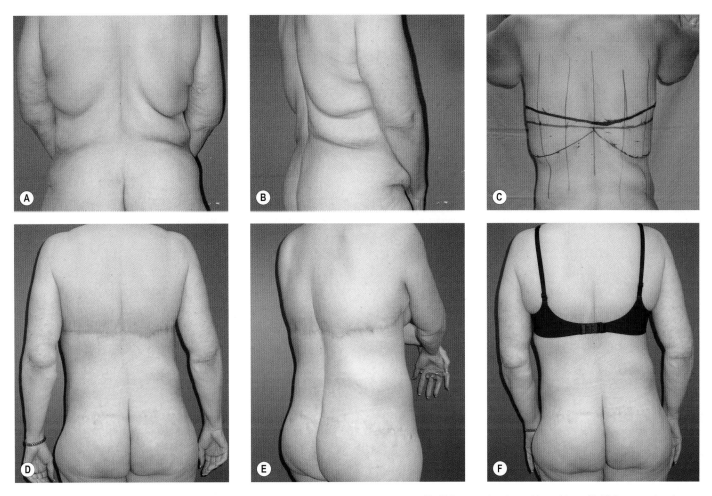

Fig. 24.6 Upper bodylift case. A 49-year-old female s/p gastric bypass following 160 lb weight loss. **(A–C)** Preoperative views with markings. **(D–F)** Postoperative views at 15 months following upper bodylift done as a second stage procedure. The patient underwent an initial staged procedure, including lower bodylift, fleur-de-lis abdominoplasty, and mastopexy. Note the final scar position hidden beneath the patient's undergarment.

Postoperative care

An ACE compressive wrap is placed in the immediate post-operative period. This may be substituted with an upper body compressive elastic garment once drains are removed. Drains are removed once outputs are <30 cc over a 24-h period. Scar therapies are begun following complete healing. If combined with brachioplasty or breast surgeries, postoperative care for these procedures is also initiated.

Outcomes, prognosis, and complications

Complications in back contouring are similar to those seen elsewhere in body contouring. More specific to upper body lifting, poor scarring, wound dehiscences

(usually near the lateral aspect of the breasts), asymmetries, and seromas are not uncommon. The majority of seromas as managed conservatively with serial aspirations. If upper bodylift procedures are performed with brachioplasty, scar contracture is possible, but is largely avoidable with sound surgical planning.

Gynecomastia and male chest contouring in the MWL patient

Basic science/disease process

Gynecomastia surgery as a whole has been increasing in popularity. Between 1992 and 2008, there has been an 211% increase in the number of men seeking gynecomastia surgery.[67] Male breast enlargement traditionally is related to gynecomastia, which is defined as the benign enlargement of male breast glandular tissue (>2 cm palpable, firm, subareolar gland and ductal tissue).[68,69] Another group of patients presenting for male breast reduction is emerging – those with pseudogynecomastia following MWL. Pseudogynecomastia is the presence of increased subareolar fat without enlargement of the glandular tissue and is a commonly seen chest deformity in the male MWL patient.

The ideal male chest is muscular, flat, with the skin-fat envelope tightly adherent to the underlying musculoskeletal anatomy. There is minimal fat or breast tissue overlying the pectoralis muscle, nor rolls extending to the upper back. However, some fullness around the nipple-areola complex representing glandular tissue does exist.[70,71] The ideal inframammary fold in men follows the contour of the inferior border of the pectoralis major muscle. The average NAC measures 28 mm in diameter and is located approximately over the fifth rib, usually at its intersection with the lateral border of pectoralis major.[72–74] The average nipple-to-sternal notch distance is 20 cm.

Characteristic changes in the chests of MWL patients demonstrates significant amounts of skin and soft tissue redundancy with deflation, along with characteristic descent of the lateral inframammary crease, lateral chest wall rolls, and pseudogynecomastia, which is characterized by increased subareolar fat without the enlargement of the breast glandular tissue.[75] The nipple is commonly descended and medialized. The areola is enlarged and reduction in size is required for an aesthetic result.[68,76]

Diagnosis/patient presentation

Males presenting with breast enlargement often suffer psychological stress, especially in patients in their teen years. Social interactions may be negatively affected and patients may be hesitant to participate in activities that involve removing their shirt.[77] Males having lost significant amounts of weight often present with sagging breasts and are unhappy with their appearance in clothing.

Gynecomastia must be differentiated from pseudogynecomastia. While pseudogynecomastia involves increased subareolar fat without enlargement of the glandular tissue, the presence of firm glandular tissue under the nipple-areola complex suggests true gynecomastia.[76]

A thorough history must include features that may suggest a pathologic etiology. A complete review of causes of true gynecomastia is beyond the scope of this chapter. As for any surgical procedure, a complete medical history, including smoking history should be obtained.

Physical examination first assesses the degree of skin excess and elasticity, glandular hypertrophy and position of the nipple. Documentation of any abnormal breast masses, the location and size of the NAC, amount of skin redundancy and ptosis, the presence or absence of a lateral chest wall roll, asymmetries, and the position and mobility of the inframammary fold is key.

The possibility of breast carcinoma must never be overlooked. Male breast cancer represents 1% of breast cancers, although it is diagnosed in only 1% of male breast enlargement.[78,79] High estrogen states predisposes to male breast cancer. Men with Klinefelter's syndrome have a 58-fold higher risk compared with nonaffected males of developing breast cancer.[80] Breast carcinoma is usually located away from the nipple areola complex and is most often unilateral. Physical examination, mammography, ultrasound, and biopsy are used to investigate masses.[69] A high index of suspicion must be maintained.

Investigations for a patient with gynecomastia involve serum testosterone, estrogen, luteinizing hormone (LH), follicle stimulating hormone (FSH), prolactin, human chorionic gonadotropin (hCG), liver, renal, and thyroid tests. Other investigations such as testicular ultrasound or CT of the abdomen should be ordered if clinical suspicion is present.

In general, physical examination and investigations should be tailored to the age and overall health of the patient. An exhaustive medical work-up need not be performed in an otherwise healthy adult with long-standing gynecomastia.[81]

Patient selection

The degree of deflation and amount of skin redundancy are assessed, along with the distance required for nipple repositioning *(Table 24.3)*. Location and mobility of

Table 24.3 Pseudogynecomastia following massive weight loss: classification and surgical options

Grade	Description	Treatment options
1.	Minimal excess skin and fat, minimal nipple areola complex (NAC) changes, inframammary fold (IMF) normal	
	a. No lateral chest wall roll	Liposuction
	b. Lateral chest wall roll present	Liposuction, direct excision of lateral chest wall roll
2.	NAC, IMF below ideal position[a], lateral chest wall roll present, minimal upper abdominal laxity	Pedicled nipple reconstruction
3.	NAC, IMF below ideal[a], lateral chest wall roll, significant upper abdominal laxity	Free-nipple graft reconstruction

[a]Ideal position of IMF = inferior border of pectoralis major. (Adapted from Gusenoff JA, Coon D, Rubin JP. Pseudogynecomastia after massive weight loss: detectability of technique, patient satisfaction, and classification. Plast Reconstr Surg 2008; 122(5):1301–1311.)

the inframammary fold is recorded. In patients with minimal skin redundancy and good skin elasticity, liposuction may be used, avoiding chest scars. Male breast tissue is classically fibrous and dense. Ultrasound-assisted liposuction techniques are ideal to break up this fibrous tissue and may lead to improved skin retraction.[15,16,63] In patients requiring debulking without significant resection of a glandular component and less skin elasticity, a two-stage procedure may be performed. Liposuction is done as a first stage, followed by a period of time to allow for skin retraction. If adequate skin retraction does not occur, a later excisional procedure may be performed.

Patients with a glandular component benefit from direct glandular excision (subcutaneous mastectomy), as liposuction will not greatly affect firm, subareolar tissues. A periareolar incision, keeping the scar in an aesthetic position provides access to the gland. It is important to leave a disk of tissue beneath the areola to prevent a sunken areola, or "dish deformity". Other complications secondary to subcutaneous mastectomy include: changes to nipple sensation, breast asymmetry, hypertrophic or keloid scarring, and nipple necrosis.[82] Liposuction may be used as an adjunct for better chest contour. Arthroscopic shavers have also been used with some success in the removal of subareolar glandular tissues.[83–85]

For patients with moderate to severe skin and soft tissue excess requiring nipple elevation, liposuction alone is not adequate. Excisional procedures that remove skin and soft tissue, while resizing and repositioning the nipple areola complex are required. A supra-areolar crescentic excision allows nipple elevation for lesser degrees of ptosis. Periareolar ("donut") skin excisions are used for larger amounts of skin redundancy and greater need for nipple elevation.[81,86] A Gore-Tex® periareolar suture may reduce the incidence of areolar spread.[77]

A technique used with good aesthetic results by the authors involves elevation of the nipple areola complex on a thin dermoglandular flap, which is transposed under a superior chest wall flap (see *Fig. 24.9*). Excision of the soft tissues under the flap thins the chest. Aggressive breast volume reduction, nipple repositioning, good scar position (around the areola and at the new inframammary fold) is possible. Lateral extension of the chest excision deals with the commonly found lateral chest roll.

An alternative method elevate the nipple areola complex in patients with extreme pseudogynecomastia is to perform a similar elliptical excision, but replace the complex as a free nipple graft (see *Fig. 24.10*). This however, may result in postoperative pigmentary changes and loss of sensation.[87]

The treatment of choice for patients requiring excision and nipple areola repositioning is an elliptical excision based on the current inframammary fold with lateral extension to treat lateral thoracic rolls.

Excision of gynecomastia with nipple repositioning utilizing the dermoglandular flap

Markings

With the patient in the standing position, the suprasternal notch, midline, breast meridian, and ribs numbers are marked *(Fig. 24.7)*. The patient is asked to flex his pectoral muscles and the lateral border is palpated and marked. The proposed new nipple location is located at the intersection between the horizontal location of

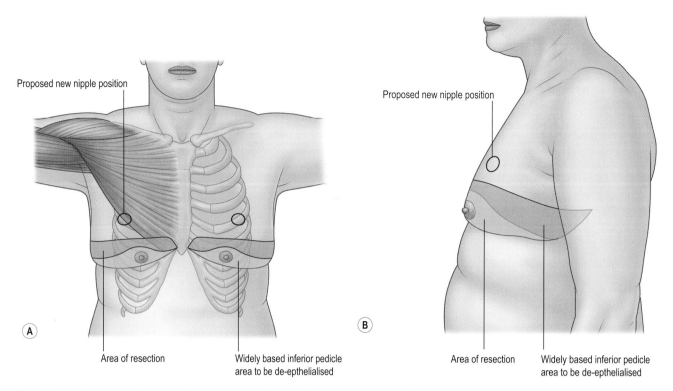

Fig. 24.7 Pseudogynecomastia after massive weight loss: excision with dermoglandular pedicle. **(A)** Markings – Anterior. The inferior margin of resection is along the existing inframammary fold. The nipple areola complex is elevated on a widely based dermoglandular pedicle. The final nipple position is determined with inferior pull on the chest wall. The intersection of the 5th rib and the lateral border of the pectoralis major muscle is the projected nipple location. **(B)** Markings – Lateral. An elliptical excision of excess skin and soft tissue is marked extending laterally to encompass the commonly found lateral thoracic roll.

the fourth or fifth rib and the lateral border of the pectoralis muscle. The superior anchor line of resection is marked corresponding to a distance of 4–5 cm inferior to the proposed nipple position. This line will determine the ultimate position of the new inframammary fold and is extended laterally, curving slightly superiorly to correct lateral chest wall laxity. The inframammary fold is marked extending laterally to meet the lateral extent of the superior resection line. A pinch test confirms acceptable tension on closure. Care must be taken to identify excessive mobility of the chest wall tissues and take into account postoperative descent of the new fold level.

Treatment/surgical technique

The wide, inferiorly based pedicle is first incised and de-epithelialized. Nipple reduction is made, using the plunger of a 20 cc syringe as a guide (estimated diameter of 23 mm). The nipple areola complex is elevated on a thin (1 cm, slightly wider at base to retain

perforators from chest wall), inferiorly-based dermoglandular pedicle. The pedicle base should be kept as wide as possible (at least 10 cm). Soft tissues deep to this flap are excised.

Superior to the excision, the skin-parenchymal flap is elevated superficial to pectoralis major fascia to the level of the clavicles. The superior flap is then pulled inferiorly to simulate closure and the superior resection line is checked for closure and resection is performed, continuing to include the lateral chest wall redundancy. The dermis of the pedicle is released with electrocautery for easier inset. The dermoglandular pedicle is then tucked under the superior flap and closure is performed, first of the SFS with absorbable sutures, followed by deep dermal and subcuticular sutures. Drains are placed bilaterally *(Fig. 24.8)*.

The nipple position is determined at the intersection of a horizontal line from the 5th rib to the lateral border of the pectoralis muscle. A 2 cm diameter areola cut-out should be made at this location; the areola spreads under tension to the correct diameter. A 10 cc syringe

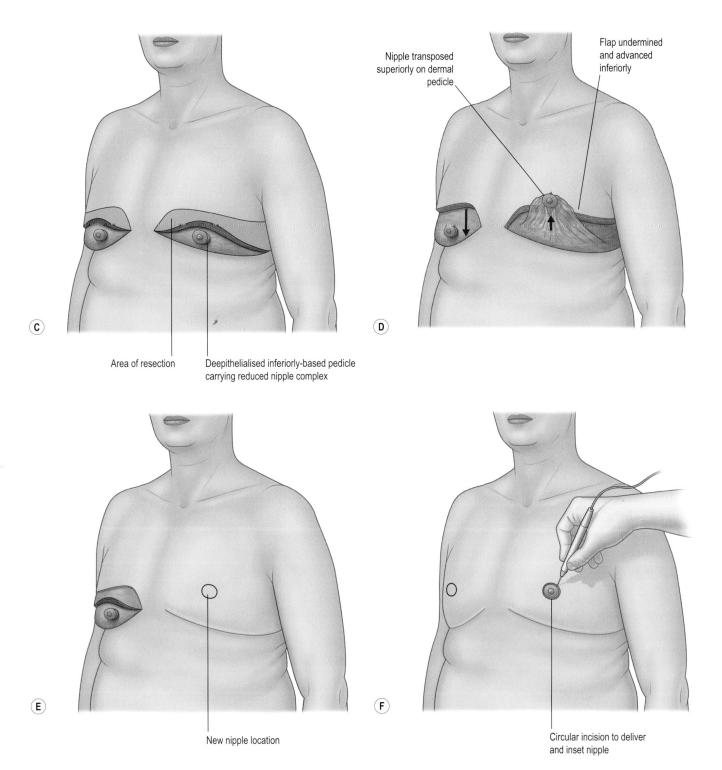

C Area of resection   Deepithelialised inferiorly-based pedicle carrying reduced nipple complex

D Nipple transposed superiorly on dermal pedicle   Flap undermined and advanced inferiorly

E New nipple location

F Circular incision to deliver and inset nipple

Fig. 24.7, cont'd **(C)** The inferiorly based dermoglandular pedicle is de-epithelialized and elevated to be approximately 1–1.5 cm thick. The tissues deep to the pedicle are excised. The superior redundancy is excised down to chest wall. **(D)** The superior and inferior edges of the resultant wound are approximated with towel clips. The de-epithelialized flap carrying the nipple areola complex is tucked under the superiorly based chest wall flap. The dermis of the pedicle may require scoring to create a sufficient edge for suturing. Braided, absorbable 2-0 sutures are used to approximate the flaps. **(E)** The new nipple location is re-checked at the intersection of the 5th rib and the lateral border of the pectoralis major muscle. The site is incised and intervening tissue removed. The nipple is brought through the new window. **(F)** Release of the periareolar dermis of the dermoglandular pedicle may be required for ease of inset.

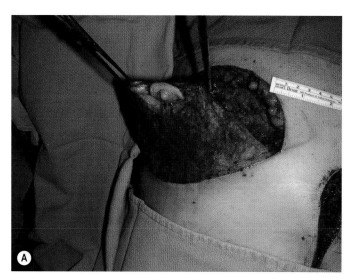
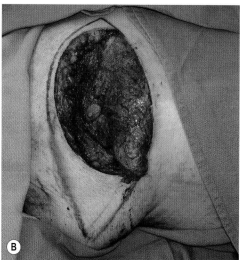

Fig. 24.8 Excisional gynecomastia with elevation of the nipple areola complex on a dermoglandular pedicle: technique. **(A)** Intraoperative view. Note elevation of the nipple areola complex on a thin inferiorly based dermoglandular pedicle. The pedicle retains a broad attachment to the chest wall. **(B)** Intraoperative view. The elliptical excision is marked and extends laterally to encompass the lateral thoracic roll. Undermining just superficial to pectoralis major fascia is performed superiorly. The dermoglandular pedicle slides under the superior chest wall flap and the nipple areola complex is delivered through a circular incision at its proposed new location. (Reprinted with permission from: Gusenoff, JA, Coon D, Rubin, JP. Pseudogynecomastia after Massive Weight Loss: Detectability of Technique, Patient Satisfaction, and Classification. *Plast Reconstr Surg.* 2008:122(5):1301–1311.)

plunger is the ideal marker for this. Care is taken to ensure a distance of 4–5 cm between the new nipple position and the position of the new inframammary fold for best aesthetics. The nipple is delivered through the window *(Figs 24.9 and 24.10)*.

The dermal layer is closed and skin glue used in substitution of subcuticular sutures. Of note, in cases that also incorporate an element of true gynecomastia, histologic analysis is recommended as atypical cellular pathology is revealed in 3%.[88]

Hints and tips

Excision of gynecomastia with nipple repositioning utilizing dermoglandular flap

- Nipple position is important. If medialized, the nipple needs to be repositioned laterally as well as superiorly. A common pitfall is placing the nipple too high or too medially.
- In the MWL patient, the areola usually requires reduction in diameter if stretched.
- When creating the dermoglandular flap that carried the nipple areola complex, the flap must be kept thin (1–1.5 cm), while maintaining a base of at least 10 cm.
- A distance of 4–5 cm should be maintained between the inferior edge of the new areola and the proposed inframammary fold scar (chest wall incision) for best appearance.

Hints and tips

Gynecomastia and male chest contouring after MWL

- Male breast enlargement may be due to true gynecomastia, pseudogynecomastia, or a combination of both. In cases of true gynecomastia, etiology must be examined and a high clinical suspicion for pathological processes maintained.
- Changes in the male chest following MWL may include skin and soft tissue redundancy, deflation, descent of the lateral inframammary crease, lateral chest wall rolls, nipple descent and medialization, areolar enlargement, and pseudogynecomastia.
- Selection of surgical technique must take into account the relative excesses of skin, fat and glandular tissue, nipple position, patient and surgeon preference, as well as the willingness of the patient to accept surgical scars in exchange for better chest contour in more severe cases.
- Large distances of repositioning of the nipple areola complex in patients with more severe deformity may be accomplished through elevation on a dermoglandular pedicle or by free nipple grafting.

Postoperative care

ACE compressive chest wrap is placed and left intact until the first follow-up visit. Drains are commonly removed at this time, when drainage is <30 cc over a 24-h period. An elastic compression garment is suggested following this.

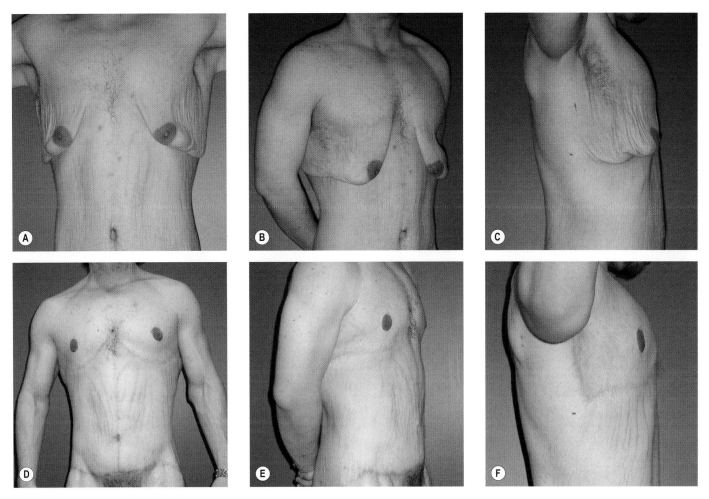

Fig. 24.9 Excisional gynecomastia with elevation of the nipple areola complex on a dermoglandular pedicle. A 26-year-old male s/p gastric bypass with 250 lb weight loss. **(A–C)** Preoperative views with markings. **(D–F)** Postoperative views at 1 year following excisional gynecomastia with elevation of the nipple areola complex on a dermoglandular pedicle, fleur-de-lis component of abdominoplasty, and medial vertical thigh lift as a second stage. The first stage was performed 5 months earlier than the second and involved a lower bodylift, panniculectomy, and brachioplasty. Note the marked improvement in chest contour with good positioning of the nipple areola complex as well as placement of the chest scars at the location of the visual inframammary fold. (Reprinted with permission from: Gusenoff, JA, Coon D, Rubin, JP. Pseudogynecomastia after Massive Weight Loss: Detectability of Technique, Patient Satisfaction, and Classification. *Plastic Reconstr Surg.* 2008;122(5):1301–1311.)

Outcomes, prognosis, and complications

As with many other body contouring procedures, wound healing problems, hematoma, seroma, and infection are all possibilities with excisional gynecomastia procedures. Other complications include: nipple loss, asymmetries, poor scarring, poor nipple position, areolar distortion (including size, shape, position), and under-resection. As the flap delivering the NAC must be significantly thinned, active smoking is considered a relative contraindication for this procedure.

Secondary procedures in upper body contouring

As seen with other body contouring procedures following MWL, recurrence of varying amounts of skin laxity may occur. Secondary procedures, including further small skin resections for improved contour may be undertaken, depending on the extent, as an office procedure, or in the operating room. In patients that have pre-existing poor skin elasticity, loosening is expected.

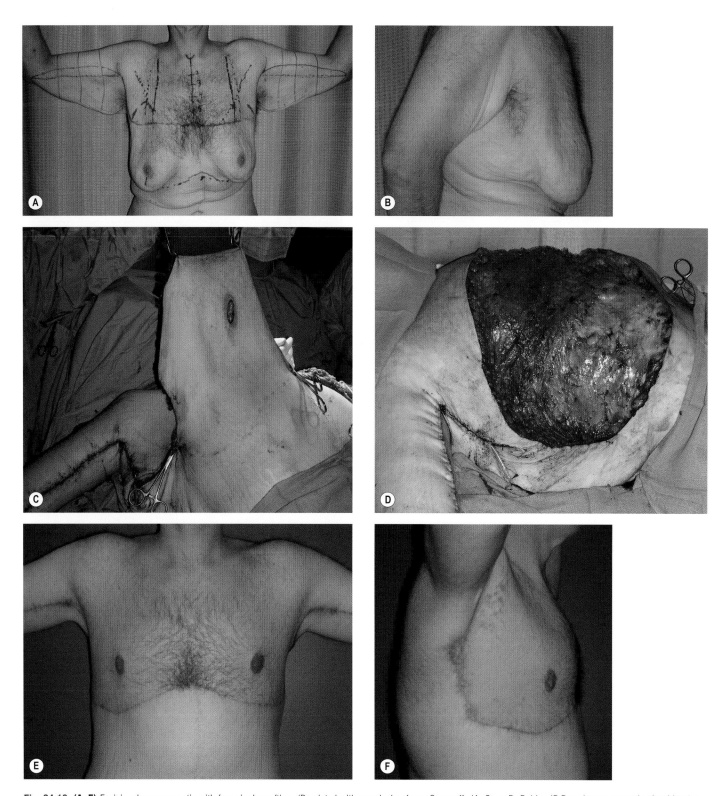

Fig. 24.10 (A–F) Excisional gynecomastia with free nipple grafting. (Reprinted with permission from: Gusenoff, JA, Coon D, Rubin, JP. Pseudogynecomastia after Massive Weight Loss: Detectability of Technique, Patient Satisfaction, and Classification. *Plastic Reconstr Surg.* 2008;122(5):1301–1311.)

Access the complete references list online at **http://www.expertconsult.com**

14. Appelt EA, Janis JE, Rohrich RJ. An algorithmic approach to upper arm contouring. *Plast Reconstr Surg.* 2006;118(1):237–246.

    An algorithmic approach to contouring the upper arm is presented with emphasis on deformities following massive weight loss. The degrees of excess of skin, skin elasticity, and relative volume of excess adiposity are considered.

21. Knoetgen J 3rd, Moran SL. Long-term outcomes and complications associated with brachioplasty: a retrospective review and cadaveric study. *Plast Reconstr Surg.* 2006;117(7):2219–2223.

    Long-term outcomes and complications of brachioplasty are presented, demonstrating a low incidence of major complications. Cadaveric study of the medial antebrachial cutaneous nerve revealed the structure penetrates the deep fascia of the forearm at 14 cm proximal to the medial epicondyle, although individual variations exist.

29. Aly A, Soliman S, Cram A. Brachioplasty in the massive weight loss patient. *Clin Plast Surg.* 2008;35(1):141–149.

35. Rubin JP. Mastopexy after massive weight loss: dermal suspension and total parenchymal reshaping. *Aesthet Surg J.* 2006;26(2):214–222.

    A safe and reproducible breast shaping technique based on the principles of dermal suspension and parenchymal reshaping are presented in the setting of the characteristic breast deformities seen following massive weight loss.

53. Colwell AS, Driscoll D, Breuing KH. Mastopexy techniques after massive weight loss: an algorithmic approach and review of the literature. *Ann Plast Surg.* 2009;63(1):28–33.

54. Rubin JP, Gusenoff JA, Coon D. Dermal suspension and parenchymal reshaping mastopexy after massive weight loss: statistical analysis with concomitant procedures from a prospective registry. *Plast Reconstr Surg.* 2009;123(3):782–789.

57. Soliman S, Rotemberg SC, Pace D, et al. Upper body lift. *Clin Plast Surg.* 2008;35(1):107–121.

    A review of techniques utilized to contour the back area following massive weight loss is presented and the differences between male and female patients is highlighted.

58. Shermak MA. Management of back rolls. *Aesthet Surg J.* 2008;28(3):348–356.

76. Gusenoff JA, Coon D, Rubin JP. Pseudogynecomastia after massive weight loss: detectability of technique, patient satisfaction, and classification. *Plast Reconstr Surg.* 2008;122(5):1301–1311.

    Male patients undergoing chest contouring procedures for deformities following massive weight loss are examined to determine satisfaction, and a classification scale is described. The technique of chest contouring with preservation of the nipple areola complex on a dermoglandular pedicle is discussed.

25

Fat grafting to the breast

Henry Wilson and Scott L. Spear

SYNOPSIS

- Autologous fat is a reconstructive workhorse when it comes to correcting mild to moderate contour deformities in reconstructed breasts.
- Fat grafting may be used safely for a variety of reconstructive indications. A variety of specific harvesting and processing techniques are available that are effective and techniques continue to evolve.
- Fat grafting for breast augmentation is effective, but its precise role in the cosmetic plastic surgeon's armamentarium is yet to be defined.
- Fat grafting to the breast is very effective at correcting commonly-encountered contour deformities.
- Fat grafting to the breast is becoming more accepted by mainstream practitioners as familiarity increases with techniques and potential complications, but it remains controversial for some indications
- Complications are minor and infrequent if a proper technique is followed.
- External pre-expansion and adipose-derived stem cells hold promise for future enhancement of the results and treatment of difficult problems.

 Access the Historical Perspective section online at
http://www.expertconsult.com

Introduction

Autologous fat grafting to the female breast has a long history surrounded by a great deal of controversy but relatively little scientific data, until recently.[1-10] Despite the paucity of high-quality published evidence and continued disagreement about the best technique, autologous lipofilling to the female breast will continue to evolve because it makes sense and it works! Like many fundamentally good ideas in plastic surgery, the concept is elegant in its simplicity: fat is removed from a location where it is not needed and used to augment body contour in an area of need or desire. To be compelling for the average practitioner, the procedure must have a reliable technique and not subject either the donor or recipient site to unacceptable risk.

This chapter will examine the current use of autologous fat grafting of the breast for a variety of indications, including filling contour irregularities and supplementing other forms of breast reconstruction after mastectomy in both the radiated and nonradiated breast. Another indication is correcting divots and other contour deficits after breast conservation therapy which included radiation treatment. Autologous fat has been used for reconstruction of the entire breast after mastectomy without requiring either an implant or a flap.[11] Fat grafting has also been described for correcting congenital anomalies of the breast such as Poland syndrome, pectus excavatum, and thoracic hypoplasia. Similarly, autologous fat can be used to correct acquired deformities of the breast other than after cancer treatment, such as might occur after previous implants or other breast surgery. The chapter concludes with an analysis of the controversy surrounding the use of autologous fat grafts for primary breast augmentation.[2,7,12–16]

Of the indications listed above, some are more widely accepted than others. The issues involving all of these applications are: cost, efficacy, acute surgical risk, interference with the diagnosis and treatment of breast cancer, and the remote possibility of increasing the risk of neoplasia. Fat grafting as a supplement to other forms of breast reconstruction after mastectomy is the most well accepted application because of its excellent risk profile, its wide adoption by many surgeons, and the absence of negative reports.

In 2005, we reported on the use of autologous fat grafting to correct contour deformities in the reconstructed breasts of 37 patients.[1] Most of the 47 treated breasts (85%) experienced worthwhile improvement from the procedure, and only 8.5% of the treated breasts experienced a significant complication (one cellulitis and three cases of fat necrosis). Based on these results, we recommended fat injection as a "safe and effective tool for improving the cosmetic result of either autologous or implant breast reconstruction".

More recently, other retrospective reviews have found similarly good results and low complication rates. In a 2007 retrospective review by Missana et al.,[3] of 74 reconstructed breasts treated with fat grafting, the authors found good–excellent results in 86.5% and moderately–good results in an additional 13.5%. Their only complications were five cases of fat necrosis. In 2009, Kanchwala et al.[6] reported on fat grafting to 110 breast reconstruction patients, finding good–excellent results in 85% and reporting no complications other than "minor contour irregularities." Reporting in 2009 on 880 patients treated over 10 years for a variety of reconstructive and cosmetic breast concerns, Delay et al.[7] noted good–excellent results in the vast majority of patients with complications, including a 3% rate of fat necrosis and less than 1% infection. None of these review articles found any correlation of fat grafting with the development of a new or recurrent breast cancer, and mammographic abnormalities were confined to calcifications that were easy for experienced radiologists to distinguish from neoplastic patterns of calcification.

An understanding of the effective use of fat grafting in principle is fundamental to the use of fat grafting for any indication. For this reason, this chapter will include a detailed discussion of the treatment of generic contour deformities of the breast for which fat grafting is indicated. Contour deformities after reconstructive breast surgery for mastectomy are relatively common, and autologous fat has become a workhorse to correct them because of its relative simplicity, low cost, and lasting results.[1,2,7] We advise the surgeon to achieve success at fat grafting for these indications, prior to considering its use in the more controversial areas of lumpectomy deformities or cosmetic augmentation.

Basic science/disease process

Adipocytes are fragile. Unlike skin, muscle or bone, fat lacks unit cohesion, which is perhaps why many early practitioners used dermal fat grafts. When fat is left attached to its overlying dermis, it is easier to work with since it can be sutured into the desired location. Oxygen diffusion prior to revascularization remains a problem, however, so such grafts must be small and are best suited to craniofacial applications where the defects are small and the vascularity is high.

Autologous fat grafting with aspirated fat uses fat in a liquid form, which permits it to be harvested and deployed with minimal incisions. It also permits its injection in precise quantities into precisely the area it is needed, at least in theory. From the procurement at the donor site to deposition in the grafted area, there are several steps in processing that must be executed successfully. Each step introduces the potential for adipocyte trauma and technical error, so attention to technique is of paramount importance.

Stem cells and radiation deformities

Adipose-derived stem cells (ADSCs) were first described in the 1920s, with early research focusing on which cells survived transplantation and became new host fat cells, which helped to characterize the process and improve the survival of fat grafts. More recently, the regenerative qualities of adipose-derived stem cells on damaged tissue were found, and they have potentially dramatic treatment implications for patients with radiation-induced injury.[20] As radiation is increasingly being used in the breast for aggressive indications, the average practitioner can be expected to encounter more and more of these deformities.

Radiation deformities are some of the most challenging problems the reconstructive breast surgeon encounters. Radiation-damaged breast tissue has a reduction of its capillary bed and is relatively hypoxic. The clinical picture is one of acute injury (radiodermatitis), followed by subcutaneous fibrosis and skin hyperpigmentation. There is substantial variability as to the extent to which an individual patient will exhibit these effects and their resolution over time. Common presenting problems after radiation include: generalized fibrosis; scar retraction at lumpectomy defects; capsular contracture around prosthetic devices, and persistent skin hyperpigmentation. Uncommonly, radionecrosis occurs, resulting in a chronic wound.

Traditionally, little in the reconstructive armamentarium has been able to address the primary problem of tissue damage. Solutions have been centered around replacement techniques: flaps to replace a retracted lumpectomy defect or eliminate an implant with surrounding capsular contracture. The promise of adipose-derived stem cells lies in their ability to reverse the fibrotic changes of radiation damage.[20] The future may bring more comprehensive solutions to breast reconstruction, such as ADSC-seeded biomaterial constructs[10] and fat grafting, combined with negative pressure external soft-tissue expansion.[11] Presently, the use of fat grafting augmented with expanded populations of ADSCs is limited to research institutions, but fat grafts harvested and processed with the traditional techniques may contain some stem cells.

Diagnosis/patient presentation

Patients present with contour deformities occurring after previous reconstructive or cosmetic breast surgery. Alternatively, a patient may request primary augmentation for hypomastia or congenital asymmetries such as tuberous breast or Poland syndrome. A potentially large patient population who may be served in the future is the post-mastectomy patient seeking total primary reconstruction with fat grafting.

Patient selection

Autologous fat grafting is indicated to restore normal contour in an area of deformity. These deformities occur commonly in breasts reconstructed with flaps or implants and also occur as undesirable sequelae of implants placed for cosmetic breast augmentation (*Table 25.1*). There follows a discussion on specific indications, with examples of each.

Contour deformity after implant reconstruction

With implant reconstructions, thin overlying tissue can lead to sharp implant borders (*Fig. 25.1*) and visible rippling (*Fig. 25.2*), both of which can be effectively softened by fat grafting. These patients are often slender with relatively little subcutaneous fat, or are patients whose mastectomy flaps were left very thin by the breast surgeon. If the implant is very mobile in a large pocket, an unnatural "trench" can form at the interface between the implant and the chest wall. This may be further accentuated medially by lateral shift of the implant when the patient is supine. Such deformities may require a combination of implant exchange to different size, capsulorrhaphy, capsular reinforcement

Table 25.1 Specific indications for fat grafting

Established indications: safe and effective	Effective and probably safe[a]	Safe but not yet proven
Flap border step-off	Deformity after lumpectomy and radiation	Primary reconstruction as the sole method[c]
Depression from fat necrosis		
Irregularities in mastectomy flap thickness	Cosmetic augmentation[b]	
Augmentation for inadequate flap volume	Augmentation deformities (rippling, visible deformities)	
Radiation deformity in flap reconstruction		
Sharp implant border (reconstruction)		
Implant rippling (reconstruction)		

[a]Detailed informed consent and IRB approval required. [b]Being evaluated in clinical trials.[11,21,22] [c]Being evaluated in clinical trials.[11]

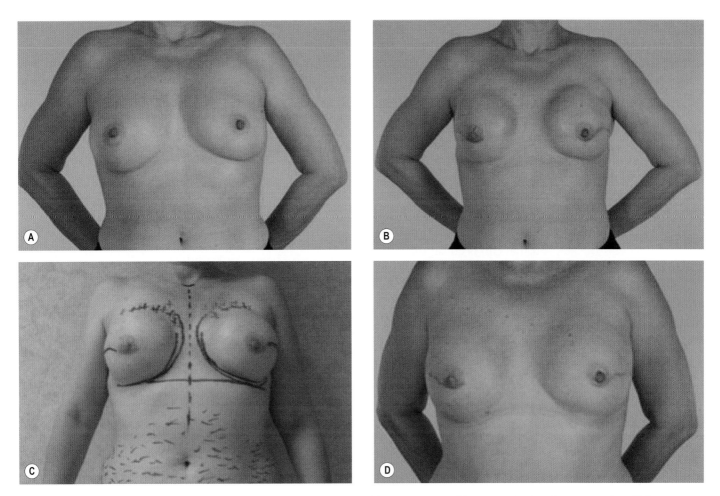

Fig. 25.1 A 55-year-old patient who underwent bilateral nipple-sparing mastectomies. **(A)** Preoperative view **(B)** postoperative view after reconstruction with tissue expanders and acellular dermal matrix illustrates typical marginal contour deformities surrounding a prosthetic device. Preoperative markings **(C)** and 3-month postoperative result **(D)** for fat grafting to margins with exchange of tissue expanders for permanent implants.

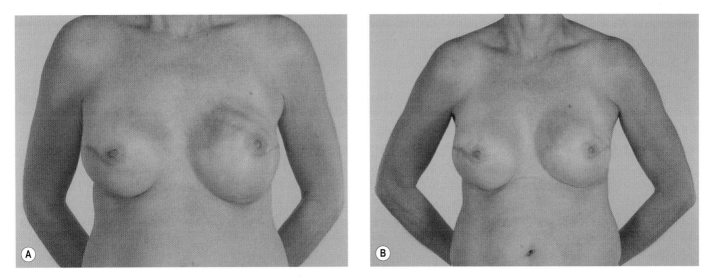

Fig. 25.2 (A) Bilateral implant reconstructions with visible implant borders superiorly on both sides and substantial rippling on the left. **(B)** 6-month postoperative results after fat grafting superior poles bilaterally (80 cc right, 50 cc left) and left inferior capsulorrhaphy. Note softening of implant contour bilaterally and resolution of visible rippling on the left.

with acellular dermal matrix, and fat grafting (see *Fig. 25.4*). These deformities are also encountered in the slender cosmetic patient, especially when implants are placed in the subglandular plane.

Contour deformity after flap reconstruction

In the case of flap reconstruction, the border of the flap is a common location for a depression, often occurring as a "step-off" where the flap ends and the normal residual tissue begins.[6] Characteristically, this deformity consists of skin flap directly over the chest wall muscle or bone, and reflects the step-off that can occur at the edge of a flap where it is inset to fill a mastectomy defect or from fat necrosis at the vulnerable edges of the reconstructive tissue *(Figs 25.3, 25.4)*. Deformities intrinsic to the flap, such as areas of fat necrosis within the substance of the flap or the periumbilical tissue in a TRAM, are also common indications and may occur within the flap substance or at the borders.

Contour deformities after implant or flap reconstructions in a radiated field

Suitable patients with radiation damage have a breast contour deformity secondary to implant or flap reconstruction after mastectomy, exacerbated by radiation changes such as those described in the radiation section above. These deformities may have components of the above step-off or intrinsic flap deformities, in addition to the tissue fibrosis, skin changes, or capsular contracture brought about by radiation *(Figs 25.5, 25.6)*. The complications of flap reconstructions that are the most difficult to correct tend to occur when the reconstruction was performed prior to the radiation.[23] These include volume loss, fat necrosis, delayed wound healing, and fibrosis. While the experience with fat grafting as an adjunct to other breast reconstructions has been largely favorable, the evidence is unclear and unconvincing, when looking specifically at the radiated breast. Radiation introduces added risks, complexities, and problems. The risks include an increased risk of infection and of nonhealing of the surgical site. The complexities include the difficulty of creating space for the fat in a badly radiation-fibrosed recipient site, and the problems are the lack of both skin elasticity

and a fertile recipient site conducive for the fat grafts to take.

A review of the literature indicates that experience with fat grafting in the radiated environment has only recently been addressed. The 2007 publication by Rigotti et al. details some cases showing dramatic improvements to both capsular contracture and impending implant exposure as a result of stem-cell enhanced autologous fat grafting.[20] In 2009, Delay et al. reported that fat grafting can improve the quality of radiation-damaged post-mastectomy skin contributing to an autologous reconstruction or permitting an implant reconstruction to be used where it may have previously been contraindicated.[7] Serra-Renom et al. reported an innovative approach to the reconstruction of radiated mastectomy defects in 2009.[24] The authors reported on 65 patients, whom they reconstructed in three stages: tissue expander placement, expander exchange for permanent implant, and nipple reconstruction. At each stage, an average of 150 cc of autologous fat was grafted to enhance the volume of the reconstruction. The authors report excellent results, with no capsular contracture or other complications. They conclude that fat grafting enhanced the reconstruction by improving the skin quality and adding subcutaneous volume to the breasts.

Lumpectomy deformities

Lumpectomy deformities of up to 10–15% of the breast volume often result in satisfactory aesthetic results.[25] The actual resected percentage, however, may often be higher with re-excisions or a desire to avoid mastectomy on the part of the patient or breast surgeon. Although oncoplastic techniques may result in very good symmetry if performed at the time of lumpectomy, they are not universally utilized or available. Accordingly, lumpectomy with radiation results in suboptimal aesthetic outcomes of up to 30% *(Fig. 25.7)*.[26] The idea of fat grafting these lumpectomy defects is very appealing because no other techniques are appropriate for most of these patients and what is missing is usually all or in part fat. Implants perform badly in a radiated environment, and flaps are often best reserved for total or sub-total mastectomy defects. The problems and challenges however, are similar as for

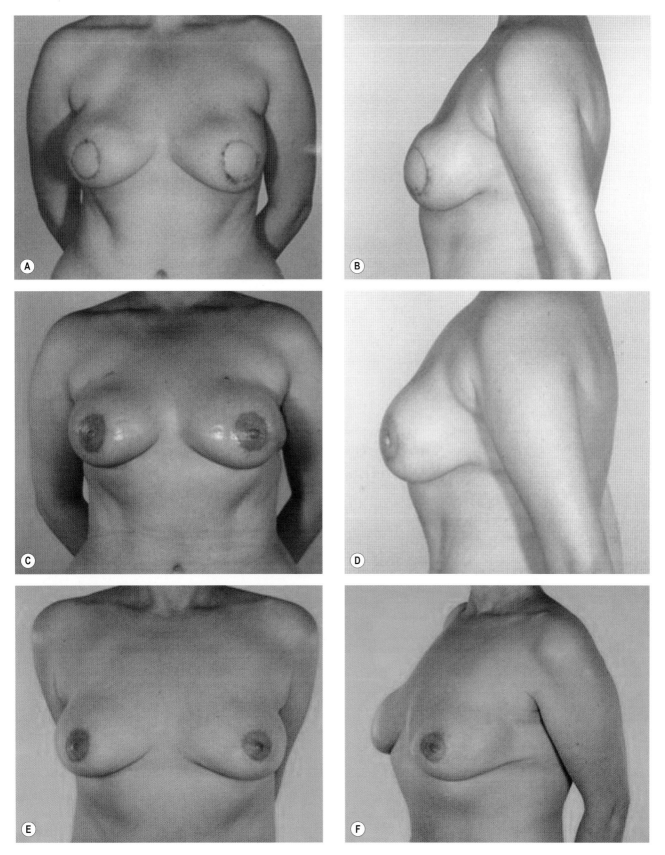

Fig. 25.3 (A,B) A 45-year-old patient with flap step-off deformities after bilateral immediate breast reconstruction with pedicled TRAM flaps. **(C,D)** 11 months after bilateral nipple reconstruction with 120 cc of fat grafting to each superior pole. **(E,F)** The same patient 7 years after fat grafting to flap step-off deformities of the superior poles bilaterally.

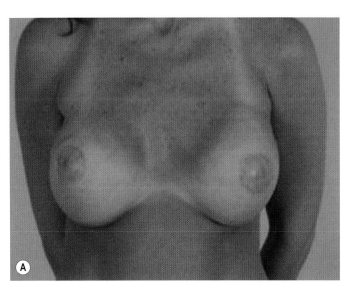
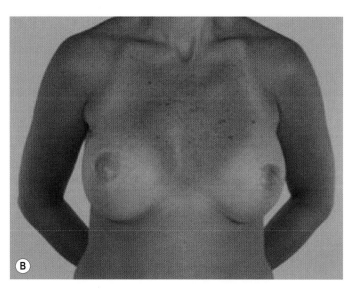

Fig. 25.4 A 33-year-old patient after with bilateral step-off deformities (most pronounced on the left) treated by fat injection. **(A)** Preoperative view 2 years after bilateral breast reconstruction with latissimus flaps and implants. **(B)** The same patient 3 years after autologous fat grafting of 170 cc to the left upper pole and 50 cc to the right upper pole.

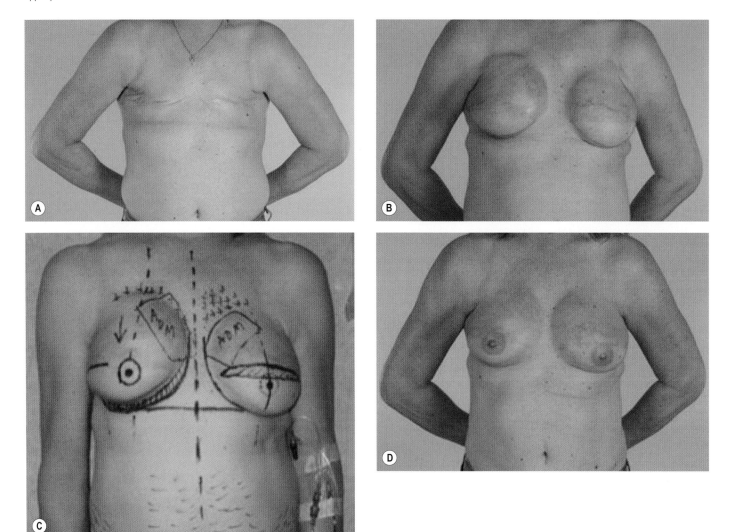

Fig. 25.5 A 51-year-old patient with history of bilateral modified radical mastectomies with postoperative radiation after each mastectomy. **(A)** Photograph shows patient preoperatively, and **(B)** 3 months after bilateral reconstruction with latissimus flaps and tissue expanders. **(C)** Preoperative view prior to bilateral exchange of expanders for implants, nipple reconstructions, and treatment of bilateral upper pole contour deformities with fat grafting and acellular dermal matrix. **(D)** 5 months after the operation.

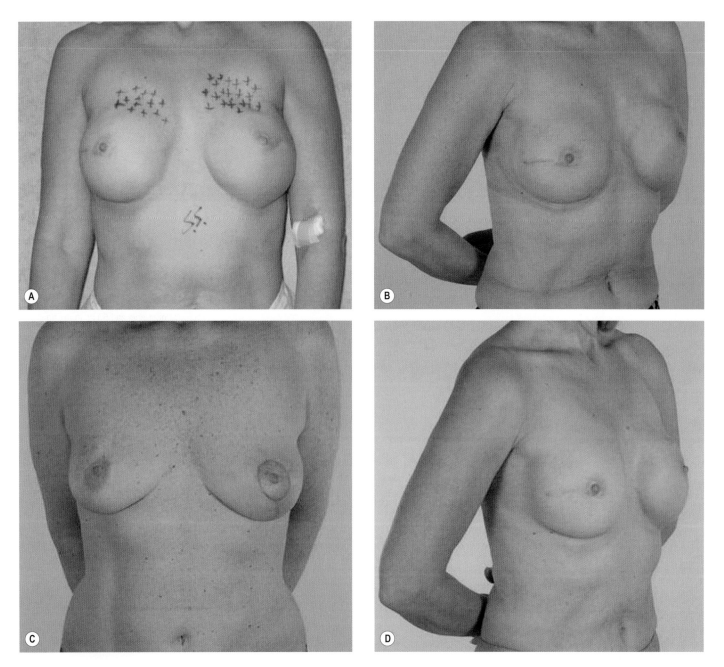

Fig. 25.6 A 55-year-old patient with a history of left breast lumpectomy and radiation 2 years prior to bilateral nipple-sparing mastectomies and subsequent tissue expander and implant reconstruction. Bilateral upper pole contour deformities **(A,B)** were treated with 35 cc right and 85 cc autologous fat injection. **(C,D)** 1 year postoperatively.

radiation after mastectomy. Fibrosis, risk of infection, and a hostile environment for grafts make the radiated lumpectomy defect an uncertain, unproven application. This is magnified by the heightened concern for monitoring and detecting local breast cancer recurrence in these patients.

There is little in the literature on lumpectomy deformities being reconstructed with autologous fat grafting. In his 2007 publication detailing the use of adipose-derived stem cells, Rigotti published impressive photographs of a patient whose radiated lumpectomy defect was dramatically improved by stem cell-enriched fat injection.[20] A 2009 report of experience by Delay et al. on 42 patients indicates that the fat grafting is valuable in the management of moderate deformities resulting from breast conservation.[7,27] The authors

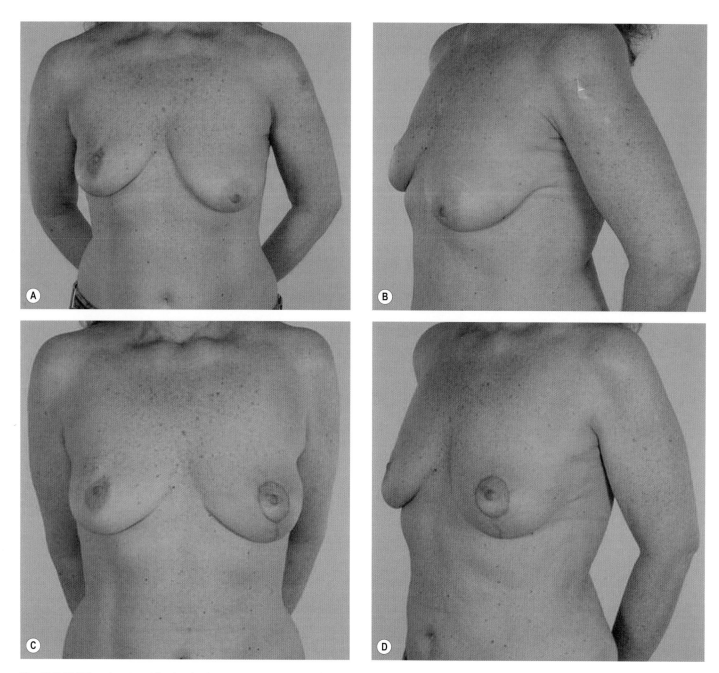

Fig. 25.7 Right breast contour deformity after breast conservation therapy. **(A,B)** Preoperative. **(C,D)** At 2 months postoperative, from fat grafting to right lumpectomy defect and left mastopexy. There has been a modest improvement in the right breast contour seen best on the oblique view.

caution that the medicolegal environment surrounding fat grafting for this indication is treacherous, however, and they use a very strict protocol involving detailed pre- and post-procedure imaging, specially trained radiologists, and management of the patient within a multidisciplinary team. Delay recommends completing the "learning curve" for fat grafting prior to using it to reconstruct radiated lumpectomy defects.[7]

Acquired breast deformities from trauma or surgery often occur in a setting without radiation damage. These patients may have problems beyond the scope of an implant correction but be unsuitable for a flap. Some may have had an implant and be unwilling to have another. For these patients fat grafting offers the possibility of an autologous correction with minimal morbidity.

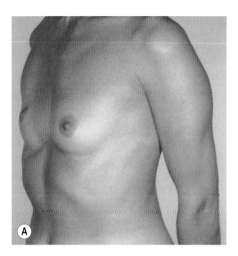 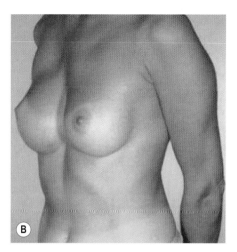 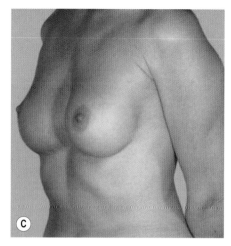

Fig. 25.8 (A) A patient with thoracic hypoplasia preoperatively. **(B)** A patient with thoracic hypoplasia after bilateral augmentation only. **(C)** 2 years after two separate procedures of fat injection to right upper pole (140 cc and 150 cc, 14 months apart).

Congenital deformities

Just as the FDA recognized that certain nonmastectomy problems were surgically comparable with those caused by cancer treatment, we recognize that some congenital and other acquired breast deformities can be and should be treated like those after mastectomy or breast conservation therapy. These include Poland syndrome, pectus excavatum, thoracic hypoplasia, tuberous breasts, and major asymmetries. Some of these patients can be treated in whole or in part by other techniques, but fat grafting brings an additional powerful tool to help solve the problem, often where nothing else is practical. This has been shown for the deformity associated with the tuberous breast.[2] It has also been demonstrated for chest wall deformities where the upper pole is beyond the reach of the implant.[1]

Poland syndrome results in absence of the pectoralis muscles and underdevelopment of the breast gland. Provided the latissimus is present, an excellent reconstructive solution involves a latissimus flap with placement of an implant.[28] Postoperative deformities in the infraclavicular hollow may occur and respond well to fat grafting. Other candidates for fat injection present with unsatisfactory reconstruction after breast implant alone, usually with contour deformities laterally accentuated by the absence of the pectoralis. The deformity resulting from Poland syndrome can also be entirely reconstructed with fat grafting,[7] but it typically requires multiple sessions of grafting.

Anterior thoracic hypoplasia is characterized by a normal pectoralis muscle and sternal position, but a unilaterally depressed chest wall with hypoplastic breast and superiorly-displaced nipple-areola complex.[29] Treatment is typically with implant alone, though residual deformities may occur and respond well to fat grafting *(Fig. 25.8)*.

Tuberous breast deformity features a constricting ring though which developing tissue herniates, resulting in an enlarged nipple-areola complex, narrow mammary base, elevation of the inframammary fold, and hypoplasia of one or more breast quadrants. Treatment depends on the presentation and may result in contour deformities that respond well to fat grafting. The tuberous breast has also been treated with fat grafting alone with impressive results.[2,7]

Primary breast augmentation

Perhaps most controversial is the use of autologous fat grafting for primary breast augmentation. While efficacy and safety are issues for all applications, here the issues are magnified. On the efficacy side, these patients are generally easily corrected with implants. With a high degree of reliability and certainty, a woman can enlarge her breast size by 200–500 cc (1 or 2 cup sizes) with a 1–2 h operation, with well known, well described, and definable risks. Regarding breast augmentation with lipofilling, however, the enlargement is less ambitious, less reliable and less certain. The authors generally describe to the patient that it is our hope and intent to increase the breast by ½ to 1 cup size. The result is clearly dependent on a number of things. The percentage of fat survival is key, but how to obtain that survival is still a work in progress. Defining the best candidate for lipo-breast augmentation is as important as the technique. Determining what type of fat to harvest, how to prepare it, where to inject it, and in what type of breast, are all important questions. Regarding safety, the questions are equally important. These women have not had breast cancer but they are at significant risk of developing breast cancer, resulting in concerns about radiographically obscuring or mimicking breast cancer. Of theoretical concern is the possibility of accelerating or inducing breast cancer in the younger at-risk women. Nevertheless, the concept of moving fat from less desirable areas such as the abdomen or thighs to more desirable areas such as a small breast is so seductive and compelling that it should be no surprise that academic-minded surgeons are studying it, entrepreneurial surgeons are marketing it, and many patients are very, very interested in it.

Safety issues apply for all of the noncancer uses of autologous fat, but they are most acute in the purely cosmetic patient. For her, the indications for correction are so elective, the other options so good, and the risk of disturbance of her normal, healthy baseline are much greater than, e.g., the previously treated cancer patient. We have had a modest experience in primary breast augmentation with fat, most of it in a funded, IRB-approved, controlled clinical trial.[21] Our experience prior to the trial in a handful of patients was mixed, with some having visually significant breast enhancement of up to 1 cup size *(Figs 25.9, 25.10)*. Others had no discernible long-term benefit, despite several hours of hard work of obtaining, processing, and infiltrating the fat in front of and behind the breast parenchyma in several different planes *(Fig. 25.11)*.

In a retrospective review published in 2007, Zheng et al. followed 66 Chinese patients treated with fat grafting for breast augmentation for an average of 37 months.[13] Fat grafts were harvested using 3 mm cannulas attached to a vacuum pump set to low negative pressure (−0.5 atm), washed with normal saline and spun in a centrifuge at 600 rpm (26 g) for 2 min to isolate the middle layer, which was used as graft. Graft injection was performed with a one-holed 3 mm cannula

through two injection sites (periareolar and inframammary), with an average of 174 mL of fat injected into each breast (101 mL subcutaneous, 73 mL subglandular). A total of 28 patients had one treatment; 21 patients were treated twice and 17 patients three times. Results were judged by three independent plastic surgeons, who noted significant improvement in 28 patients (42.4%); improvement in 24 patients (36.4%); and no improvement in 14 patients (21.2%); 27 patients (40.9%) were very satisfied; 26 patients (39.4%) were satisfied; and 13 (19.7%) were unsatisfied with the results. The only complications noted were fat necrosis or cyst formation in 11 patients (16.7%), none of which interfered with the final contour of the breast.

In another study published in 2008 of purely cosmetic breast augmentation with fat injection, Yoshimura et al. treated 40 Japanese patients using a protocol designed to increase the percentage of adipose-derived stem cells (ADSCs) in the grafted fat.[14] Adipose tissue was harvested using a 2.5 mm (inner) diameter cannula and conventional liposuction machine, after which half of the harvested fat was either washed and placed upright (25% of patients) or centrifuged unwashed at 700 g for 3 min (75% of patients). The other half of the liposuction aspirate was used to isolate the stromal vascular fraction in order to combine it with the fat to be grafted, a 90 min procedure designed to enhance the population of ADSCs in the fat graft. Injection was performed with 150 mm long 18-gauge needles into one of four injection sites (two periareolar, two inframammary) to distribute fat "on, around and under the mammary glands and also into the pectoralis muscles." An average of 273 mL of fat was grafted into each breast during a procedure that required, on average, over four hours. Results were measured by increase in chest circumference, which was between 4 and 8 cm at 6 months, corresponding to a 100–200 mL increase in the volume of each breast mound or "two to three brassiere cup sizes". The authors state that "almost all" of the patients were satisfied with their enlarged breasts but did not quantify this and also did not have a separate panel to judge the results subjectively. MRI detected cysts in two patients and mammography found two patients with microcalcifications at 24 months.

In 2008, Zocchi and Zuliani reported on 181 patients for breast augmentation with fat grafting.[30] They injected processed fat into the retroglandular and periglandular

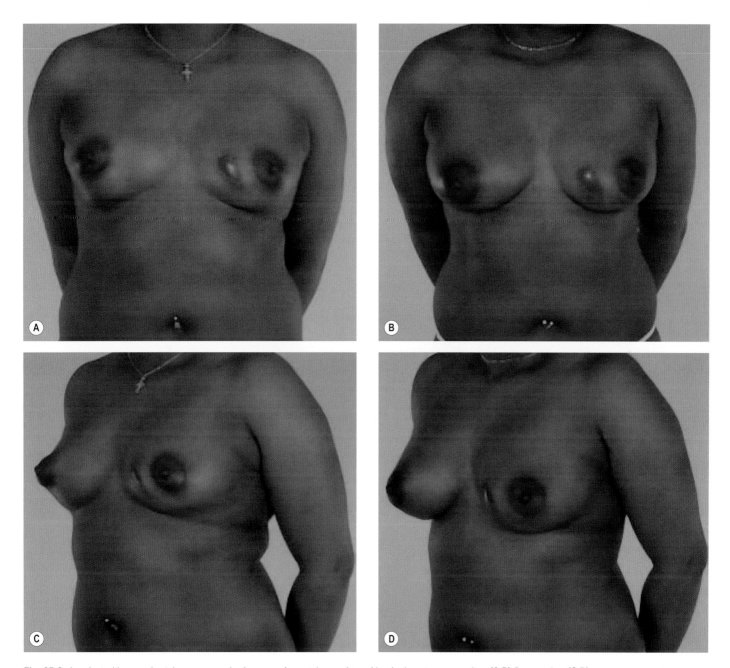

Fig. 25.9 A patient with approximately a one cup size increase after autologous fat grafting for breast augmentation. **(A,B)** Preoperative. **(C,D)** 1 year postoperative view after one session of 300 cc of fat grafting to each breast.

subcutaneous plane, using a disposable 2 mm cannula with a single hole for harvesting with negative pressure generated by a 60-mL syringe. Fat is "processed" only by vibration of the upright syringes on a special vibrating table to stratify the fat into layers. Fat is then reimplanted into the above planes using special 2 mm cannulas: a flexible 27 cm-long one for the retroglandular plane and a stiffer 25 cm-long one for the

subcutaneous plane. They injected an average of 325 mL or 375 mL of fat into each breast (two different numbers are reported in their article) and also utilized an external breast expansion device (BRAVA, Miami, FL) in some patients. The authors state that some patients did not comply with external expansion but do not reveal how many. Rating the aesthetic results, 38 patients (23%) judged them as excellent; 128 (72%) as good; 10 (6%)

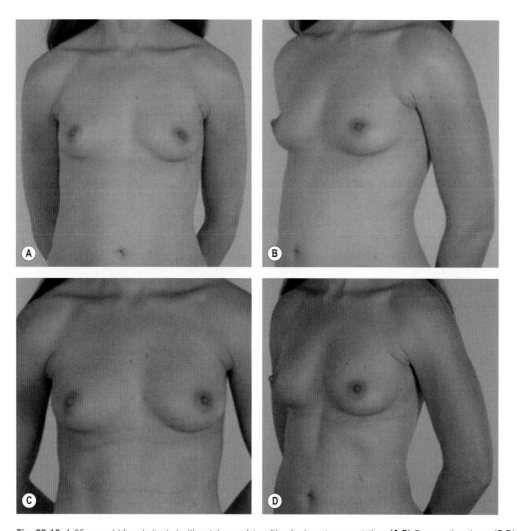

Fig. 25.10 A 35-year-old female treated with autologous fat grafting for breast augmentation. **(A,B)** Preoperative views. **(C,D)** 6-month postoperative views. A total of 280 cc on each side was used in the following locations: 50 cc to each pectoralis muscle, 100 cc in each subglandular plane, and 130 cc subcutaneously.

as fair; and five (3%) as insufficient. The surgeon judged them as excellent in 23 cases (13%); good in 123 (69%); fair in 25 (12%); and insufficient in 10 (6%). The authors state that an average of 55% of grafted volume persisted at 1 year but do not state how this was measured. Complications were not quantified, except to say they were "minimal and temporary" and that microcalcifications were found in some patients. While this study reports on a relatively large number of patients, it is mostly an informal report of cases.

With little quality data having been published on breast augmentation with fat grafting,[5] several clinical trials have been started in the United States to better study the issue. Autologous fat grafting for cosmetic augmentation is currently being performed under research protocols in Miami,[11] Washington, DC[21] and New Orleans.[22] Each is of prospective design featuring 3D photographic analysis preoperatively and postoperatively, and the patients will be followed for years to determine the long-term results and complications. The first results of the Miami study are being reported as this chapter is being written, and the results are encouraging.

Breast augmentation patients should not be at risk for breast cancer because of a strong family history, and it is preferred that they have no personal history of significant benign breast disease. They must also have sufficient donor sites to support at least two stages of fat harvest of several hundred cubic centimeters of fat during each session. Preoperative MRI is recommended as a baseline as well as a preoperative mammogram if the patient is aged 40 or over. Finally, a frank discussion

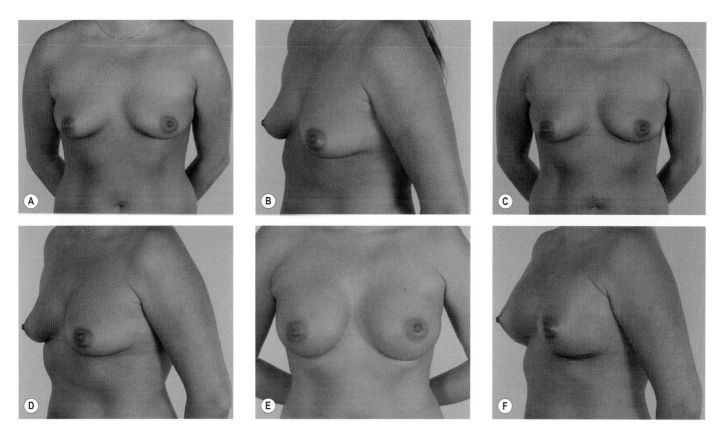

Fig. 25.11 (A) Preoperative anterior view of a patient who experienced essentially no discernible benefit from fat grafting for breast augmentation. **(B)** Preoperative oblique view. **(C)** Postoperative anterior view of the patient 1 year after 165 cc autologous fat grafting to each breast. **(D)** 1-year postoperative oblique view after grafting. **(E)** Anterior view of the patient 1 year postoperatively from bilateral prosthetic augmentation with 339 cc silicone implants. **(F)** 1-year postoperative oblique view after implants.

with the patient about potential implications of fat grafting for cancer screening must occur, and a detailed informed consent should be included. We recommend that the surgeons performing breast augmentation with autologous fat grafting do so under Institutional Review Board oversight.

If and when the issues of efficacy and safety have been settled, the other issues that remain are efficiency and practicality. If a breast augmentation with an implant can be done easily in 60–90 min at a cost of, e.g., US$4000, then a breast augmentation with autologous fat cannot take 6 h and still remain affordable for both the patient and the surgeon. This is especially the case if the reliability of graft-take remains uncertain.

Total breast reconstruction

For the most ardent advocates of fat grafting of the breast, the next great opportunity is reconstructing the entire breast with autologous fat injections. The authors have never personally done this, but total breast reconstruction for the patient with post-mastectomy or congenital absence of the breast is possible. Although there have been no formally published results on this, anecdotal cases have been reported at meetings and on websites by researchers involved in clinical trials.[11] Clearly, this requires a high level of commitment, motivation and expertise on the part of both the surgeon and the patient.

Treatment/surgical technique

The defect is analyzed, using as much information as is available, including preoperative photographs, the contralateral normal breast, the original operative note and pathology reports. The latter is especially valuable when reconstructing lumpectomy defects, since it typically contains a specimen weight, which can be used to plan the graft volume. Informed consent is obtained.

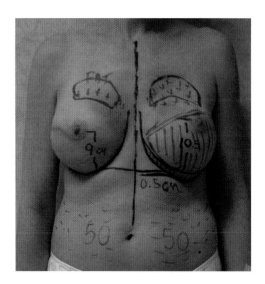

Fig. 25.12 Preoperative marking of the patient in *Figure 25.2*. Areas for autologous fat grafting are denoted by the blue outline with "+" signs superiorly on each breast. The patient has also been marked for the left capsulorrhaphy.

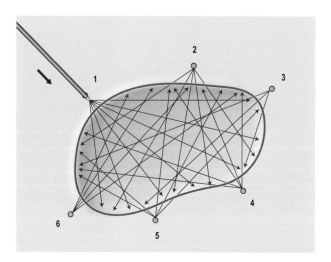

Fig. 25.13 Top view with defect borders marked with the bold line. Multiple criss-crossing tunnels across a typical small contour deformity, with six separate injection sites located at the periphery (1–6). Each tunnel may receive different amounts of graft along its length depending on the needs of the area and amounts already grafted by previous tunnels originating from other injection sites.

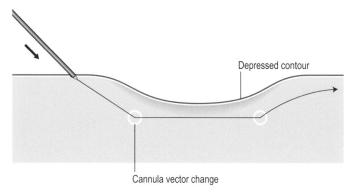

Fig. 25.14 This illustration depicts a typical contour depression viewed from the side, with the cannula positioned at the top left near the injection site. Note the changes in directional vector the cannula must undergo as it traverses the bottom of the defect concavity. These depend on a rigid cannula and sometimes releasing underlying tethering scar tissue.

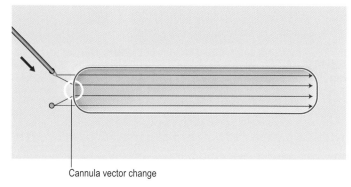

Fig. 25.15 Multiple longitudinal vectors used to treat longitudinal depressions (such as the edge of a flap or implant). Note vector change to permit multiple parallel treatment tunnels from a minimum of injection sites.

Estimates of volume to be grafted are made to assist with determining what volume to harvest from the donor site.

The patient is marked in the standing position (*Fig. 25.12*), when areas of contour irregularity can be most clearly seen because of shadows created by overhead lighting. This most important step ensures that areas noticeable while standing are not overlooked when the patient is supine with powerful surgical lights overhead that obscure shadows. The surgeon estimates the amount of fat needed for grafting and marks

appropriate donor sites. After fat harvest and processing per the surgeon's preference, grafting is performed in a manner appropriate to the deformity being treated. Depressions are treated with multiple tunnels in a cross-hatch fashion (*Figs 25.13, 25.14*), while ridges and rippling respond best to a few long tunnels below the longitudinal depression (*Fig. 25.15*). Depressed areas with substantial scarring from fat necrosis or radiation damage may benefit from scar release with specialized cannulas that have cutting edges (*Fig. 25.16*). Care must be exercised when using these instruments – their effect

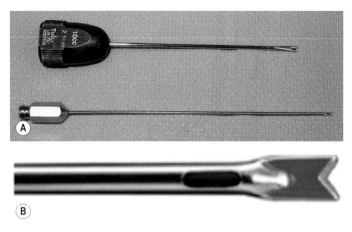

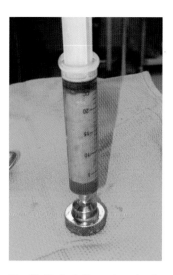

Fig. 25.16 V-shaped dissectors (©Tulip, Byron Medical, with permission).

Fig. 25.17 Aspiration syringe standing upright. Note aqueous layer below aspirated fat and oil layer above aspirated fat.

can be quite destructive to an implant and catastrophic near a flap pedicle.

Multiple locations are selected as graft insertion sites. This may be as few as 4–8 around a lumpectomy defect or as many as 20 for breast augmentation. A blunt-tipped cannula attached to a 3 mL syringe is used to inject small volumes of fat during the withdrawal phase of the cannula movement. The cannula is passed repeatedly in a radial pattern from each injection site, with the goal being an interwoven mesh pattern of graft deposition at multiple levels. For breast augmentation, it is important to attempt to stay within the subcutaneous plane and not within breast parenchyma during graft injection. Additional volume for augmentation may be grafted into the subglandular, intramuscular and submuscular planes. Minimal "molding" is performed externally; the emphasis should be on correct and even graft deposition during cannula withdrawal. When the goal volume is reached, the injection sites are closed with adhesive strips and conforming dressing applied to the breast.

Notes on harvesting and processing fat

Appropriate donor site selection includes any area that has sufficient fat to donate, typically the abdomen, hips and thighs. The site selected can be based on ease of harvest and patient preference, since no studies have demonstrated superiority of different sites in graft survival.[31]

Standard liposuction infiltration is performed with a dilute epinephrine-containing solution to minimize

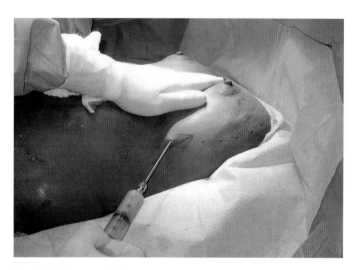

Fig. 25.18 Processed fat is grafted into the patient, in this case for breast augmentation.

blood loss. To harvest the fat, all that is needed is an appropriate cannula attached to a means of suction and a collection container. Most practitioners use a 3 mm multi-hole cannula to harvest fat intended for use in the breast. Next, the aspirated fat is refined by removing oil, blood and infiltrate fluid. The simplest method of this is to allow the aspiration syringe to stand for 10–15 min *(Fig. 25.17)*.[32] Finally, the processed fat is reinjected *(Fig. 25.18)* to the intended recipient site using a specialized injection cannula. Sydney Coleman, MD, was the earliest recent practitioner to codify and publish reliable

Fig. 25.19 Coleman aspiration cannula (©Byron Medical, with permission).

steps, so his method is detailed below, followed by alternative methods that have been used successfully by other practitioners.

Coleman's method

Coleman advocates using a cannula of his design, which has a blunt tip and two adjacent holes *(Fig. 25.19)*. This is connected to a 10 mL syringe to which modest suction is applied when the surgeon's ring and small fingers pull back on the plunger. As the cannula is pushed through the harvest site, a combination of the curetting action of the cannula and the negative pressure pulls fat into the syringe. When the syringe is full, it is disconnected from the cannula, capped at the Luer connector end with a sterile cap and the plunger is removed. The open end of the syringe may be covered with a Tegaderm (3M) to maintain sterility of syringe contents after plunger removal.[33] The syringe is placed into a sterile sleeve in a small centrifuge *(Fig. 25.20)*. Other syringes are added, and the centrifuge spins the contents at 3000 rpm for 3 minutes.

After centrifugation, the syringe contents have been separated by density. The upper level of oil (ruptured adipocytes from aspiration) is removed by pouring it off and then removing any remainder with absorbent wicks of Telfa (Kendall). The bottom, densest level contains blood as well as infiltrate and is removed by briefly removing the cap and allowing it to drain. Using a Luer-to-Luer connector *(Fig. 25.21)*, the prepared fat is transferred into 3-mL syringes ready for injection into the recipient site.

Alternative methods

Critics of Coleman's method point to the multiple small harvest syringes and two-hole cannula as unnecessarily time-consuming. Other practitioners therefore

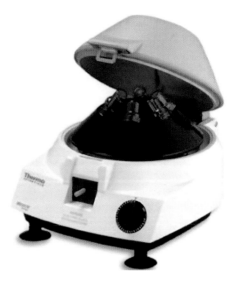

Fig. 25.20 Small centrifuge (Photo courtesy of Thermo Fisher Scientific, Inc. Reprinted with permission.)

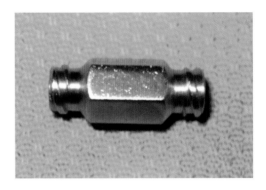

Fig. 25.21 Luer-to-Luer connector (©Tulip, Byron Medical, with permission).

use larger syringes and multi-hole cannulas available from Tulip Products™ or a modified liposuction set-up with a fat trap,[34,35] along with a cannula with multiple (10–12) holes to speed the process. A simple method of straining the fat is by using a sterilizable kitchen strainer *(Fig. 25.22)* to remove the aqueous and oil layers or standing the syringe up to allow the layers to separate as described above. The fat is then quickly (to prevent desiccation) transferred to a large syringe (using a sterile spoon or scalpel handle), from which point it is distributed to the smaller 3 cc or 1 cc syringes (using a Luer-to-Luer or 3-way connector) for grafting back into the patient.

The harvesting and processing of fat is now being commercialized, with specialized systems available in the United States and elsewhere, which simplify many

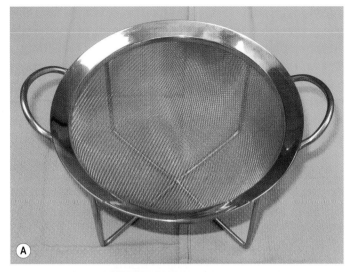

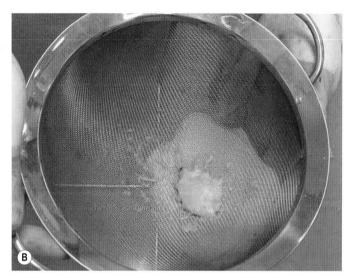

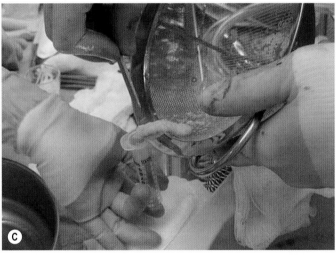

Fig. 25.22 (A) Sterilizable kitchen strainer. **(B,C)** A small amount of prepared fat after straining and washing (i). Note folded gauze against the fat beneath the strainer; this quickly wicks moisture from the strained graft. (ii) Prepared fat is transferred to a 10 cc syringe for injection.

of the steps and provide "one-stop shopping" for the equipment necessary. These systems, such as those available from LipiVage® *(Fig. 25.23)*, Lipokit™ *(Figs 25.24, 25.25)*, and Cytori™ *(Fig. 25.26)*, promise substantial time savings for grafting. These systems provide standardization and simplicity and eliminate the need to collect the proper instruments, sometimes from several sources, to have an effective set-up. Drawbacks are that they are largely unproven and their cost is high.

Injection technique

Different cannulas are used for injection to those for harvesting. Typically, the injection cannula is a blunt cannula with a single hole for precise fat deposition

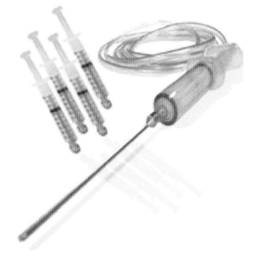

Fig. 25.23 LipiVage® fat harvest system. (©Genesis Biosystems, with permission).

(Fig. 25.27) and is available in different lengths and flexibilities. The cannula has a Luer connector for fitting to a syringe containing processed fat. If scarring is present and needs to be released, a sharp cannula is used selectively *(Fig. 25.16)*. An 11 blade may be used to create the 2 mm hole for introduction of the injection cannula, which is advanced through an area of the intended fat grafting. As the cannula is withdrawn, slow and even pressure on the syringe plunger deposits a fine cylinder of fat into the tunnel created by introduction of the cannula.

The proper technique of depositing an even layer of fat one-handed during cannula withdrawal is a skilled practice. Some practitioners use an IV extension tubing to technically separate the process, permitting an assistant to focus only on plunger pressure while they focus on a slow and even cannula withdrawal.[14] It is here also that the fat preparation technique may have implications for the consistent deposition of the grafted fat. The compression that results from a high-speed centrifuge or the existence of connective tissue clumps may create an obstacle to the even flow of grafted fat through the injection cannula. This leads some practitioners to prefer one preparation technique over another. Open straining permits removal of aspirated connective tissue clumps, and a low-speed centrifuge technique (Spingraft™) packs the fat less tightly. Because increased pressure can sometimes clear a clump from the cannula, resulting in sudden focal overgrafting, it is best to avoid this situation entirely by stopping the procedure to clear a stoppage.[36]

The protocol of the senior author of this chapter (Spear) in a current clinical trial of breast augmentation with autologous fat at Georgetown is as follows. Low-pressure vacuum aspiration is used with a 3-hole cannula to harvest fat from selected sites. Fat is transferred to 10 cc syringes for centrifuging, after which

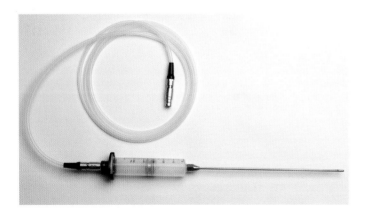

Fig. 25.24 Lipokit 60 cc syringe with suction tubing. (©Medi-Khan, with permission).

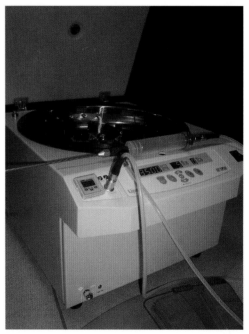

Fig. 25.25 Lipokit centrifuge (©Medi-Khan, with permission).

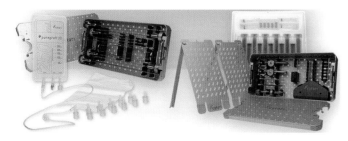

Fig. 25.26 Cytori Puregraft 250 (©Cytori Therapeutics Inc, with permission).

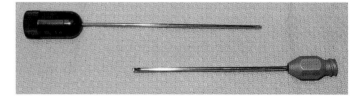

Fig. 25.27 Injection cannulae by Tulip (1.4 mm) and Byron (2 mm) (© Byron Medical, with permission).

oil is decanted from the top and the aqueous component is poured out of the bottom of the syringe. Using periareolar and inframammary access incisions and a single-hole 2 mm cannula, fat is infiltrated into three planes: the subcutaneous, subglandular, and intramuscular. The exact amounts of grafting to each of these planes vary with the patient.

Brava

An exciting recent enhancement of fat grafting technique is the addition of external pre-expansion prior to and after grafting. The Brava device (Brava LLC, Miami, FL) was initially developed as an external breast tissue expander whose goal was nonsurgical breast augmentation.[37] The device consists of two semirigid polyurethane domes that are placed over each breast and seal at its periphery with silicone gel-filled donut bladders (*Fig. 25.28*). A small pump maintains 20 mmHg of negative pressure inside the domes, which are worn continuously for 10 h a day for a minimum of 10 weeks, if the device is used alone. One cup size increase can reasonably be expected, with the increase in size being maintained over time. The limited permanent size increase and compliance difficulties temper its more widespread use.

On the other hand, the device causes a temporary increase in the size of the breasts, past what can be expected to be maintained, due to swelling. This is effectively an expansion of the scaffold of soft tissues that comprise the breast, and is thought to have a salutary

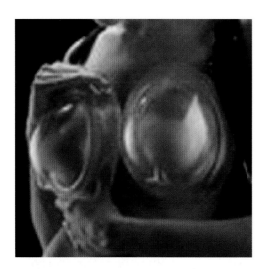

Fig. 25.28 BRAVA device (©BRAVA LLC, with permission).

effect on fat graft survival. When used before autologous fat grafting for breast augmentation or reconstruction (for this indication, only 3–4 weeks is needed), it is thought to increase both the volume possible to graft and graft survival percentage. Studies are presently underway to quantify these effects,[21,22] and initial results are encouraging.[16] If proven effective and reproducible, this technique may transform autologous breast reconstruction into a previously-impossible minimally-invasive procedure for patients.

Postoperative care

Skin closure of the 2 mm access slits may be with fine suture or adhesive strips, and a loosely supportive breast garment is fitted with cotton fluffs over grafted areas. Cool compresses reduce swelling and the patient is encouraged to minimize arm movements for a week. The donor site is treated with a compressive garment similarly to any area of liposuction.

Acute swelling can be expected for 1–2 weeks but may persist for months. If a contour deformity remains after swelling has resolved, we recommend waiting at least 6 months prior to attempting another round of grafting. Physical examination and radiographic follow-up follow the same schedule as for any other breast surgery.

> **Hints and tips**
>
> - Use fat grafting on reconstructive contour deformities early in your experience, preferably while already performing a different procedure requiring general anesthesia.
> - Basic instrumentation and techniques work well, are inexpensive, and provide an easy way to get started.
> - Overgraft less if fat is centrifuged during processing.
> - Appropriate patient expectations are important. Impressive results are possible, but may require more than one session of grafting.

Outcomes, prognosis, and complications

Patient outcomes

Refer to the before and after pictures (*Figs. 25.1–25.11*) given for each of the indications listed above.

Graft survival

Early practitioners, using free *en bloc* fat grafts, noted substantial resorption of their free fat grafts and tried various measures to prevent this, such as transplanting fascia with the fat[38] or cutting the graft into several pieces.[39] Early reports of graft survival ranged from 25% to 50%, so early practitioners began to advocate the practice of overgrafting.[40,41] The modern method of transplanting fat by injecting it has not altered this recommendation, though there seems to be no consensus as to how much overgrafting should be done.

Graft survival percentage varies with the methods used to aspirate, prepare and transplant the fat. It also varies with respect to the destination of the graft, with fat grafted into well-vascularized muscle surviving at a higher rate than fat grafted into a relatively oxygen-poor environment such as a depressed breast contour from fat necrosis of a TRAM flap. Some recent authors define the amount of overgrafting that should be performed in the breast; for example, Emmanuel Delay, grafting into reconstructed breasts, writes that he plans on 30% resorption rate and advocates overgrafting by 40%. Kanchwala et al.[6] recommend overgrafting by no more than 10% to avoid fat necrosis and subsequent calcifications. Our experience supports overgrafting amounts in these approximate ranges for contour deformities. Preparation method matters: fat processed with washing and straining needs more overgrafting than centrifuged fat. Until more specific research is performed on the subject, there is no substitute from the personal experience of beginning conservatively. We recommend that judicious overgrafting should be performed early in a surgeon's experience until one acquires a "feel" for how much overgrafting should be performed based on the technique being used and the quality of the recipient bed. Reconstructive contour deformities in nonradiated fields lend themselves well to this early experience.

Complications

There are risks in any surgical procedure, and autologous fat grafting to the female breast is no exception. Major complications are rare, and the ones reported in the literature are often the result of procedures being performed by poorly-trained practitioners.[42,43] Even when properly performed, however, there are certain events which occur with enough regularity to be highlighted in the informed consent.

Mammographic abnormalities[44–49] are relevant in patients who have not had mastectomy. After breast augmentation with fat grafting, the most commonly seen abnormalities are calcifications. These come in the form of either coarse or fine microcalcifications and are thought to be the result of areas of fat necrosis. They can usually be readily distinguished from suspicious patterns by an experienced radiographer; those that cannot should be biopsied. Mammography can also detect oil cysts, which may also be palpable on exam. Preoperative mammography is recommended prior to autologous fat grafting to the breast for augmentation for comparison purposes in the event of any abnormality developing later. With respect to interference with breast cancer detection, the ASPS Fat Graft Task Force concluded, in its 2009 report: "Based on a limited number of studies with few cases, there appears to be no interference with breast cancer detection; however, more studies are needed to confirm these preliminary findings."[5]

Liponecrotic cysts or oil cysts, occur in areas of walled-off liquefaction necrosis. These can be multiple and small or, on occasion, quite large. A cyst is effectively treated by surgical excision. Their development probably correlates with improper technique of inadequately distributing the grafted fat – or attempting to graft too much fat into a particular area.[50,51] In his experience of 880 patients, Delay reports that approximately 15% of his patients developed oil cysts on mammogram.[7]

Infection may occur after fat injection and typically presents as painful swelling with erythema, warmth, and sometimes fever. The outcome of infection is variable, with reports of both loss of the grafted fat[1] and no effect on the results,[7] but abscess formation with sepsis has been reported in the literature.[52]

Persistent swelling. If swelling persists for over 2 months, it may signal the development of fat necrosis or a liponecrotic cyst. The index of suspicion for either of these complications is higher with higher volumes of grafted fat. Watchful waiting is the best course of action, since early imaging studies can be expected to show nonspecific inflammation. If a cyst is suspected, it may be detected with ultrasound.

Neoplasia risk is perhaps theoretical. The same qualities of adipose-derived stem cells that make them regenerative (such as angiogenesis) might be shown in the future to increase the risk of breast cancer for the patient. In a literature review encompassing 283 patients undergoing fat grafting to the breast for cosmetic and reconstructive purposes, the ASPS Fat Graft Task Force report identified two cases of breast cancer.[5] One was in an area of the breast that was not grafted, and one was in an area potentially grafted, but there was no delay in diagnosis or treatment.[2] Only further study will prove or disprove any correlation between fat grafting and the development of subsequent breast cancer; until that time, the risk of neoplasia must be classified as unknown.

Secondary procedures

Fat grafting may need to be repeated, and it is often necessary to do so *(Fig. 25.29)*. A recent retrospective review of 110 patients who underwent fat grafting for contour deformities in reconstructed breasts found that 55% of the patients required more than one session to satisfactorily correct the deformities.[6] More sessions can be expected in hostile environments such as irradiated fields.[20] Additional sessions may also be required for breast augmentation, depending on the goals of the patient, since there is a limit to how much fat can be

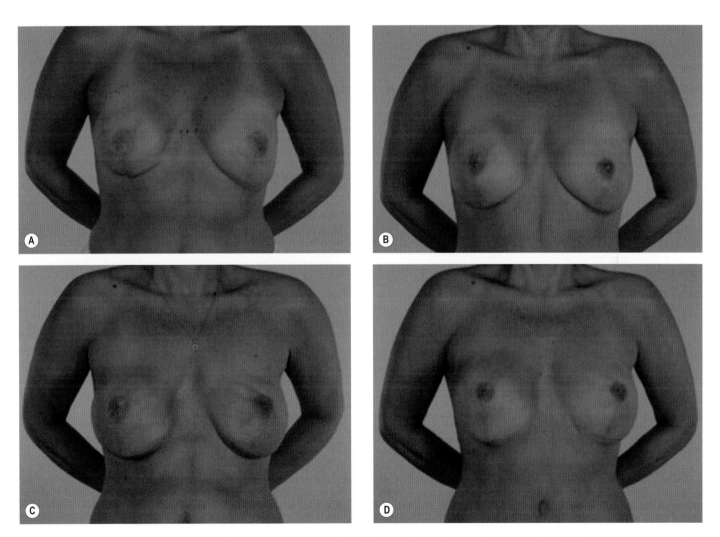

Fig. 25.29 This 49-year-old patient underwent multiple sessions of autologous fat grafting after bilateral nipple-sparing mastectomies with tissue expander reconstructions. **(A)** At 9 months after bilateral immediate breast reconstruction with tissue expanders. **(B)** The same patient 3 months after bilateral exchange of tissue expanders for 560 cc gel implants and fat grafting to superior poles; 80 cc right and 40 cc left. **(C)** At 4 months postoperative view after bilateral exchange to 650 cc gel implants and 75 cc fat grafting to the superomedial and inferomedial quadrants bilaterally. **(D)** At 9 months after bilateral breast scar revisions and fat grafting of 35 cc to each upper pole.

realistically grafted into each breast at one time to expect reasonably good take of the graft. This limit varies patient-to-patient and is probably higher in patients who have undergone external pre-expansion.

Conclusions

Autologous fat grafting to the female breast is here to stay and will continue to evolve as practitioners continue to refine the technique and discover new applications of the grafted adipocyte. Established indications include contour deformities in breasts reconstructed by a variety of methods. No longer are practitioners debating whether fat grafting works; what is being discussed is the appropriate role of the more controversial indications, such as breast augmentation or total breast reconstruction. The next decade is likely to see more established protocols for these indications, as well as further progress defining the potential therapeutic power of adipose-derived stem cells.

 Access the complete reference list online at **http://www.expertconsult.com**

1. Spear S, Wilson H, Lockwood M. Fat injection to correct contour deformities in the reconstructed breast. *Plast Reconstr Surg.* 2005;116(5): 1300–1305.

    This article helped initiate the recent resurgence in interest in fat grafting to the breast and remains a good overview of real-world results and typical complications.

2. Coleman SR, Saboeiro AP. Fat grafting to the breast revisited: safety and efficacy. *Plast Reconstr Surg.* 2007;119(3):775–785.

    This comprehensive review with impressive results furthered the call to legitimize fat grafting to the breast and reverse the ASPS's 1987 condemnation of the practice.

3. Missana MD, Laurent I, Barreau L, et al. Autologous fat transfer in reconstructive breast surgery: indications, technique and results. *Eur J Surg Oncol.* 2007;33(6):685–690.

5. Gutowski K. Current applications and safety of autologous fat grafts: a report of the asps fat graft task force. *Plast Reconstr Surg.* 2009;124: 272–280.

    The ASPS Fat Graft Task Force reports the results of a critical appraisal of the current literature on indications for autologous fat grafting and the risks associated with it.

6. Kanchwala SK, Glatt BS, Conant EF, et al. Autologous fat grafting to the reconstructed breast: the management of acquired contour deformities. *Plast Reconstr Surg.* 2009;124(2):410–418.

7. Delay E, Garson S, Tousson G, et al. Fat injection to the breast: technique, results, and indications based on 880 procedures over 10 years. *Aesthetic Surg J.* 2009;29(5):360–376.

9. Mizuno M, Hyakusoku H. Fat grafting to the breast and adipose-derived stem cells: recent scientific consensus and controversy. *Aesthetic Surg J.* 2010;30(3):381–387.

    An accessible current review article covering complications and adipose-derived stem cells.

20. Rigotti G, Marchi A, Galie M, et al. Clinical treatment of radiotherapy tissue damage by lipoaspirate transplant: a healing process mediated by adipose-derived adult stem cells. *Plast Reconstr Surg.* 2007;119:1409.

    A landmark article reporting on the efficacy of adipose-derived stem cells at reversing radiation damage to the breast.

24. Serra-Renom JM, Del Olmo JM, Serra-Mestre JM. Fat grafting in post mastectomy breast reconstruction with expanders and prosthesis in patients who have received radiotherapy: formation of new subcutaneous tissue. *Plast Reconstr Surg.* 2010;125(1):12–18.

42. Hyakusoku H, Ogawa R, Ono S, et al. Complications after autologous fat injection to the breast. *Plast Reconstr Surg.* 2009;123(1):360–370.

Index

*Note: **Boldface** roman numerals indicate volume. Page numbers followed by f refer to figures; page numbers followed by t refer to tables; page numbers followed by b refer to boxes.*

Note: **Boldface** *roman numerals indicate volume. Page numbers followed by f refer to figures; page numbers followed by t refer to tables; page numbers followed by b refer to boxes.*

*Note: **Boldface** roman numerals indicate volume. Page numbers followed by f refer to figures; page numbers followed by t refer to tables; page numbers followed by b refer to boxes.*

*Note: **Boldface** roman numerals indicate volume. Page numbers followed by f refer to figures; page numbers followed by t refer to tables; page numbers followed by b refer to boxes.*

Note: **Boldface** roman numerals indicate volume. Page numbers followed by f refer to figures; page numbers followed by t refer to tables; page numbers followed by b refer to boxes.

*Note: **Boldface** roman numerals indicate volume. Page numbers followed by f refer to figures; page numbers followed by t refer to tables; page numbers followed by b refer to boxes.*

Note: **Boldface** roman numerals indicate volume. Page numbers followed by f refer to figures; page numbers followed by t refer to tables; page numbers followed by b refer to boxes.

Note: **Boldface** *roman numerals indicate volume. Page numbers followed by f refer to figures; page numbers followed by t refer to tables; page numbers followed by b refer to boxes.*

*Note: **Boldface** roman numerals indicate volume. Page numbers followed by f refer to figures; page numbers followed by t refer to tables; page numbers followed by b refer to boxes.*

Note: **Boldface** *roman numerals indicate volume. Page numbers followed by f refer to figures; page numbers followed by t refer to tables; page numbers followed by b refer to boxes.*

Note: **Boldface** roman numerals indicate volume. Page numbers followed by f refer to figures; page numbers followed by t refer to tables; page numbers followed by b refer to boxes.

Note: **Boldface** *roman numerals indicate volume. Page numbers followed by f refer to figures; page numbers followed by t refer to tables; page numbers followed by b refer to boxes.*

Note: **Boldface** *roman numerals indicate volume. Page numbers followed by f refer to figures; page numbers followed by t refer to tables; page numbers followed by b refer to boxes.*

Note: **Boldface** roman numerals indicate volume. Page numbers followed by f refer to figures; page numbers followed by t refer to tables; page numbers followed by b refer to boxes.

*Note: **Boldface** roman numerals indicate volume. Page numbers followed by f refer to figures; page numbers followed by t refer to tables; page numbers followed by b refer to boxes.*

Note: **Boldface** *roman numerals indicate volume. Page numbers followed by f refer to figures; page numbers followed by t refer to tables; page numbers followed by b refer to boxes.*

*Note: **Boldface** roman numerals indicate volume. Page numbers followed by f refer to figures; page numbers followed by t refer to tables; page numbers followed by b refer to boxes.*

Note: **Boldface** *roman numerals indicate volume. Page numbers followed by f refer to figures; page numbers followed by t refer to tables; page numbers followed by b refer to boxes.*

*Note: **Boldface** roman numerals indicate volume. Page numbers followed by f refer to figures; page numbers followed by t refer to tables; page numbers followed by b refer to boxes.*

Note: **Boldface** roman numerals indicate volume. Page numbers followed by f refer to figures; page numbers followed by t refer to tables; page numbers followed by b refer to boxes.

*Note: **Boldface** roman numerals indicate volume. Page numbers followed by f refer to figures; page numbers followed by t refer to tables; page numbers followed by b refer to boxes.*

Note: **Boldface** roman numerals indicate volume. Page numbers followed by f refer to figures; page numbers followed by t refer to tables; page numbers followed by b refer to boxes.

Note: Boldface roman numerals indicate volume. Page numbers followed by f refer to figures; page numbers followed by t refer to tables; page numbers followed by b refer to boxes.

Note: **Boldface** roman numerals indicate volume. Page numbers followed by f refer to figures; page numbers followed by t refer to tables; page numbers followed by b refer to boxes.

Note: **Boldface** *roman numerals indicate volume. Page numbers followed by f refer to figures; page numbers followed by t refer to tables; page numbers followed by b refer to boxes.*

Note: **Boldface** roman numerals indicate volume. Page numbers followed by f refer to figures; page numbers followed by t refer to tables; page numbers followed by b refer to boxes.

Note: **Boldface** roman numerals indicate volume. Page numbers followed by f refer to figures; page numbers followed by t refer to tables; page numbers followed by b refer to boxes.

Note: **Boldface** *roman numerals indicate volume. Page numbers followed by f refer to figures; page numbers followed by t refer to tables; page numbers followed by b refer to boxes.*

Note: **Boldface** *roman numerals indicate volume. Page numbers followed by f refer to figures; page numbers followed by t refer to tables; page numbers followed by b refer to boxes.*

Note: **Boldface** roman numerals indicate volume. Page numbers followed by f refer to figures; page numbers followed by t refer to tables; page numbers followed by b refer to boxes.

Note: Boldface roman numerals indicate volume. Page numbers followed by f refer to figures; page numbers followed by t refer to tables; page numbers followed by b refer to boxes.

*Note: **Boldface** roman numerals indicate volume. Page numbers followed by f refer to figures; page numbers followed by t refer to tables; page numbers followed by b refer to boxes.*

Note: **Boldface** roman numerals indicate volume. Page numbers followed by f refer to figures; page numbers followed by t refer to tables; page numbers followed by b refer to boxes.

*Note: **Boldface** roman numerals indicate volume. Page numbers followed by f refer to figures; page numbers followed by t refer to tables; page numbers followed by b refer to boxes.*

Note: **Boldface** *roman numerals indicate volume. Page numbers followed by f refer to figures; page numbers followed by t refer to tables; page numbers followed by b refer to boxes.*

Note: **Boldface** roman numerals indicate volume. Page numbers followed by f refer to figures; page numbers followed by t refer to tables; page numbers followed by b refer to boxes.

*Note: **Boldface** roman numerals indicate volume. Page numbers followed by f refer to figures; page numbers followed by t refer to tables; page numbers followed by b refer to boxes.*

*Note: **Boldface** roman numerals indicate volume. Page numbers followed by f refer to figures; page numbers followed by t refer to tables; page numbers followed by b refer to boxes.*

Note: **Boldface** roman numerals indicate volume. Page numbers followed by f refer to figures; page numbers followed by t refer to tables; page numbers followed by b refer to boxes.

*Note: **Boldface** roman numerals indicate volume. Page numbers followed by f refer to figures; page numbers followed by t refer to tables; page numbers followed by b refer to boxes.*

Note: **Boldface** *roman numerals indicate volume. Page numbers followed by f refer to figures; page numbers followed by t refer to tables; page numbers followed by b refer to boxes.*

*Note: **Boldface** roman numerals indicate volume. Page numbers followed by f refer to figures; page numbers followed by t refer to tables; page numbers followed by b refer to boxes.*

*Note: **Boldface** roman numerals indicate volume. Page numbers followed by f refer to figures; page numbers followed by t refer to tables; page numbers followed by b refer to boxes.*

*Note: **Boldface** roman numerals indicate volume. Page numbers followed by f refer to figures; page numbers followed by t refer to tables; page numbers followed by b refer to boxes.*

Note: **Boldface** roman numerals indicate volume. Page numbers followed by f refer to figures; page numbers followed by t refer to tables; page numbers followed by b refer to boxes.

*Note: **Boldface** roman numerals indicate volume. Page numbers followed by f refer to figures; page numbers followed by t refer to tables; page numbers followed by b refer to boxes.*

*Note: **Boldface** roman numerals indicate volume. Page numbers followed by f refer to figures; page numbers followed by t refer to tables; page numbers followed by b refer to boxes.*

Note: **Boldface** *roman numerals indicate volume. Page numbers followed by f refer to figures; page numbers followed by t refer to tables; page numbers followed by b refer to boxes.*

*Note: **Boldface** roman numerals indicate volume. Page numbers followed by f refer to figures; page numbers followed by t refer to tables; page numbers followed by b refer to boxes.*

Note: **Boldface** *roman numerals indicate volume. Page numbers followed by f refer to figures; page numbers followed by t refer to tables; page numbers followed by b refer to boxes.*

Note: **Boldface** *roman numerals indicate volume. Page numbers followed by f refer to figures; page numbers followed by t refer to tables; page numbers followed by b refer to boxes.*

Note: **Boldface** *roman numerals indicate volume. Page numbers followed by f refer to figures; page numbers followed by t refer to tables; page numbers followed by b refer to boxes.*

*Note: **Boldface** roman numerals indicate volume. Page numbers followed by f refer to figures; page numbers followed by t refer to tables; page numbers followed by b refer to boxes.*

Note: **Boldface** roman numerals indicate volume. Page numbers followed by f refer to figures; page numbers followed by t refer to tables; page numbers followed by b refer to boxes.

Note: **Boldface** roman numerals indicate volume. Page numbers followed by f refer to figures; page numbers followed by t refer to tables; page numbers followed by b refer to boxes.

Note: **Boldface** roman numerals indicate volume. Page numbers followed by f refer to figures; page numbers followed by t refer to tables; page numbers followed by b refer to boxes.

Note: **Boldface** roman numerals indicate volume. Page numbers followed by f refer to figures; page numbers followed by t refer to tables; page numbers followed by b refer to boxes.

*Note: **Boldface** roman numerals indicate volume. Page numbers followed by f refer to figures; page numbers followed by t refer to tables; page numbers followed by b refer to boxes.*